Vision: coding and efficiency

Vision: coding and efficiency

edited by

COLIN BLAKEMORE

Waynflete Professor of Physiology
University of Oxford

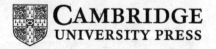

CAMBRIDGE UNIVERSITY PRESS
Cambridge, New York, Melbourne, Madrid, Cape Town, Singapore, São Paulo

Cambridge University Press
The Edinburgh Building, Cambridge CB2 8RU, UK

Published in the United States of America by Cambridge University Press, New York

www.cambridge.org
Information on this title: www.cambridge.org/9780521364591

© Cambridge University Press 1990

First published 1990
First paperback edition 1993

A catalogue record for this publication is available from the British Library

Library of Congress Cataloguing in Publication data
Vision: coding and efficiency/edited by C. Blakemore.
    p. cm.
ISBN 0 521 36459 0 (hbk)   0 521 44769 0 (pbk)
1. Vision. 2. Visual perception. I. Blakemore, Colin.
QP475.V574 1990
599′.01823–dc20   89–37311CIP

ISBN 978-0-521-36459-1 hardback
ISBN 978-0-521-44769-0 paperback

Transferred to digital printing 2008

Contents

Contributors

M. Alpern
  W. G. Kellog Eye Center
  University of Michigan Medical Center
  1000 Wall Street
  Ann Arbor MI 48105, USA
Atkinson
  Visual Development Unit
  Department of Experimental Psychology
  Downing Street
  Cambridge CB2 3EB, UK
H. B. Barlow
  Physiological Laboratory
  Downing Street
  Cambridge CB2 3EG, UK
C. Blakemore
  University Laboratory of Physiology
  Parks Road
  Oxford OX1 3PT, UK
T. J. Bossomaier
  Centre for Visual Sciences
  Australian National University
  Canberra, Australia
O. J. Braddick
  Visual Development Unit
  Department of Experimental Psychology
  Downing Street
  Cambridge CB2 3EB, UK
D. G. Brown
  Office of Science & Technology
  Center for Devices & Radiological Health, FDA
  Rockville MD 20857, USA
A. E. Burgess
  Department of Radiology
  University of British Columbia
  10th Avenue & Heather Street
  Vancouver B.C. Canada V5Z 1M9
D. C. Burr
  Laboratorio di Neurofisiologia del CNR
  Via S. Zeno 51
  56127 Pisa
  Italy

C. R. Cavonius
  Institut für Arbeitsphysiologie
  Ardeystrasse 67
  Postfach 1508
  D-4600 Dortmund 1, F R Germany
B. Chen
  Department of Psychology C–009
  University of California
  San Diego
  La Jolla, CA 92093–0109
T. E. Cohn
  School of Optometry
  University of California
  Berkeley CA 94720, USA
A. M. Derrington
  Department of Physiological Sciences
  The Medical School
  The University of Newcastle upon Tyne
  Framlington Place
  Newcastle-upon-Tyne NE2 4HH, UK
O. Estévez
  Academic Medical Centre
  Department of Medical Informatics
  Meibergdreef 15
  1105 AZ Amsterdam–Zuidoost
  The Netherlands
D. J. Field
  Physiological Laboratory
  Downing Street
  Cambridge CB2 3EG, UK
R. D. Freeman
  Group in Neurobiology
  360 Minor Hall
  University of California
  Berkeley CA 94720, USA
B. S. Garra
  Clinical Center
  National Institutes of Health
  Bethesda MD 20892, USA

R. Gemperlein
    Zoologisches Institut der Universität
    Luisenstrasse 14
    D 8000 Munchen 2, F R Germany
M. J. Hawken
    Centre for Neural Science
    Department of Psychology
    New York University
    4 Washington Place
    NY 10003, USA
R. F. Hess
    Department of Ophthalmology
    McGill University
    Royal Victoria Hospital
    687 Pine Avenue West, Montreal
    Canada H3A 1A1
A. A. Hughes
    National Vision Research Institute
    386 Cardigan Street
    Carlton
    Victoria 3053, Australia
M. F. Insana
    University of Kansas Medical Center
    Kansas City KS 66103, USA
R. J. Jennings
    Office of Science & Technology
    Center for Devices & Radiological Health, FDA
    Rockville MD 20857, USA
D. Kersten
    Walter S. Hunter Laboratory of Psychology
    Brown University
    Providence RI 02912, USA
T. D. Lamb
    Physiological Laboratory
    Downing Street
    Cambridge CB2 3EG, UK
M. F. Land
    Department of Biological Sciences
    University of Sussex
    Falmer
    Brighton Sussex BN1 9QG, UK
S. B. Laughlin
    Department of Zoology
    Downing Street
    Cambridge CB2 3EJ, UK
W. R. Levick
    John Curtin School of Medical Research
    GPO Box 334, Canberra City
    ACT 2601 Australia
D. I. A. MacLeod
    Department of Psychology, C-009
    University of California
    San Diego CA 92093-0109, USA

P. A. McNaughton
    Physiology Group
    Biomedical Sciences Division
    King's College London
    Strand, London WC2R 2LS
R. Malach
    Center for Neurosciences
    The Weizman Institute of Science
    Rehovot 76100, Israel
D. E. Mitchell
    Department of Psychology
    Dalhousie University
    Halifax
    Nova Scotia, Canada B3H 4J1
G. I. Mitchison
    Physiological Laboratory
    Downing Street
    Cambridge CB2 3EG, UK
J. D. Mollon
    Department of Experimental Psychology
    Downing Street
    Cambridge CB2 3EB, UK
M. C. Morrone
    Laboratorio di Neurofisiologia del CNR
    Via S. Zeno 51
    56127 Pisa
    Italy
K. T. Mullen
    Department of Ophthalmology
    McGill University
    Royal Victoria Hospital
    687 Pine Avenue West, Montreal
    Canada H3A 1A1
K. Nakayama
    Psychology Department
    Harvard University
    33 Kirkland Street
    Cambridge MA 02138, USA
I. Ohzawa
    Group in Neurobiology
    360 Minor Hall
    University of California
    Berkeley CA 94720, USA
J. Olavarria
    Division of Biology 216–76
    California Institute of Technology
    Pasadena CA 91125, USA
C. W. Oyster
    The University of Alabama at Birmingham
    School of Optometry, The Medical Center
    Department of Physiological Optics
    UAB Station
    Birmingham AL 35294, USA

A. J. Parker
  University Laboratory of Physiology
  Parks Road
  Oxford OX1 3PT, UK
R. Paul
  Zoologisches Institut der Universität
  Luisenstrasse 14
  D 8000 Munchen 2, F R Germany
D. G. Pelli
  Institute for Sensory Research
  Syracuse University
  Merrill Lane
  Syracuse NY 13244-5290, USA
J. D. Pettigrew
  Department of Physiology
  Neuroscience Laboratory
  University of Queensland
  St. Lucia
  Queensland 4067, Australia
V. S. Ramachandran
  Brain and Perception Project
  Department of Psychology, 0109
  University of California at San Diego
  9500 Gilman Drive
  La Jolla, CA 92093-0109, USA
Azriel Rosenfeld
  Center for Automation Research
  University of Maryland
  College Park MD 20742, USA
A. W. Snyder
  Optical Sciences Centre
  Institute of Advanced Studies
  The Australian National University
  Canberra Australia
A. Steiner
  Zoologisches Institut der Universität
  Luisenstrasse 14
  D 8000 Munchen 2, F R Germany
A. Stockman
  Department of Psychology, C-009
  University of California
  San Diego CA 92093-0109, USA
L. N. Thibos
  Optometry School
  Indiana University
  Bloomington IN 47405, USA

I. D. Thompson
  University Laboratory of Physiology
  Parks Road
  Oxford OX1 3PT, UK
D. I. Vaney
  Vision, Touch and Hearing Research Centre
  University of Queensland,
  St Lucia,
  Queensland 4067, Australia
A. Van Meeteren
  TNO Institute for Perception
  P.O. Box 23
  3769 ZG Soesterberg
  Kampweg 5 The Netherlands
R. C. Van Sluyters
  School of Optometry
  University of California
  Berkeley CA 94720, USA
R. F. Wagner
  Office of Science & Technology
  Center for Devices & Radiological Health, FDA
  Rockville MD 20857, USA
A. B. Watson
  Perception & Cognition Group
  NASA Ames Research Center
  Moffett Field CA 94035, USA
R. J. Watt
  Department of Psychology
  University of Stirling
  Stirling, Scotland, UK.
G. Westheimer
  Division of Neurobiology
  Department of Molecular and Cell Biology
  211 Life Sciences Addition
  University of California
  Berkeley, CA, 94720, USA
M. G. Yoon
  Department of Psychology
  Dalhousie University
  Halifax
  Nova Scotia Canada B3H 4J1
S. Zeki
  Department of Anatomy & Development Biology
  University College London
  Gower Street
  London WC1E 6BT, UK

Preface

By the end of the nineteenth century the mood of sensory physiology was marvellously mechanistic. Sir Charles Bell and Johannes Müller set the scene in the 1830s with their evidence for a direct and automatic link between the stimulation of particular sensory nerves and the resulting perceptions; but even then there was a dissenting voice. In volume 3 of his *Treatise on Physiological Optics* Hermann von Helmholtz drew attention to many problems in a simplistic interpretation of the relation between sensory messages and perception. He pointed out that 'without any change of the retinal images, the same observer may see in front of him various perceptual images in succession'. 'We are not simply passive to the impressions that are urged on us, but we *observe*.' Equally, the generalities of experience that we can express in single words correspond to an infinity of precise patterns of sensory stimulation: 'the species "table" includes all individual tables and expresses their common peculiarities'. Helmholtz concluded that the processes underlying perception were essentially inductive, learned, but below the level of consciousness: 'by their peculiar nature they may be classed as *conclusions*, inductive conclusions unconsciously formed'.

No wonder that Helmholtz's revolutionary views were anathema to many physiologists and philosophers of the time. They flew in the face of the prevailing notion of the innate basis of knowledge and experience, which linked such heavyweights as Ewalt Hering and Immanuel Kant. But Helmholtz's appeal to the inferential, learned nature of perception echoed the much earlier views of the empiricist philosophers, most especially George Berkeley, and presaged the ideas of the buoyant new field of cognitive psychology.

Perception may be inferential, but how does it *work*? There are in our heads only nerves to do the job. As Helmholtz put it: 'what similarity can be imagined between the process in the brain that is concomitant with the idea of a table and the table itself? Is the form of the table to be supposed to be outlined by electric currents?' Such a question is, of course, still the central one in visual science. Perception has to be achieved by a network of nerves. But as signalling devices, nerves seem hopelessly ill-equipped: their poor electrical properties force most of them to transmit messages in the form of all-or-nothing impulses; and with a maximum rate of impulses of only a few hundred per second, nerves have a ridiculously narrow dynamic range. Yet we can see a light when our retinas catch only a few quanta; we can discriminate hundreds of colours with only three photopigments in our cones; we can detect a vernier offset or a disparity between the images in the two eyes of just seconds of arc; and we can reconstruct the whole three-dimensional richness of the world from the tiny, flat images in our eyes.

The modern approach to this problem has its origins in the blossoming of information theory and cybernetics in the 1940s. The major problem was seen in terms of the need for the eyes to provide appropriate information to the brain to support the performance of perception. Keffer Hartline, recording from single nerve axons teased from the optic nerve of the frog and the horseshoe crab *Limulus*, provided the first quantitative description of the relationship between a light stimulus and the responses of neurons. Though he did much to establish the deterministic relations between light and neural response, under some conditions his records showed that these responses were not entirely reliable, for the same weak light would sometimes elicit an impulse and sometimes not. Many years later, Hartline's collaborator Floyd Ratliff pointed out that the properties of *Limulus* nerve fibres could be described by a sigmoid 'frequency-of-response' curve, plotting the probability of a particular number of impulses being produced by a light of increasing intensity, in much the same way that a 'frequency-of-seeing' function can be used to characterize the variability of response of a human observer. Indeed, for some fibres in the *Limulus* optic nerve, the statistical fluctuations of response were very well predicted in terms of the response being generated by only two absorbed quanta, with all the variability in neuronal response being due to quantal fluctuation in the stimulus itself.

Hartline himself emphasized another finding: if a spot of light is enlarged beyond the ommatidium generating the response being recorded, the magnitude of that response declines. This phenomenon of lateral inhibition was the first example of active coding in the characteristics of a visual neuron. It makes the single optic nerve fibre a detector of local contrast. Thus it provides both increased efficiency (because it partly removes the effect of overall illumination and makes better use of the limited dynamic range of impulse generation) and a form of coding (because lateral inhibition 'tunes' the optic fibre to detect light only at one particular restricted position in the visual field).

In 1943, while Hartline was starting his classical work at the Rockefeller Institute in New York, Horace Barlow, who had just completed a degree in Physiology at Cambridge, England, worked for a short time with William Rushton, recording impulses from the giant fibre of the earthworm. At that time Rushton was interested in the mechanism of impulse generation. A decade later both he and Barlow were passionately involved in the study of vision. In 1946, when Barlow had finished his medical degree at Harvard, he worked with Kohn and Walsh on the visual sensations produced by intense magnetic fields and on the effects of light on the sensitivity of the human eye to electric stimulation. On his return to take his medical degree in Cambridge, England, Edgar (Lord) Adrian, Professor of Physiology suggested that he should work on eye movement, following up Talbot and Marshall's suggestion that tremor may be important in 'sharpening' the central representation of the visual image. Barlow never submitted that work as a Ph.D. thesis; but he published it and it was the first step in his commitment to a career in vision research.

By 1949, Barlow had started to apply Ragnar Granit's microelectrode technique to the study of ganglion cells in the frog retina. Even that early work bore Barlow's characteristic stamp of imagination combined with quantitative rigour. He was the first to describe lateral inhibition in a vertebrate retina (shortly before Steve Kuffler's first account of it in the cat) and did a thorough study of spatial summation.

But for me, the Discussion section of Barlow's classical paper on the frog retina (*Journal of Physiology*, **119**, 58–68, 1953) was its most remarkable contribution. He chose not to interpret his results in conventional academic terms but to speculate on the meaning of the messages in the optic nerve for the behaviour of the frog. Here was the first attempt to describe the signals of sensory nerves in terms of both the behavioural needs of the animal and the salient features of the retinal image. Barlow's suggestion that one class of frog ganglion cell was ideally suited to the detection of movement and another to the location of a fly at tongue's length clearly anticipated the 'bug detectors' and feature analysis of Lettvin, Maturana, McCulloch and Pitts's famous paper 'What the frog's eye tells the frog's brain', published six years later.

Barlow was invited by Kuffler to visit the Willmer Institute at Johns Hopkins University, where he worked on the cat retina with the impressive team that Kuffler had gathered there – Richard Fitzhugh, Ken Brown and Torsten Wiesel. Barlow brought with him his interest in the cybernetic approach and the various possible sources of 'noise' in the retina, which might limit visual thresholds. Those questions became incorporated in the three well-known papers of 1957 by Barlow, Fitzhugh and Kuffler, on the spontaneous, maintained activity of retinal ganglion cells, on the change in organization of receptive fields during dark adaptation, and on the absolute threshold of single ganglion cells. In the same year Richard Fitzhugh, undoubtedly influenced by his young collaborator from Cambridge, wrote, in a paper on 'The statistical detection of threshold signals in the retina' (*Journal of General Physiology*, **40**, 925–48, 1957), that 'the problem of the analysis of a nerve-fiber message by the brain is similar to the engineering problem of detection of a signal in a noisy communication channel'. He used Tanner and Swets's principle of statistical detection (*Transactions of the IRE Professional Group on Information Theory*, PGIT-4, 213–21, 1954) to describe optic nerve fibres in terms of their efficiency as communication channels.

Barlow returned to Cambridge, where his ideas about efficiency and coding developed over the following five years. When he went on leave to the University of California at Berkeley in 1962, he and Richard Hill were forced (by the lack of facilities for keeping cats) to indulge in a little comparative physiology, and they recorded from ganglion cells in the rabbit retina. To their surprise, this retina was quite different from the cat's and had a variety of cell types that was even greater than in the frog. As David Hubel and Torsten Wiesel at Harvard were describing the sensitivity of neurons in the cat striate cortex to the orientation of lines and edges, Barlow and Hill were finding cells in the rabbit retina that responded selectively to the *direction* of motion of images. It was typical of Barlow, with his long-standing interest in the psychology of perception, that he immediately linked the properties of such cells to phenomena of human perception – the movement after-effect and the whole range of figural after-effects (a subject that he tackles again in his chapter in this book).

In 1964 Barlow moved to a Professorship in the School of Optometry in Berkeley, where he stayed for nine enormously productive years. His interests in dark adaptation and the reliability of ganglion cells continued, mainly through his collaboration with Bill Levick, but in addition he developed his ideas about the encoding of the visual scene. I had the pleasure and the privilege of working under his supervision as a graduate student. We set up a laboratory for work on the cat's visual cortex and in the summer of 1966, during the visit of Jack Pettigrew, then a medical student working in Peter Bishop's department in Sydney, we found binocularly-driven neurons that were selectively sensitive to the disparities of retinal images and hence seemed to be encoding the relative distances of objects from the eyes.

Like Helmholtz, Barlow questioned the way in which the brain can become capable of making inferences about the world. Helmholtz had opted for empiricism: 'Doubtless, the reactions of natural objects to our senses are those that are most frequently and generally perceived. For both our welfare and convenience they are of the most powerful importance.' Hubel and Wiesel had earlier suggested that the striking properties of neurons in the cat's cortex (orientation selectivity, binocularity, columnar organization) were already present at the time of natural eye-opening, presumably established on the basis of genetic instructions. In 1971, Barlow and Pettigrew challenged this opinion with evidence that no cells were really orientation selective in the absence of visual experience. There followed a period of, shall we say, spirited debate, ending in a compromise that sees the visual cortex as firmly pre-determined in its basic organization but with mechanisms of activity-dependent synaptic plasticity that are now universally accepted and still the subject of intensive study. Barlow's 1975 review (*Nature*, **258**, 199–204, 1975), written at the height of the controversy, was a remarkably objective and balanced assessment of this important problem.

Since his return to the Physiological Laboratory,

Cambridge, and to a Fellowship at his undergraduate college, Trinity, Barlow has continued to move with the trends of vision research and in many cases to cause them. His current interest in the multitude of accessory visual areas in the cerebral cortex has led him to speculate about the general function of the cortex and its role in intelligence. He has written about language, about the nature of inductive inference and even about consciousness (with the clarity of an active scientist, rather than as an amateur philosopher).

Horace Barlow's support for others in the field, especially young researchers trying to establish their own reputations, is well known to all his friends. He encouraged David Marr, for instance, as he developed the new and influential computational approach to vision and helped him in many ways as he struggled to finish his remarkable book *Vision* (San Francisco: W. H. Freeman and Company, 1982) while fighting leukemia. Barlow too has embraced the computational approach which, in Marr's words, considers vision to be 'the *process* of discovering from images what is present in the world, and where it is'. This attitude is, indeed, a natural extension of the notion that visual neurons must encode and represent efficiently to the brain those aspects of the retinal image that are rich in information about the nature of the visual world.

The efficiency of coding in the visual system is the subject of this book, which is based on a conference held in Cambridge to honour Horace Barlow in his 65th year. When Horace found out about plans for a celebration he wanted, at first, to stop it; not just out of modesty, but mainly because he didn't want people to think that he was about to retire! With agreement that the word 'retirement' should not enter into the vocabulary of the occasion, Horace finally acquiesced.

The book ranges over all the major topics within visual science – the organization of the visual pathway, the function of the visual areas of the cortex, the detection of light, contrast, colour, movement and distance, dark and light adaptation, the development and plasticity of vision, the computational approach. The authors are leaders in their respective fields. All of this would not be particularly surprising, but for one fact. Every contributor to this book has studied or worked with Horace Barlow, or has been a close colleague, happy to acknowledge his or her debt to Barlow. There could be no better tribute to the extraordinary breadth of Barlow's own contribution and his influence on others.

Colin Blakemore
Oxford

Reply

Scientific papers usually have a short section of acknowledgements at the end (in small print) which says (if you're lucky) who really had the ideas and who really did all the work. On this occasion it would be appropriate to start off with these acknowledgements, in large print, but there is a difficulty, for if I were to tell you who was really responsible for all the work attributed to me I would have to go back far before my research days and it would become an autobiography as long as this book itself. I can recall hundreds of detailed episodes that gave me the confidence to continue being inquisitive: parents who did not brush a question aside but took the trouble to answer it, or at least acknowledge that it was interesting; friends and colleagues who shared my curiosity so that we dug around together for the answers; teachers whose eye was not on the current page of the textbook but on their pupil's mind and understanding; and institutions that responded to my aspirations, sometimes in spite of my inability to fill in forms and other such impediments. I suspect that anyone's list of those who have helped them on the path of science would always be very long, and it would mean little to give my list here without going into details about the particular people and situations involved. All the same it is very sad that the people whose help is so important rarely learn what they have done or how much they have been appreciated.

However I must somehow play the role of 'senior scientist', now that Colin Blakemore has made me into one by organising the meeting at Cambridge, so I shall regale you with some stories about times long past. When I started as a graduate student in Cambridge under E.D. (later Lord) Adrian there was no equipment money for the likes of me, so we had to use whatever we could find. To record eye-movements, I duly found and cannibalised an old 35 mm movie camera in a beautiful mahogany case, added my own optics and motor drive (it only had a handle originally), devised a system for immobilising the subject's head and delivering a small drop of mercury to his cornea, and found a subject or two willing to undergo torture in the cause of science. But I needed film. I was apprehensive about asking the lab superintendent for this because he has just told me, when I had recently asked him for tuppence-worth of pins for the undergraduate's experimental practical class, that he had 'given them plenty last year'. However there was nothing for it so I went to him again and asked him to order the minimum possible quantity of film, 20 ft I think. He immediately said 'We get no discount for that quantity, the Prof. always orders 1000 ft at a time, and I don't want to have to repeat this order for you every week or so'. So I took 1000 ft, and somewhere in Physiology stores there must be about 950 ft of ageing 35 mm movie film. It taught me the very important lessons that you should always find a precedent for what you ask, and that resistance to a budgetary item is a non-monotonic function of its size.

I got another budgetary lesson a little later when I wanted to try repeating some of Hartline's observations on the frog retina. I had told Adrian that I wanted to do this but he had not been very encouraging; he had just said 'I wouldn't do that – Hartline's a very clever chap you know'. That made it more difficult to get the equipment together, so I wrote him what I thought was a very tactfully worded letter asking for £10 to buy war surplus electronic junk sufficient for the job. It was obviously too tactfully worded, for I got the letter back the next day with 'What is this? An application for leave of absence or something?' scrawled on the back.

After this first unsuccessful grant application I decided to go ahead anyway, and drove my car up to

Lisle Street where the junk shops were. Pat Merton and the people at the National Hospital in Queen's Square were experts on what was available, and with their help £10 was quite enough to fill my car with a power supply, oscilloscope, and numerous valves and other components, including of course solder and soldering iron (i.e. about 100 lbs weight, at an average of 10p per lb, which was how they sold it). The car was a British Salmson without any top, but I had picked a nice day and started to drive back to Cambridge. Now the car had a peculiarity: its wheels were held on with single large brass nuts, and as I only had a small adjustable spanner to tighten these, they tended to work loose. On the way back I detected the 'thud-thud-thud' that indicated a loose wheel, and after putting it off as long as possible, reluctantly drew off the road. It was getting dark, the car lights were not too good, it was starting to rain, and furthermore the spanner and jack were *under* the 100 lbs of equipment, but I could not avoid unloading it all onto the verge of the road. After re-tightening the wheel-nut, I reloaded the stuff in too great a hurry – and as a result I had to return to the spot a week later to recover a resistor that was an essential part of my illuminating circuit.

Eventually I got the whole set-up more or less working, and as it happened R. Granit was on a visit to Cambridge about that time and Adrian brought him into my lab. I had just dropped my best electrode on to the floor, and since I had no other I rather despondently lowered it on to the retina again. At that point Granit and Adrian came in and we chatted for a minute or two while I showed them what I was doing. Then Granit pulled on his cigar and emitted a dense puff of smoke; it drifted between the light and the preparation, which obligingly gave a massive off-response. That was very satisfactory, since he had just been saying he didn't think my electrodes would work, even if I didn't drop them on the floor.

In those days there was not much money or equipment, but you didn't have to spend much time begging for it either. Earlier this year there was some correspondence in *Nature* about fraud in science; one short contribution, which probably contained a higher density of truth than anything else in the whole issue, just said 'Isn't it amazing how *little* fraud there is, considering the lies we all have to tell in our grant applications'. Anybody who has read a proposal for one of our present government's white elephants, an Interdisciplinary Research Centre, will know just what he meant.

The popular image of a scientist is that of a lonely and somewhat isolated genius, but in fact science is almost always an intensely social activity – as those who marry scientists quickly discover. Hundreds of people, many of whom have contributed to this book, have taught me facts, given me ideas, or removed some of my misconceptions. It would be invidious to mention names, but in my long experience I have learned what are the 5 most important characteristics of a good colleague, and I shall tell you them.

(1) He or she must tell you when you're wrong. When you've risen above the Associate Professor level most people are convinced that you think yourself infallible. Of course they're right, but it's annoying that they tell everybody else when you're wrong and won't tell you. As soon as the truth of this basic situation dawned on me I became addicted to computers, for they report your errors as fearlessly as Bill Levick.

(2) The ideal colleague must tell you you're wrong without actually stopping you doing the experiment you're just planning. With some colleagues things stop dead when the idea is killed; with others the argument and discussion is such fun that the experiment gets forgotten. I think this was why I only published one paper (actually his first joint-authored paper, I think) with William Rushton.

(3) The ideal colleague must constantly convert a theoretical argument into an experimental prediction: 'You say X is so, therefore Y should happen'. This is the most basic step in all of science, but it's a rare ability to constantly make that step; most of us either waste our time basking in the brilliant sunshine of theory, or just *love* fiddling with the equipment. Come to think of it, there's a third category: those who spend all their time writing grant applications.

(4) The ideal colleague must have read all the literature you cannot be bothered to read, must understand the historical development of the subject accurately and dispassionately, and whenever necessary must exaggerate the importance of your own role in it.

(5) Any colleague of any sort has to tidy up the lab after you've made a mess of it.

The relation between the written record of science and how it is actually done is rather interesting. Important scientific facts and ideas spend very little of their lives as the sole property of their ostensible author. Before they are crystallised in print, they exist in corridor arguments and tea-room discussions among colleagues, and their essence rapidly dissolves again from the printed page to modify arguments, discussions, and plans for future experiments. Furthermore, the message that comes off the page and has an influence is often quite different from what the author intended. Although we pretend to worship *facts*, the real life of science lies in these free-floating *ideas*: it may not have been exactly what he meant, but Eddington said 'Never believe a fact until it has been confirmed by theory'; new facts make no sense without fitting them together with old facts, and then what matters is whether they change people's ideas.

All of us who have been involved in vision research over the past decade or so have had the good fortune to be involved in an exciting enterprise where facts and ideas have interacted frequently, so the scene has been ever-changing. It's hard for me to imagine being anything other than a scientist, and the continual possibility of these interactions has prevented me wanting to be anything else.

But it's the interactions with people that keep one's spirits up. The meeting of which this book is the record was extraordinarily cheering for me. Let me illustrate this by referring to the diametrically opposite opposite experience, which most scientists must have had at some time or other. You write a paper with immense expenditure of time, effort, and pain, and then when it has been submitted, refereed, modified,

accepted, and finally published, you see and hear nothing more at all: in spite of the launch, there is no splash, no wave, no indication of whether the paper sank without trace or is drifting unheeded somewhere in the ocean of science. Well, for me the meeting was the exact opposite of that experience; it created collossal euphoria and the feeling that it has all been worthwhile. I wish there was a way of transferring back to authors of worthy but unsung papers a fraction of this euphoria: should we start a charity that issues a bottle of champagne for every genuine, duly-refereed, paper that is published?

I have had marvellous support from teachers, colleagues, collaborators and institutions, and I would like to thank them all and tell them how much they have been appreciated, especially Colin Blakemore who organised the meeting.

Horace Barlow
Cambridge

Acknowledgements

This book is based on a conference held at the Physiological Laboratory, University of Cambridge. Without the permission of Professor Ian Glynn and the support of many other members of staff in the Physiological Laboratory, the meeting would have been impossible. In particular, Jo Brown, Horace Barlow's secretary, Clive Hood, senior technician in Fergus Campbell's laboratory, and Margaret Twinn, secretary to Professor Glynn, gave a great deal of practical help. Special thanks go to Sue Saunders of the University Laboratory of Physiology, Oxford, who not only dealt with most of the practical arrangements for the conference but also nursed this book through its complicated gestation. King's College and Trinity College, Cambridge, provided accommodation and entertainment for the participants and the conference was generously supported by grants from:

British Telecom Research Laboratories
Cambridge University Press
King's College, Cambridge
T.F.C. Frost Charitable Trust
Trinity College, Cambridge
The Admiralty Research Establishment
The European Office of the US Air Force
The Physiological Society
The Royal Society
The Ulverscroft Foundation
The Worshipful Company of Spectacle Makers

Concepts of coding
and efficiency

1

The quantum efficiency of vision

D. G. Pelli

How did you come to be interested in quantum efficiency?

H. B. Barlow: I was an undergraduate and doing Part II Physiology [at Cambridge University in the early 1940s]. I was directed to R. A. Fisher's book [1925, *Statistical Methods for Research Workers*]. The idea of statistical inference seemed relevant to understanding what the brain was doing. . . . It gave an objective handle to something the brain did rather well.

[August 27, 1987]

Attempts to understand the quantum efficiency of vision have resulted in three distinct measures of efficiency. This chapter shows how they fit together, and presents some new measurements. We will show that the idea of equivalent input noise and a simplifying assumption called 'contrast invariance' allow the observer's overall quantum efficiency (as defined by Barlow, 1962a) to be factored into two components: transduction efficiency (called 'quantum efficiency of the eye' by Rose, 1948) and calculation efficiency (called 'central efficiency' by Barlow, 1977).

When light is absorbed by matter, it is absorbed discontinuously, in discrete quanta. Furthermore, it is absorbed randomly; the light intensity determines only the probability of absorption of a quantum of light, a photon (Einstein, 1905). This poses a fundamental limit to vision; the photon statistics of the retinal image impose an upper limit to the reliability of any decision based on that retinal image. An observer's overall *quantum efficiency F* is the smallest fraction of the corneal quanta (i.e. quanta sent into the eye) consistent with the level of the observer's performance (Barlow, 1958b, 1962a). (This is closely analogous to Fisher's (1925) definition of the efficiency of a statistic.) Surprisingly, the overall quantum efficiency of vision is very variable, and much smaller than best estimates of the fraction of photons absorbed by the photoreceptors in the retina.

At all reasonable luminances the fraction of corneal photons that excite photoreceptors is almost certainly quite constant. Barlow (1977) concluded that for rods it must be in the range 11% to 33% (for 507 nm light). This is independent of the size and duration of the signal, and independent of the background luminance, up to extremely high luminances. Yet, Barlow (1962b) had previously shown (see Fig. 1.1) that the highest overall quantum efficiency of vision is

only 5%, and *that* only for a small brief spot on a very low luminance background. Figure 1.1 shows that increasing the background luminance reduces the overall quantum efficiency by many orders of magnitude.

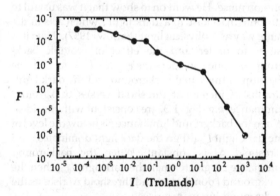

Fig. 1.1. Overall quantum efficiency versus retinal illuminance (in scotopic Trolands) for detecting a 46′ diameter spot presented for 86 ms on a uniform background at 15° in the nasal field. Replotted from Barlow (1962b).

Figure 1.2 shows that the overall quantum efficiency is strongly dependent on both the area and duration of the spot. But, if the fraction of photons that excite photoreceptors is constant, why should the experimental conditions so dramatically affect the quantum efficiency?

The question still lacks a full answer, but this chapter will present a framework that will allow simple threshold measurements to distinguish between two classes of explanation for the variation in efficiency. The key idea is the notion of an observer's equivalent input noise, which is analogous to Barlow's (1956, 1957) dark light.

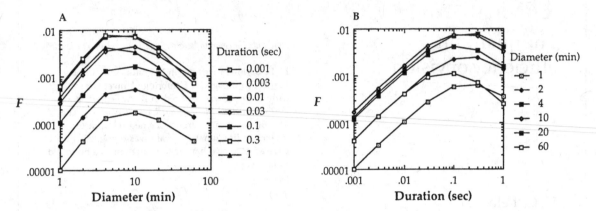

Fig. 1.2A and B. Overall quantum efficiency versus spot diameter and duration on a uniform background of 3.4 cd/m². Replotted from Jones (1959).

Barlow (1956) pointed out that Hecht, Shlaer & Pirenne's (1942) estimate of the fraction of photons absorbed was really only a lower bound, because there might be noise in the visual system which added to the photon noise. He went on to show that it was useful to attribute that noise to a 'dark light', which acts in the same way as a physical light (Barlow, 1957). Thus it is easier to understand the effect of scotopic backgrounds if one considers the *effective background* to be the sum of the actual background and the dark light. Graphs of increment threshold versus background luminance, e.g. Fig. 1.3, are consistent with this idea. When the background luminance I is below the level of the dark light I_{dark} then the dark light dominates, and threshold ΔI is constant. When the background luminance I is greater than the dark light I_{dark} then the background I dominates, and threshold ΔI rises as the background luminance rises.

Fortunately for our night vision, the dark light is very small (0.0028 td in Fig. 1.3) and is negligible at any luminance well above absolute threshold. However, it turns out that contrast thresholds in noise behave in an analogous way. At high luminances we usually don't worry about photon noise, but it is increasingly common to artificially add luminance noise to the display, typically by adding a random number to each pixel of an image. One can then measure threshold as a function of the amplitude of the noise. This approach is reminiscent of Barlow's dark light measurements. In fact, this sort of measurement is routine in electrical engineering, where it is called equivalent input noise measurement (e.g. Mumford & Schelbe, 1968). Equivalent input noise measurement dates back at least to the 1940s, and probably much before (North, 1942; Friis, 1944).

Consider traditional equivalent noise measure-

ment. Suppose we are setting up an audio system. We have a record player, or some other audio signal source which inevitably has some noise. Suppose we know how much noise the source has. Now we want to choose an audio amplifier to amplify our signal. We want to choose an amplifier that has very little noise, so that it will reproduce the signal faithfully. Even the best amplifier has some noise. However, we don't want to buy an unnecessarily expensive low-noise amplifier, since it's enough for the amplifier's noise to be small relative to the noise already in our audio source. How shall we evaluate the amplifier? We could just measure the noise at the amplifier's output, but that would not be directly comparable with the noise in our original audio source. Or we could open the

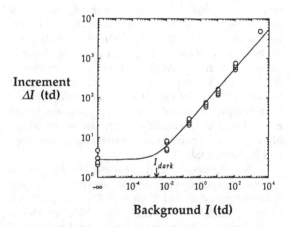

Fig. 1.3. Threshold increment ΔI for a small brief spot as a function of background luminance I, both in scotopic Trolands. The smooth curve represents the relation $\Delta I \propto (I + I_{dark})^{0.5}$, where $I_{dark} = 0.0028$ td. Replotted from Barlow (1957).

amplifier up and measure the noise at some point inside. But where? Nearly all electrical components generate noise.

Figure 1.4 illustrates the standard procedure, which is to measure the output noise level when a series of calibrated noise levels are applied to the input of the amplifier. Figure 1.5 shows a typical set of results, showing output noise level versus input noise level. Both scales are logarithmic, and are calibrated in deciBels. Noise should be described by its spectral density N, which is the power per unit bandwidth. In this example it has units of Watts per Hertz. The meters in Fig. 1.4 measure power, in Watts. The power spectral density N is calculated by dividing the measured power by the bandwidth, in Hertz, of the

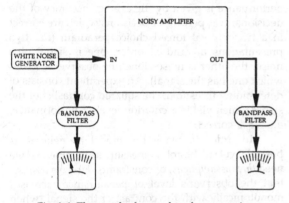

Fig. 1.4. The standard procedure for measuring equivalent input noise. The noise level (power spectral density) is measured at the input and output of the amplifier, at many levels of white noise input (Mumford & Schelbe, 1968). Power spectral density is measured by the combination of a bandpass filter and power meter.

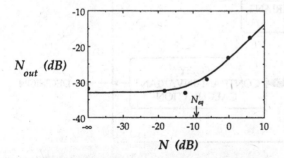

Fig. 1.5. Results from the experiment in Fig. 1.4: output noise level versus input noise level. Both decibel scales are relative to 1 μW/Hz. The smooth curve represents the relation $N_{out} \propto N + N_{eq}$, where N_{eq} is −9 dB re 1 μW/Hz.

filter preceding the meter. *White noise* has the same spectral density at all frequencies of interest.

In general, both the amplifier gain and the output noise power spectral density are frequency dependent, so measurements like those in Fig. 1.5 are made at each of many frequencies, by changing the center frequency of the bandpass filters. However, we will ignore the complication of frequency dependence for now, and come back to it later. The noise measured at the output contains contributions from both the external noise and the intrinsic noise of the amplifier. Low external noise levels are insignificant compared to the intrinsic noise, so the curve is flat at low external noise levels. At high external noise levels the *external* noise N dominates so the curve rises with a log–log slope of 1, indicating proportionality. The knee of the curve occurs when the effect of the external noise is equal to that of the intrinsic noise. That input noise level is called the *equivalent input noise* N_{eq}.

The smooth curve in Fig. 1.5 represents a simple relation. Output noise level is proportional to the sum of external and equivalent noise levels.

$$N_{out} \propto N + N_{eq} \qquad (1)$$

Noises add for the same reason that variances add; the variance of the sum of two independent random variables is the sum of the variances of each variable. The proportionality constant and N_{eq} were determined so as to provide a maximum likelihood fit by Eq. 1 to the data. The value of N_{eq} is indicated by an arrow on the horizontal axis at the knee of the curve. The curve is asymptotically straight on either side of the knee and N_{eq} is the horizontal coordinate of the intersection of the two limiting lines. Note that N_{eq} is independent of the amplifier gain. With a higher gain the curve would be shifted higher on these logarithmic axes, but the horizontal position would be unchanged.

We have just measured the amplifier's intrinsic noise by finding its equivalent input noise. Figure 1.6, which illustrates this idea schematically, is a conceptual model of the situation we saw in Fig. 1.4. This is a *black-box* model, intended to model the input and output behavior of the system under study, without regard for its internal construction. The noisy amplifier is conceived to be made up of a hypothetical noiseless amplifier with a built-in noise generator at its input. The required internal noise level to match the intrinsic noise of the actual amplifier is called the *equivalent input noise*.

Thus we can measure the intrinsic noise by finding an equivalent input noise. This is sometimes called 'referring the amplifier's noise to its input'. Essentially the same approach can be applied to vision. Indeed, this is analogous to Barlow's (1957) dark light measurements. By a similar analogy we can apply this idea to the contrast domain.

In order to measure the observer's equivalent input noise we need an output power meter. For this we will use the observer's squared contrast threshold, since it is well known that the squared contrast threshold is proportional to the noise level at the display (e.g. Stromeyer & Julesz, 1972; Pelli, 1981). The idea here is that, instead of building our own power meter, we use one that is already built into the visual system under study.

Figure 1.7 shows the model for the human observer. Like Fig. 1.6, this is a black-box model, intended to correctly model the behavior, but not the internal construction, of the observer. The stimulus to the observer is the sum of signal and noise. The signal

is present to provide a dependent measure analogous to output noise level, as we'll see below. Note the fat arrows. They indicate transmission of a spatiotemporal function, a time-varying image, which could be represented by a three-dimensional array of numbers. For example the signal might be a flickering grating or a television program. The black-box model has an equivalent input noise ('contrast-invariant noise') which adds to the stimulus. We will call the sum of the stimulus and the equivalent input noise the *effective stimulus*. Finally, there is a transformation, 'calculation', which somehow reduces the spatiotemporal *effective* stimulus down to a simple decision, such as 'yes' or 'no', which can be represented by a single number, as indicated by the thin arrow. The observer's task is to detect the signal. The observer's level of performance is given by the average accuracy of the decisions, e.g. percent of decisions which are correct in a two-interval forced choice paradigm (i.e. two presentations in random order, one is signal plus noise, the other is noise alone; the observer is asked which one has the signal). An experiment consists of determining threshold, the squared contrast c^2 of the signal which yields a criterion level of performance, e.g. 75% correct.

In order to make the model as general as possible, yet still be able to measure its parameters, we need *three assumptions*, or constraints. First we assume that the observer's level of performance increases monotonically with the contrast of the signal (when everything else is fixed). This guarantees that there will be a unique threshold. Secondly, as indicated on the diagram by the prefix *contrast-invariant*, we assume that the calculation performed is independent of the

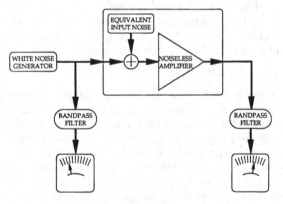

Fig. 1.6. A black box model for the noisy amplifier in Fig. 1.4.

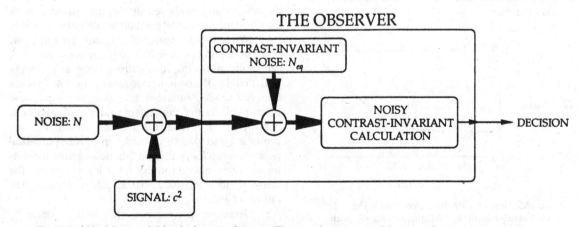

Fig. 1.7. A black box model for the human observer. The stimulus consists of the sum of noise with nose level N and a signal with a squared contrast c^2. The fat arrows indicate transmission of a time-varying image. The thin arrow indicates transmission of a scalar, the observer's decision.

contrast of the effective stimulus, which is its immediate input. Together, assumptions 1 and 2 are a linking hypothesis. They imply that the observer's squared contrast threshold (which we can measure) is proportional to the effective noise level (which is inaccessible). Thirdly, we assume that the equivalent input noise is independent of the amplitude of the input noise and signal, or at least that it too is contrast-invariant, independent of the contrast of the effective image. These assumptions allow us to use two threshold measurements at different external noise levels to estimate the equivalent noise level. In effect, the assumptions state that the proportionality constant and the equivalent noise N_{eq} are indeed constant, independent of the contrast of the effective image. These three assumptions are just enough to allow us to make psychophysical measurements that uniquely determine the parameters of our black-box model. Our model makes several testable predictions, as will be discussed below.

I should point out too, that while this model is required in order to measure the equivalent input noise (and 'transduction efficiency'), we will see below that the model is not required for measurement of either the 'calculation' or overall quantum efficiency of the observer, as these latter measurements are assumption-free. Those measures are assumption-free partly because each can be determined from a single threshold measurement. Measurement of an observer's equivalent noise level requires two threshold measurements and a linking hypothesis (our black-box model) to relate the two measurements.

Note that we have redefined *equivalent input noise* from its usual meaning in which it reflects all the noise in the system under study, to now only reflect noise that can be described by a contrast-invariant input noise. This subtlety is irrelevant in many simple systems, such as the linear amplifier in Figs. 1.4 and 1.6, where all the internal noise is contrast-invariant, but in general nonlinear systems can have an internal noise that is contrast-dependent (Legge, Kersten & Burgess, 1987; Ahumada, 1987). However, our model does allow the calculation to be noisy, provided the calculation is still contrast-invariant. This means that any noise introduced within the calculation would have to be proportional to the effective noise level at the input of the calculation. This would happen, if, for example, the observer used a randomly chosen receptive field on each trial to detect the same signal (Burgess & Colborne, 1988). Using the terminology of Lillywhite (1981), 'additive' noise (independent of the effective noise) is assigned by our model to the contrast-invariant noise, and 'multiplicative' noise (proportional to the effective noise) is assigned to the noisy calculation. From here on, *equivalent input noise* refers solely to the contrast-invariant input noise of our black box model in Fig. 1.7.

A wide range of models are consistent with our black box because they are contrast-invariant, e.g. all the ideal receivers derived by Peterson, Birdsall & Fox (1954) for various kinds of signal (known exactly or only statistically) in white noise, the uncertainty model shown by Pelli (1985) to provide a good model for many aspects of visual contrast detection and near-threshold discrimination, and the ideal discriminators of Geisler & Davila (1985).

Some popular models for detection, e.g. ones incorporating a high fixed threshold, are *not* scale invariant and are incompatible with our black-box model. However, these models are also incompatible with the empirical effects of noise (Pelli, 1981, 1985) and criterion effects (Nachmias, 1981). The desirable aspects of high-threshold-like behavior can arise from scale invariant models (Pelli, 1985) so incompatibility with such models is not a cause for worry.

Figure 1.8A shows a grating in white noise. The luminance of each pixel has an added random variation. In my experiments, these variations are dynamic and uncorrelated over space and time. That is what is meant by *white noise*. I measured contrast thresholds for the grating at many different noise levels, keeping the mean luminance of the display constant. Figure 1.8B illustrates another way to do this experiment, using a random dot display, such as used by Rose (1957) and van Meeteren & Boogaard (1973). A random-dot display models the way that photons are absorbed in the retina. The random-dot display in Fig. 1.8B appears very similar to the additive-noise display in Fig. 1.8A, but now the display consists solely of white dots on a black background, and the grating simply modulates the probability of occurrence of the dots. The most common random-dot display is the image intensifier, which is used to see at night (van Meeteren & Boogaard 1973).

Once detected by the photocathode . . . photons can be made visible as bright specks on an image screen by electronic amplification. When the detected photon flux is sufficiently high, these specks combine in space and time to form a normal, smooth image. At lower light levels in object space, however, the detected photon flux can be so small that the corresponding specks are visible as such, especially when the amplification is high.

Many people have used such displays to 'bypass early levels of processing'. Barlow (1978) discussed,

the demonstration by French, Julesz, Uttal and

A

B

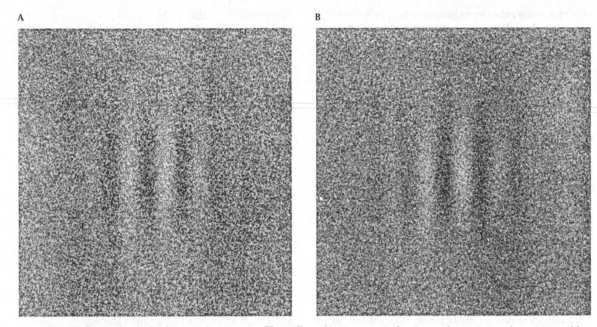

Fig. 1.8. Two ways to display a grating in noise. These illustrations are static, but in a real experiment the noise would be dynamic. The signal is a sinusoidal grating with 0.4 contrast, vignetted by a circularly symmetric Gaussian with a space constant of 1.5 grating periods, i.e. $s(x, y) = 0.4 \exp(-[(x+y)/1.5]^2) \sin(2\pi x)$. The main difference between these displays is that in A the variance is independent of the signal, and in B it is dependent, proportional to the expected luminance at each point. A. An additive display: each cell is the sum of signal and independent noise. The reflectance of each halftone cell is $(1 + s(x, y) + X_{x,y})L_{av}$, where $X_{x,y} = \pm 0.3$ is a random sample from a binomial distribution, determined independently for each cell, and the mean luminance corresponds to a 50% reflectance, $L_{av} = 0.5$. B. A random-dot display: each cell is a sample from a Poisson distribution whose mean is modulated by the signal. The reflectance of each halftone cell in the image is $X_{x,y}/11$, where $X_{x,y}$ is a random sample from a Poisson distribution with mean $11(1 + s(x, y))L_{av}$. The Poisson distribution was approximated by the sum of 11 samples from a binomial distribution yielding 1 with probability $(1 + s(x, y))L_{av}$ and 0 otherwise.

others that patterns composed largely of random dots provide an opportunity to probe intermediate levels of processing in the visual system. The dots which compose the pattern are, it is suggested, reliably transduced and transmitted by the lower levels, and the limitations of performance result from the ways in which the nervous system can combine and compare groups of these dots at the next higher level.

It turns out that we can analyze both kinds of experiment (Figs. 1.8A and B) in the same way: the contrast threshold of the grating as a function of the spectral density of the noise (Pelli, 1981). Figures 1.8A and B show that although the methods of generation of the two kinds of display are quite different, the two displays look very much alike when they have the same noise level and luminance.

Since each experiment is done at a constant average luminance, it is convenient to define our measures of signal and noise in terms of the *contrast function*, which is a normalized version of the luminance function,

$$c(x, y, t) = \frac{L(x, y, t)}{L_{av}} - 1 \qquad (2)$$

where (x, y, t) is a time and place on the display and L_{av} is the mean luminance (Linfoot, 1964). A complete set of definitions and a formal derivation of the theoretical results of this chapter appear in Appendix A.

Power spectral density N is the contrast power per unit bandwidth. Imagine filtering the image with a narrowband filter with unit gain in the passband. The *contrast power* of the filtered image is c_{rms}^2, the mean of the square of the contrast function. The ratio of the power to the bandwidth is an estimate of the power spectral density of the original image at the center frequency of the filter.

Figure 1.9 presents a typical set of results obtained with displays like those in Fig. 1.8. It shows the squared contrast threshold for a 4 c/deg grating in the presence of a noise background. The vertical scale is the contrast threshold. The horizontal scale is the noise level. All of the points are within two standard errors of the smooth curve. The curve represents proportionality of squared contrast threshold to the sum of the external noise and the equivalent noise.

$$c^2 \propto N + N_{eq} = N_{ef} \qquad (3)$$

At *low* noise levels the squared contrast threshold is nearly constant. At *high* noise levels the threshold rises in proportion to the noise level. This entire experiment can be summarized by Eq. 3 and its two fitted parameters: the observer's equivalent input noise N_{eq} (which we want to know) and the proportionality constant (which is not of interest here).

In the same way that earlier we talked of the *effective* luminance being the sum of the stimulus light and the dark light, we will now speak of the *effective* noise level N_{ef} being the sum of the displayed noise and the observer's equivalent noise.

It may not be obvious that Eq. 3 is dimensionally correct, nor why the contrast is squared. We are interested in squared contrast (i.e. contrast power), rather than contrast, because we are dealing with independent random quantities, so their variances add, and variance is proportional to the square of the amplitude. Recall that N represents power spectral density, which is proportional to the contrast power of the noise. c^2 is proportional to the contrast power of the signal. Thus, Eq. 3 basically says that the contrast

power of the signal at threshold is proportional to the contrast power of the effective noise.

In our notation, upper case symbols like N are generally proportional to squared contrast and lower-case symbols like c are generally proportional to contrast.

Equation (3) is the principal prediction of our model. The model explicitly assumes that the performance is independent of the overall contrast of the effective image, so at a constant level of performance the squared contrast of the signal is proportional to the effective noise level, $c^2 \propto N_{ef}$. Equation (3) is not as direct as the analogous Eq. (1) used in electrical engineering because we cannot directly measure the observer's 'output' noise. Instead we measure a squared contrast threshold and assume that it is proportional to the observer's effective noise level (the 'output' noise). Equation (3) is obeyed by *every* published record or contrast threshold versus noise level at a constant luminance (Pelli, 1981).

Consider Figure 1.10, which shows thresholds for detection of a 4 c/deg grating at two luminances, 3.3 and 330 cd/m² (pupil size was not measured). Both conditions are well fit by Eq. 3. The effect of luminance on the two parameters is interesting. In the absence of noise the threshold is higher at the lower luminance. However, as the noise level increases, the curves eventually converge, so that at high noise level, the

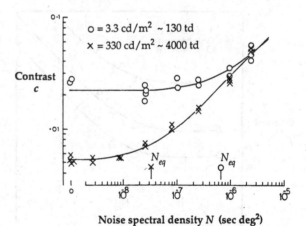

Fig. 1.10. Contrast threshold for a grating in noise at two luminances: 3.3 cd/m² and 330 cd/m² (about 130 and 4000 td, respectively). The smooth curve represents Eq. 3. The signal was a vertical 4 c/deg grating with a Gaussian envelope with a horizontal space constant of 2°, a vertical space constant of 5°, and a time constant of 70 ms. The noise was white up to 66 c/deg horizontally, 6.6 c/deg vertically, and 50 Hz temporally. From Pelli (1981).

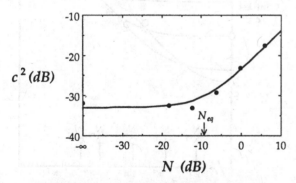

Fig. 1.9. Squared contrast threshold (in dB) versus noise level (in dB re 1 µs deg²). The smooth curve represents the relation, $c^2 \propto N + N_{eq}$, where N_{eq} is −9 dB re 1 µs deg². Note that a deciBel is one tenth of a log unit change in *power*. Thus there are 10 dB per decade of squared-contrast and noise level, since they are both proportional to power.

hundred-fold change in luminance does not affect the contrast threshold. The two curves converge because they have the same proportionality constant. The only effect of the hundred-fold luminance increase is to reduce the equivalent noise level.

Figure 1.11 shows data from Nagaraja (1964), as re-analyzed by Pelli (1981), for detecting a disk on a uniform background of 0.34 cd/m^2 (pupil size was not measured). Each curve is for a different disk size: 5.7', 14.7', 32'. As one would expect, the smaller disks have higher thresholds. However, remarkably, all the disk sizes yield virtually the same estimate of the equivalent noise level.

Figure 1.12 shows data from van Meeteren & Boogaard (1973), as re-analyzed by Pelli (1981), for detecting a 4.5 c/deg sinusoidal grating on a random dot display. Each curve is for a different luminance: 0.035, 0.35, and 3.5 td. The curves tend to converge at higher noise level. Note that the equivalent noise level is higher at lower luminance.

Figure 1.13 shows data from van Meeteren (1973), as re-analyzed by Pelli (1981), for detecting a 2.2 c/deg sinusoidal grating on a random dot display. Each curve is for a different luminance: 0.0013, 0.013, 0.13, 1.3, and 13 td. Again, the curves tend to converge at higher noise level, and the equivalent noise level is higher at lower luminance.

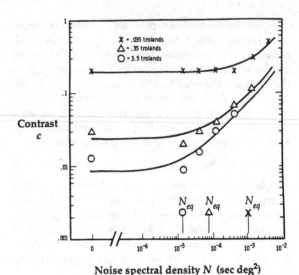

Fig. 1.12. Contrast threshold for a 4.5 c/deg grating on a random dot display at three luminances: 0.035, 0.35, and 3.5 td. The smooth curve represents Eq. 3. From Pelli (1981), who re-analyzed data from van Meeteren & Boogaard (1973). (The relatively poor fit at zero noise is probably due to the fact that these data were collected using a different apparatus, long after the other measurements.)

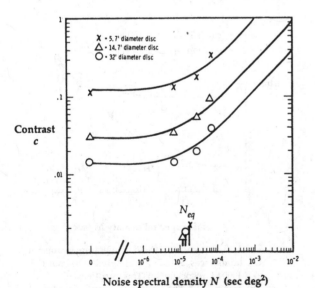

Fig. 1.11. Contrast threshold for a disk in noise. The disk diameter was 5.7', 14.7', or 32' on a 0·34 cd/m^2 background (about 7 td). The smooth curve represents Eq. 3. From Pelli (1981), who re-analyzed data from Nagaraja (1964).

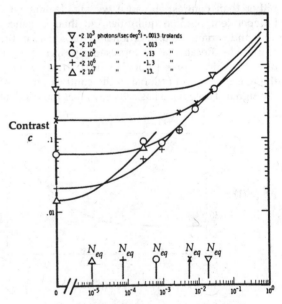

Fig. 1.13. Contrast threshold for a 2.2 c/deg grating at 7° nasal field on a random dot display at luminances of 0.0013, 0.013, 0.13, 1.3, and 13 td. The smooth curve represents Eq. 3. From Pelli (1981), who re-analyzed data from van Meeteren (1973).

Since all we care about in these graphs is the equivalent noise level, it is easy to summarize them all in a single graph. The various plotted symbols in Fig. 1.14 show the equivalent noise level for each experiment, versus the retinal illuminance, in Trolands. (Where necessary, pupil size was estimated from standard tables, Wyszecki & Stiles, 1967. Data are also included from Pelli, 1983, which will be described below.) Note that the data are quite orderly. At each luminance the equivalent noise levels are all nearly the same. As luminance increases the equivalent noise level decreases, in inverse proportion, as indicated by the slope of minus one.

It is interesting to compare the equivalent noise with photon noise, since photon noise may be an important component of the observer's equivalent noise. To make this comparison we need to calculate what noise level would result from full utilization of a given photon flux. The formula is

$$N_{\text{photon}} = \frac{1}{J_{\text{photon}}} \tag{4}$$

where J_{photon} is the photon flux (in photons per deg^2 sec) and N_{photon} is the *corneal-photon noise*, i.e. the noise level corresponding to use of all the photons, in contrast power per unit band width, in (c/deg)^2 Hz (see Appendix A). N_{photon} is the lowest possible equivalent noise level at retinal illuminance J_{photon}.

Figure 1.14 shows the corneal-photon noise N_{photon} as a solid line. This corresponds to absorbing 100% of the corneal photons. Obviously the corneal-photon noise is much too low to account for the equivalent noise of the observers. Real observers fail to use all the photons and have additional sources of noise (Barlow, 1977), so their equivalent noise is higher than N_{photon}. If only 10% of the photons are absorbed, then, by the reciprocal relation between photon flux and noise level, the noise level will be ten times higher. That is shown as the middle line. Finally, if only 1% of the photons are absorbed, then the noise level will be 100 times higher, which is shown as the upper line. Note that most of the data points lie between the 1% and 10% lines. That means that these equivalent noise estimates can be accounted for by the absorbed-photon noise, if we are prepared to assume that somewhere between 1% and 10% are absorbed. (Or, alternatively, we could talk about the fraction that excite photoreceptors, and the exciting-photon noise.) Although the data points come from a variety of experiments by different laboratories, there is surprisingly little scatter.

The largest deviation occurs at 252 td, for the Pelli (1983) data, for which most of the points are clustered around the $10N_{\text{photon}}$ line, corresponding to 10% absorbed. Part of the reason for the discrepancy is that only these data have been corrected for the modulation transfer of the optics of the eye, so the plotted equivalent noise level is that at the retina. Whether the discrepancy among data points in Fig. 1.14 is real would be best determined by new experiments spanning the entire luminance range.

The data of van Meeteren (1973) are from the periphery and mostly at scotopic luminances so they mostly reflect rod activity; whereas the rest of the data are for foveal viewing, mostly at photopic luminances and thus mostly reflect cone activity. Even though Fig. 1.14 includes two receptor systems the data points are all consistent with a fairly constant fraction of photon absorption (1% to 10%), with little or no effect of background luminance, or parameters of the signal. Incidentally, this conclusion is consistent with that of the original authors, though the analysis presented here differs in important ways from that made by van Meeteren *et al.* (see Discussion).

At the beginning of this chapter we noted that we expect the fraction of photons absorbed to be constant, unlike the observer's overall quantum

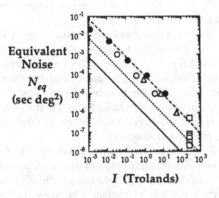

Equivalent
Noise

N_{eq}

(sec deg^2)

I (Trolands)

△   Nagaraja (1964)
●   van Meeteren (1973)
○   van Meeteren & Boogaard (1973)
□   Pelli (1983)
—— N_{photon}
······ $10\,N_{photon}$
– – $100\,N_{photon}$

Fig. 1.14. Equivalent noise levels from Fig. 1.11 to 1.13 and from Pelli (1983). (The figure also includes more data of Nagaraja, 1964, as re-analyzed by Pelli, 1981, for a 14.7′ disk at luminances of approximately 0.9 and 50 td.) The lines show the equivalent noise level corresponding to use of 100% of the corneal quanta (solid line), 10% (finely dashed line), and 1% (coarsely dashed line).

efficiency, which is known to depend strongly on experimental conditions (e.g. Barlow's data in Fig. 1.1). Unfortunately, although the data in Fig. 1.14 span a wide range of conditions, they do not include the conditions used by Barlow (1962b) to measure quantum efficiency (Fig. 1.1).

The observer's equivalent input noise can only come from *two* sources, absorbed-photon noise, and neural noise. Neural noise arises in virtually all neural elements of the visual system from photoreceptor to cortex. Noise is ubiquitous in most physical systems. However, at least in man-made systems, it is a hallmark of good engineering that the dominant noise occurs at the first stage (e.g. North, 1942). This is achieved by having a high enough gain in each stage so that the noise of the first stage dwarfs the noise added in at each subsequent stage. North (1942) suggested that it would be useful to compare the equivalent input noise of sensitive radio receivers with the unavoidable thermal noise in the radio's antenna (the radio's input), and called this the radio's 'noise factor'. We will take a similar approach, comparing the observer's equivalent input noise with the unavoidable photon noise, and call it the observer's 'transduction efficiency'. (As we will see later, Rose (1948a) invented transduction efficiency, and though he did not point out the parallel to North's noise factor, he did acknowledge many discussions with North, who was also at RCA. Rose was developing sensitive television cameras; North was developing sensitive television receivers. Both were evaluating the sensitivity of their creations on an absolute scale.)

All of this will hopefully have convinced the reader that the observer's equivalent noise level is an interesting empirical quantity. Now we will need some definitions. The following narrative will emphasize an intuitive explanation for the equivalent noise idea that allows us to factor quantum efficiency into two components. Appendix A presents a parallel but more formal derivation.

For convenience, instead of referring to the contrast of the signal, it will be useful to refer to its contrast energy E, which is proportional to the squared contrast (see Appendix A; Pelli, 1981; Watson, Barlow & Robson, 1983).

Now let us consider several stages in the visual process. First consider the object, a luminance function at the visual field, or its image, a retinal illuminance function at the retina. In either case, it contains a target pattern with a certain contrast and thus a certain contrast energy. Similarly, the experimenter may introduce noise, e.g. by randomly varying the luminance of each pixel. Or, of course,

there may be no noise at all. It is most convenient to describe an image by its contrast function (see Appendix A). The signal-to-noise ratio is the ratio of the signal contrast energy E to the noise level N, as shown in the upper left entry in Table 1.1. If there is no display noise, then the signal-to-noise ratio is infinite, as shown in the lower left entry.

The next stage that we can consider in the visual process is to imagine the image, instead of being a continuous luminance or illuminance function, as being a discontinuous collection of discretely absorbed photons. Call this the *photon* image. Knowing the retinal illuminance, we can calculate how much corneal-photon noise there will be (i.e. corresponding to absorption of 100% of the corneal photons). The photon noise adds to any noise in the contrast image, so the signal-to-noise ratio is $E/(N + N_{photon})$. If there is no display noise then the signal-to-noise ratio is just E/N_{photon}.

So far we have only considered the stimulus, without taking the observer into account at all. Now consider the *effective* image. We define the effective image as the sum of the original image (expressed as a contrast function) and the observer's equivalent input noise. The signal-to-noise ratio of the effective image is $E/(N + N_{eq})$. If there is no display noise then the signal-to-noise ratio is just E/N_{eq}.

Note that the absorbed-photon noise does not appear in the signal-to-noise ratio of the effective image in Table 1.1. The observer's equivalent noise already includes all the photon noise and any contrast-invariant neural noise. Besides, we do not know how much absorbed-photon noise there is in the observer's eye, because we do not know precisely what fraction of the photons is absorbed.

Finally, we can measure the observer's performance, which is the final result of the visual processing. We can calculate a signal-to-noise ratio d'^2 from the observer's percent of correct responses, or hit and false alarm rates (see Appendix A for definition of d').

A very important point is that these signal-to-noise ratios define the best possible performance with the information available at that stage (approximately; see 'signal-to-noise ratio' in Appendix A for a minor qualification.) Since the visual system cannot add information as the image goes through these various stages in the visual system, the signal-to-noise ratio can only go down. The ratio of the signal-to-noise ratios of any two stages is the *efficiency* of the transformation relating the two stages (Tanner & Birdsall, 1958).

Figure 1.15 shows the last three stages: the photon image, the effective image, and the perform-

Table 1.1. *Signal-to-noise ratios at four stages in the visual process.*
See Appendix A for definitions.

	Image	Photon image	Effective image		Performance
In general:	$\dfrac{E}{N}$ $\geqslant$	$\dfrac{E}{N + N_{\text{photon}}}$ $\geqslant$	$\dfrac{E}{N + N_{\text{eq}}}$	$\geqslant$	d'^2
When $N = 0$:	∞ $\geqslant$	$\dfrac{E}{N_{\text{photon}}}$ $\geqslant$	$\dfrac{E}{N_{\text{eq}}}$	$\geqslant$	d'^2

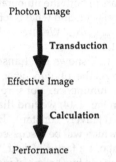

Fig. 1.15. Three stages of visual processing, and the
efficiencies (in bold) of the transformations that relate
them. For simplicity the diagram assumes no display
noise, $N = 0$.

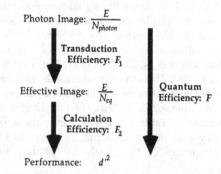

Fig. 1.16. The signal-to-noise ratios and efficiencies
corresponding to Fig. 1.15.

ance, and names for the transformations that relate
them. *Transduction* transforms the photon image (a
physical stimulus) into an effective image (an internal
effect), i.e. it substitutes the observer's equivalent
input noise for the corneal-photon noise. This just
makes the image noisier, because the equivalent noise
reflects the failure to use all the corneal photons and
the addition of neural noise. It includes all of the
observer's contrast-invariant noise. *Calculation* transforms the noisy effective image into a decision, such as
'yes' or 'no'. The appropriate calculation depends on
the signal and task. Our visual system, under our
conscious guidance, reduces the spatiotemporal effective image (which could be represented by a large
three-dimensional array of numbers) down to a single
number, the decision, which is manifest as the
observer's *performance*. The visual system's algorithm
for making its decision may or may not be optimal, and
may be constrained physiologically (e.g. by range of
available receptive field sizes) and intellectually (e.g.
by task complexity), and may vary from trial to trial.

Figure 1.16 shows the signal-to-noise ratios of
the three stages, and the efficiencies of the transformations that relate them:

Transduction efficiency F_1, in the absence of
display noise ($N = 0$), measures how efficiently the

visual system converts the photon image, which is just
a stimulus, into the effective image, which incorporates the equivalent noise of the visual system (Pelli,
1981). This efficiency will be less than 1 if there is any
increase in noise, either because of incomplete capture
of the photons, or because of introduction of neural
noise (or both). It might seem that 'transduction
efficiency' ought to be defined physiologically, as a
ratio of quantum bumps to incident photons. This is
not a conflict. The black-box approach can be applied
equally well to a cell as to an observer. We merely have
to specify the input and output. We would naturally
take the photoreceptor's input to be the incident light
flux, and its output to be the bump count, which will
yield the desired definition. Future research, comparing transduction efficiency of photoreceptor, retinal
ganglion cell, and observer could reveal how our low
equivalent noise level is achieved.

Calculation efficiency F_2 measures how efficiently
the visual system converts the effective image into
performance (Barlow, 1978; Pelli, 1981; Burgess, Wagner, Jennings & Barlow, 1981). This tells us how good a
statistician our visual system is, how efficiently do we
make decisions on the basis of noisy data? Calculation
efficiency, like transduction efficiency, may be applied
physiologically, but is not interesting for cells with

linear responses because it merely measures how well the stimulus and receptive field match.

Quantum efficiency F, in the absence of display noise ($N = 0$), measures the whole thing, how efficiently the visual system converts the photon image into performance (Barlow, 1958b, 1962a). (This is closely analogous to Fisher's (1925) definition of efficiency of a statistic, presumably reflecting Barlow's early interest in Fisher's approach.)

Figure 1.16 shows the signal-to-noise ratios (in the absence of display noise), and the symbols which represent the efficiencies. The efficiency of the first transformation is F_1, the efficiency of the second transformation is F_2, and the overall efficiency is F. Finally, Table 1.2 lists the formulas for the efficiencies, which are just ratios of signal-to-noise ratios. Each entry in Table 1.2 is the ratio of two entries in the bottom row of Table 1.1. For example, transduction efficiency is the ratio of the signal-to-noise ratios of the effective image, E/N_{eq}, and the photon image, E/N_{photon}.

The beauty of these definitions is that the quantum efficiency is just the product of the transduction and calculation efficiencies.

$$F = F_1 F_2 \qquad (5)$$

At the beginning of this chapter we saw that quantum efficiency varies over a very wide range, even though intuitively one might have expected it to be constant. Now that we can factor quantum efficiency into two components, we would like to know how much each varies.

Let us look at transduction efficiency first. We

Table 1.2. *Transduction, calculation, and quantum efficiencies.* Note that $F = F_1 F_2$. In general (when N is not constrained to be zero), the calculation efficiency is $F_2 = d'^2/(E/(N + N_{eq}))$.

	Transduction	Calculation	Quantum
When $N = 0$:	$F_1 = \dfrac{E/N_{eq}}{E/N_{photon}}$	$F_2 = \dfrac{d'^2}{E/N_{eq}}$	$F = \dfrac{d'^2}{E/N_{photon}}$

can see that, by its definition in Table 1.2, the signal energy appears in both the numerator and denominator, so it cancels out, and what is left is just the ratio of two noises, N_{photon}/N_{eq}. We already have the necessary data in Fig. 1.14.

Figure 1.17 shows the transduction efficiency, i.e. the ratio of the photon noise to the equivalent noise, at each luminance. Not surprisingly, given our comments on Fig. 1.14, we find that the transduction efficiency is relatively constant. Excluding the Pelli (1983) data, which will be discussed below, the entire variation is about a factor of four, yet the luminance ranges over nearly five orders of magnitude. Thus the variation is slight. Bear in mind too, that these experiments were conducted by different authors using various methods and that there are some uncertainties such as estimated pupil size, and accuracy of the noise and luminance calibrations.

We expect the fraction of photons absorbed to be constant, unlike the observer's overall quantum efficiency, which is known to depend strongly on experimental conditions, such as the signal area and duration and the background luminance (e.g. Figs. 1.1 and 1.2). However, Nagaraja's data show no effect of the disk size on the transduction efficiency. Unfortunately, although the data in Fig. 1.14 span a wide range of conditions, they do not include the conditions used by Barlow (1962b) to measure quantum efficiency (Fig. 1.1), so we cannot factor Barlow's measurements, to determine whether the enormous variation in quantum efficiency is due to variation of just transduction or calculation efficiency.

Over the years, various authors have measured calculation efficiencies, but, unfortunately, most of the experiments have been done with static noise, so they are not relevant here (Pelli, 1981; Burgess *et al.*, 1981). Another obstacle is that most of the experiments that one would like to use for such a calculation, such as those by van Meeteren, allowed unlimited viewing of the stimulus, so that we cannot sensibly calculate the contrast energy of the stimulus.

So far we have examined the dependence of the observer's equivalent noise on luminance. We have

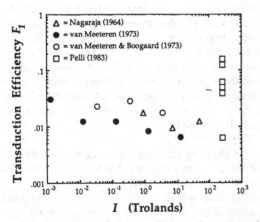

Fig. 1.17. The transduction efficiency, F_1, computed from the data in Fig. 1.14.

not yet stopped to ask what is the spatiotemporal spectrum of this noise, $N(f_x, f_y, f_t)$. At first this might seem unanswerable, since, as pointed out before, we cannot measure the observer's equivalent noise directly; we can only measure its effect on the contrast threshold. However, we can take advantage of the phenomenon of the critical band (i.e. spatiotemporal frequency channels) whereby the threshold for a flickering grating is only affected by noise frequencies close to the signal frequency, in both spatial frequency (Greis & Rohler, 1970; Stromeyer & Julesz, 1972; Henning, Hertz & Hinton, 1981; Pelli, 1981) and temporal frequency (Pelli & Watson in Pelli 1981; Mandler & Makous, 1984). As a result, an equivalent noise measurement made with a flickering grating provides an estimate of the equivalent noise level in the vicinity of the spatiotemporal test frequency.

Referring back to Fig. 1.4, the output of the noise amplifier is analogous to the observer's noisy effective image, and the subsequent bandpass filter and power meter are analogous to the observer's spatiotemporal frequency channel and squared contrast threshold. A key point is that we do not need to know the bandwidth of the filter or channel, because that only affects the measured power by a constant proportionality factor (provided the spectrum is smooth over the bandwidth of the filter), and we only need to know the output power to within a proportionality factor (see Eqs. 1 and 3).

In this way, Pelli (1983) measured the spatiotemporal spectrum of the equivalent noise at 300 td. The results are shown in Fig. 1.18. The spectrum is flat (within experimental error) at about $10N_{photon}$ (i.e. corresponding to a transduction efficiency of 10%) except for a great rise at very low spatiotemporal frequency (0 c/deg, 0 Hz). Similar data (not shown) have been collected on a second observer and for the same observer six months later, after a complete re-calibration of the system.

The observer looked through a 1 mm artificial pupil, so the eye of the observer could be assumed to be diffraction limited (Campbell & Gubisch, 1966), allowing calculation of the retinal contrasts of the signal and noise as a function of spatial frequency. The plotted equivalent noise level is at the retina, which is most directly comparable to the photon noise, since the photon noise arises at the retina and thus is white (has a flat spatiotemporal spectrum) at the retina, but not at the visual field. Other methodological details are presented in Appendix B.

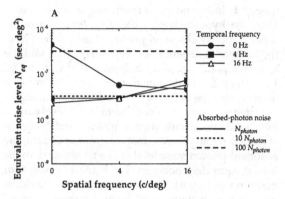

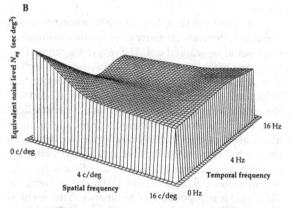

Fig. 1.18. A. The equivalent noise level at the retina as a function of spatiotemporal frequency at 252 td. Nine spatiotemporal frequencies were tested, all the combinations of 0, 4, and 16 c/deg and 0, 4, and 16 Hz. All signals were vignetted by a Gaussian with a width (and height) at 1/e of 0.75° and a duration of 0.75 s. The 95% confidence interval about each equivalent noise estimate is about ±0.3 log units. See Appendix B for methods. The data are from Pelli (1983). B. A smooth surface has been fit to the nine data points, and is shown in perspective. The floor seen at the edges represents the corneal-photon noise level N_{photon}.

Discussion

The source of the equivalent input noise

Absorbed-photon noise and neural noise are both sources for the observer's equivalent noise, but does one type dominate? Absorbed-photon noise $N_{absorbed}$ has only one degree of freedom, the fraction of photons absorbed, otherwise it is fully determined. It is inversely proportional to luminance, and, because photon absorptions are uncorrelated over space and time, it is independent of spatiotemporal frequency. Thus the hypothesis that the observer's equivalent noise is mostly absorbed-photon noise predicts both the luminance dependence seen in Fig. 1.14, and the spatiotemporal frequency independence seen in Fig. 1.18 (except for the deviation at the origin). Since noise levels cannot be negative – there is no such thing as negative variance – the equivalent noise level cannot be less than the absorbed-photon noise level. Since the absorbed-photon noise is frequency-independent, the absorbed-photon noise level can be no higher than the lowest equivalent noise level in Fig. 1.18 (except for measurement error). Thus the large rise in equivalent noise at low spatiotemporal frequency *must* be neural noise.

It is difficult to make a clear prediction for neural noise, as it depends on many physiological details that have yet to be worked out. However, we can make a few comments, making the simplifying assumption that at its site of origin the neural noise is independent of luminance. Neural noise that arises at a site distal to the site of light adaptation would act as a dark light and would become insignificant at luminances much above absolute threshold. Neural noise that arises at a site central to the site of light adaptation (i.e. after the contrast gain control, Rose, 1948a; Shapley, 1986) would produce an equivalent input noise (at the visual field) that is independent of luminance. This predicts that the low-frequency mountain seen in Fig. 1.18 is independent of luminance. Increasing the luminance would reveal more and more of the neural-noise mountain, as the absorbed-photon-noise sea was drained away. Reducing the luminance would eventually submerge the neural-noise under the rising sea of photon-noise.

The fact that at most spatiotemporal frequencies the observer's equivalent noise level can be accounted for (at least tentatively) by the absorbed-photon noise implies that the visual system exhibits that hallmark of good engineering that we described earlier in the context of man-made amplifiers and radio receivers. For the absorbed-photon noise to dominate the observer's equivalent noise implies that the gains at each stage of the visual system are high enough to amplify the absorbed-photon noise to exceed any contrast-invariant neural noise introduced at later stages. In the same way, the intrusion of neural noise at low spatiotemporal frequency implies that the gain is not high enough at those frequencies. It is well known that the visual system has very low sensitivity at low spatiotemporal frequency (Robson, 1966), probably as a side effect of light adaptation. All together this suggests that the familiar 'low-frequency

cut' of the contrast sensitivity function, i.e. the relatively low sensitivity at low spatiotemporal frequencies is due to a higher equivalent noise level at those frequencies, due to the intrusion of neural noise above the absorbed-photon noise level.

The Rose–de Vries law

The finding of a fairly constant transduction efficiency in Fig. 1.17 is not a complete surprise, since when the overall quantum efficiency is constant, it is simplest to expect the component transduction and calculations efficiencies to be constant too. The Rose–de Vries law, $c \propto I^{-0.5}$ is equivalent to the statement that quantum efficiency is constant (provided that threshold is at a fixed d'; Rose, 1942, 1948a; de Vries, 1943; Barlow, 1977). The violations of the Rose–de Vries law (e.g. Fig. 1.1) seem to be more the exception than the rule. Thresholds for flickering gratings follow the Rose–de Vries law up to at least 1000 td (van Nes, Koenderink, Nas & Bouman, 1967; Kelly, 1972). Banks, Geisler, & Bennet (1987) show that, with respect to the retinal image (which is blurred by the eye's optics), the observer's overall quantum efficiency is independent of spatial frequency from 5 to 40 c/deg, from 3.4 to 340 cd/m^2, if the spatial-frequency gratings have a fixed number of cycles. However, quantum efficiency does depend on the number of cycles in a grating because of the inefficiency of 'probability summation' (Robson & Graham, 1981; Watson, Barlow & Robson, 1983; Banks, Geisler & Bennet, 1987).

The Rose–van Meeteren paradigm

We have chosen to present the ideas in this chapter in a logical progression, not in historical order. Now it is time to go back and point out where Rose's (1942, 1946, 1948a, b, 1957, 1977) ideas fit in the structure we have erected.

The early papers on quantum efficiency of vision (before 1956) all assumed that the definition of quantum efficiency as a psychophysical property was self evident, and defined it only implicitly, by their method of measuring it. There is no difficulty in understanding what Rose (1942, 1946, 1948a, b, 1957) meant when he made the first determinations of the quantum efficiency of a video camera and photographic film – signal-to-noise ratio out $(E/N)_{out}$ over signal-to-noise ratio in $(E/N)_{photon}$ – but it is not obvious how to apply this to the eye. As Barlow (1958b) pointed out, in the case of the eye one might wish to say *quantum efficiency* is

the fraction of quanta sent through the pupil which are 'effectively absorbed' by the photosensitive materials subserving the mechanism under consideration, but a difficulty arises in deciding what to understand by the words 'effectively absorbed'. In the case of rhodopsin a quantum can be absorbed without bleaching the molecule, and even if bleaching occurs it is by no means certain the rod is always activated. Further, if the rod is activated it is still not certain that this information is successfully transmitted to the place where the threshold decision is made.

Barlow (1956, 1962a, b) went on to give the definition of overall quantum efficiency used here, which amounts to computing the output signal-to-noise ratio from the observer's performance, $(E/N)_{out} = d'^2$. However, that was not what Rose (1948a, 1957) had in mind.

As we will see below, Rose's (1948a) 'quantum efficiency of the eye' is what we have here dubbed the *transduction efficiency*, so it is not surprising that his efficiencies (roughly 5%, independent of background luminance, in rough agreement with Fig. 1.17) were very different from Barlow's, which fall precipitously with background luminance, as seen in Fig. 1.1. In fact, this confusion of two fundamentally different measures bearing the same name has persisted for thirty years. While Jones (1959), Barlow (1962b), Cohn (1976), and Geisler & Davila (1985) measured quantum efficiency, Rose (1948a, 1957), Sturm & Morgan (1949), Nagaraja (1964), van Meeteren (1973), van Meeteren & Boogaard (1973), and Engstrom (1974) all measured what is here called transduction efficiency, though everyone claimed to be measuring 'quantum efficiency'. It is the purpose of this chapter to point out that both measures are important, and that it would be most informative to measure both over a wide range of conditions.

As discussed earlier, the paradigm advocated here for measuring the observer's equivalent noise level or transduction efficiency (and first used by Nagaraja, 1964) is to measure thresholds at more than one noise level, assuming contrast invariance. The contrast-invariance assumption implies that at threshold the two (or more) conditions will differ only in the overall contrast of the effective image.

The Rose–van Meeteren paradigm is to measure thresholds at more than one luminance (Rose, 1957; van Meeteren & Boogaard, 1973; Engstrom, 1974), implicitly assuming *luminance invariance*, i.e. assuming that the observer's performance depends solely on the contrast function of the effective image, independent of its luminance. In this approach, noise is added to the brighter display (i.e. at the higher luminance) to equate threshold with that of the dimmer display. The luminance-invariance assumption implies that this

will equate the effective noise levels of the two displays, so that at threshold the two conditions will differ only in luminance, having identical effective (contrast) images. This paradigm lends itself particularly well to experiments in which the dimmer display has no noise (i.e. continuous) and the brighter display is a random dot display. The transduction efficiency is just the ratio of dot flux (on the bright display) to corneal photons (on the dim display). (This assumes that the bright display is sufficiently bright and noisy that the observer's equivalent input noise is negligible, which is easily achieved in practice.) However, as we have seen in Figs. 1.12 and 1.13, it is possible to analyze even these experiments by the Nagaraja paradigm, if several noise levels (dot fluxes) are used at one luminance. (This requires using neutral density filters to compensate for the increase in brightness as the dot flux is increased.)

The idea that vision is usually photon-noise limited has been widely discounted, as a result of dramatic violations of the Rose–de Vries law, $c \propto I^{-0.5}$ (Rose, 1942, 1948a; de Vries, 1943; e.g. Aguilar & Stiles, 1954; Barlow, 1958, 1962b). However, a constant transduction efficiency, by itself, does not require that the Rose–de Vries law be obeyed. Unfortunately, Rose's methods of measuring transduction efficiency forced him to make overly strong assumptions about the observer. Initially, Rose (1948a) boldly assumed that *all* thresholds have the same effective signal-to-noise ratio. The later, more sophisticated, Rose–van Meeteren paradigm requires only the luminance-invariance assumption, i.e. the assumption that thresholds for the same pattern at two different luminances have the same effective signal-to-noise ratio. (More precisely, they need the three assumptions of the Nagaraja paradigm, substituting luminance-invariance of performance for contrast-invariance of performance.) However, even this weaker assumption, when combined with the assumption of constant transduction efficiency, implies the Rose–de Vries law, $c \propto I^{-0.5}$, which is not generally true, so this approach cannot disentangle luminance-dependent variations of transduction and calculation efficiencies. In this chapter we use only the Nagaraja paradigm with its contrast-invariance assumption, which is consistent with all published measurements of threshold versus noise level at a constant luminance (Pelli, 1981). The Nagaraja paradigm can be used to determine, for example, whether the variation of overall quantum efficiency seen in Fig. 1.1 is due to variation of transduction or calculation efficiency (or both).

Future work

Extensive measurements of transduction and quantum efficiency are planned, both to re-analyze Barlow's (1962b) result shown in Fig. 1.1, and to examine the spatiotemporal spectrum at many luminances, to study the luminance-dependence of neural noise.

It will be important to test the model of Fig. 1.7. As noted before, the main prediction of the model is Eq. 3, $c^2 \propto N + N_{eq}$, which is widely confirmed (Pelli, 1981; Burgess *et al.*, 1981; Legge, Kersten & Burgess, 1987). But note that this equation must apply at any threshold criterion d'. This implies that the psychometric function, the growth of d' with contrast, must be contrast invariant too, i.e. when threshold is raised by external noise, the psychometric function must shift along the log contrast axis without changing shape. For gratings in dynamic white noise, this prediction has been confirmed by Pelli (1981), disconfirmed by Kersten (1984), and reconfirmed by Thomas (1985). More work is warranted.

Summary

The overall quantum efficiency of human vision is strongly dependent on many stimulus parameters. Quantum efficiency refers only to the stimulus and the observer's performance. However, in analogy to Barlow's notion of dark light, which is in the intensity domain, we can measure an observer's equivalent noise in the contrast domain. With this, and the contrast-invariance assumption, we can define and measure the signal-to-noise ratio at an intermediate stage in the visual process: the *effective* image, which includes the observer's equivalent noise. Introducing this intermediate stage allows quantum efficiency to be factored into two components: transduction and calculation efficiencies. This is derived formally in Appendix A. It appears that the transduction efficiency is quite stable, in the range 1% to 10%, over most conditions, confirming Rose (1948a).

While all these measures can be studied as a function of any experimental variation, it is particularly informative to study them as a function of spatiotemporal frequency. This is because the existence of spatiotemporal frequency channels (i.e. critical bands) allows us to interpret the variation in equivalent noise level N_{eq} with spatiotemporal frequency directly as the spatiotemporal spectrum $N_{eq}(f_x, f_y, f_t)$ of the equivalent noise. Preliminary results at 252 td indicate that the equivalent noise is dominated by absorbed-photon noise (corresponding to absorption of 10% of corneal photons) at all spatiotemporal frequencies in the range 0 to 16 c/deg and 0 to 16 Hz, except for very low spatiotemporal frequencies (near 0 c/deg, 0 Hz, i.e. signals that change slowly in space and time) where the equivalent noise is much higher, and therefore is of neural origin.

Appendix A:
Quantum efficiency is the product of transduction and calculation efficiencies $F = F_1 F_2$

This sequence of definitions is organized as a derivation, beginning with the physical stimulus, and ending with the factoring of quantum efficiency into transduction and calculation efficiencies.

L_{av} is the *mean luminance*, averaged over space and time.

$L_{SN}(x, y, t)$ is the *luminance function* of the image over space and time on a signal-plus-noise presentation. Note that because the noise is random, the luminance function is random, different on each presentation, drawn from an ensemble of possibilities.

$c_{SN}(x, y, t)$ is the *contrast function* of the image over space and time on a signal-plus-noise presentation (Linfoot, 1964),

$$c_{SN}(x, y, t) = \frac{L_{SN}(x, y, t)}{L_{av}} - 1$$

$s(x, y, t)$ is the *signal* expressed as a contrast function over space and time,

$$s(x, y, t) = \langle c_{SN}(x, y, t) \rangle$$

where the angle brackets $\langle \ \rangle$ indicate the ensemble average, across all possible instances (to average away the noise).

$n(x, y, t)$ is the *noise* expressed as a contrast function over space and time,

$$n(x, y, t) = c_{SN}(x, y, t) - s(x, y, t)$$

E is the contrast energy (i.e. integrated square contrast) of any contrast function, usually of the signal,

$$E = \int_{-\infty}^{\infty} \int_{-\infty}^{\infty} \int_{-\infty}^{\infty} s^2(x, y, t) \, dx \, dy \, dt$$

(Pelli, 1981; Watson, Barlow & Robson, 1983).

$N(f_x, f_y, f_t)$ is the *power spectral density* of the noise, i.e. contrast power per unit two-sided bandwidth at spatiotemporal frequency f_x, f_y, f_t.

$$N(f_x, f_y, f_t) = \left\langle \lim_{X,Y,T \to \infty} \frac{1}{XYT} \right.$$

$$\left. \times \left| \int_{-T/2}^{T/2} \int_{-Y/2}^{Y/2} \int_{-X/2}^{X/2} n(x, y, t) \, e^{-i\pi(xf_x + yf_y + tf_t)} \, dx \, dy \, dt \right|^2 \right\rangle$$

When $N(f_x, f_y, f_t)$ is constant over the band of interest, it will often be called simply the *noise level N*. Note that this definition uses *two-sided* bandwidth, including positive and negative frequency. A filter passing frequencies between 30 and 40 Hz also passes frequencies between -30 and -40 Hz and thus has a two-sided bandwidth of $10 + 10 = 20$ Hz. In vision, unlike audition, we deal with noise varying in one, two, or three dimensions (though this chapter deals only with three), and we need this two-sided definition of N in order to make the expression for signal-to-noise ratio (see below) independent of the number of dimensions (Pelli, 1981).

c_{rms}^2 is the *contrast power* (i.e. the mean square contrast) of the noise,

$$c_{rms}^2 = \langle n^2(x, y, t) \rangle$$

or, more generally, if we don't want to assume the noise is stationary,

$$c_{rms}^2 = \left\langle \lim_{X,Y,T \to \infty} \frac{1}{XYT} \int_{-T/2}^{T/2} \int_{-Y/2}^{Y/2} \int_{-X/2}^{X/2} n^2(x, y, t) \, dx \, dy \, dt \right\rangle$$

Note that, by Rayleigh's theorem (Bracewell, 1978), the integral of the power spectral density over all frequencies yields the contrast power,

$$c_{rms}^2 = \int_{-\infty}^{\infty} \int_{-\infty}^{\infty} \int_{-\infty}^{\infty} N(f_x, f_y, f_t) \, df_x \, df_y \, df_t$$

E/N is the *signal-to-noise ratio*, a dimensionless quantity that determines the levels of performance for detection of any known signal with energy E in white noise with power spectral density N (Peterson, Birdsall & Fox, 1954). (Note that in audition, where the noise is always one-dimensional, the signal-to-noise ratio is usually written as $2E/N_0$, where $N_0 = 2N$, e.g. Tanner & Birdsall, 1958; Green & Swets, 1974, Eq. 6.37.)

d'^2 is the smallest signal-to-noise ratio consistent with the observed level of performance (Tanner & Birdsall, 1958),

$$d'^2 = \left(\frac{E}{N} \right)_{ideal}$$

In terms of the usual performance measures this works out to

$$d' = \begin{cases} \sqrt{2} \, z[P_{2afc}(c)] & \text{if task is two-alternative forced} \\ & \text{choice} \\ z[P_{yn}(c)] - z[P_{yn}(0)] & \text{if task is yes–no} \end{cases}$$

for a known signal in white noise (Elliott, 1964), where $P_{2afc}(c)$ is the proportion correct (at contrast c) in a two-alternative forced choice task, $P_{yn}(c)$ is the hit rate and $P_{yn}(0)$ is the false alarm rate in a yes–no task, and $z[P]$ represents the inverse cumulative normal, i.e.

$$P = \frac{1}{\sqrt{(2\pi)}} \int_{-\infty}^{z} e^{-u^2/2} \, du$$

N_{eq} is the *equivalent input noise level* of the observer, i.e. the noise that would have to be added at the display to model the observer as noise-free (Pelli, 1981; Ahumada & Watson, 1985; Ahumada, 1987). However, that is not measurable without some assumptions about the observer, so we re-define the equivalent noise as a parameter of the black-box model in Fig. 1.7. This model predicts that the squared contrast will be proportional to the sum of the noise and the equivalent noise,

$$c^2 \propto N + N_{eq}$$

Empirically we determine the observer's equivalent noise level by fitting this equation to our data (Nagaraja, 1964; Pelli, 1981).

N_{ef} is the *effective noise level* of the observer and display,

$$N_{ef} = N + N_{eq}.$$

The *effective image* is the sum of the stimulus $c_{SN}(x, y, t)$ and the observer's equivalent input noise. It has a signal-to-noise ratio of $E/(N + N_{eq})$.

N_{ideal} is the maximum noise level consistent with the observed level of performance,

$$N_{ideal} = \frac{E}{d'^2}$$

J represents the mean event flux of a Poisson process, e.g. photons per $deg^2 sec$. The noise level of a Poisson process is the inverse of the flux (Papoulis, 1965; Pelli, 1981),

$$N = \frac{1}{J}$$

This statement is strictly true only for a uniform original image, or a very low contrast signal. However, it is an extremely useful simplification, and a good approximation as long as the signal contrast is not too high. The simplification is required because, unfortunately, the signal-to-noise ratio E/N does not fully determine detectability of a known signal in Poisson noise (which is signal-dependent), as it does in white noise (which is independent of the signal). However, calculations show that if the signal contrast is less than 20%, $|s(x, y, t)| < 0.2$, then, for two-alternative forced-choice detection of a known signal in Poisson noise, the discrepancy between E/N and the best possible performance, $d'^2 = 2z^2[P_{2afc}]$, is at most $\pm 0.5\,dB$, which is negligible when one considers that contrast thresholds are generally measured with a standard deviation of $1\,dB$ at best (also see Geisler & Davila, 1985).

J_{eq} is the minimum photon flux consistent with the measured equivalent noise level,

$$J_{eq} = \frac{1}{N_{eq}}$$

J_{ideal} is the minimum event flux consistent with the observed level of performance,

$$J_{ideal} = \frac{1}{N_{ideal}}$$

J_{photon} is the corneal photon flux.
N_{photon} is the noise level corresponding to the corneal photon flux,

$$N_{photon} = \frac{1}{J_{photon}}$$

J_{ef} is the minimum event flux consistent with the effective noise level,

$$J_{ef} = \frac{1}{N_{ef}}$$

The (corneal) *photon image* is the spatiotemporal pattern of absorption that would result if all corneal photons were absorbed. It is a sum of many delta functions (each representing one photon absorption) as a function of space and time. It has a signal-to-noise ratio of $E/(N + N_{photon})$.

Efficiency of any transformation is the ratio of the signal-to-noise ratios before and after (Tanner & Birdsall, 1958),

$$\frac{(E/N)_{out}}{(E/N)_{in}}$$

Transduction efficiency F_1 is the fraction of the corneal quanta required to account for the observer's equivalent input noise level (Nagaraja, 1964; Pelli, 1981),

$$F_1 = \frac{J_{eq}}{J_{photon}}$$

or, equivalently,

$$F_1 = \frac{E/N_{eq}}{E/N_{photon}}$$

which, in the absence of display noise ($N = 0$), is the observer's efficiency, from photon image to effective image (Rose, 1948a; Pelli, 1981). Rose called it the 'quantum efficiency of the eye'. Transduction efficiency, like the equivalent noise, is only measurable in the context of a model like that of Fig. 1.7, with its three assumptions (mainly contrast-invariance, in the Nagaraja paradigm, or luminance invariance, in the Rose–van Meeteren paradigm; see Discussion).

Calculation efficiency F_2 is the smallest fraction of the effective number of Poisson events on a random dot display consistent with the observed level of performance,

$$F_2 = \frac{J_{ideal}}{J_{ef}}$$

or, equivalently, it is the observer's efficiency, from effective image to response,

$$F_2 = \frac{d'^2}{E/N_{ef}}$$

(Barlow, 1977, 1978; Pelli, 1981; Burgess et al. 1981; Legge, Kersten & Burgess, 1987). Barlow (1977) defined calculation (which he called 'central') efficiency in terms of J and N, not J_{ef} and N_{ef}, but this is an insignificant difference when the noise level is high, $N \gg N_{eq}$, as is usually the case when calculation efficiency F_2 is measured. In Barlow's form, calculation efficiency can be measured without any assumptions.

Quantum efficiency F is the smallest fraction of the corneal quanta consistent with the observed level of performance (Barlow, 1958b, 1962a),

$$F = \frac{J_{ideal}}{J_{photon}}$$

or, equivalently, it is the observer's efficiency, from photon image to response,

$$F = \frac{d'^2}{E/N_{photon}}$$

Quantum efficiency can be measured without any assumptions. Note that this definition of F makes sense only when there is no display noise, $N = 0$, in which case the effective noise equals the equivalent noise, $N_{ef} = N_{eq}$, and

$$F = F_1 F_2$$

which is what we set out to prove.

Appendix B:
Methods for Fig. 1.18

Procedure

A PDP-11/23 computer synthesized the signal and ran all the trials. The noise was always on and was at constant noise level throughout each trial.

Threshold was measured by the method of two-interval forced-choice, with feedback. Each trial consisted of two intervals, announced by a voice synthesizer (Intex talker), 'One . . . two'. The signal was presented during one or the other of the two intervals, pseudo-randomly determined. Then the observer indicated, by button push, which interval he thought contained the signal. The talker acknowledged the response ('one', 'two', or 'cancel') and gave feedback ('right' or 'wrong').

The QUEST staircase procedure determined the contrast of the signal on each trial, presenting the signal at the current maximum-probability estimate of threshold for that condition (Watson & Pelli 1983). After 40 trials, QUEST provided the maximum likelihood estimate of threshold (82% correct), based on the observer's responses. Each threshold was measured twice, and their average was used in subsequent analyses.

The observers

Two observers participated, one emmetrope and one well-corrected myope. Viewing was monocular. The observer sat in a light-proof booth, and viewed the display through a 1 mm pupil and a 550 nm narrowband filter (and the optical correction, if any). The position of the observer's head was maintained by a bite bar covered with dental impression compound, heat-molded to the observer's bite. The bite bar, in turn, was attached to a two-axis tool holder which allowed the observer's head to be moved horizontally and vertically relative to the fixed artificial pupil. The artificial pupil was carefully centered on the observer's pupil.

The display

Sinusoidal gratings were displayed using a television-like raster on a cathode-ray tube as described by Graham, Robson & Nachmias (1978). The screen was 30 cm wide and 20 cm high. Room lights were turned off to minimize intraocular scattered light. The screen displayed 100 frames per second, otherwise the space-average luminance in the absence of a signal, was constant throughout each experiment.

Noise

The noise was generated by a custom-designed Schottky TTL computer card which plugged into the PDP-11/23 bus. A 33 bit shift register was given exclusive–or feedback so as to produce a maximal-length sequence of states before repeating (Lipson, Foster & Walsh 1976, Peterson & Weldon, 1972).

Each clock cycle shifted the EXCLUSIVE OR of three of the bits into bit 1. The clock rate could be programmed to any rate up to 40 MHz. There were $2^{33} - 1 \sim 10^{10}$ clock cycles before the feedback shift register sequence repeated: 3.6 minutes at a 40 MHz clock rate. One bit of the register drove an output producing one sample per clock cycle, either +1 or −1 volt, changing pseudorandomly at the beginning of each clock cycle. These samples were uncorrelated, and had a mean of 0 volts. This analog output was attenuated by a programmable attenuator and added to the signal at the display. The samples were uncorrelated, so the noise spectrum was nearly flat up to half the sample rate. The noise was free-running, not synchronized to the frames of the display or signal presentations, making it very unlikely that the observer could benefit by any memory of the previous noise cycle, more than 3 minutes ago. The noise was attenuated by a computer-controlled passive attenuator (FORESIGHT dB Attenuator), with a $75\,\Omega$ characteristic impedance. The attenuator directly drove a coaxial cable with a $75\,\Omega$ characteristic impedance terminated in its characteristic impedance at the display, where it was added to the signal. This arrangement resulted in a very flat transfer function; the gain was down by only 1 dB at 10 MHz.

Display calibration

The display (Joyce Electronics) exhibited no significant nonlinearity up to contrasts of 90%. The linearity was checked at the beginning of every experimental session by the simple expedient of counterphase flickering a sinusoidal grating at a rate above critical flicker fusion, and confirming that the display appeared uniform. Second harmonic distortion would produce a static grating of twice the original spatial frequency.

The display's luminance was 275 td. Because the display was viewed through a 550 nm narrowband filter, the luminance was computed from a radiance measurement by a radiometer which was NBS traceable (UDT 161), using the identity

$$1\,\text{lumen} = 4.1 \times 10^{15}\,\text{quanta (555 nm)/s}$$

(The photopic efficiency at 550 nm is negligibly different from that at 555 nm, i.e. 0.995 versus 1.)

The Modulation Transfer Function (MTF) of the display $H(f_x)$ was measured by drifting a sinusoidal grating past a microphotometer (Schade, 1958). The microphotometer consisted of a photometer (UDT 161) which measured the light passed through a 1 mm aperture in the image plane of a 5:1 microscope objective (N.A. 0.11, Rolyn 80.3044), giving a 0.2 mm-wide collection area in the plane of the phosphor. All spatial frequencies were drifted at 1 Hz so as to produce the same temporal frequency in the measuring system, to avoid confounding the spatial MTF of the display with the temporal MTF of the photometer. This calibration was checked at low spatial frequency (where the MTF is essentially flat) by very slowly drifting a low-spatial-frequency square wave at a nominal contrast of 20%, measuring the luminance in the center of the bright and dark bars, and calculating the contrast,

$$c = (L_{max} - L_{min})/(L_{max} + L_{min}),$$

with good agreement with the above procedure.

Noise calibration

It was not practical to directly measure the spatiotemporal spectrum of the noise. Therefore indirect methods were used. The method of generation of the noise produces a white spectrum (before attenuation and display). Since the attenuator Modulation Transfer Function (MTF) is flat over the relevant bandwidth the noise spectrum is proportional to the square of the display MTF:

$$N(f_x, f_y, f_t)/N(0, 0, 0) = H^2(f_x, f_y, f_t)$$

Since I have already measured the spatial MTF in the preceding section, all I need to do now is to measure $N(0, 0, 0)$, the noise level near zero spatiotemporal frequency.

The concept of *noise-equivalent bandwidth* is helpful in calibrating noise level. For a filter it is defined as follows. Imagine a bandpass filter with a passband gain equal to the peak gain of the actual filter, and zero gain outside the passband. Suppose we apply a white noise input to both the actual and the hypothetical filters. The equivalent bandwidth of the actual filter is defined as the bandwidth the hypothetical filter has to have in order to pass the same total noise power as the actual filter. Similarly we can consider any noise spectrum to be the result of passing white noise through some filter, and define the equivalent bandwidth of the noise as the noise-equivalent bandwidth of the imputed filter.

I calibrated the noise level at the display by measuring the output power of a narrowband spatiotemporal filter which accepted the display as its input. This procedure is a direct application of the definition of spectral density: the power passed by a narrowband filter divided by its equivalent bandwidth. The filter was synthesized by using a photometer to average light from a large aperture (4 cm by 8 cm). The photometer output was low-pass filtered (30 Hz cut off) and sampled by a 14-bit analog-to-digital converter at 100 Hz (once per frame). The computer smoothed these data by calculating the running average of the 10 most recent samples. Thus each smoothed sample represents the average luminance over an area of known width (4 cm) and height (8 cm) and duration (10 frames = 100 ms). These smoothed samples are the output of the synthesized spatiotemporal filter, whose input is the display. The filter has a (two-sided) noise-equivalent bandwidth of 1/(width × height × duration), centered on zero frequency. The contrast power c_{rms}^2 of the smoothed photometer readings, divided by the noise-equivalent bandwidth of the filter yields an estimate of the noise level near zero frequency.

Acknowledgements

These ideas have developed over the last 12 years, and, though largely equivalent to the combination of what I presented in my 1981 Ph.D. dissertation and at the 1983 meeting of the Association for Vision and Ophthalmology, the notation and explanations have advanced significantly. Among the many people who provided helpful discussion, I would particularly like to thank Al Ahumada and Horace Barlow (on rigor of the analysis), Dan Kersten, Gordon Legge, Gary Rubin, and Beau Watson (on clarity), Dwight North and Al Rose (on their work at RCA), and Bob Wagner (on R. A. Fisher). I thank Dan Horne for locating the translation of Einstein (1905) and John Perrone for showing me how to produce Fig. 1.18B. This work was supported during 1978–9, by MoD contract 'Spatial noise spectra and target detection/recognition' to F. W. Campbell, and, during 1982–8, by National Institutes of Health Biomedical Research Grant to Syracuse University and National Eye Institute grant EY04432 to me. This chapter was written while on a sabbatical from Syracuse University to visit the Vision Group at the NASA Ames Research Center.

References

Aguilar, M. & Stiles, W. S. (1954) Saturation of the rod mechanism of the retina at high levels of stimulation. *Optica Acta*, **1**, 59–65

Ahumada, A. J. Jr & Watson, A. B. (1985) Equivalent-noise model for contrast detection and discrimination. *J. Opt. Soc. Am. A*, **2**, 1133–9.

Ahumada, A. J. Jr (1987) Putting the visual system noise back in the picture. *J. Opt. Soc. Am. A*, **4**, 2372–8.

Banks, M. S., Geisler, W. S. & Bennet, P. J. (1987) The physical limits of grating visibility. *Vision Res.*, **27**, 1915–24.

Barlow, H. B. (1956) Retinal noise and absolute threshold. *J. Opt. Soc. Am.*, **46**, 634–9.

Barlow, H. B. (1957) Increment thresholds at low intensities considered as signal/noise discrimination. *J. Physiol.*, **136**, 469–88.

Barlow, H. B. (1958a) Temporal and spatial summation in human vision at different background intensities. *J. Physiol.* **141**, 337–50.

Barlow, H. B. (1958b) Intrinsic noise of cones. *Visual Problems of Colour*. National Physical Laboratory Symposium, pp. 615–30. London: HMSO.

Barlow, H. B. (1962a) A method of determining the overall quantum efficiency of visual discriminations. *J. Physiol.*, **160**, 155–68.

Barlow, H. B. (1962b) Measurements of the quantum efficiency of discrimination in human scotopic vision. *J. Physiol.*, **160**, 169–88.

Barlow, H. B. (1977) Retinal and central factors in human vision limited by noise. In *Vertebrate Photoreception*, ed. H. B. Barlow & P. Fatt. New York: Academic Press.

Barlow, H. B. (1978) The efficiency of detecting changes of density in random dot patterns. *Vision Res.*, **18**, 637–50.

Bracewell, R. N. (1978) *The Fourier Transform and Its Applications*, New York: McGraw-Hill.

Burgess, A. E. & Colborne, B. (1988) Visual signal detection IV – observer inconsistency. *J. Opt. Soc. Am.*, (in press).

Burgess, A. E., Wagner, R. F., Jennings, R. J. & Barlow, H. B. (1981) Efficiency of human visual signal discrimination. *Science*, **214**, 93–4.

Campbell, F. W. & Gubisch, R. W. (1966) Optical quality of the human eye. *J. Physiol. (Lond.)*, **186**, 558–78.

Cohn, T. E. (1976) Quantum fluctuations limit foveal vision. *Vision Res.*, **16**, 573–9.

Einstein, A. (1905) Über einen die Erzeugung und Verwandlung des Lichtes betreffenden heuristischen Gesichtspunkt. *Annal. Physik*, **17**, 132–48. Translation by Arons, A. B., & Peppard, M. B. (1965) Einstein's proposal of the photon concept – a translation of the *Annalen der Physik* paper of 1905. *American Journal of Physics*, **33**, 367–74.

Elliott, P. B. (1964) Tables of *d'*. In *Signal Detection and Recognition by Human Observers*, ed. J. A. Swets. New York: John Wiley.

Engstrom, R. W. (1974) Quantum efficiency of the eye determined by comparison with a TV camera. *J. Opt. Soc. Am.*, **64**, 1706–10.

Fisher, R. A. (1925) *Statistical Methods for Research Workers.* Edinburgh: Oliver and Boyd.

Friis, H. T. (1944) Noise figures of radio receivers. *Proceedings of the IRE*, **32**, 419–22.

Geisler, W. S. & Davila, K. D. (1985) Ideal discriminators in spatial vision: two-point stimuli. *J. Opt. Soc. Am. A*, **2**, 1483–97.

Graham, N., Robson, J. G. & Nachmias, J. (1978) Grating summation in fovea and periphery. *Vision Res.*, **18**, 815–26.

Green, D. M. & Swets, J. A., (1974) *Signal Detection Theory and Psychophysics*. Huntington, NY: Krieger.

Greis, U. & Rohler, R. (1970) Untersuchung der subjektiven Detailerkennbarkeit mit Hilfe der Ortsfrequenzfilterung. *Optica Acta*, **17**, 515–26. (A translation by Ilze Mueller with amendments by D. G. Pelli, 'A study of the subjective detectability of patterns by means of spatial-frequency filtering' is available from D. G. Pelli, Institute for Sensory Research, Syracuse University, Syracuse, NY 13244, USA.)

Hecht, S., Shlaer, S. & Pirenne, M. H. (1942) Energy, quanta, and vision. *J. Gen. Physiol.*, **25**, 819–40.

Henning, G. B., Hertz, B. G. & Hinton, J. L. (1981) Effects of different hypothetical detection mechanisms on the shape of spatial-frequency filters inferred from masking experiments: I. noise masks. *J. Opt. Soc. Am.*, **71**, 574–81.

Jones, R. C. (1959) Quantum efficiency of human vision. *J. Opt. Soc. Am.*, **49**, 645–53.

Kelly, D. (1972) Adaptation effects on spatio-temporal sine-wave thresholds. *Vision Res.*, **12**, 89–101.

Kersten, D. (1984) Spatial summation in visual noise. *Vision Res.*, **24**, 1977–90.

Legge, G. E., Kersten, D. & Burgess, A. E. (1987) Contrast discrimination in noise *J. Opt. Soc. Am. A*, **4**, 391–404.

Lillywhite, P. G. (1981) Multiplicative intrinsic noise and the limits to visual performance. *Vision Res.* **21**, 291–6.

Linfoot, E. H. (1964) *Fourier Methods in Optical Image Evaluation.* New York: Focal Press.

Lipson, E. D., Foster, K. W. & Walsh, M. P. (1976) A versatile pseudo-random noise generator. *IEEE Transactions on Instrumentation and Measurement*, **25**, 112–16.

Mandler, M. & Makous, W. (1984) A three channel model of temporal frequency perception. *Vision Res.*, **24**, 1881–7.

van Meeteren, A. (1973) *Visual Aspects of Image Intensification.* Report of the Institute for Perception, TNO. Soesterberg, The Netherlands.

van Meeteren, A. & Boogaard, J. (1973) Visual contrast sensitivity with ideal image intensifiers. *Optik*, **37**, 179–91.

Mumford, W. W. & Schelbe, E. H. (1968) *Noise Performance Factors in Communication Systems*. Dedham, MA: Horizon House–Microwave Inc. (See chapter 4.)

Nachmias, J. (1981) On the psychometric function for contrast detection. *Vision Res.*, **21**, 215–33.

Nagaraja, N. S. (1964) Effect of luminance noise on contrast thresholds. *J. Opt. Soc. Am.*, **54**, 950–5.

van Nes, F. L., Koenderink, J. J., Nas, H. & Bouman, M. A. (1967) Spatiotemporal modulation transfer in the human eye. *J. Opt. Soc. Am.*, **57**, 1082–8

North, D. O. (1942) The absolute sensitivity of radio receivers. *RCA Review*, **6**, 332–44.

Papoulis, A. (1965) *Probability, Random Variables, and Stochastic Processes*. New York: McGraw–Hill Book Co.

Pelli, D. G. (1981) Effects of visual noise. PhD thesis. Cambridge: University of Cambridge (unpublished).

Pelli, D. G. (1983) The spatiotemporal spectrum of the equivalent noise of human vision. *Invest. Ophthal. and Vis. Sci. (Suppl.)*, **4**, 46.

Pelli, D. G. (1985) Uncertainty explains many aspects of visual contrast detection and discrimination. *J. Opt. Soc. Am.*, **2**, 1508–32.

Peterson, W. W., Birdsall, T. G. & Fox, W. C. (1954) Theory of signal detectability. *Transactions of the IRE PGIT*, **4**, 171–212.

Peterson W. W. & Weldon E. J. Jr (1972) *Error-Correcting Codes*. Second Edition. Cambridge, Mass: MIT Press.

Robson, J. G. (1966) Spatial and temporal contrast-sensitivity functions of the visual system. *J. Opt. Soc. Am.*, **56**, 1141–2.

Robson, J. G. & Graham, N. (1981) Probability summation and regional variation in contrast sensitivity across the visual field. *Vision Res.*, **21**, 409–18.

Rose, A. (1942) The relative sensitivities of television pickup tubes, photographic film, and the human eye. *Proc. IRE*, **30**, 293–300.

Rose, A. (1946) A unified approach to the performance of photographic film, television pickup tubes, and the human eye. *Journal of the Society of Motion Picture and Television Engineers*, **47**, 273–94.

Rose, A. (1948a) The sensitivity performance of the human eye on an absolute scale. *J. Opt. Soc. Am.*, **38**, 196–208.

Rose, A. (1948b) Television pickup tubes and the problem of vision. *Advances in Electronics*, **1**, 131–66.

Rose, A. (1957) Quantum effects in human vision. *Advances in Biological and Medical Physics*, **5**, 211–42. (See the bottom paragraph on page 237.)

Rose, A. (1977) Vision: human versus electronic. In *Vertebrate Photoreception*, eds. H. B. Barlow & P. Fatt. New York: Academic Press.

Schade, O. H., Sr (1958) A method of measuring the optical sine-wave spatial spectrum of television image display devices. *Journal of the Society of Motion Picture and Television Engineers* **67**, 561–6.

Shapley, R. (1986) The importance of contrast for the activity of single neurons, the VEP and perception. *Vision Res.*, **26**, 45–61.

Stromeyer, C. F. & Julesz, B. (1972) Spatial frequency masking in vision: critical bands and spread of masking. *J. Opt. Soc. Am.*, **62**, 1221–32.

Sturm, R. E. & Morgan, R. H. (1949) Screen intensification systems and their limitations. *The American Journal of Roentgenology and Radium Therapy* **62**, 617–34.

Tanner, W. P., Jr. & Birdsall, T. G. (1958) Definitions of d' and η as psychophysical measures. *J. Acoust. Soc. Amer.* **30**, 922–8.

Thomas, J. P. (1985) Effect of static noise and grating masks on detection and identification of grating targets. *J. Opt. Soc. Am. A*, **2**, 1586–92.

de Vries, H. L. (1943) The quantum character of light and its bearing upon threshold of vision, the differential sensitivity and visual acuity of the eye. *Physica*, **10**, 553–64.

Watson, A. B., Barlow, H. B. & Robson, J. G. (1983) What does the eye see best? *Nature*, **302**, 419–22.

Watson, A. B. & Pelli, D. G. (1983) QUEST: A Bayesian adaptive psychometric method. *Perception and Psychophysics* **33**, 113–20.

Wyszecki, G. & Stiles, W. S. (1967) *Color Science*. New York: John Wiley and Sons Inc.

2
Coding efficiency and visual processing

S. B. Laughlin

Improving the efficiency of vision brings distinct advantages. Improved spatial resolution and the better detection of small intensity differences allows an animal to resolve more objects and to see objects at a greater distance. These improvements in accuracy and resolution extend both the range and the richness of perception, so providing a greater return for an animal's investment in eye and brain. It follows that coding efficiency, that is the accuracy and fidelity with which information is gathered by the eye, and transmitted and processed by neurons, is an important biological factor. Consequently, the need for efficiency must shape visual processing, and considerations of efficiency can guide our understanding of vision (e.g. Hecht, Shlaer & Pirenne, 1942; Rose, 1972; Barlow, 1964). The dictates of coding efficiency are illustrated by our work on the blowfly retina (Laughlin & Hardie, 1978; Laughlin, 1981; Srinivasan, Laughlin & Dubs, 1982; Laughlin, Howard & Blakeslee, 1987). Both our experimental–theoretical approach to retinal coding in the blowfly, and our major conclusions have recently been reviewed (Laughlin, 1987; 1989). In this article I will briefly summarise our arguments and explore some of the general implications of the finding that retinal circuits are designed to promote coding efficiency.

The constraints imposed upon vision by the properties of natural images and the construction of neurons are readily apparent in the retina. A detailed optical image is projected onto the photoreceptors and transformed into the first neural image – the distribution of receptor potentials across the photoreceptor mosaic. The properties of natural signals and photoreceptors severely limit the amplitude of the signal in this electrical 'image'. Most natural objects are rendered visible by small changes in the reflection and transmission of ambient light. Thus vision depends upon the detection of small changes in relative intensity (i.e. small changes in contrast) about an average or background light level. Over 24 hours the background level changes by at least eight orders of magnitude, and even between dawn and dusk, the variation is about four orders of magnitude (e.g. Martin 1983). By comparison, the dynamic range of fly photoreceptors is 70 mV, being limited by factors such as ionic reversal potentials. With a wide daily range of input amplitudes to be accommodated to this limited response range, it is not surprising that, at any one time, the amplitude of the fluctuation in electrical signal across the receptor mosaic is small. For a blowfly, the mean contrast of natural images is 0.4 (Laughlin, 1981) and this corresponds to a change in receptor potential of approximately 10 mV. Thus at any one background intensity, most of the image detail is contained within a narrow band of receptor response. Such small receptor signals are prone to contamination by the intrinsic noise generated in neural circuits, and it is logical to devote the first stage of processing to noise protection. The effects of the noise added during neural processing are reduced by amplifying the signal at the earliest opportunity. Amplification of the signal alone increases the signal to noise ratio. The fly retina is designed to maximise the amplification of signals at the photoreceptor synapse. To boost the permissible level of amplification, and so improve the reliability of the coded signal, the fly adheres to principles of retinal coding first suggested by Horace Barlow (1961a,b,c).

Barlow observed that a single nerve cell can only transmit a limited amount of information per unit time. This finite information capacity is set by biophysical factors, such as the maximum rate of generating action potentials, random fluctuations in action potential rate, reversal potentials, noise and membrane time constants. Given a limited information capacity, it is advantageous to efficiently pack information from the retinal image into neurons. One way of improving efficiency is to remove those components of the signal that convey little or no information. This prevents the wastage of neural information capacity. The cell's limited repertoire of responses is devoted to the meaningful components of the signal, so allowing the cell to code the essential pictorial detail with greater accuracy. Barlow pointed out that information theory (Shannon & Weaver, 1949) provides an appropriate theoretical framework for evaluating the proposition that retinal coding promotes the efficient use of limited neural resources. For example, information theory identifies worthless signal components as redundancy. These redundant parts of the signal convey no additional information because they can be predicted from the worthwhile bits. Barlow observed that lateral inhibition, as found in the compound eye of *Limulus* (Hartline, 1969) and in the centre–surround organisation of bipolar and ganglion cell receptive fields, removes redundancy (e.g. Attwell, 1986). In areas where the brightness of the image is constant, inhibition and excitation are equal and no signal is generated. The lateral inhibitory network only responds where intensity changes; i.e. lateral inhibition selects high spatial frequencies and edges. A similar argument holds for signals that vary in time. The delayed or slower inhibition that generates transient neural responses is the temporal equivalent of lateral inhibition. It selects those components of the signal that change in time and attenuates those redundant components that remain constant. Barlow's proposition that retinal antagonism, i.e. the counteracting forces of inhibition and excitation, strip away redundancy to promote coding efficiency is an attractive one, but is it compelling? To provide additional support for his argument, one must show that retinal processing is designed to strip away redundancy effectively, and demonstrate that, if redundancy were not removed, vision would be impaired. The favourable anatomy and physiology of insect compound eyes has allowed us to produce such arguments. Our analysis confirms that the promotion of coding efficiency is a major function of visual processing in the retina, and that redundancy reduction is an essential part of this process.

Coding efficiency in the fly retina

There are a number of factors that enable us to analyse coding in the fly retina with the accuracy that is required to develop and test quantitative hypotheses of function. The fly photoreceptors are arranged in optical modules, with a set of eight anatomically identified and physiologically characterised cells sampling each point in space (rev. Hardie, 1986). The photoreceptors sampling a single point project to a single neural module. This contains a well defined population of interneurons whose connectivity has been defined to the level of the number of synapses connecting each type of identified receptor axon and interneuron (rev. Shaw, 1984). A sub-class of the second order neurons in the module, the large monopolar cells (LMCs), are amenable to intracellular recording. Like the photoreceptors, and the analogous bipolar cells of the vertebrate retina, their responses are graded: action potentials are rarely seen (Järvilehto & Zettler, 1973). LMC response amplitudes of 40–50 mV and stable recordings lasting for more than an hour are not uncommon. These recordings are made in essentially intact preparations, and the graded nature of photoreceptor and LMC responses simplifies the analysis of signal and noise. Such favourable experimental conditions allow one to describe the transfer of signal and noise from photoreceptors to LMCs by comparing the responses of the two cell types to identical stimuli.

Early in our studies (Laughlin & Hardie, 1978) we found that the transfer of signal from fly photoreceptor to LMC resembled the transfer of signal from cone to bipolar cell, as observed in the retinas of lower vertebrates (rev. Werblin, 1973). In both the fly and the vertebrate retina the photoreceptors and second order neurons communicate via graded potentials. Moreover, the second order neurons exhibit antagonistic response components which are not present in the individual photoreceptor. The antagonism is both spatial and temporal, generating spatially opponent centre–surround receptive fields and transient responses. Furthermore, the bipolars and the LMCs have a smaller dynamic range than the photoreceptors, indicating that the signal is amplified during transfer. The antagonistic processes keep the narrower response window of the second order cells centred upon the mean level of receptor response. This enables the second order neuron to respond to fluctuations in intensity over a wide range of background light levels. A major difference between the vertebrate and the fly retina is that the bipolar cells are segregated into ON and OFF types, whereas a light adapted LMC codes increments and decrements of intensity with equal facility.

On the basis of this comparison, Roger Hardie and I suggested that the similarities between the second order cells indicated a common function for the two types of retina (Laughlin & Hardie, 1978). These common properties could be so important for retinal function that they had to be incorporated into eyes that were constructed according to different plans. We observed that, in the fly retina, two major transformations occur as the signal passes from photoreceptor to LMC. The background component of the receptor signal is subtracted away, and the residue is amplified. These transformations match the response of the LMC to the incoming receptor signal so that the range of signals expected at any one background intensity makes full use of the LMC dynamic range. It is relatively simple to see why subtraction and amplification are advantageous. The LMC has a limited information capacity. Its 50 mV dynamic range is contaminated by noise and this restricts the number of discriminable signals that it can transmit. The object of coding is to pack as much pictorial information as possible into the LMC. But, at any one background intensity, the contrast signals generated by natural objects generate response fluctuations of a few millivolts and these fluctuations are superimposed on a larger background signal. The narrow band of contrast signals contains most of the pictorial information. To pack the pictorial information into the LMCs, one must amplify the narrow band of signals generated by objects to fill the LMC response range. This maximises the signal to noise ratio. However, if one also amplifies the background component of the receptor response, the LMC is easily saturated. When one removes the background component, the signals from objects can be amplified to fill the LMC dynamic range. This simple role for subtraction and amplification is in accord with Barlow's suggestions about redundancy reduction and coding efficiency.

The proposal that retinal coding is designed to promote efficiency is substantiated by a detailed analysis of the processes of subtraction and amplification. First consider subtraction. The role of subtraction is to remove the background component. How should the retina estimate the background level? This is not a trivial problem because factors such as shading generate uneven patterns of illumination. The appropriate value of background intensity will change across the retina and must, therefore, be estimated locally. Just how localised should this estimate be? One approach is to invoke redundancy. The local mean at a given point on the retina is estimated from its surroundings. If one weights the values one takes from the surroundings so that they provide a good estimate of the signal expected at a particular point then this estimate is a prediction. Predictable components of the signal are, by definition, redundant.

When one subtracts away the prediction from the signal received at that point, the amplitude of the signal is greatly reduced but no information is lost. This predictive coding technique was developed to compress image data into smaller amplitude signals so that pictures could be more economically and efficiently transmitted and stored (rev. Gonzalez & Wintz, 1977).

Does the fly retina exploit redundancy when deriving the local mean? We used the established theory to see if the fly retina used predictive coding (Srinivasan *et al.*, 1982). We found that the retinal area used to derive the prediction should depend on the light intensity. At high intensities the photoreceptor signal is reliable and the nearest neighbours provide a satisfactory estimate of the local mean. As intensity falls, photon fluctuations lead to a decline in the signal to noise ratio in the photoreceptors, consequently more receptors must be used to derive a reliable estimate. Translating this finding into physiological terms, predictive coding in space should be implemented by centre–surround antagonism in the receptive field. The surround predicts the signal expected at the centre and this is subtracted from the centre response. The surround should be narrower and stronger at high light levels and become weaker and more diffuse at low levels. The theory of predictive coding gives the sensitivity profile of the surround required at each intensity, so providing an exact test for the hypothesis that the surround mechanism is designed to remove this particular form of redundancy.

Our measurements (Srinivasan *et al.*, 1982) showed that in fly LMCs the surround extended and weakened at low intensities but it was always too wide to give the best prediction of the signal at the centre. The wider surround may be necessary to take account of unpredictable movements in the retinal image. Predictive coding can also be implemented in time, much as it is implemented in space. The temporal transients in the LMC response represent the removal of a time average of the previous input. We found that the time course of the LMC response has precisely the intensity dependence necessary for predictive coding in time. This matching of time constant to intensity demonstrates that retinal antagonism is designed to remove redundancy. The removal of the redundant local mean promotes coding efficiency by reducing the amplitude of the signal to be coded within the confines of the interneuron's dynamic response range.

Following subtraction, one amplifies the remaining signal to fill the response range of the second order cell. Again it is desirable to match the form of coding to the nature of the image. If the gain of amplification is too small, the extremes of LMC response will hardly ever be used and it is advantageous to increase the gain to improve the detectability of small signals. When the gain is too great the large signals will saturate the LMC and be lost. A neat compromise is to have a gain that is high for small signals and lower for larger ones (Laughlin & Hardie, 1978). Moreover, if the small signals are more commonly encountered than the large ones, one can taper off the gain in proportion to the probability of encountering that particular amplitude of signal at the input. With the gain matched to probabilities in this way, the non-uniform probability density of input signal amplitudes is turned into a uniform probability density of signal levels in the interneuron (e.g. Laughlin, 1981). This means that all of the neuron's response levels are used equally often, and the gain has been adjusted to make full use of the cell's dynamic response range. As with redundancy reduction, this matched gain strategy follows from the application of information theory and is used in digital picture processing. Measurements of the statistical distribution of contrast in natural scenes, as viewed by the fly, and of the relationship between LMC response amplitude and contrast, show that amplification is matched to probability (Laughlin, 1981; Laughlin et al., 1987). Thus the combination of information theory and physiological measurement again demonstrates that retinal processing has been designed to maximise the amplification of the signal, within the constraint of a limited dynamic range. Amplification improves coding efficiency by reducing the deleterious effects of the intrinsic noise.

Where is the intrinsic noise that subtraction and amplification supposedly suppress? In theory, the matching of subtraction and amplification to image properties is advantageous when a finite amount of noise is added somewhere in the neural pathway, and when this added noise degrades perception. Under these conditions, the amplification of the signal before it encounters the noise will improve the performance of the visual system. Note that, because the added neural noise must degrade perception, amplification and redundancy removal will not be effective when the incoming photoreceptor signal is heavily contaminated with noise. One might expect different strategies for the optimum coding of rod signals, but these still take into account the known limitations of neural processing such as synaptic non-linearity (Attwell et al., 1987). Returning to vision at high intensities, it has been possible to identify a source of intrinsic noise in the fly retina that is potentially a serious impediment

to visual acuity, and is reduced in effect by amplification. This is the noise generated at the site of amplification: the synapses from photoreceptor to second order cell.

Measurements of signal to noise ratios in photoreceptors and LMCs (Laughlin et al., 1987) indicate that, at high light levels, more than 50% of the noise in LMCs has been added during the passage of the signal from the site of phototransduction to the LMC membrane. This added noise is equivalent to a contrast of about 0.01, a value that is of the same order as the lowest detectable contrast of a moving grating of optimum velocity and spatial wavelength (Laughlin et al., 1987; Eckert, 1973). The added noise can be identified in the power spectrum by prominent high frequency components, and these are associated with synaptic transmission from photoreceptor to LMC. How is this synaptic noise suppressed by an amplification process that involves an increase in synaptic activity? Assume that the major sources of synaptic noise are the random processes associated with transmitter release and the activation of post-synaptic channels. In this case the noise level depends upon the amount of transmitter released, and hence the number of channels activated at the post-synaptic membrane. However, the number of active channels also determines the post-synaptic membrane potential. Thus in the simplest system, where all changes in post-synaptic potential result from changes in conductance at the one type of synapse, the amplitude of synaptic noise is a fixed function of the post-synaptic response level. Under this condition the signal to noise ratio for synaptic transmission is increased when a given pre-synaptic input produces a larger post-synaptic response. In other words, maximising the amplification of the signal at the synapse improves the signal to noise ratio for synaptic transmission. This argument is supported by using a simple model of synaptic transmission (Falk & Fatt, 1972) to derive the signal to noise ratio (Laughlin et al., 1987). The model also shows the synapse should use a large quantity of transmitter (and/or transmitter vesicles) to carry the signal. Fly photoreceptors are probably designed to recruit large numbers of vesicles, because each photoreceptor makes over 200 synapses with each LMC (Shaw, 1984).

The observation that synaptic amplification improves the signal to noise ratio for transmission provides a concrete reason for maximising amplification, and hence for removing redundancy and for matching amplification to input levels. The argument is as follows. We have observed that the photoreceptors portray the details of the retinal image as small fluctuations in potential across the receptor mosaic. This fragile neural image is prone to contamination by noise. Receptors communicate via chemical synapses and these are potent sources of noise. Consequently, the receptors must be carefully interfaced to the second order cells to minimse the inescapable effects of synaptic noise. Synaptic noise is minimised by amplification, but amplification is constrained by the dynamic range of response: hence the need for redundancy removal and the requirement for a matched gain. Note that the constraints invoked for this functional interpretation are common to many retinae, both vertebrate and invertebrate.

In summary we have vindicated Barlow's suggestion (Barlow, 1961a,b,c) by showing that the fly retina is designed to strip away redundancy, and that redundancy reduction minimises a serious impediment to vision, synaptic noise at the photoreceptor terminals. The importance of redundancy reduction in retinal coding has been independently confirmed by applying information theory to human colour vision (Buchsbaum & Gottschalk, 1983). The luminance channel and the two opponent chromatic channels inferred from psychophysical studies are extremely effective at removing the correlated (and hence redundant) components that are introduced by overlaps between the spectral sensitivity functions of the three cone types. In the fly we have also found a second strategy that improves the efficiency of retinal coding, the matching of the gain of amplification to the expected amplitude distribution of the incoming signal. Again, this strategy has psychophysical parallels. It has been argued that our ability to judge lightness is matched to the statistical distribution of intensity levels. We sacrifice the ability to judge rare extremes to gain a better resolution of the commonplace moderate levels (Richards, 1982).

Coding efficiency – a guiding principle in visual processing?

To what extent are the dictates of coding efficiency confined to the retina? Let us first examine the case that coding efficiency is a peculiarly retinal consideration. In the vertebrate eye the optic nerve is a bottleneck for information transfer from retina to brain. The retina has to compress information into a limited number of ganglion cells, hence the need for neural interactions that promote coding efficiency. This argument may well be true for ganglion cells, but it is not a compelling one for second order neurons such as bipolars. The second order cells of the fly retina code the receptor input extremely efficiently but in the insect eye there is no bottleneck – several second order cells are devoted to every spatial sampling point on the retina (rev. Shaw, 1984). Rather the requirement for efficiency is imposed by the nature of photoreceptors and the nature of neurons. Receptors generate small signals, neurons have a limited dynamic range of response, and synaptic transmission introduces noise. One can also argue that the retina's job is to enhance the picture presented to the brain by removing all the useless parts and expanding the remainder. Such enhancement is advantageous because, as argued above, boosting the signal in the retina will reduce the effects of intrinsic noise in the brain.

Now consider the counter argument, namely that coding efficiency is advantageous at all levels of neural processing. One can consider two types of argument, analogous to the design of computer software and hardware. The software argument suggests that concise descriptions are easier to operate upon, and less likely to give ambiguous descriptions of objects. In other words, one is more likely to see what is out there when one has stripped away all the obscuring redundancy. Moreover, objects are identifiable precisely because they are, at the retinal level, redundant. As Barlow put it (1961c, p. 365) 'The features of the sensory input which are recognised, or discriminated from each other, appear to be the very features which enable sensory messages to be compressed.' In other words, objects are identifiable because they are composed of related parts. Thus, stripping away these correlations (i.e. removing the redundancy) leads to the concise, and hence logical description of objects (Barlow, 1961c). Like many of Barlow's arguments this has the ring of eternal truth, but it has not, to my knowledge, provided a unique and compelling explanation for a particular high level visual process.

The second argument for the general relevance of coding efficiency is one that considers the hardware. Processing is carried out by neurons, and neurons suffer from a limited dynamic range and intrinsic noise. In many situations a given circuit will work more accurately when information is coded efficiently, because, as we have seen with LMCs, efficiency promotes accuracy. Thus, as the nervous system evolves, the small changes in circuitry that promote coding efficiency will be selected for because they increase the accuracy of the existing hardware. Better accuracy results in lower thresholds, and an increase in the number of objects resolved.

At least two types of higher order visual interneuron show properties that will enhance accuracy. Both change their sensitivity to accommodate a wide range of input levels within their response range. Many of the cells encountered in the striate cortex of the cat adapt to the prevailing contrast of stimuli (Albrecht, Farrar & Hamilton, 1984). When exposed to low or zero contrast, the sensitivity to contrast (i.e. the slope of the curve relating response amplitude to stimulus contrast) is high. Thus small contrast changes are monitored accurately. When subjected to sustained higher contrasts, the sensitivity to contrast falls to prevent saturation of the response. This process of adaptation to contrast should improve accuracy within the constraint of a limited dynamic response range and intrinsic noise. Moreover, simulation suggests that such local adaptation to contrast is an effective means of delineating the boundaries between objects (Osorio, Snyder & Srinivasan, 1987).

A similar adaptation process has been examined in an identified pair of movement sensitive neurons in the fly, the H1 cells (Maddess & Laughlin, 1985). This unique pair of neurons responds to movements from front to back in the contra-lateral eye (rev. Hausen, 1984). The sensitivity to stimulus velocity decreases in the presence of sustained and vigorous movement. This adaptation process is localised to the stimulated region of the receptive field, and it prevents the neuron from saturating. Adaptation helps maintain operations in the region of the response range where H1 is most sensitive to changes in velocity about the mean level. Thus adaptation promotes coding efficiency by matching the sensitivity of the cell to the prevailing stimulus conditions. Note again that this adaptation process could have evolved because it promotes the accuracy of an existing function, the coding of velocity.

However, the adaptation process has changed H1's properties in a manner that profoundly influences the way in which it codes retinal flow fields (Maddess & Laughlin, 1985). H1 now codes velocity relative to a mean level, i.e. it codes velocity contrast. Moreover, because adaptation is a local process, H1 will be driven most effectively by the areas of the image where velocity changes suddenly. There are neurons in the same region of the fly brain that are extremely effective at performing figure ground discriminations on the basis of relative motion (Egelhaaf, 1985), and Horridge (1987) has championed the view that locally adapting motion detecting neurons play a crucial role in discriminating objects in a moving world. Given the importance of coding relative motion, and the ability of locally adapting networks to detect moving boundaries, it is possible that coding efficiency has promoted the evolution of more sophisticated motion detecting networks in the fly. We can postulate that, to improve the accuracy of

relatively simple motion detecting cells, such as H1, the input elements evolved the ability to adapt. The matrix of locally adapting input elements is now extremely effective at picking out discontinuities in the flow field, and forms an excellent substrate for the evolution of neurons that localise moving boundaries. Thus coding efficiency may be a guiding principle in vision, not only for understanding the function of circuits, but in the sense that it provides the selective advantage for evolutionary change. The changes dictated by coding efficiency will add new orders of complexity to existing systems and so predispose them for more sophisticated operations.

In the examples that we have considered, two factors have improved coding efficiency. In the striate cells and in H1, adaptation of the response adjusted sensitivity to take account of the previous history of stimulation. As we have seen, such dynamic changes accentuate discontinuities and novelty, such as boundaries. Secondly, we have seen the advantages to be gained by tailoring coding to the statistical structure of the incoming data. In fly LMCs, the sensitivity to contrast is matched to the expected distribution of input amplitudes and antagonism is matched to the signal to noise ratio. It follows that sampling and processing in the visual system may often be matched to the statistical structure of the data. For example, Hughes (1977) argues that the uneven distribution of ganglion cells across the vertebrate retina matches sampling to the structure of an animal's visual world in order to prevent redundancy, in the form of over-sampling. The clustering of ganglion cells in a visual streak accommodates the decreasing angular dimensions of objects as they recede towards the horizon. Similarly the radial decrease in density from a central fovea matches the sampling mosaic to the blur introduced by forward motion. If, at higher levels, efficiency continues to demand ever more complicated forms of response adaptation, and more sophisticated matches between response properties and image statistics, then natural selection may inevitably generate concise and unambiguous descriptions of objects. Thus our considerations of retinal coding efficiency, and of adaptation in higher order neurons, has resurrected Barlow's intriguing idea by suggesting that evolutionary pressures have enabled the hardware of the visual system to bootstrap the software. Neural coding efficiency may well promote new, economical, and hence logical representations of images that facilitate recognition and we might be well advised to look again at the adaptability of higher order responses, both from a physiological and an evolutionary point of view.

References

Albrecht, D. G., Farrar, S. B. & Hamilton, D. B. (1984) Spatial contrast adaptation characteristics of neurones recorded in the cat's visual cortex. *J. Physiol.* (Lond.), **347**, 713–39.

Attwell, D. (1986) Ion channels and signal processing in the outer retina. *Quart. J. Exp. Physiol.*, **71**, 497–536.

Attwell, D., Borges, S., Wu, S. M. & Wilson, M. (1987) Signal clipping by the rod output synapse. *Nature*, **328**, 522–4.

Barlow, H. B. (1961a) Possible principles underlying the transformations of sensory messages. In *Sensory Communication*, ed. W. A. Rosenblith, pp. 217–34. Cambridge, Mass: MIT Press.

Barlow, H. B. (1961b) Comment – three points about lateral inhibition. In *Sensory Communication*, ed. W. A. Rosenblith, pp. 782–6. Cambridge, Mass: MIT Press.

Barlow, H. B. (1961c) The coding of sensory messages. In *Current Problems in Animal Behaviour*, ed. W. H. Thorpe & O. L. Zangwill, pp. 331–60. Cambridge: Cambridge University Press.

Barlow, H. B. (1964) The physical limits of visual discrimination. In *Photophysiology*, vol. II, ed. A. C. Giese. New York: Academic Press.

Buchsbaum, G. & Gottschalk, A. (1983) Trichromacy, opponent colours coding and optimum information transmission in the retina. *Proc. Roy. Soc. Lond.*, **B220**, 89–113.

Eckert, H. (1973) Optomotorische Untersuchungen am visuellen System der Stubenfliege *Musca domestica*. *Kybernetik*, **14**, 1–23.

Egelhaaf, M. (1985) On the neuronal basis of figure–ground discrimination in the visual system of the fly. III. Possible input circuitries and behavioural significance of the FD-cells. *Biol. Cybern.*, **52**, 267–80.

Falk, G. & Fatt, P. (1972) Physical changes induced by light in the rod outer segment of vertebrates. In *Handbook of Sensory Physiology*, vol. VII/1, ed. H. J. A. Dartnall, pp. 200–44. Berlin–Heidelberg–New York: Springer.

Gonzalez, R. C. & Wintz, P. (1977) *Digital Image Processing*. Reading, Mass: Addison–Wesley.

Hardie, R. C. (1986) The photoreceptor array of the dipteran retina. *Trends Neurosci.*, **9**, 419–23.

Hartline, H. K. (1969) Visual receptors and retinal interaction. *Science*, **164**, 270–8.

Hausen, K. (1984) The lobula-complex of the fly: structure, function and significance of visual behaviour. In *Photoreception and Vision in Invertebrates*, ed. M. A. Ali, pp. 523–59. New York: Plenum Press.

Hecht, S., Shlaer, S. & Pirenne, M. (1942) Energy, quanta and vision. *J. gen. Physiol.*, **25**, 819–40.

Horridge, G. A. (1987) The evolution of visual processing and the construction of seeing systems. *Proc. Roy. Soc. Lond.*, **B230**, 279–92.

Hughes, A. (1977) The topography of vision in mammals of contrasting life style: comparative optics and retinal organisation. In *Handbook of Sensory Physiology*, vol. VII/5, ed. F. Crescitelli, pp. 613–756. Berlin–Heidelberg–New York: Springer.

Järvilehto, M. & Zettler, F. (1973) Electrophysiological–histological studies on some functional properties of visual cells and second-order neurons of an insect retina. *Z. Zellforsch.*, **136**, 291–306.

Laughlin, S. B. (1981) A simple coding procedure enhances a neuron's information capacity, *Z. Naturforsch.*, **36c**, 910–12.

Laughlin, S. B. (1987) Form and function in retinal processing. *Trends Neurosci.*, **10**, 478–83.

Laughlin, S. B. (1989) Coding efficiency and design in visual processing. In *Facets of Vision*, ed. D. G. Stavenga & R. C. Hardie, pp. 213–34. Berlin–Heidelberg–New York: Springer.

Laughlin, S. B. & Hardie, R. C. (1978) Common strategies for light adaptation in the peripheral visual systems of fly and dragonfly. *J. Comp. Physiol.*, **128**, 319–40.

Laughlin, S. B., Howard, J. & Blakeslee, B. (1987) Synaptic limitations to contrast coding in the retina of the blowfly *Calliphora*. *Proc. Roy. Soc. Lond.*, **B231**, 437–67.

Maddess, T. & Laughlin, S. B. (1985) Adaptation of the motion sensitive neuron H1 is generated locally and governed by contrast frequency. *Proc. Roy. Soc. Lond.*, **B 225**, 251–75.

Martin, G. R. (1983) Schematic eye models in vertebrates. *Prog. Sensory Physiol.*, **4**, 43–81.

Osorio, D., Snyder, A. W. & Srinivasan, M. V. (1987) Bi-partitioning and boundary detection in natural scenes. *Spatial Vision*, **2**, 191–8.

Richards, W. A. (1982) A lightness scale from image intensity distributions. *Applied Optics*, **21**, 2569–82.

Rose, A. (1972). *Vision: Human and Electronic*. New York: Plenum Press.

Shannon, C. E. & Weaver, W. (1949) *The Mathematical Theory of Communication*. Urbana: University of Illinois Press.

Shaw, S. R. (1984) Early visual processing in insects. *J. Exp. Biol.*, **112**, 225–51.

Srinivasan, M. V., Laughlin, S. B. & Dubs, A. (1982) Predictive coding: a fresh view of inhibition in the retina. *Proc. Roy. Soc. Lond.*, **B216**, 427–59.

Werblin, F. S. (1973) The control of sensitivity in the retina. *Sci. Am.*, **228**, 70–9.

3
Statistical limits to image understanding

D. Kersten

Introduction

Many visual decisions are fundamentally statistical in nature. This can be because of noisy physical processes such as quantum fluctuations (Rose, 1948; Barlow, 1962), or the indeterminacy of the environmental causes of the images on the eye's retinae. The problem with noisy imaging is that a single source can give rise to many images. The challenge is to integrate image information in such a way as to discount the noise. The problem with indeterminacy of the environmental causes of the image is that there are too many possible scene descriptions that could have given rise to the image data. If one can find a statistical description of a visual task, one can often devise an observer that handles both of these types of uncertainty optimally. This *ideal observer* is one that makes optimal use of the data available, given a statistical description of the task, and a criterion to satisfy (e.g. minimal classification error). The ideal observer comprises a quantitative computational theory for a given task, in the sense of Marr (1982), and as such is an abstract model of the information processing requirements of the task, independent of the particular algorithm or implementation. The statistical approach to understanding biological vision, thus, involves three parts: (1) formulate the statistically optimal observer for a visual task; (2) devise a biological or psychophysical model of performance; (3) compare experimental data to ideal and model. Typically, one compares the biological model with the data, leaving out an analysis of the statistical requirements imposed by the task as specified by an ideal observer. By comparing biological performance to the ideal, it is sometimes possible to partition out the inherent informational limits to a task apart from the limits imposed by the algorithm or hardware (Barlow, 1977; Geisler, 1984).

There are now a number of examples of the ideal observer approach to quantum efficiency (Pelli, Chapter 1; Geisler, 1984), pattern detection (Burgess *et al.*, 1981; Watson *et al.*, 1983; Kersten, 1984), symmetry detection (Barlow & Reeves, 1979), and graphical perception (Legge *et al.*, 1989), among others. Classical signal detection theory (e.g. van Trees, 1968) provides the theoretical underpinning for understanding optimal models that relate to human performance. These studies primarily have to do with human visual capacity defined in terms of the image representation. The purpose of this chapter is to illustrate how the idea of an ideal observer can be extended to the image understanding problems involving the estimation of scene parameters from images. First, the statistical theory of the problem will be presented. This will be related to the deterministic regularization framework suggested by Poggio *et al.* (1985). Statistical modeling tools known as Markov Random Fields (MRFs) will be introduced and applied to an example in which the material reflectance of a surface has to be estimated from luminance data. This problem is called reflectance estimation, and is closely related to the perceptual phenomena of color and lightness constancy. It provides a simple case of the cooperative estimation of two independent scene causes to image intensity changes. In most real implementations, performance limitations also occur as a result of the algorithmic tools available. An example of an associative learning estimator for shape from shading will be described that is optimal subject to the constraint that it is linear. Recent progress in analog parallel computation, for which the linear associator is an example, illustrates relationships that exist between ideal observers, algorithms and possible neuronal networks (Koch et al., 1986).

Scene properties from images

It has become clear in the last couple of decades that one of the profound problems of human vision is how we reliably estimate low level scene properties such as shapes, distances, movements and material characteristics of objects from data consisting of luminance values as a function of space and time (Fig. 3.1). On the one hand, when we consider any particular source of visual information, the image data often underconstrains the solution of a scene property. That is, there are many interpretations of the world that could give rise to the same image. On the other hand, the problem of how to satisfy multiple constraints is not straightforward either, and can lead to non-linear formulations. This problem occurs in two forms. One can have multiple cues that have to be integrated to yield a unique scene property (e.g. depth from stereo and motion parallax information), or the estimate of one kind of scene property (e.g. illumination) can affect the estimate of another (e.g. reflectance). The latter problem will be illustrated in the section below on reflectance estimation. The statistical approach has the potential for providing a framework for these problems which is both computationally and biologically useful.

Let the image and scene parameters be represented discretely by vectors, **i** and **s**, respectively:

$$\mathbf{i} = (i_1, i_2, \ldots, i_n)$$
$$\mathbf{s} = (s_1, s_2, \ldots, s_m) \tag{1}$$

where m is not, in general, equal to n. Image parameters could be as simple as the intensities as a function of position and time, or could be some derived image cue or feature, such as a filtered image, or edge map. The scene parameters could be a list of surface material or lighting attributes, for example a scene based edge map marking surface reflectance discontinuities or orientation discontinuities. The computer graphics or *forward optics* problem of calculating an image vector, **i** from a scene representation **s** can be represented by:

$$\mathbf{i} = \mathbf{As}, \tag{2}$$

where **A** may be a non-linear operator. Modeling image formation is non-trivial (Foley & Van Dam, 1982), but from a mathematical point of view, imaging is well-defined. Given a representation of the scene, and a model of image formation, the image can, in principle, be computed. However, the *inverse optics* problem, of computing **s** from **i**, given **A**, is often ill-posed in the sense that there is not a unique **s** which satisfies the equation. Additional constraints have to be imposed in order to force a unique solution. One mathematical approach to the study of ill-posed

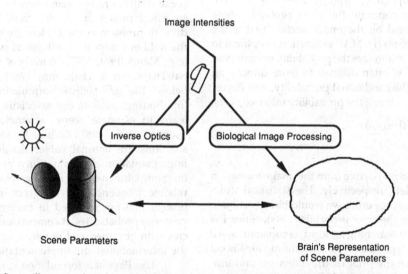

Fig. 3.1. This figure illustrates the relationship between the inverse optics problem and biological image processing. The ideal observer in one case estimates the probability of scene parameters conditional on the image intensities, and in the other computes the probability of the brain's representation (or homologues) of these scene characteristics conditional on the image intensities. The scene parameters could include: material properties, lighting conditions, motion, and shapes of surfaces.

problems is *regularization theory* which has been proposed as a framework to unify many of the computational problems of early vision (Poggio *et al.*, 1985).

In regularization theory, one incorporates a suitable constraint operator, **P**, which, together with a choice of norms, $||\cdot||$, serves to constrain the search for **s**. One approach is to find **s** that minimizes

$$||\mathbf{As}-\mathbf{i}||^2+\lambda||\mathbf{Ps}||^2. \tag{3}$$

For example, for discrete linear regularization, **s** and **i** are vectors, **A**, **P** matrices, and the norm is vector length. The form of the constraint operator is usually arrived at by a combination of heuristics, mathematical convenience and experiment. One example from motion measurement is to assume velocity flow fields are smooth almost everywhere. This heuristic can be quantified by using a discrete Laplacian constraint operator on the desired velocity field (Hildreth, 1983). If the imaging operator, **A** is linear, then equation (3) is a quadratic form in **s**, and thus convex with no local minima. A solution can be found with standard techniques such as gradient descent.

How can scene-from-image problems be formulated statistically? One approach to solving the inverse problem is Bayesian estimation, and in particular *maximum a posteriori* estimation (MAP) (Bolle & Cooper, 1984; Geman & Geman, 1984; Marroquin, 1985). Let the *posterior* probability of the scene description conditional on the image be $p(\mathbf{s}|\mathbf{i})$. The computational goal is then to compute the most probable scene vector, conditional on the image vector, that is the mode or peak of $p(\mathbf{s}|\mathbf{i})$. MAP estimation is optimal in the sense that it minimizes the probability of error (van Trees, 1968). It is often difficult to write directly an expression for the conditional probability, and Bayes' rule enables us to break the probability into two parts:

$$p(\mathbf{s}|\mathbf{i})=\frac{p(\mathbf{i}|\mathbf{s})p(\mathbf{s})}{p(\mathbf{i})}, \tag{4}$$

where $p(\mathbf{i}|\mathbf{s})$ and $p(\mathbf{s})$ derive from the image formation and scene models, respectively. The statistical structure of the scene properties we would like to estimate are specified by the *prior* probability, $p(\mathbf{s})$. Since **i** is held fixed, while searching for **s**, $p(\mathbf{i})$ is constant. MAP estimation is equivalent to maximum likelihood estimation when the prior distributions are uniform. Given certain assumptions, MAP estimation is equivalent to regularization theory. If we assume

$$\mathbf{i}=\mathbf{As}+noise, \tag{5}$$

where the noise term is multivariate Gaussian with a constant diagonal covariance matrix, then

$$p(\mathbf{i}|\mathbf{s})=k\,e^{-((\mathbf{i}-\mathbf{As})^{\mathrm{T}}(\mathbf{i}-\mathbf{As}))/2\sigma_n^2} \tag{6}$$

where k is a normalization constant. Superscript T indicates transpose, so $\mathbf{x}^{\mathrm{T}}\mathbf{x}$, for example, is the inner product. Further, suppose $p(\mathbf{s})$ is multivariate Gaussian:

$$p(\mathbf{s})=k\,e^{-\mathbf{s}^{\mathrm{T}}\mathbf{Bs}}, \tag{7}$$

and **s** is adjusted to have zero mean. By substituting (6) and (7) in (4) and taking the logarithm, maximizing $p(\mathbf{s}|\mathbf{i})$ is equivalent to minimizing:

$$(\mathbf{As}-\mathbf{i})^{\mathrm{T}}(\mathbf{As}-\mathbf{i})+\lambda\mathbf{s}^{\mathrm{T}}\mathbf{Bs}, \tag{8}$$

where λ is a Lagrange multiplier equal to the ratio of the noise to scene variance. If the data are noise-free, MAP estimation is equivalent to minimizing

$$\mathbf{s}^{\mathrm{T}}\mathbf{Bs} \tag{9}$$

for those **s** that satisfy

$$\mathbf{i}=\mathbf{As}. \tag{10}$$

For vector length norms, the MAP formulation (8) gives the cost function (3) if the image and scene are represented by discrete vectors, and when $\mathbf{B}=\mathbf{P}^{\mathrm{T}}\mathbf{P}$.

Expressing regularization theory in terms of MAP estimation has several advantages. The constraint term can, in principle, be based on verifiable scene statistics rather than heuristics. Finding a good statistical model of natural scene parameters is a difficult problem in itself. Here we may benefit from the field of computer synthesis of naturalistic scenes (e.g. Mandelbrot, 1977; Fournier *et al.*, 1982; Magnenat-Thalmann & Thalmann, 1987). As we will see below, the probabilistic formulation also provides input/output pairs to use associative algorithms that learn to estimate scene parameters from images (Kersten *et al.*, 1987; Knill & Kersten, 1990). These solutions are optimal subject to an algorithmic or implementation constraint, such as a linear approximation. Ultimately we may be able to deal with the relative frequencies of incorrect interpretations of images that are reflected in multiple modes of the posterior probabilities. A comparison of ideal frequencies with observed will require a knowledge of both the informational and implementation constraints.

The Bayesian formulation can be extended to multiple image cues and scene representations where the posterior distribution is given by

$$p(\mathbf{s}_1,\mathbf{s}_2,\ldots,\mathbf{s}_m|\mathbf{i}_1,\mathbf{i}_2,\ldots,\mathbf{i}_n) \tag{11}$$

where s_j represents a particular scene representation, and j indexes the type (e.g. shape, reflectance values, reflectance discontinuities, etc.). i_j represents image cues, such as intensity, color, or higher level features such as discontinuities at various scales, or texture measurements. The problem, of course, is that it is difficult enough to formulate a posterior probability function, and quite another matter to compute statistics, such as modes or means, on it. An example of using multiple image cues (image intensities and edges) to cooperatively compute texture, motion and stereo depth discontinuities is found in Poggio *et al.* (1988).

We should note that one could formulate alternative goals to MAP estimation. One could minimize the least squared error or calculate the posterior mean, which can be more appropriate for certain tasks (Marroquin, 1985). It is tempting think of the MAP solution in terms of an ideal adaptation to inferring the environment from image data, based on ontogenetic or phylogenetic experience. Although appealing, the frequency interpretation of probability, in this case, is a weaker motivation than one would like. Because of the high dimensionality of the spaces under consideration, the frequency of correct solutions is exceedingly small. It retains some appeal, however, with the Markov Random Field assumption to be elaborated below where the probability of being locally right is a reasonably large number. The frequency interpretation is then important from the point of view of verifying the scene model by actually gathering statistics. On the other hand, even without a frequency interpretation a logical response is a special case of selecting the most probable response (Cox, 1946). Also, certain forms of maximum entropy are equivalent to MAP estimation (Frieden, 1983).

As mentioned above, when the image formation process is linear, and the prior distribution Gaussian, the cost function is convex, and thus standard techniques, such as gradient descent, can be used to find the global minimum; however, linear methods are extremely restrictive. They do not handle discontinuities, or general multiple constraint interactions, essential to understanding vision. Recent work has shown how the MAP formulation can be extended to solving non-convex cost functions involving discontinuities and multiple constraints (Geman & Geman, 1984). An example below shows an application of the MAP approach to the non-linear reflectance estimation problem.

Markov Random Fields and energy functions

How can we find suitable priors or constraints, $p(\mathbf{s})$? One of the strengths of the statistical approach is in the programming, and ultimately, the testing of constraints. One would like to have modeling tools that extend the traditional smoothness constraints, such as spatial derivatives (e.g. Laplacian) or power spectrum descriptions. Markov Random Fields (MRFs) are a generalization of Markov Chains beyond one dimension, and include other discrete image characterizations (above) as special cases. Although we will not explore the potential here, MRFs are not restricted to second order statistical relations. The conditional probabilities of site values in a MRF depend only on a predefined neighborhood structure:

$$p(s_i|s_j, i \neq j) = p(s_i|s_j, j \subset N_i)$$
$$p(s_1, s_2, \ldots, s_n) > 0 \tag{12}$$

where N_i is the neighborhood of i. An example of a neighborhood would be the four nearest neighbors. (See Geman & Geman, 1984, for a general description of a neighborhood system). Although MRFs are not necessarily restricted to local neighborhoods, this is where they are especially convenient. There are several reasons why local MRF descriptions provide a useful language for characterizing spatial interactions in vision. One is that many of the low-level constraints in both images and scenes are fairly local; and even when they are not, data structures can be devised that express global constraints as pair-wise local ones at a coarse spatial scale. This can be used to form a hierarchical ordering of constraints useful for efficient computation. Another reason, as we will see below, is that local neighborhoods are well suited to multiple local computations in parallel. Although we cannot draw a literal comparison, neuronal computations are limited by the spatial spread of dendrites, which may account for the need for multiple cortical maps to deal with constraints over large regions of visual space (Barlow, 1986). Even when the region over which one brings together spatial information is large, the interactions between elements of the computed representation may still be local, but at a coarse topographic scale or on a non-topographic representation. This is analogous to a Hough transform for line detection (Duda & Hart, 1973). We will also see below how the MRF formalism is useful both for scene modeling, and for finding likely scenes causing the image. Although there are theoretical advantages to continuous formulations of surface costraints (Blake & Zisserman, 1987), Markov Random Fields provide a formalism to incorporate symbolic as well as metric information.

There are several problems with the Markov Random Field characterization as stated in (12). Although it is straightforward to calculate local conditional probabilities of a MRF from the global joint distribution (via Bayes' rule), it can be difficult to go the other way. Further, from a modeling point of view, it is not at all easy to guess appropriate local conditional probabilities based on observations of global samples. Fortunately, the MRF formulation is equivalent to a Gibbs distribution (Besag, 1972). That is, for a given neighborhood system, the random variable corresponding to **s**, is a MRF if and only if

$$p(\mathbf{s}) = \frac{1}{Z} e^{-U(\mathbf{s})/T} \qquad (13)$$

where $U(\mathbf{s})$ is a posterior or global energy function, T is the temperature, and Z is a normalizing constant. $U(\mathbf{s})$ is a sum of local potentials defined on *cliques*, where a clique is either a single site, or a subset of sites such that each member is a neighbor of the others. The local potentials embody prior knowledge or assumptions about scene properties. Maximizing probability is equivalent to minimizing energy. The temperature parameter is a useful tool for adjusting the width of the distribution. In conjunction with a sampling algorithm (see below), if the temperature is held constant, one can generate samples, if zero one can find local modes, and if gradually lowered, compressing the distribution improves the odds of finding a global model. The latter procedure is *simulated annealing*. These terms reflect the connections between statistical physics and parallel computation that have been exploited recently in a number of papers (Hopfield, 1982; Hinton & Sejnowski, 1983; Smolensky, 1986).

One consequence of the MRF–Gibbs equivalence is that the local conditional probabilities can be expressed in terms of local potential functions, for example

$$p(s_i \mid s_j, j \subset N_i) = \frac{1}{Z_i} e^{-1/T \sum_{j \subset N_i} \phi(s_i, s_j)} \qquad (14)$$

where $\phi(\cdot)$ is a local potential function defined over pair-wise cliques, and Z_i is the normalizing constant. The theory generalizes to more complex interactions; however, even nearest neighbor pair-wise interactions permit considerable flexibility. The linear constraint operator, **B** of (8) is just a special case corresponding to quadratic potentials.

Our problem is composed of two tasks: devise suitable local potentials corresponding to $p(\mathbf{s})$, and maximize the posterior distribution $p(\mathbf{s} \mid \mathbf{i})$. For both of these tasks, we can make use of Geman and Geman's *Gibbs Sampler*. First, the Gibbs Sampler provides a way of generating sample scenes from the local potentials which allows us to generate and verify our scene model. Second, because the posterior distribution, $p(\mathbf{s} \mid \mathbf{i})$ is itself a MRF, we can use simulated annealing to draw samples from the posterior distribution that get closer to the global mode as the temperature decreases.

In order to generate scene samples, a scene vector **s**' is initially set to some random set of values. Then for a given iteration, each site of **s**' is updated by sampling from the local conditional probability defined by (14). That is the values of the neighbors determine a 'hat' from which we draw the sample. In fact, the updating can be asynchronous, that is occur in any order. As the number of iterations gets large, the probability of **s**' approaches $p(\mathbf{s})$. Temperature is held fixed (e.g. at 1) throughout. Generating samples provides one way of exploring synthesis of natural scene properties based on local spatial constraints.

Given the scene and image formation model, how can we find the scene vector that maximizes the posterior probability? Because of MRF–Gibbs equivalence, we look for **s** that minimizes

$$U_P(\mathbf{s}) = (\mathbf{i} - \mathbf{As})^{\mathrm{T}}(\mathbf{i} - \mathbf{As})/2\sigma^2 + U(\mathbf{s}) \qquad (15)$$

for image formation with Gaussian noise. A direct search for the mode is computationally prohibitive for even small images. Further the posterior energy may, in general, have a rugged topography, precluding strict descent methods such as gradient or Hopfield descent for finding the global minimum. In order to reduce the likelihood of getting stuck in a local valley or pit, there are a number of tricks that are described below. The idea of an image formation constraint, the use of local potentials to model scene synthesis and algorithms for finding modes of the posterior probability are probably best illustrated in the context of a specific example.

Reflectance and illuminance estimation

The visual system seems to try to represent an object's surface properties in a way that is invariant to changes in the imaging environment. In particular, it is useful to represent surface material in such a way as to be invariant with respect to the illumination. This problem is difficult because it requires that the image intensity changes be parsed according to cause. Intensity changes can be due to: occlusion of one object by another, shape change, illumination change, and material reflectivity or texture change. The computation of 'intrinsic images' corresponding to the various scene causes of the image has been a problem of interest in computer vision for over a decade (Barrow & Tenenbaum, 1978). One problem is that the estimation of one cause, such as illumination, affects the estimation of another, say reflectance. One requires techniques that can cooperatively couple various estimates of these intrinsic images. The potential of MRFs can be illustrated with the example of reflectance estimation.

Of particular interest to us is the fact that human observers seem to be rather good at estimating material reflectance (the ratio of reflected to incident light) despite intensive, spatial and wavelength changes of the light falling on the surface. (Plummer & Kersten, 1988). In addition, the visual system also has some capacity to estimate illumination. To understand how well we estimate reflectance and illuminance involves investigating ideal observers for the task. This, in turn, means formulating and testing statistical models of natural reflectance, and image formation. Consider the following model for monocular achromatic image formation

$$L(x, y) = R(x, y)I[\mathbf{n}(x, y), \mathbf{v}(x, y), \mathbf{e}(x, y)] + \text{noise}(x, y) \tag{16}$$

where $L(x, y)$, $R(x, y)$, and I are luminance, reflectance and effective illumination, respectively. The effective illumination is a function of surface orientation $\mathbf{n}$, viewpoint $\mathbf{v}$, and illumination $\mathbf{e}$. Estimating R from L is the reflectance estimation problem. In general, this may require the simultaneous computation of the effective illuminance. This is an example of cooperative interaction between estimates of scene representations. Often, but not always, the discontinuities in $R(x, y)$ coincide with those due to changes in surface orientation; thus, reflectance and effective illumination are not necessarily independent and knowledge of one can augment the solution of the other. We will take a simpler approach in this example, and assume flat surfaces with an independent illumination.

To make the problem concrete, consider the following example made familiar by the work of Land (Land, 1983; Land & McCann, 1971). Imagine pieces of paper are cut from sheets of various reflectances, arranged on a flat surface and then illuminated, to produce an achromatic 'mondrian' (top three pictures of Fig. 3.2). As observers of natural images, we effortlessly take the image data $L(x, y)$ and make fairly

good judgments of the relative reflectance values $R(x, y)$. One manifestation of our ability to estimate reflectance is lightness constancy. Under certain conditions, we are quite insensitive to the illuminance change, which has led to some classical lightness illusions (cf. Cornsweet, 1970). Several models of lightness perception exist in the literature (see Hurlbert, 1986, for a review; Grossberg, 1983). However, illumination information is not necessarily discarded. Even when we do notice the difference in brightness, due to the illumination, and lightness constancy *per se* fails, we are still good at inferring the causes of the brightness differences. This ability probably involves both low- and high-level processing. We will attempt to construct a reflectance and illumination map from the image using simple constraints. Our ability to estimate such maps exists despite the fact that we have one equation and two unknowns per position. There are infinite combinations of reflectance and illumination which could give rise to one image. Additional constraints are needed.

In order to minimize the probability of error, the ideal observer's goal is to maximize the conditional probability of the estimated reflectance and illumination map conditional on the image data, L, available. This requires: that the solution is constrained by the image formation equation (2); and statistical models of what reflectances and illuminations are usually like.

Specifically, we require two scene models – one for reflectance and one for illumination. The estimates are then coupled via the image formation equation. Ideally, the probability of the simulated reflectance and illumination maps should match environmental probabilities. Although an exact match would, in general, require a complete theory of natural scenes, we can construct a 'toy world', in which our observer will be ideal. Further, the statistical assumptions used in this toy world are, in principle, verifiable. As more information becomes available, the scene model may be improved independent of modifications to the algorithm.

One characteristic of reflectances is that they are, to a first order approximation, piece-wise constant. That is, nearby reflectances tend to be similar unless they are different, in which case they are markedly different, that is, there are edges. Although we do occasionally have to cope with sharp shadows, illumination changes, especially due to extended sources, are usually smoother than reflectance changes. Thus, for the moment, assume that nearby illumination values tend to be alike, but usually do not have edges. Qualitatively, these constraints are the same as those used in all extant lightness algorithms.

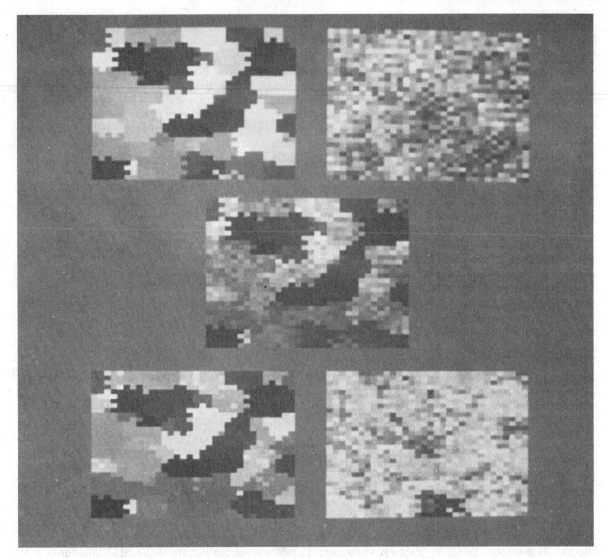

Fig. 3.2. The upper panels show Markov Random Field samples generated with a Gibbs Sampler at a constant temperature of 1 for the smoothed Ising potential (left), and a quadratic potential (right). The left and right panels are the results of models of piece-wise constant reflectances and smooth illuminations, respectively. The center panel is the image data, and is the product of the upper panels. It represents the image formation constraint that image intensities are the product of reflectance and illumination maps. The computational problem is, given the data in the center panel, factor the image into its original reflectance and illumination functions. The results of one simulation are shown in the two lower panels. The left and right panels are estimates of the original reflectance and illumination, respectively.

The above rules can be quantified in terms of local conditional probabilities defining a Markov Random Field. The reflectance model was chosen to have a 'smoothed Ising' potential function (Geman & McClure, 1985)

$$V_R(s_i, s_j) = \begin{cases} \dfrac{-\alpha}{1 + (s_i - s_j)^2/\beta} & \text{for } j \in N_i \\ 0 & \text{otherwise} \end{cases} \quad (17)$$

The conditional distribution for the illumination is similar except that the potential function is quadratic

$$V_I(s_i, s_j) = \begin{cases} (s_i - s_j)^2/\sigma & \text{for } j \in N_i \\ 0 & \text{otherwise} \end{cases} \quad (18)$$

The conditional probability of a site value, for both MRFs, depends only on the values of the eight nearest neighbors in neighborhood, N_i. The models of reflectance and illumination differ in how they weight differences between central and neighborhood pixels. This is represented by the local potentials, shown in Fig. 3.3. Abrupt changes are very unlikely for the illumination potential, but likely for the reflectance potential.

The top left panel in Fig. 3.2 shows a piece-wise constant quasi-sample generated by relaxation from this MRF process. (True samples are arrived at after an infinite number of iterations, and are in fact constant for this potential). The top right panel in Fig. 3.2 shows a quasi-sample for the illumination model produced by the quadratic local potential.

Recall that Bayes' rule says that we can maximize the probability of getting the right reflectance and illumination if we maximize the products of the probability of the image data conditional on the scene and the probability of the scene. Since the reflectance and illumination processes are independent, the joint probability of the reflectance and illumination maps is equal to their product:

$$p(\mathbf{R} \& \mathbf{I} \mid \mathbf{L}) = p(\mathbf{L} \mid \mathbf{R} \& \mathbf{I}) p(\mathbf{R} \& \mathbf{I}) / p(\mathbf{L}) \propto p(\mathbf{L} - \mathbf{RI}) p(\mathbf{R}) p(\mathbf{I})$$
$$(19)$$

A simulation was carried out as follows. Reflectance and illumination maps were generated using the Gibbs Sampler and the local characteristics given by the smoothed Ising and quadratic potentials with $T = 1$. The pictures consisted of 32×32 pixels with 32 levels for each pixel. The reflectance and illumination maps were multiplied together and a small amount of white Gaussian noise was added to produce the image. The reflectance and illumination maps were estimated using 300 iterations of simulated annealing,

going from a temperature of 4 to 0.49. In simulated annealing, temperature parameter, T in (13), is initially set high to expand the distribution. Then one iterates through the picture, generating samples from the local conditional posterior probability. The temperature is gradually lowered, thereby compressing the distribution function. The annealing process reduces the probability of getting stuck in local energy minima, by allowing for occasional energy increases, which, for example, gradient descent does not. Lowering the temperature lowers the likelihood of popping out of energy minima. However, for the conditions of this example simulation, there was very little change in energy after 20 iterations. Other simulations using the Gibbs Sampler at zero temperature indicate that this energy landscape is fairly smooth. During an iteration, L_i is measured, then each reflectance (R_i) and illumination pixel (I_i) was updated by drawing a sample from the local posterior distribution defined by:

$$p(R_i, I_i \mid L_i, R_j, I_j : j \in N_i) \qquad (20)$$
$$\propto \exp\left(-\frac{1}{T}\left\{\frac{(L_i - R_i I_i)^2}{2\sigma^2} + \sum_{j \in N_i} [V_I(I_i - I_j) + V_R(R_i - R_j)]\right\}\right)$$

Fig. 3.4 schematically represents the Gibbs Sampler algorithm for sampling from the posterior local characteristics.

The resulting reflectance and illumination estimates are shown in the bottom left and right panels of Fig. 3.2, respectively. Although the restored reflectance pattern does resemble the original, it is not perfect. This can be due to one of two possibilities. Either these results represent a local minimum, or the global minimum is the wrong answer, in which case the ideal estimator gives the wrong answer. When we know the right answer, we can actually check whether the minimum found is lower than the energy for the correct answer. The reflectance map shown does in fact constitute a lower minimum than the right answer. Confusing regions in the reflectance and illumination map is analogous to mistaking a patch of high reflectance for a spotlight or a black surface for a shadow. This natural illusion occurs occasionally in everyday viewing.

This example is meant to be an illustration of the philosophy behind a statistical approach to image understanding. To see practical results will require considerably more sophistication for both scene representation and modeling, image formation and algorithms. One possible extension to scene modeling is to construct MRFs with higher order neighborhoods to produce prescribed power spectra that may do a better job of modeling illumination gradients (Woods, 1976).

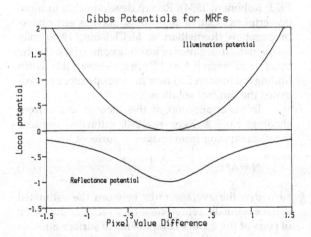

Fig. 3.3. The illumination and reflectance potentials are quadratic (equation 18) and smoothed Ising functions (equation 17), respectively.

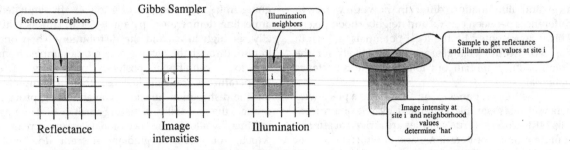

Fig. 3.4. The Gibbs Sampler measures the neighborhood values of the reflectances and illuminations corresponding to the ith site. The neighborhoods, in this case, are the eight nearest neighbors on a square lattice. (The neighborhood values are initially arbitrary). These measured neighborhood values, together with the image intensity data at site i determine a local conditional probability distribution represented by the hat. A sample consisting of reflectance and illumination values is drawn from the hat to replace the old values at site i. If simulated annealing is used, the distribution represented by the hat is gradually compressed by a temperature parameter, T, over the course of successive iterations.

To extend this approach to sharp shadows or transparency may require prior models of contours, as well as intensive processes, where the contour processes serve to break the neighborhood relations of the intensive processes (Geman & Geman, 1984). When line processes are introduced, the energy terrain can become very bumpy. One trick that seems to help is constraint relaxation, where the image formation constraint is tightened gradually. For simulated annealing, if T is lowered slowly enough, the scene will converge to the MAP estimate. In practice, 'slowly enough' is too slow. Depending on the problem, good results can often be obtained with relatively fast annealing schedules. An algorithm related to the Gibbs Sampler with annealing is the Boltzmann machine which uses the Metropolis sampling algorithm (Hinton & Sejnowski, 1983). The Metropolis algorithm is a special case of the Gibbs Sampler with relaxation, for binary valued pixels.

Sub-optimal linear models

So far, we have considered a formulation of the ideal observer independent of the algorithm or hardware. It is useful to consider suboptimal observers that are optimal except that they are constrained to compute an approximation in a particular way. For example, the energy topography, could be sculpted by a particular associative learning algorithm. The probabilistic model of scenes provides input/output pairs to use associative algorithms that can learn to estimate scene parameters from images (Kersten *et al.*, 1987; Hurlbert & Poggio, 1988; Lehky & Sejnowski, 1988; Knill & Kersten, 1990). This becomes particularly

interesting when it is difficult to compute the posterior distribution, and we have a complete description of the prior distribution and the image formation model. We may not be able to directly address the optimality of the learning algorithm, but we may find out whether a given architecture is capable of computing the desired map to within some desired degree of accuracy. For example, suppose **A** and **B** in equation (8) are linear, but unknown. Then, the generalized inverse of **A**, $\mathbf{A}^\star$, is the matrix (in general, rectangular) mapping **i** to **s**, which minimizes the squared error over the set of training pairs $\mathbf{s}_k$, $\mathbf{i}_k$. With training, this approaches the MAP estimate when **A** is linear and the prior distribution and noise are Gaussian. $\mathbf{A}^\star$ can be estimated by associative learning over the training set using Widrow–Hoff error correction. (Duda & Hart, 1973; Kohonen, 1984). Recent developments in more powerful associative algorithms, such as error back-propagation (Rumelhart & McClelland, 1986) may broaden the usefulness of learning constraints. On the other hand, even if **A** and **B** are non-linear, it is worth finding out how well a linear inverse operator approximates the optimal solution.

In an application of this idea to shape from shading, Knill & Kersten (1990) estimated pseudo-inverse mapping from images to surfaces

$$\mathbf{N} = \mathbf{A}^\star \mathbf{L}, \tag{21}$$

such that the average error between the estimated surface normals, represented by a vector **N** (made up of pairs of the x and y components of surface normals at each spatial location), and the real surfaces was minimized. The image formation constraint was based on a Lambertian model, with a known point source illumination, and assumed constant reflectance

$$L(x,y) \propto \mathbf{n} \cdot \mathbf{e} \qquad (22)$$

(see equation 16). Rather than image intensities, luminance at each point, normalized by the average value, was used as image data. When the imaging function is linear and the distribution of $\mathbf{N}$ is Gaussian, the optimal mapping is linear. For shape from shading, neither of these conditions holds. A linear mapping may, however, be near optimal. If the sample surfaces are randomly drawn from the prior distribution, $p(\mathbf{N})$; span its space, and the images are calculated using the Lambertian image formation function, the derived mapping is the best linear estimate of the mean of $p(\mathbf{N}|\mathbf{L})$. The actual form of the distribution need not be known, as it is implicitly defined by the set of sample surfaces. An optimal mapping for a particular space of surfaces may thus be learned through appropriate selection of samples.

Given pairs of sample surfaces and images, the Widrow–Hoff algorithm was used to derive a linear mapping between them which minimizes the mean squared error between estimated and real surfaces

$$\mathbf{A}_{k+1}^{\star} = \mathbf{A}_k^{\star} + \varrho(\mathbf{N}_k - \mathbf{A}_k^{\star}\mathbf{L}_k)\mathbf{L}_k^{\mathsf{T}}. \qquad (23)$$

where $\mathbf{A}^{\star}$ is the mapping being learned. The term in parentheses is the error between estimated and actual values of $\mathbf{N}_k$. Iterative application of this rule to example vectors, $\mathbf{N}_k$ and $\mathbf{L}_k$, *with appropriate relaxation of the learning constant*, ϱ, (typically $1/k$) will result in a convergence of $\mathbf{A}^{\star}$ to the desired mapping.

One could either use examples of real surfaces as the training set, or draw them from a statistical model of surfaces. The latter approach avoids the data collection problems of using real surfaces, and has the advantage of providing a tool for analyzing the performance of the shape from shading estimator. Because of the potential usefulness of fractal models to describe surfaces (Pentland, 1986), a statistical fractal model was used to generate surfaces for the training set. If the surface statistics are assumed to be spatially invariant, the linear estimators of surface normal in the x and y directions are just convolution filters as applied to the normalized luminance values of the image. The filters learned were spatially oriented bandpass filters. Fig. 3.5 shows results of an original and reconstructed surface. In general, simulations showed that the linear approximation worked well for a wide range of surfaces, including non-fractals.

Discussion

The ideal image understander that has been presented is a MAP estimator. If the scene constraints can be modeled as a Markov Random Field, then the ideal image understander is embodied by an energy function. Of course, having an energy function is just a start, because, in general, it can be very difficult to locate global minima. Many of the current popular neural network algorithms can be interpreted as MAP estimators of various sorts (Golden, 1988). Neural models, such as Hopfield nets which use strict descent, can settle at local minima. This raises an interesting perceptual issue. Introducing the ideal or MAP observers makes it clear that there are two ways of making perceptual mistakes. Some mistakes, or illusions, may not be due to non-optimal biological algorithms or hardware. The MAP observer may get the wrong answer too. That is, there may be illusions which never go away, no matter how smart we become, or how well our robots can understand images when optimally matched to the uncertainties of the environment. On the other hand, local minima may be the reason for human mistakes. In principal, the ideal observer provides a baseline by telling us how probable local minima are relative to ideal, for a given energy landscape. What makes these kinds of comparisons difficult in practice, is that they depend on the representation used to describe the environment our brain is trying to model. Further, accurate modeling of the statistics of scene morphology may be an unrealistic goal. This is where both neurophysiology and psychophysics may be useful in developing insights into the nature of perceptual approximations to scene representations.

The statistical approach suggests a change of emphasis. When modeling complex perceptual tasks, we often place our attention on finding an algorithm that will at least work and account for the data. One problem is that at a certain level of detail, there may be too many possible models that give the same input/output relations. The probabilistic approach emphasizes research into statistical models of image formation and scene synthesis. Although heuristics were used to derive the MRF models in the examples above, the scene models are testable, independent of the algorithm. This is analogous to the modeling of image statistics via measurements of the autocorrelation function for natural images with a view to arriving at an explanation for lateral inhibition (Srinivasan *et al.*, 1982).

Understanding our perceptual representations of scene properties involves understanding both

42   D. Kersten

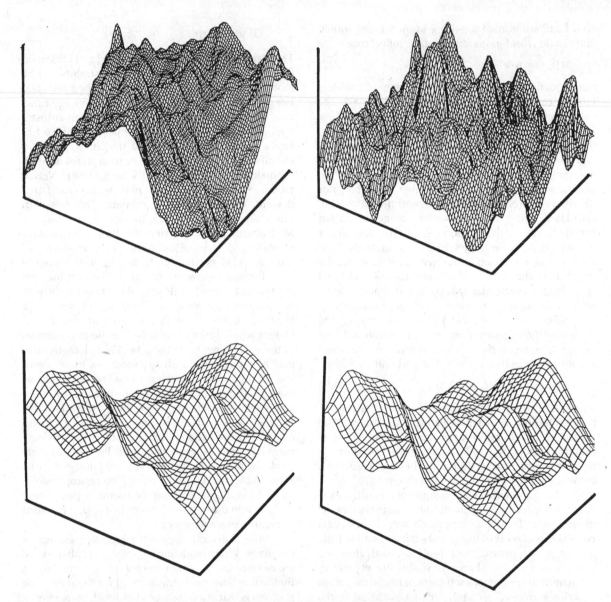

Fig. 3.5. The upper and lower left panels show original fractal surface height as a function of $x - y$ position. The upper left panel represents a surface with a higher fractal dimension than the lower left one. The upper and lower right panels show reconstructions computed from the image intensities of the surfaces on the left. These reconstructions are calculated from a linear suboptimal Bayesian shape-from-shading estimator. The estimates are computed using convolution filters that operate on the normalized luminance values to find the x and y components of the surface normal at each point. The reconstructions do a good job of capturing topographic features, such as hills and valleys; however, the fact that low spatial frequency information in the surface depths is lost, can be seen by comparing the upper left and right plots.

scenes and their biological homologues (Fig. 3.1). Thus, there are really two models of scene representation to consider. One is determined by natural optics and scene morphology. To model adequately the ideal

observer in this world may be an unrealistic goal. We can treat biological perceptual systems as suboptimal adaptations to this environment. The degree of optimality are determined by factors having less to do with informational limits, but rather with other factors such as biological hardware, phylogenetic history, and motor requirements. But, we can also consider our own perceptual model of scenes. Our perceptual model could be defined as being isomorphic to that synthetic environment in which we are optimal observers for a given task. Our long range goal would be to model this environment. We will not have completely understood vision until we can account for both ecological scene constraints, their perceptual relations, and the optimality of the relation between the two.

Acknowledgements

This work was supported by the National Science Foundation under grant NSF BNS 87-8532 and BSRG PHS2 S07 RR07085 and has benefited considerably from discussions with David Knill and Richard Golden.

References

Barlow, H. B. (1962) A method of determining the overall quantum efficiency of visual discriminations. *J. Physiol.*, **160**, 155–68.

Barlow H. B. (1977) Retinal and central factors in human vision limited by noise. In *Photoreception in Vertebrates*. ed. H. B. Barlow & P. Fatt. New York: Academic Press.

Barlow H. B. (1986) Why have multiple cortical areas? *Vision Res.*, **26**, 81–90.

Barlow H. B. & Reeves B. C. (1979) The versatility and absolute efficiency of detecting mirror symmetry in random dot displays. *Vision Res.*, **19**, 783–93.

Barrow H. G. & Tenenbaum, J. M. (1978) Recovering intrinsic scene characteristics from images. In *Computer Vision Systems*, ed. A. R. Hanson & E. M. Riseman, New York: Academic Press.

Besag J. (1972) Spatial interaction and the statistical analysis of lattice systems. *J. Royal Stat. Soc.* **B**, **34**, 75–83.

Blake A. & Zisserman A. (1987) *Visual Reconstruction*. Cambridge, Mass: The MIT Press.

Bolle R. M. & Cooper, D. B. (1984) Bayesian recognition of local 3-D shape by approximating image intensity functions with quadric polynomials. *IEEE Trans. Patt. Anal. and Machine Intell.*, **PAMI-6**, 418–29.

Burgess A. E., Wagner R. F., Jennings R. J., & Barlow, H. B. (1981) Efficiency of human visual signal discrimination. *Science*, **214**, 93–4.

Cornsweet, T. N. (1970) *Visual Perception*. New York: Academic Press.

Cox, R. T. (1946) Probability, frequency and reasonable expectation. *American Journal of Physics*, **14**, 1–13.

Duda, R. O. & Hart, P. E. (1973) *Pattern Classification and Scene Analysis*. New York: John Wiley & Sons.

Foley J. D. & Van Dam A. (1982) *Fundamentals of Interactive Computer Graphics*. Reading, Mass: Addison-Wesley.

Fournier, A., Fussell, D., & Carpenter L. (1982) Computer rendering of stochastic models. *Graphics and Image Processing*, **25**, 371–84.

Frieden, B. R. (1983) Unified theory for estimating frequency-of-occurrence laws and optical objects. *J. Opt. Soc. Am.*, **73**, 927–38.

Geisler, W. S. (1984) Physical limits of acuity and hyperacuity. *J. Opt. Soc. Am. A*, **1**, 775–82.

Geman, S., & Geman, D. (1984) Stochastic relaxation, Gibbs distributions, and the Bayesian restoration of images. *Trans. Patt. Anal. and Machine Intell.*, **PAMI-6**, 721–41.

Geman, S. & McClure, D. E. (1985) Bayesian image analysis: an application to single photon emission tomography. *Stat. Comp. Sect., Proc. Am. Stat. Assoc.*, 12–18.

Golden R. (1988) A unified framework for connectionist systems. *Biol. Cybern.*, **59**, 109–20.

Grossberg, S. (1983) The quantized geometry of visual space: the coherent computation of depth, form, and lightness. *Behavioral and Brain Sciences*, **6**, 625–92.

Hildreth, E. C. (1983) *The Measurement of Visual Motion*. Cambridge, Mass: M.I.T. Press.

Hinton, G. E. & Sejnowski, T. J. (1983) Optimal perceptual inference. In *Proceedings IEEE Conference in Computational Vision and Pattern Recognition*.

Hopfield, J. J. (1982) Neural networks and physical systems with emergent collective computational abilities. *Proc. Natl. Acad. Sci. USA*, **79**, 2554–8.

Hurlbert A. (1986) Formal connections between lightness algorithms. *J. Opt. Soc. Am. A*, **3**, 1684–93

Hurlbert, A. C. & Poggio, T. A. (1988) Synthesizing a color algorithm from examples. *Science*, **239**, 482–5.

Kersten, D. (1984) Spatial summation in visual noise. *Vision Res.*, **24**, 1977–90.

Kersten, D., O'Toole A., Sereno, M., Knill D., & Anderson, J. A., (1987) Associative learning of scene parameters from images. *Applied Optics*, **26**, 4999–5006.

Knill D. C. & Kersten D. (1990) Learning a near-optimal estimator for surface shape from shading. *Computer Vision, Graphics and Image Processing*, **50**, 75–100.

Koch, C., Marroquin, J., & Yuille, A. (1986) Analog 'neuronal' networks in early vision. *Proc. Natl. Acad. Sci. USA*, **83**, 4263–7.

Kohonen, T. (1984) *Self-Organization and Associative Memory*. Berlin, New York: Springer-Verlag.

Land, E. H. (1983) Recent advances in retinex theory and some implications for cortical computations: color vision and the natural image. *Proc. Natl. Acad. Sci. USA*, **80**, 5163–9.

Land E. H. & McCann J. J. (1971) Lightness and retinex theory. *J. Opt. Soc. Am.*, **61**, 1–11.

Legge G. E., Gu, Y. & Luebker, A. (1989) Efficiency of graphical perception. *Perception and psychophysics*, **46**, 365–74.

Lehky, S. R. & Sejnowski, T. J. (1988) Network model of shape from shading: neural function arises from both receptive and projective fields. *Nature*, **333**, 452–4.

Magnenat-Thalmann, N. & Thalmann, D. (1987) *Image Synthesis: Theory and Practice*. Tokyo: Springer-Verlag.

Mandelbrot, B. B. (1977) *Fractals: Form, Chance and Dimension*. San Francisco: W. H. Freeman and Company.

Marr, D. (1982) *Vision*. San Francisco: W. H. Freeman and Company.

Marroquin J. L. (1985) *Probabilistic Solution of Inverse Problems*. M.I.T. Tech. Rep. 860.

Pentland A. (1986) Shading into texture. *Artificial Intelligence*, **29**, 147–70.

Plummer D. J. & Kersten D. (1988) Estimating reflectance in the presence of shadows and transparent overlays. Annual meeting of the Optical Society of America, November.

Poggio, T., Torre V., & Koch C. (1985) Computational vision and regularization theory. *Nature*, **317**, 314–19.

Poggio T., Gamble E. B., & Little J. J. (1988) Parallel integration of vision modules. *Science*, **242**, 436–40.

Rose A. (1948) The sensitivity performance of the human eye on an absolute scale. *J. Opt. Soc. Am.*, **38**, 196–208.

Rumelhart, D. E., McClelland, J. L. & the PDP Research Group (1986) *Parallel Distributed Processing*. Cambridge, Mass: MIT Press.

Smolensky, P. (1986) Information processing in dynamical systems: foundations of harmony theory. Chapter 6 in Rumelhart *et al.* (1986).

Srinivasan, M. V., Laughlin, S. B. & Dubs, A. (1982) Predictive coding: a fresh view of inhibition in the retina. *Proc. Roy. Soc. Lond.*, **B216**, 427–59.

van Trees H. L. (1968) *Detection, Estimation and Modulation Theory*, Vol. I. New York: John Wiley & Sons.

Watson A. B., Barlow H. B. & Robson J. G. (1983) What does the eye see best? *Nature*, **31**, 419–22.

Woods J. W. (1976) Two-dimensional Markov spectral estimation. *IEEE Trans. Info. Theory*, **IT–22**, 552–9.

4
The theory of comparative eye design

A. W. Snyder, T. J. Bossomaier and A. A. Hughes

Introduction

Perhaps the most fascinating and yet provocative aspect of vision is the manner in which eyes adapt to their environment. There is no single optimum eye design as physicists might like, but rather a variety of different solutions each dictated by the animals lifestyle, e.g. the 'Four-eyed fish', *Anableps anableps*, with one pair of aerial pupils and a second pair of aquatic pupils (Walls, 1942). This unique fish, which patrols the water surface, dramatizes the extreme plasticity of optics in adapting to a particular subset of the environment. The animal's life style within an environment obviously shapes many properties of the retina such as the distribution and types of rods, cones and ganglion cells (Walls, 1942; Hughes, 1977; Lythgoe, 1979). Furthermore, it is probable that the grand strategy of early visual information processing is also an adaptation to the particular world in which we live, i.e. a world of objects rather than the infinitely unexpected. We develop this perspective after considering the optical design of eyes.

Our first objective here is to show that elementary ideas of physics and information sciences can give insight into eye design. In doing so we stress the comparative approach. Only by studying diverse eyes, of both the simple and compound variety can we appreciate the common design principles necessary to apply meaningfully concepts from physics to biology. Accordingly, we try to explain observations such as: (a) the optical image quality is often superior to the photoreceptor grain; (b) the resolving power of falconiforms and dragonflies is proportional to their head size; (c) the cone outer segment diameter of diverse hawks that differ enormously in head size is fixed at about $2\,\mu m$; (d) cone mosaics (and probably associated neural arrays) are nearly crystalline in foveas but highly disordered in deep sea fish and undergrowth dwellers like cockroaches; (e) many photoreceptors function as optical waveguides; (f) the photosensitive membrane is organized differently in different classes of photoreceptor.

Before commencing, we single out Barlow's 1964 paper on the physical limits of visual discrimination and his follow up 20 years later (Barlow, 1986) as striking examples of how elementary ideas of physics can lead to a rich insight into visual biology.

Interrelation of optical image quality and the retinal grain

The classical approach to answering how the optical image is matched to the retinal grain is to take the optical image quality as a 'given' and assume that the retinal grain adjusts itself accordingly. Ignoring noise, the solution is to sample at each node and antinode of the highest spatial frequency ν_0 passed by the optics where, for a circular pupil,

$$\nu = D/\lambda, \tag{1}$$

with D the minimum pupil diameter in bright light (when considering diural photoreceptors) and λ the wavelength of light in vacuum. Taking $\Delta\phi$ to be the angular spacing between sampling centres, then $\Delta\phi = \lambda/2D$ for a square lattice (Nyquist, 1924), while for a hexagonal lattice (Snyder & Miller, 1977)

$$\Delta\phi = \lambda/D\sqrt{3} \tag{2}$$

which corresponds to 19 samples within an Airy disc

(rev. Snyder, Bossomaier & Hughes, 1987). Animals with both compound and simple eyes that are active in brilliant sunlight and that are nearly stationary relative to their specific prey come close to satisfying this condition (Horridge, 1977; Wehner, 1981; Miller, 1977). *However, such eyes are the exception! Outside of foveas and throughout the entire region of eyes without foveas, the retina undersamples the optical image.* By modifying the sampling spacing to account for photon noise in dim conditions (Snyder, Laughlin & Stavenga, 1977) and in the presence of relative motion (Snyder, 1977), it was concluded that the grain should be more coarse (rev. Snyder, 1979). Numerous compound eyes fit this description (Horridge, 1977; Wehner, 1981).

In the above analysis we assume that the retinal grain must be matched to a given optical image. While this is plausible for compound eyes, because of intimate relation between the facets and the rhabdomeric photoreceptors, it is unlikely for simple eyes as discussed below.

Matching the optics to the retinal grain in simple eyes

It is clear from comparative surveys that the biological life style sets the retinal grain of simple eyes (Walls, 1942; Duke-Elder, 1958; Hughes, 1977), while it is the optical image quality that is moulded to this grain. Indeed, the 6 mm pupil of a human sized falcon eye is more nearly diffraction limited (Shlaer, 1972) than our eyes at 2 mm (Campbell & Gubisch, 1966). Thus the classical aberrations need not pose a problem. This is just one of numerous examples showing that the optical image quality is highly adaptive.

Accepting that the optical image quality is the flexible element, then how should it be moulded to the retinal grain? If it were not for noise, the optimum solution is to have the optics matched to the retinal grain as expressed by eq. (2). While improving the image quality beyond matched conditions sharpens the point spread function, this leads to interpolation errors or 'blind' spots in a mixed retina of rods and cones – both of which are manifestations of aliasing in the spatial frequency domain. However, in the presence of noise, improving the optical image quality beyond that of the matched condition leads to enhanced contrast sensitivity but at the cost of the aliasing errors discussed above. Thus, the most suitable optical image quality is determined by a tradeoff between the advantage of increased contrast sensitivity on one hand, weighed against the disadvantage of errors due to aliasing on the other hand.

Snyder, Bossomaier & Hughes (1986) used information theory to determine the best optical image for a given retinal grain in bright daylight. The theory finds the maximum number of different pictures a cone array can produce assuming a hypothetical object world composed of a grain equal to that of the photoreceptor matrix, i.e. finding the maximum number of pictures at the animals subjective resolution (rev. Snyder, Bossomaier & Hughes, 1988; Bossomaier & Snyder, 1986).

Information theory suggests that eyes should undersample by about 50% as shown by the solid curve of Fig. 4.1. The results are consistent with data for the rat, cat and snake as compiled from source material by Snyder, Bossomaier & Hughes (1986) but not the human fovea. However, the analysis assumes an achromatic retina and an integration time set by cones, whereas the human fovea is dichromatic with the capacity for a protracted fixation time. Optimizing the optics for either of these capabilities decreases the amount of undersampling. Of course, it also remains possible that foveas are designed according to a criterion different from information, e.g. threshold detection of the highest resolvable frequency, $\nu = \nu_s$, leading to the broken curve of Fig. 4.1.

The garter snake provides the most direct test of the theory in an all-cone retinal region. First, it is a retina of nearly uniform density, so that the same considerations apply approximately at all retinal positions. More important, the snake pupil is about half the diameter of man's pupil in bright light, yet image quality is only about one-tenth as good (Land & Snyder, 1985). In other words, there is no pressure for diffraction-limited optics in this snake. Nevertheless, the optical image quality is about three times better than that required to match the cone mosaic. This strategy is consistent with the theory presented here.

Barlow (1979) has suggested that hyperacuity implies interpolation by the visual pathways whereby the cortex has a finer grain than the retina. If this were true, then hyperacuity would decline with increased undersampling (Snyder, 1982) basically because of the comparative 'blind spots' discussed above. However, when the noise is sufficiently large, undersampling is again advantageous (Bossomaier, Snyder & Hughes, 1985).

Prediction that the individual cones are visible through the natural pupil

If the retinal cones undersample the optical image by a sufficient amount, then it should be possible to view individual cones directly through the natural optics of

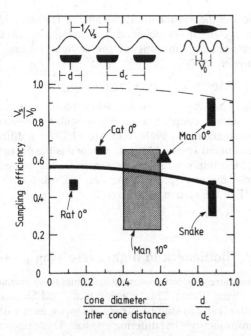

Fig. 4.1. Theoretical optimum sampling efficiency (unbroken curve) derived from information theory compared with the biological data in Snyder, Bossomaier & Hughes (1986). The figure assumes that cone inner segments are equal in diameter, that is, small values of d/d_c result from a high rod and cone density. The dashed curve gives the minimum optical image quality to detect a grating of frequency v_s.

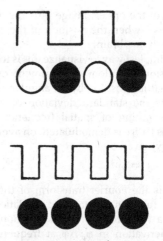

Fig. 4.2. The highest frequency that the cone mosaic can resolve is half that of the mosaic itself (above). To observe the cone mosaic, however, requires that the eye's cut-off frequency must be greater than the cone mosaic frequency, or the cones and spaces will not be resolved (below).

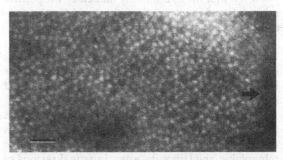

Fig. 4.3. Ophthalmoscopic appearance of the retina of garter snake just beyond the optic disc (dark circular sector indicated by arrow on right). The scale on this photograph represents 1°. This photograph was developed to a medium contrast and printed on normal (grade 2) paper to preserve the contrast of the original image.

the eye. For this condition, the optics need to be at least twice as good as when matched (i.e. the cones must undersample by at least 50%) so that each cone is, say, at a minimum while the intervening space between the cones is at a maximum of the grating intensity (Fig. 4.2). Following this logic, Land & Snyder (1985) clearly viewed the cone mosaic of a live garter snake using a standard hand held ophthalmoscope. Indeed, Fig. 4.3 provided the first definitive cone map in a vertebrate eye. Subsequently, similar results were found in the frog (Jagger, 1985) but the frog does not exhibit the same clarity as the garter snake. The near perfect clarity of the cone mosaic though a standard hand-held opthalmoscope suggests that the optical image quality of the garter snake is greatly superior to its retinal grain i.e. in excess of about 4 c/deg. Using a double pass technique, Land & Snyder (1985) found that the MTF was about 35% at the highest spatial frequency (2.1 c/deg) that can be unambiguously resolved by the cone matrix which is consistent with the required image quality.

Necessity for regular sampling mosaics

The sampling lattice is nearly crystalline in the 'foveal' regions of animals that rely primarily on vision (Engström, 1963; Horridge, 1977; Miller, 1977), whereas significant disorder exists in nocturnal types, e.g. bottom dwelling fish (Engström, 1963).

An explanation for this phenomena was first advanced by French, Snyder & Stavenga, (1977) who showed that disorder is equivalent to a deterioration in the quality of the optical image plus the addition of random noise, when the position of the samplers is not known by the brain.

The simplest way to visualize this is to consider a one-dimensional random displacement of samplers from their lattice position by an angular amount ϕ_p, where ϕ_p is the standard deviation of a Gaussian process. A grating of spatial frequency ν viewed through this lattice is demodulated, on average, by an amount $M(\nu)$ given by

$$M(\nu) = e^{-2(\pi\phi_p\nu)^2} \tag{3}$$

where M^2 is the Fourier transform of the Gaussian probability function of standard deviation ϕ_p, e.g. leading to a 10% reduction in modulation for a 10% standard derivation in $\phi_p/\Delta\phi$ at frequency $\nu = \nu_s = 1/\Delta\phi\sqrt{2}$, with $\Delta\phi$ the centre to centre sampler spacing and ν_s the maximum frequency resolved by the one-dimensional array. This result shows clearly that disorder has the same effect as optical blur and holds whether or not the brain is aware of the precise position of the samplers. Thus, were it not for photoreceptor noise, ultimately limited by the particle nature of light, exact reconstruction would be theoretically possible as it is also in the presence of optical blur.

If the brain is *unaware of the precise position of the samplers*, then white noise of amplitude $[1 - M^2(\nu)]^{1/2}$ is distributed over all spatial frequencies, i.e. all power lost in the demodulation of eq. (3) is redistributed uniformly into a broad band of spatial frequencies.

Presumably the existence of a slight randomness in the lattice of cones (Hirsch & Hilton, 1984) is unintentional, so that there is significant pressure for minimizing any lattice disorder. In retinal regions of high convergence, it remains possible to have slight disorder at the cone level with comparative regularity of receptive fields.

Lastly, we note that both hexagonal as well as square lattices exist. While hexagonal lattices minimize the number of cones per unit area, the logic for square arrays is not immediately apparent. Perhaps it is a strategy for having equal coverage of spectral types, consistent with that of certain fish (Lythgoe, 1979).

Point spread function

Armed with the above result for cone disorder, we have a simple description of the on-average point spread function, PS, of the optical system given by

$$PS \simeq e^{-2.77(\phi/\Delta\varrho)^2} \tag{4}$$

within the Gaussian approximation (rev. Snyder, 1979) where the PS function is normalized to unity at maximum, ϕ is the angular displacement and $\Delta\varrho$ is the width of the PS function at half height. The half width parameter $\Delta\varrho$ is obtained by convolving all the characteristic functions of the system leading to (Snyder, 1977)

$$(\Delta\varrho)^2 = \Delta\varrho_o^2 + \Delta\varrho_r^2 + (\Delta\varrho_i)^2 + (\Delta\varrho_m)^2 \dots \tag{5}$$

where $\Delta\varrho_o$, $\Delta\varrho_s$, $\Delta\varrho_i$ and $\Delta\varrho_m$ are the blurring effects of the optics, sampling aperture, irregular matrix and movement respectively, e.g. $\Delta\varrho_o = \lambda/D$ for a diffraction limited system, $\Delta\varrho_r \simeq d/f$ where d is the diameter of the sampling capture region and f the posterior nodal distance (pnd) of the eye, $\Delta\varrho_i = 3\pi\phi_p/4$. The MTF of the system M is given as

$$M \simeq e^{-3.56(\nu\Delta\varrho)^2} \tag{6}$$

Bottleneck to higher resolving power

It is interesting to investigate the limits to an animal's resolving power. This question motivated Snyder & Miller (1977) to study a variety of hawks, each with a similar life style but differing eye size. These birds are assumed to have the greatest pressure for high resolving power on one hand but with the constraint of economy of eye size (weight) on the other hand.

In birds we expect the highest resolving power for a given eye size of length L. Now, resolving power, RP, is proportional to pupil diameter, D, and also the grain of the cone matrix, of angular extent L/d, where d is the cone centre to centre spacing. Thus,

$$RP \propto D \propto L/d \tag{7}$$

For a fixed eye length L, the RP can be increased by simultaneously increasing the pupil D and decreasing the cone separation d. Snyder & Miller (1977) found two interesting results in hawks: firstly, the centre to centre cone spacing within the deep fovea of all hawks was about 1.9 μm, based both on fresh and fixed preparations done also in parallel with similar preparations of man and monkey to insure proper normalization. This first result would appear to imply that 1.9 μm in hawk represents some fundamental limit (discussed below) because the bird eye could be made significantly shorter and hence lighter by simply decreasing the cone spacing instead of extending the length of the eye. This disadvantage could partly be compensated for by the fact that the deep foveal pit acts as the negative element in a telephoto lens system to optically extend the eye (Snyder & Miller, 1977; Williams & McIntyre, 1980; Barlow, 1981). The second finding of Snyder & Miller (1977) was that the bright light pupil diameter scaled with head size – a design consistent with a diffraction limited eye as dictated by eq. (7). This is in sharp contrast to Barlow's (1961) prediction that hawk pupils scale proportional to $\sqrt{D}$ due to the limitations of chromatic aberrations (see Barlow, 1986). Perhaps the oil droplets narrow the spectral content of light, thus mitigating such aberrations.

Photoreceptor optics

The optical properties of photoreceptors, e.g. arrangement, orientation, shape, size, refractive index and membrane properties, influence absorption and establish many specialized functions (Snyder and Menzel, 1975; Van Hateren, 1985), e.g. directional sensitivity to the Stiles–Crawford effect (Snyder & Pask, 1973). Rhabdomeric photoreceptors, in particular, display the richness of possibilities as is discussed elsewhere (Snyder & Menzel, 1975; Snyder, 1979). Furthermore, photoreceptor optics are closely related to the study of optical waveguides, the theory of which is now well developed (Snyder & Love, 1983). Here we consider several general questions.

Why photoreceptors function as light guides
Because photoreceptors are composed of membrane material they are more dense than the sounding medium and can contain light by total internal reflection. While the situation offers the potential for improved optical isolation from neighbouring photoreceptors, it would nonetheless appear that the main advantage of light guiding is economy of photopigment for a given photon capture (Snyder & Laughlin, 1975). This, for example, is consistent with the conical shape of cone outer segments. Thus, waveguide effects are probably a by-product of an attempt to minimize the volume of photopigment (Snyder, 1979). To illustrate this concept, consider the maximum length photoreceptors (outer segments) can be if they are pressed together in a continuous sheet. They cannot be too long or else the contrast sensitivity is reduced by defocus. We have examined this question by using an electromagnetic analysis of absorption, but the results are clearly seen by the classical Rayleigh expression for tolerance to defocus. This predicts a maximum outer segment length l_{os} of

$$l_{os} = \frac{8\lambda}{\pi}\left(\frac{f}{D}\right)^2 \tag{8}$$

where f is the pnd of the eye. Thus, the outer segment length depends on the F-number, f/D, of the eye. All eyes within one strategy that are scaled according to this size, e.g. hawks, should have cone outer segments of equal length, whereas different strategies, like man and falcon, have different lengths, l_{os}. This

argument is best tested in animals with foveas where the cones are narrow and thus forced to be comparatively long for enhanced light capture. Taking $\lambda = 550$ nm and the pupil diameter D in bright light, gives $l_{os} = 65 \,\mu m$ for the human outer segments and $34 \,\mu m$ for the outer segments of a falcon with a man sized eye which is a reasonable approximation to the measured values of $40 \,\mu m$ and $25 \,\mu m$ respectively (Snyder & Miller, 1977; Miller, 1977). The theory is in even better agreement for the very short cone outer segments of garter snake. In other words, light guiding is unnecessary for preventing defocus in the bright light (when D is small).

Limitation of diffraction to absorption
Finally, we note that outer segments become inefficient absorbers below a certain diameter because of diffraction effects. The fraction η of light propagating within the narrow inner segments is given by (Snyder & Love, 1983, p. 341)

$$\eta \simeq 1 - 1/V^2 \tag{9}$$

(for $V \geqslant 1$), where $V = \pi d (n^2 - n_s^2)^{1/2}/\lambda$, with n, n_s the refractive index of the outer segment and surround respectively and d is the outer segment diameter. Unfortunately, V is highly sensitive to the difference $n - n_s$ in refractive index and this difference is difficult to measure. Kirschfeld & Snyder (1976) circumvented this difficulty by measuring the effect of mode propagation on birefringence in the rhabdomers of the fly *Musca* and found that the fly rhabdomere 1–6, of diameter about $2 \,\mu m$, had $V \approx 2.3$ at $\lambda \approx 5.50$ nm corresponding to 80% light flow within the photoreceptor. Because of the extreme sensitivity of V to the difference in refractive index $\eta - \eta_s$, each photoreceptor must be evaluated on an individual basis to determine V and hence η of eq. (9).

Light loss due to diffraction is minimized in outer segments with a circular cross section (Snyder & Zheng, 1986). Diffraction also causes optical coupling between photoreceptors that are physically separated (Snyder, 1972; Snyder & Menzel, 1975).

In summary, the macroscopic shape and optical properties of photoreceptors are consistent with economy of photopigment for a given light capture, while the photoreceptor length is approximately the maximum tolerable for defocus in bright light (smallest pupil) based on a thin sheet of photopigment.

Photoreceptive membrane

We have been discussing the macroscopic properties of the photoreceptor. However, the arrangement of photoreceptor membrane determines the light capture and polarization sensitivity of the photoreceptor and physical principles lead to insight here also: Snyder & Laughlin (1975) found that the absorbing dipoles are oriented in the membrane to provide photoreceptors with the maximum absorption to *unpolarized* light in all animals including those that rely on polarized light detection. Furthermore, Kirschfeld & Snyder (1975) found that the microvillus membrane of *Musca* is significantly more crystalline than the membrane of pig outer segments (Liebman & Entise, 1974).

Technological insights inspired by visual systems

While we have emphasized how the concepts of physics and information sciences provide insight into comparative eye design, we should be aware also that the applied sciences have borrowed ideas from animal eyes, e.g. 'polarizing' fibres for various optical devices (Fig. 4.4 and Snyder & Ruhl, 1983) and no doubt strategies for robotic and machine vision from the neural principles of the visual pathways (Marr, 1980).

A unifying perspective of visual processing

In conclusion it is tempting to speculate on the more macroscopic aspects of design, e.g. on the strategy of early visual information processing. We begin with some general observations to gain perspective.

The notion that eye design can be anticipated by compiling comprehensive data of the visual environment is obviously wrong. Comparative surveys show, e.g. that even eye position, as well as retinal and neural topography are highly variant among those animals that share the same habitat. Examples are numerous, many discussed in Hughes (1977). Clearly, it is the life style of an animal within a particular visual environment and not its habitat that sets these design parameters. On the other hand, the neural architecture is roughly invariant among diverse animals, i.e. they have similar anatomical packaging and similar physiology with the possibility that only the proportion of cells and unit classes vary among animals. Thus, it would appear that animals want essentially the same thing from the visual environment, but the degree and scale with which it is wanted varies. One universality in common with virtually all animals is their need for object detection so perhaps the neural architecture is moulded in some fashion to this task – the more highly developed animals requiring more sophisticated information about objects for their

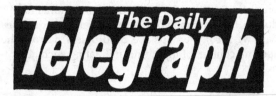

Fig. 4.4. Copy of 1983 newspaper article. Reproduced with permission from *The Daily Telegraph*.

ultimate recognition. It would seem apparent that one primary task of the visual pathway is to code attributes of objects.

The limitation of a finite brain is manifest. Eyes view only a subset of the visual world and process this subset selectively according to specialization that reflects their life style. There is clearly a drive for economical neural strategies so we anticipate efficient coding of object attributes.

Following this logic, Snyder & Barlow (1988) identify two essential goals of the brain — one to simplify the recognition of objects, the other to report objects with the utmost economy. These two principles provide a unifying perspective of visual processing and one that is consistent with perceptual data.

Simplification of object recognition

Visual processing is more rapid and efficient if the brain has expectations about what is to be seen. It would be plausible for these expectations to be incorporated into perceptual mechanisms during the course of evolution. The structure and sequence of visual processing would then be determined by these expectations, which should reveal themselves as illusions in unnatural situations. Natural scenes, as distinguished from the infinity of contrived scenes, are composed of discrete objects. It is such attributes of objects as they occur in the natural world, that should be structured into visual processing. Most of these attributes are well known to artists because they have had to master them to create the illusion of the three-dimensional world on a two-dimensional surface.

By making assumptions about the world, the brain is vulnerable to errors in artificial situations. This is consistent with various illusions and also strongly suggests that colour vision has evolved for gaining attention and rapidly labelling objects that would otherwise be quite visible to an achromatic eye by virtue of their luminance borders (Snyder & Barlow, 1988).

Economy of object reporting
While the brain might accelerate its formulation of the percept by incorporating expectations about object attributes, the report of this percept might also be hastened by economy principles. It is the objects themselves that are important to an animal, not the object attributes processed by the brain to formulate the percept. Artists know that object attributes are not apparent even after careful inspection; the viewer sees the object itself instead. Thus, the brain reports only the object, suppressing conscious information about the attributes used to find it. The reason, Snyder & Barlow (1988) suggest, is for economy of object reporting.

Neurobiological evidence for object coding
Recently, Osorio, Snyder & Srinivasan (1987) argue like Marr (1980) that the two primary object attributes are boundaries and internal structure. Encoding these two attributes exclusively into two channels is thus maximally efficient in that the natural world is represented by a small number of highly-active channels rather than dispersing such information over many channels (Osorio, Snyder & Srinivasan, 1987).

Striking evidence for this bi-partitioning exists in the locust medulla where there are two classes of cells – one non-linear cell class ideally suited for detecting boundaries, the other class suitable for filling in the region between the boundaries (Osorio, Snyder & Srinivasan, 1987). While no equivalent subdivision of cells has been identified in the visual pathways of vertebrates, it remains possible that the simple cortical cells are the 'filling in' class discussed above. Thus, both the presumed local Fourier processing strategy attributed to simple cells (Robson, 1983) and their possible role in removing spatial redundancy (Bossomaier & Snyder, 1986) may merely be by-products of the more global bi-partitioning strategy as also may be the fact that the neural image is made to look like the object under suprathreshold conditions (Snyder & Srinivasan, 1979), i.e. the optical blur is compensated (Georgeson & Sullivan, 1975). Biological perspective is essential for identifying the primary motivation for a particular strategy from the various by-products. We are reminded of one of the more eloquent passages in the pages of the visual sciences:

A wing would be a most mystifying structure if one did not know that birds flew. One might observe that it could be extended a considerable distance, that it had a smooth covering of feathers with conspicuous markings, that it was operated by powerful muscles, and that strength and lightness were prominent features of its construction. These are important facts, but by themselves they do not tell us that birds fly. Yet without knowing this, and without understanding something of the principles of flight, a more detailed examination of the wing itself would probably be unrewarding. I think that we may be at an analogous point in our understanding of the sensory side of the central nervous system. We have got our first batch of facts from the anatomical, neurophysiological, and psychophysical study of sensation and perception, and now we need ideas about what operations are performed by the various structures we have examined. For the bird's wing we can say that it accelerates downwards the air flowing past it and so derives an upward force which supports the weight of the bird; what would be a similar summary of the most important operation performed at a sensory relay?

(Barlow, 1961).

References

Barlow, H. B. (1961) Possible principles underlying the transformations of sensory messages. In *Sensory Com-munication*, ed. W. Rosenbligh, pp. 217–34. Boston: MIT Press.

Barlow, H. B. (1979) Reconstructing the visual image in space and time. *Nature*, **279**, 189–90.

Barlow, H. B. (1981) Critical limiting factors in the design of the eye and visual cortex. The Ferrier Lecture, *Proc. Roy. Soc. London.*, B212, 1–34.

Barlow, H. B. (1986) Why can't the eye see better. In *Visual Neuroscience*, ed. J. D. Pettigrew, K. J. Sanderson & W. R. Levick, pp. 3–19. Cambridge: Cambridge University Press.

Bossomaier, T. R. J., Snyder, A. W., & Hughes, A. (1985) Irregularity and aliasing: solution? *Vision Res.*, 25, 145–7.

Bossomaier, T. R. J., & Snyder, A. W. (1986) Why spatial frequency processing in the visual cortex. *Vision Res.*, 26, 1307–9.

Campbell, F. W. & Gubisch, R. W. (1966) Optical quality of the human eye. *J. Physiol. (Lond.)*, 186, 558–78.

Duke-Elder, W. S. (1958) *System of Ophthalmology*, Vol. 1, In The Eye in Evolution. London: Henry Kimpton.

Engström, K. (1983) Cone types and cone arrangements in teleost retinae. *Acta. Zool. (Stockh.)* 44, 179–243.

French, A. S., Snyder, A. W. & Stavenga, D. G. (1977) Image-degradation by a non-uniform retinal mosaic. *Biol. Cybern.*, 27, 229–33.

Georgeson, M. A. & Sullivan, G. D. (1975) Contrast sensitivity: deblurring in human vision by spatial frequency channels. *J. Physiol. (Lond.)*, 252, 627–56.

Hirsch, J. & Hilton, R. (1984) Quality of the primate lattice and the limits of spatial vision. *Vision Res.*, 24, 347–55.

Horridge, G. A. (1977) The compound eyes of insects. *Sci. Am.*, 237, 108–20.

Hughes, A. (1977) The topography of vision in mammals. In *Handbook of Sensory Physiology*, Vol. VII/5, ed. F. Crescitelli, pp. 613–756. Berlin: Springer-Verlag.

Jagger, W. S. (1985) Visibility of photoreceptors in the intact living eye of the cane toad. *Vision Res.*, 25, 729–31.

Kirschfeld, K. & Snyder, A. W. (1975) Waveguide mode effects, birefringence and dichroism in fly photoreceptors. In *Photoreceptor Optics*, ed. A. W. Snyder & R. Menzel. Berlin: Springer-Verlag.

Kirschfeld, K. & Snyder, A. W. (1976) Measurement of a photoreceptor's characteristic waveguide parameter. *Vision Res.*, 16, 775–8.

Land, M. F. & Snyder A. W. (1985) Cone mosaic observed directly through natural pupil of live vertebrate. *Vision Res.*, 25, 1519–23.

Liebman, P. A. & Entise, G. (1974) Lateral diffusion of visual pigment in photoreceptor disc membrane. *Science*, 185, 457–9.

Lythgoe, J. N. (1979) *The Ecology of Vision*. Oxford: Clarendon Press.

Marr, D. (1980) *Vision*. San Francisco: W. H. Freeman.

Miller, W. H. (1977) Interocular filters. In *Handbook of Sensor Physiology*, Vol. VII/5, ed. F. Crescitelli. Berlin: Springer-Verlag.

Nyquist, H. (1924) Certain factors affecting telegraph speed. *Bell Systems Tech. J.*, 3, 324–46.

Osorio, D., Snyder, A. W. & Srinivasan, M. V. (1987) Bi-partitioning of natural scenes in early vision. *Spatial Vision* (in press).

Robson, J. G. (1983) Frequency domain visual processing. In *Physical and Biological Processing of Images*, ed. O. J. Braddick & A. C. Sleigh, pp. 73–87. Berlin: Springer-Verlag.

Schlaer, R. (1972) An eagle's eye, quality of the retinal image. *Science*, 176, 920–2.

Snyder, A. W. (1972) Coupled-mode theory for optical fibres. *J. Opt. Soc. Am.*, 62, 1278–83.

Snyder, A. W. (1977) Acuity of compound eyes. *J. Comp. Physiol.*, 116, 161–82.

Snyder, A. W. (1979) The physics of vision in compound eye. In *Handbook of Sensory Physiology*, Vol. VII/6A, ed. H. Autrum. Berlin: Springer-Verlag.

Snyder, A. W. (1982) Hyperacuity and interpolation by the visual pathways. *Vision Res.*, 22, 1219–20.

Snyder, A. W. & Barlow, H. B. (1988) Revealing the artist's touch. *Nature*, 331, 117–18.

Snyder, A. W. & Bossomaier, T. J. (1986) Optical image quality and cone mosaic. *Science*, 231, 499–501.

Snyder, A. W., Bossomaier, T. J. & Hughes, A. (1986).

Snyder, A. W. & Laughlin, S. B. (1975) Diochroism and absorption by photoreceptors. *J. Comp. Physiol.*, 100, 101–6.

Snyder, A. W., Laughlin, S. B. & Stavenga, A. G. (1977) Information capacity of eyes. *Vision Res.*, 17, 1163–75.

Snyder, A. W. & Love, J. D. (1983) *Optical Waveguide Theory*. London: Chapman and Hall.

Snyder, A. W. & Menzel, R. (1975) Photoreceptor optics. In *Photoreceptor Optics*. Berlin: Springer-Verlag.

Snyder, A. W. & Miller, W. H. (1977) Photoreceptor diameter and spacing for highest resolving power. *J. Opt. Soc. Am.*, 67, 696–8.

Snyder, A. W. & Miller, W. H. (1978) Telephoto lens system of falconiform eyes. *Nature*, 275, 127–9.

Snyder, A. W. & Pask, C. (1973) The Stiles-Crawford effect – explanation and consequences. *Vision Res.*, 13, 1115–37.

Snyder, A. W. & Ruhl, F. (1983) New single-mode single polarisation fibre. *Electronics Letters*, 19, 185–6.

Snyder, A. W. & Srinivasan, M. V. (1979) Human Psychophysics: functional interpretation of contrast sensitivity curve. *Biol. Cybern.*, 32, 9–17.

Snyder, A. W. & Xue-heng, Zheng (1986) Optical fibres of arbitrary cross-section. *J. Opt. Soc.*, 3, 600–9.

Van Hateren, J. H. (1985) The Stiles–Crawford effect in the eye of the blowfly. *Vision Res.*, 25, 1305–15.

Walls, G. L. (1942) *The vertebrate eye and its adaptive radiation*. New York: Hafner.

Wehner, R. (1981) Spatial vision in arthropods. In *Handbook of Sensory Physiology*, Vol. VII/6C, ed. H. Autrum, pp. 288–551. Berlin: Springer-Verlag.

Williams, D. S. & McIntyre, P. (1980) The principal eyes of a jumping spider have a telephoto component. *Nature*, 288, 578–80.

Efficiency of the visual pathway

5

The design of compound eyes

M. F. Land

Introduction

In 1952, Barlow wrote a paper in which he spelled out the implications of the diffraction limit for compound eyes, where the small size of each lens makes diffraction a much more severe problem than it is in eyes like our own with a single large lens. This paper, modestly entitled 'The size of ommatidia in apposition eyes', contained a sentence which seemed to me when I first read it as a graduate student wonderfully immodest. He wrote, 'Imagine the problems concerned in designing an eye for an insect', and then went on to work out the relation between the resolution of a compound eye and its size, and the size of its component parts. People in those days rarely thought like that; it was one thing to try to sort out an organ's function, but quite another to set about its design. A generation before genetic engineering made such ideas almost commonplace, Barlow's assertion that one could understand natural structures at that kind of level seemed exciting and pleasingly impious.

It is because we understand the behaviour of light so well that it is possible to entertain such ideas about eyes. For livers and kidneys, or even ears and noses, no correspondingly exact body of knowledge exists to permit a thorough analysis of the physical constraints on their design. Thus it is possible to attribute function to structure with more precision in the eye than in any other sense organ; and to a comparative physiologist one of the beauties of studying eyes is the confidence one has that differences between eyes are important. As Gordon Walls put it, 'everything in the vertebrate eye means something' (Walls, 1942). I hope to show in this chapter that he could have omitted the word 'vertebrate'.

Since Barlow's pioneering paper, many others have turned their hand to eye design. Barlow himself published an excellent review, 'The physical limits of visual discrimination' in 1964. The question of differences between the attainable resolution of simple and compound eyes was taken up again by Kirschfeld (1976), and an important new idea was introduced by Snyder, Stavenga & Laughlin (1977) who showed how eye design could be optimized, in terms of the information obtained from the image, for any given light intensity. Much useful comparative information, in general confirming these theoretical ideas, was provided by Horridge (1978), and the whole subject of the physics of insect vision was exhaustively reviewed by Snyder in 1979. Unknown to Barlow, his study did have a distinguished antecedent. In 1894 Mallock published a remarkable paper on 'Insect sight and the defining power of composite eyes' in which he stated with admirable clarity how diffraction affects both the size and resolution of compound eyes. His paper seems never to have penetrated the vision literature, until it was rediscovered by de Vries (1956).

In this chapter I want to do two things. First to recapitulate some of Barlow's arguments relating to the way diffraction prevents compound eyes from attaining what we would regard as respectable resolution without becoming implausibly large; and second to present some of the ways that insects try to get round this problem by carefully 'tailoring' the distribution of resolution across their eyes to fit their behavioural needs.

The resolving power of compound eyes

The effects of the diffraction limit

The feature of an eye that ultimately limits its ability to resolve detail is the size of the lens. This is because the larger the lens the smaller is the diffraction pattern that it produces; large telescopes resolve better than small ones. The diffraction pattern due to a point source, the Airy disc, has a radius (r) from its centre to the first dark ring given by

$$r = 1.22\lambda/D \qquad \text{radians,} \qquad (1a)$$

or a width (w) at half maximum intensity of

$$w = \lambda/D \qquad \text{radians} \qquad (1b)$$

where λ is the wavelength and D the aperture diameter. The Rayleigh criterion, used in astronomy, assumes that two point sources can be separated if the image of one falls on the first dark ring of the image of the other, so that they are resolvable if their angular separation exceeds 1.22 λ/D. Applying this to a bee, with lenses only 25 μm in diameter, gives a resolution limit of 0.024 radians, or 1.4°, when λ is 0.5 μm. For our own eyes, with daylight pupil diameters of 2.5 mm, the limit is 100 times smaller, 0.84 minutes of arc. A slightly more modern version of the same thing has it that the highest spatial frequency transmitted by a lens is given by D/λ (cycles per radian), but the result is essentially the same. Compound eyes are limited by the small sizes of their lenses to resolution that we would regard as very poor. Mallock (1894) puts it nicely: 'The best of the eyes . . . would give a picture about as good as if executed in rather coarse wool-work and viewed at a distance of about a foot'.

The resolution of an eye is not just a matter of optics. However good the image there must be an adequate density of receptor elements for that image to be exploited fully. In eyes like ours this presents no difficulty; the bigger the eye the better the diffraction image and the greater the number of receptors available to receive it. In apposition compound eyes, however, the two determinants of resolution are in conflict. The larger the individual lenses – and hence the better the image – the fewer their number in an eye of a given size, and hence the fewer the number of receptors available to exploit the overall image. Given that there is a conflict, then, between 'optical' and 'anatomical' resolution, the question arises: what is the right answer to it? This, and the related question of how this answer changes as the eye itself varies in size, were the main subjects of Barlow's 1952 paper.

(The word 'apposition' needs an explanation. It means that each element – an ommatidium – consists of a lens and a group of receptors whose photosensitive parts all image the same region of space. Adjacent ommatidia image adjacent regions of space. Individual images are inverted, but this is irrelevant as there is effectively only one receptive element in each ommatidium, and the overall image, dictated by the geometry of the eye as a whole, is erect (Fig. 5.1). The 'neural superposition' eyes of dipteran flies behave optically like ordinary apposition eyes, even though the inverted images in each ommatidium are partially resolved by separate receptors. Optical superposition eyes, however, such as are found in nocturnal moths and beetles, embody quite different optical principles, (Kunze, 1979; Land, 1985) and most of the following discussion does not apply to them.)

In a spherical apposition compound eye the angle between adjacent ommatidia ($\triangle\phi$) must be the angle subtended by adjacent lenses at the centre of the eye (Fig. 5.1). That is:

$$\triangle\phi = D/R \qquad \text{(radians)} \qquad (2)$$

where D is the lens diameter and R the eye radius. As we have seen already, the finest resolvable periodic structure in the image in each ommatidium has a spatial frequency of D/λ, or a period of λ/D radians. An eye organized to detect the finest grating-like detail provided by the optics would need to sample it in such a way that two detectors are available for each period – one for the dark and one for the light bar. This is true

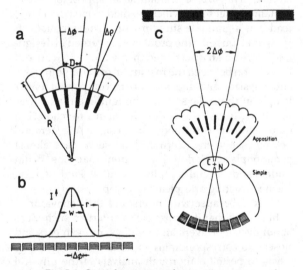

Fig. 5.1. Optical geometry of apposition compound eyes. (a) The inter-ommatidial angle $\triangle\phi$ is equal to the facet diameter (D) divided by the eye radius (R); this is usually similar to the acceptance angle $\triangle\varrho$. (b) Distribution of intensity (I) in the Airy disc. The diffraction-limited image is fully sampled when $2\triangle\phi$ is equal to the half-width (w). The radius (r) of the 1st dark ring is 1.22 times the half-width. (c) The finest grating that a simple or a compound eye can resolve has a period of $2\triangle\phi$, where $\triangle\phi$ is the inter-ommatidial or inter-receptor angle. (b) and (c) are based on Kirschfeld (1976).

even when the detectors lie behind separate lenses, as in apposition eyes (Fig. 5.1). This means that:

$$2 \triangle \phi = \lambda/D \tag{3}$$

Combining equations (2) and (3) to eliminate the inter-ommatidial angle $\triangle \phi$ gives:

$$D^2 = \lambda R/2, \text{ or } D \propto \sqrt{R} \tag{4}$$

The diameters of individual facets should be proportional to the square root of eye radius, or in a non-spherical eye to some other linear dimension.

Barlow argued that if this relation held between insects with different eye sizes, then this would constitute a proof that diffraction was indeed the limiting factor in compound eye design. He examined the eyes of 27 diurnal hymenopteran insects from the University Museum of Zoology in Cambridge, ranging in size from a 1 mm chalcid wasp to a 60 mm tropical bee. The eyes ranged from 0.2 to 5 mm in height, and the individual facets from 8 to 36 μm in diameter. The full results are shown in Fig. 5.2. They do indeed fit the anticipated square-root relation, and thus confirm that diffraction must be a prime ingredient in compound eye design. More recently Wehner (1981) surveyed all arthropod groups with apposition eyes, including the extinct trilobites, and found that an approximate square-root relation between eye size and lens size holds across the whole phylum.

The size of apposition eyes

Similar arguments lead to some remarkable conclusions concerning the relation between resolution and eye size. Mallock (1894) was the first to point out that a compound eye with resolution similar to our own (about 1 minute of arc) would have ridiculous dimensions. He estimated a radius of 19 feet! The reason for this can be seen if we again combine equations (2) and (3), but this time eliminating the lens diameter D. The result is:

$$R = \lambda/(2 \triangle \phi^2) \tag{5}$$

The reader is invited to insert a value of $\triangle \phi$ of 1 minute (0.0003 radians) and see what happens to R.

Kirschfeld (1976) pointed out that our eyes only have 1 minute resolution in the foveal region, and that away from the line of sight it falls off drastically. Incorporating this into a more realistic apposition eye design reduces the size of the eye dramatically. Kirschfeld's final version is shown in Fig. 5.3, and it now has a diameter of about 1 metre. It is still absurdly large, however, compared with the simple eye equivalent with a diameter of 2 cm. An intuitively simple reason for the difference between the two types of eye can be seen by considering what happens when the acuity of

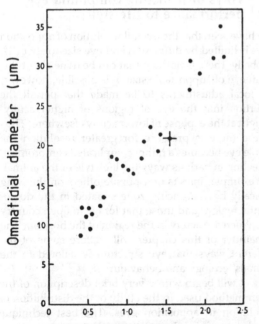

Fig. 5.2. Relation of ommatidial diameter and eye height, for 27 diurnal hymenopterans (Barlow, 1952).

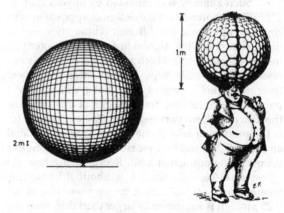

Fig. 5.3. Two attempts to realize a compound eye with the same resolution as the human eye. The eye on the left has a resolution of 1 minute all over. Mallock (1894) estimated a radius of 19 feet (6 m). The eye on the right has the same distribution of resolution as the human eye, with the finest resolution only in the 'fovea'. The size is greatly reduced, but it is still impracticable. Each 'facet' represents 10^4 actual lenses. Both figures from Kirschfeld (1976) with permission.

each type is doubled. In a simple eye all that is required is a doubling of the size of the eye, whilst the distance between receptors in the retina stays the same. In an apposition compound eye, however, not only must the size of each lens double, to improve the diffraction limit by a factor of two, but the number of lenses along the row must also double to make use of the doubled acuity. Hence the square term in Equ. (5).

Sensitivity and the eye parameter

Diffraction may not be the only reason for the presence of large lenses in compound eyes. The light available to the receptors also depends on the facet diameter, and Barlow (1952) considered 'that insects living where the light is feeble might sacrifice acuity for sensitivity by having large ommatidia'. On the whole, arthropods move over to a superposition type of eye, which is inherently more sensitive, when living in dim conditions, but there are exceptions. The crepuscular dragonfly *Zyxomma* has lenses about three times wider than would be expected on the basis of diffraction alone (Horridge, 1978), as does the crepuscular butter-fly *Melanitis* (Nilsson *et al.*, 1988). *Limulus*, which lives in murky water and has nocturnal habits, has lenses with a diameter of 0.3 mm, more than 100 times larger than Equ. (4) would suggest for an eye with an inter-ommatidial angle of about 6°. It is clear that a complete explanation of apposition eye design must take both sensitivity and resolution into account.

Such a theory was provided by Snyder *et al.* in 1977. They showed how the design of apposition eyes could be optimized for different illumination condi-tions, to produce the highest 'information content', a measure that combined both acuity and the number of resolvable grey-scale steps. I do not intend to review their ingenious argument here, but I will borrow a particularly useful idea that came out of that analysis: the idea of the 'eye parameter' (p). The eye parameter is the product of lens diameter and inter-ommatidial angle, $p=D\triangle\phi$, and it is a measure of how close the eye comes to the diffraction limit. Reorganizing Equ. (3) gives: $p=D\triangle\phi=\lambda/2$. Since λ is about 0.5 μm, this means that at the diffraction limit p should be about 0.25 μm. If it is substantially larger than this, then the eye is indeed sacrificing resolution for sensitivity. The relation expected between p and the illumination con-ditions that different animals inhabit is given in Fig. 5.4, which shows that over the whole 'daylight' range p stays close to its minimum value, but that as back-ground luminances fall below about 10 cd/m² p begins to rise very rapidly. These predictions do accord well with what is found in practice. For most diurnal insects with apposition eyes p is typically in the range 0.3 to 0.5 μm (Horridge, 1978) – just on the right side of

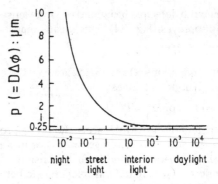

Fig. 5.4. The magnitude of the eye parameter (p) in compound eyes designed to work optimally at different light intensities. Below about 10 cd/m² p becomes large, implying that larger facets are needed for a given inter-ommatidial angle. Based on Snyder (1979).

the diffraction limit. In crespuscular insects it rises to around 1 μm, in deep-sea amphipods it lies between 1 and 20 μm, and in *Limulus* it is about 30 μm, indicating adaptation to a very dark environment (Fig. 5.4).

Ways of matching compound eye performance to life-style

We have seen that the overall resolution of apposition eyes is limited by diffraction and eye size to about 1°. Globally, there is nothing that can be done about this in an eye of supportable size. It is possible, however, for local adjustments to be made that permit the insertion into the eye of regions of higher acuity, bought at the expense of lower acuity elsewhere. Thus where there is pressure for greater resolution the whole eye becomes a rather complicated compromise, reflecting in various ways the life-style of the animal. For example, insects that pursue others on the wing typically have an acute zone situated in the dorso-frontal region, and those that forage in open country often increase acuity in the region of the horizon. The remainder of this chapter will explore some of the different ways that eye structure is tailored to the animals' ecology and behaviour.

I will begin with a very brief description of the main method used in the study of the distribution of resolution in apposition eyes. The best technique involves mapping the position of the 'pseudopupil' on the eye surface, as the eye is viewed from different directions. The pseudopupil is typically a black dot that appears to move across the eye as the observer moves around the animal (Fig. 5.5 d&e). The dot is black because it indicates the ommatidia that are imaging – and therefore absorbing light from – the observer. This in turn means that the line joining the pseudopupil to the observer's eye is the direction of sight of the ommatidium marked by the pseudopupil. By rotating a microscope around the animal on a

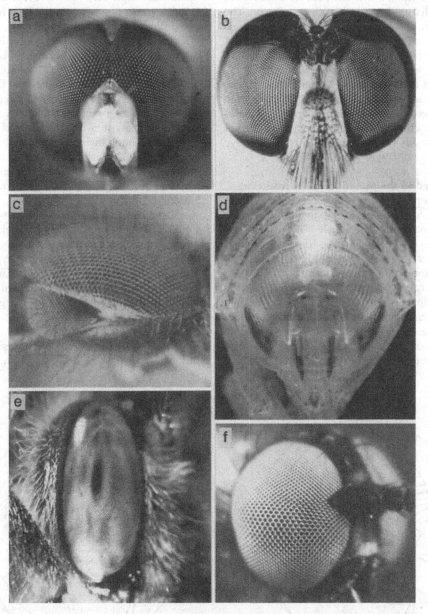

Fig. 5.5. Six examples of arthropods in which the resolution varies across the eye. (a) *Syritta* male. A small hover-fly with an acute zone (large facets) pointing dorso-frontally. The eyes of the female do not meet in front, and the facets are of equal size. (b) Frontal acute zone, used by both sexes for catching prey, in a large robber-fly (*Neoaratus*) (c) Completely divided eye in a male bibionid fly (*Dilophus*). The female has only the small-facetted part. (d) Divided eye in the deep-water amphipod *Phrosina*, showing a binocular pseudopupil in the lower eyes. Both sexes have double eyes. (e) Eye of a bee (*Amegilla*) from the side, showing the greatly elongated vertical pseudopupil. The elongation results from the vertical magnification (small $\Delta\phi$s) of the region around the equator. (f) An empid fly, with a horizontal band of large facets used to view the water surface over which they catch prey. (c) and (f) courtesy of Dr Jochen Zeil.

goniometer, and mapping the changing position of the pseudopupil on the eye, the direction of view of each ommatidium can be established. This map, of angle versus position, is then the basis for working out inter-ommatidial angles, axis densities, and so on. The only problem with this method is that some eyes are so dark that it is not possible to see the pseudopupil. A variant can then be used in which the head is illuminated from inside, with a light-guide for example; the receptors' tips then become self-luminous, and this 'antidromic' pseudopupil appears light rather than dark, but its geometrical properties are the same as before (Franceschini & Kirschfeld, 1971). For further details of methods the reader should read Horridge (1978), Stavenga (1979) or Land (1985).

Eyes used in the pursuit of other insects

There are two reasons why an insect might wish to chase another: to mate it or to eat it. In many species of insect the male pursues the female in forward flight, and catches her on the wing. This is true for houseflies and many other dipterans (Dietrich, 1909; Land, 1985) and also for drone honey bees (Praagh *et al.*, 1980). In most of these cases there is a dorso-frontal region in the eye of the male where the resolution is better (Fig. 5.5a and 5.6), and there is no corresponding region in the female eye. (The word 'fovea' is often used to describe such regions, but G. A. Horridge's term 'acute zone' is better, because it doesn't have the literal

meaning of a 'pit' which is only appropriate to some vertebrate retinas). It is this acute zone that images the female during pursuit. The difference in inter-ommatidial angle between these regions in males and female eyes can be large. In the little hoverfly *Syritta pipiens* the male 'shadows' the female, remaining out of sight, and $\triangle\phi$ in his acute zone is only 0.6°, whereas in the equivalent region of her eye $\triangle\phi$ is 1.6° (Collett & Land, 1975). In terms of sampling densities (ommatidial axes per square degree) this is a sevenfold difference. In all these cases, facet diameters are larger where inter-ommatidial angles are smaller, as Equ. (3) predicts. In *Syritta* the lenses of the male acute zone are 40 μm in diameter compared with 16–20 μm in the female. The larger lenses create the paradoxical impression of a coarser mosaic in the male than the female, but in *angular* terms it is of course finer (Fig. 5.5a&b).

In males that form swarms – bibionid flies and simuliid midges for example – the male acute zone is directed dorsally, and may be so exaggerated that it completely dwarfs the rest of the eye (Zeil, 1983). There is a real division between the two parts of the eye, not a smooth graduation as in *Syritta* (Fig. 5.5a,c). In simuliids not only are the lenses larger in the acute zone, the receptors themselves are so elongated that they reach right down to the roof of the mouth. Kirschfeld (1979) points out that the task of detecting a tiny object against the dusk sky is one that involves

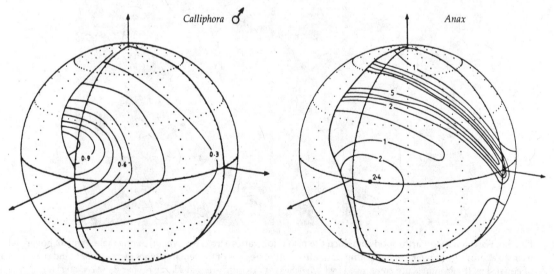

Fig. 5.6. Distribution of resolution in the visual fields of the left eyes of a male blow-fly (left) and a large dragon-fly (right). The contours show the numbers of ommatidial axes per square degree of visual field, and the arrows point forwards (left) dorsally and laterally. In *Calliphora* the semi-circular acute zone points forwards and slightly upwards: the chasing direction. In *Anax* there is a strip-like dorsal acute zone concerned with prey-capture, and a weaker one pointing forwards, along the line of flight. Data from Land & Eckert (1985) and Sherk (1978).

high sensitivity as well as good resolution, and the long receptors certainly suggest that the eye design is one that maximizes both. In the deep sea rather similar conditions occur, where many animals rely for either mate-finding or food on the ability to sight small targets in the dim down-welling light. The only animals in this fauna with good apposition compound eyes are the hyperiid amphipods (Fig. 5.5d), and they often have double eyes that are strikingly similar to those of swarming flies (Land, 1981).

Insects that capture others for food usually have acute zones similar to those concerned with sexual pursuit, but here they are present in both sexes. The broad frontal acute zones of robber-flies (Fig. 5.5b) were beautifully illustrated by Dietrich (1909), and the even more impressive acute zones of dragonflies (Fig. 5.6) by Sherk (1978). Sherk found a particularly inter-esting situation in the large aeshnid dragonflies. These have a dorsally-directed wedge-shaped sector of very large facets, and pseudopupil mapping showed that in this region inter-ommatidial angles had values as low as 0.25°, probably the smallest of any insect. However, unlike the roughly circular acute zones of other predatory insects – mantids for example (Rossel, 1980) – these high acuity regions form a strip which lies along the great circle passing through the lateral poles of the eye and a point 60° above the anterior pole (Fig. 5.6). These dragonflies hunt by 'trawling' through the air, looking for insects against the sky above. With such a technique there is no point in having an acute zone extending very far in the fore-and-aft direction; all that is needed is a bar of high acuity across the dorsal field that will pick up a target, very much like the line on a radar scanner. The forward flight of the animal itself provides the scanning motion.

Eyes of foraging insects

The eyes of nectar-feeding and foliage-eating flying insects show a consistent but rather complicated dis-tribution of resolution. Bees, butterflies and acridid grasshoppers all show variation in resolution in both horizontal and vertical directions. Figure 5.7 shows the pattern of inter-ommatidial angles in a typical butterfly. Going from front to back, the horizontal inter-ommatidial angles ($\triangle\phi$) decrease from about 1.4° to 3.1°, whilst vertical values of $\triangle\phi$ change little, remaining around 1.3° to 1.5°. However, going from top to bottom of the eye there are large changes in vertical $\triangle\phi$ values, which rise to 2° at the poles from their minimum value in the region of the eye's equator; these are not matched by changes in horizontal $\triangle\phi$. In other words, horizontal acuity decreases from front to back, and vertical acuity decreases above and

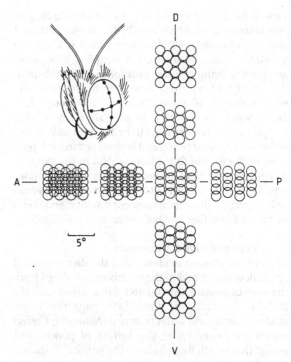

Fig. 5.7. The packing of receptive fields of adjacent ommatidia in the Australian butterfly *Heteronympha merope*. The dark-adapted acceptance angle ($\Delta\varrho$, Fig. 5.1a) is close to 1.9° everywhere, but vertical and horizontal inter-ommatidial angles vary in a characteristic way from front to back and from the equator to the poles as described in the text.

below the horizon. This pattern is virtually identical in foraging bees (Fig. 5.5e), where the extra ommatidia involved in magnifying the horizon cause the pseudopupil to be elongated vertically, and give the whole eye an oval shape. A thorough study of the resolution of the eyes of honey bees was made by Seidl (1982), and a summary is given in Land (1989).

It makes sense that an animal which flies forward is mainly interested in objects in front. Equally, if it lives in open country, the objects it feeds on will be located not far from the horizon – close to the eye's equator – rather than in the top and bottom of the field of view. It may simply be that the variations in resolution across these insects' eyes reflect the relative importance to the animal of different parts of the environment. The front-to-back differences, however, may have another component to them which is related to the blurring effect of motion. We are all familiar with the difficulty of seeing anything close from the win-dow of a moving train, and of the way this problem increases towards the side, compared with the clear view in the direction of motion. Insects, flying close to vegetation, will experience much the same effect, and one way of dealing with the lateral blur is simply to have a lower density of receptors sampling it. Suppose an insect is flying at 2 m/s past foliage 0.5 m distant, then in the 10 ms integration time of the receptors each point in the image will have moved through 2.3°. There would be nothing to be gained by having receptor separations smaller than this, and indeed this is the sort of value for $\triangle \phi$ that is observed in the lateral parts of the eyes of flying insects. Not in the front, of course, because there the image is more or less stationary. As the blur is horizontal, not vertical, one would only expect a reduction in horizontal acuity, and this is just what butterflies and bees seem to show (Fig. 5.7).

Eyes of flatland arthropods

Perhaps the clearest evidence that the distribution of resolution is matched to the environment comes from the eyes of animals that inhabit flat interfaces. Crabs that live on sand and mud flats, bugs like water striders (*Gerris*) and water boatmen (*Notonecta, Corixa*) which live on or under the surface of ponds, and empid flies which fly just above the surface all show a very strong development of vertical resolution around the horizon. In these animals the part of the visual field of greatest interest is virtually one-dimensional,

and the eye structure reflects this to a much greater degree than in the case of ordinary foragers.

The water bugs are particularly interesting. In *Notonecta*, a predator which hangs from the surface looking upwards, the eye has *two* strips of high acuity, one looking just above the surface, into air, and the other looking at the underside of the surface, through the water (Schwind, 1980). Because of refraction at the water surface, these strips are separated by about 40°, with a low resolution region between them (Fig. 5.8a). Interestingly, there is a fish, *Aplocheilus lineatus*, which also exploits the surface film, and which has two horizontal 'visual streaks' of high ganglion cell density, imaging the upper and lower views of the surface (Munk, 1970). Bugs like *Gerris* that live just above the surface also have an impressive horizontal acute zone (H-U. Dahmen, personal communication), but in this case only one, because refraction prevents them seeing the underside of the surface layer. In the water bugs these acute zones are not visible in the sizes of the facets on the eye surface, and they can only be found by mapping the pseudopupil. However, in some empid flies, which cruise a few mm above the water surface, again looking for drowning insects, there is a high acuity band which is marked by larger facets (Fig. 5.5f).

Figure 5.8b, from Zeil *et al.* (1986), shows how

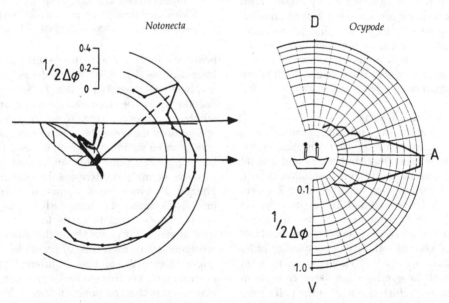

Fig. 5.8. Variation of vertical resolution in the back-swimmer and the ghost crab. The former has two horizontal acute zones that image both the aerial and the under-water views of the surface. The latter has a single intense acute zone which images the horizon. Units are cycles per degree (see Figure 5.1c). A, D and V are anterior, dorsal and ventral. Data from Schwind (1980) and Zeil *et al.* (1986).

vertical resolution varies with altitude in the ghost crab *Ocypode*, which lives on sand flats. The eyes are vertically elongated cylinders, and there is a very obvious belt of elevated resolution, about 30° in height, which includes the horizon and the flat shore surface below it. In the crabs like *Carcinus* that inhabit more three-dimensional rocky shores the horizon belt is nothing like so pronounced. Vertical values of $\Delta \phi$ in *Ocypode* are about 0.5°, almost four times smaller than the horizontal values. Zeil *et al.* make the ingenious suggestion that this magnification of the horizon strip provides a basis for a rangefinding system that uses the angle of declination from the eye to the feet of the target animal as a basis for distance estimation. Clearly such a system can only work properly on an absolutely flat substrate.

The three categories of 'visual tailoring' just listed are probably not the only ones, but they do seem to cover the majority of apposition eyes, apart from the roughly spherically symmetrical eyes of slow-moving vegetarians, and others for whom vision is not at a premium. The one or two oddities that I know of tend to confirm the overall pattern. For example there are certain flies (Phoridae) that parasitize ants, and track them from above; these, uniquely, have enlarged facets in the *lower* part of the eye (R. H. L. Disney, personal communication). Such exceptions do seem to be fairly rare.

Conclusions

It is amazing to me that the apposition compound eye has survived as the dominant optical arrangement in insects and crustaceans. D-E. Nilsson comments that 'It is only a small exaggeration to say that evolution seems to be fighting a desperate battle to improve a basically disastrous design' (Nilsson, 1989), and that really summarizes the thrust of this chapter. The pressure for space has produced some very interesting compromises, bending the eye to fit the animal's needs. None of this would be necessary, however, if arthropods had switched from compound to simple eyes, where good resolution does not require impossible size. They never did, even though simple eyes of sorts are present – and one would think available for conversion – in both the larval eyes and the dorsal ocelli of adults. Evolution seems to have been quite perversely conservative here; unless of course we have all missed something.

References

Barlow, H. B. (1952) The size of ommatidia in apposition eyes. *J. Exp. Biol.*, **29**, 667–74.

Barlow, H. B. (1964) The physical limits of visual discrimination. *Photophysiology*, **2**, 163–202.

Collett, T. S. & Land, M. F. (1975) Visual control of flight behaviour in the hoverfly *Syritta pipiens* L. *J. Comp. Physiol.*, **99**, 1–66.

Dietrich, W. (1909) Die Facettenaugen der Dipteren. *Z. Wiss. Zool.*, **92**, 465–539.

Franceschini, N. & Kirschfeld, K. (1971) Les phénomènes de pseudopupille dans l'oeil composé de *Drosophila*. *Kybernetik*, **9**, 159–82.

Horridge, G. A. (1978) The separation of visual axes in apposition compound eyes. *Phil. Trans. Roy. Soc. Lond.*, **B285**, 1–59.

Kirschfeld, K. (1976) The resolution of lens and compound eyes. In *Neural Principles in Vision*, ed. F. Zettler & R. Weiler, pp. 354–70. Berlin: Springer.

Kirschfeld, K. (1979) The visual system of the fly: physiological optics and functional anatomy as related to behaviour. In *The Neurosciences 4th Study Program*, ed. F. O. Schmitt & F. G. Worden, pp. 297–310. Cambridge Mass: MIT Press.

Kunze, P. (1979) Apposition and superposition eyes. In *Handbook of Sensory Physiology* VII/6A, ed. H. Autrum, pp. 441–502. Berlin: Springer.

Land, M. F. (1981) Optics of the eyes of *Phronima* and other deep-sea amphipods. *J. Comp. Physiol.*, **145**, 209–26.

Land, M. F. (1985) The eye: optics. In *Comprehensive Insect Physiology Biochemistry and Pharmacology*, vol 6, ed. G. A. Kerkut & L. I. Gilbert, pp. 225–75. Oxford: Pergamon Press.

Land, M. F. (1989) Variations in the structure and design of compound eyes. In *Facets of Vision*, eds. R. C. Hardie & D. G. Stavenga, pp. 90–111, Berlin: Springer.

Land, M. F. & Eckert, H. (1985) Maps of the acute zones of fly eyes. *J. Comp. Physiol.*, A. **156**, 525–38.

Mallock, A. (1894) Insect sight and the defining power of composite eyes. *Proc. Roy. Soc. Lond.*, B55, 85–90.

Munk, O. (1970) On the occurrence and significance of horizontal band-shaped retinal areae in teleosts. *Vidensk Meddr. dansk naturh. Foren.*, **133**, 85–120.

Nilsson, D-E. (1989) The evolution of compound eyes. In *Facets of Vision*, ed. R. C. Hardie & D. G. Stavenga, pp. 30–73. Berlin: Springer.

Nilsson, D-E., Land, M. F. & Howard, J. (1988) Optics of the butterfly eye. *J. Comp. Physiol.*, A. **162**. 341–66.

Praagh, J. P. van, Ribi, W., Wehrhahn, C. & Wittman, D. (1980) Drone bees fixate the queen with the dorsal frontal part of their compound eyes. *J. Comp. Physiol.*, **136**, 263–6.

Rossel, S. (1980) Foveal fixation and tracking in the praying mantis. *J. Comp. Physiol.*, **139**, 307–31.

Schwind, R. (1980) Geometrical optics of the *Notonecta* eye:

adaptations to optical environment and way of life. *J. Comp. Physiol.*, **140**, 59–68.

Seidl, R. (1982) Die Sehfelder und Ommatidien-Divergenzwinkel von Arbeiterin, Königin und Drohn der Honigbiene (*Apis mellifica*). Doctoral Thesis, Darmstadt: Technischen Hochschule (unpublished).

Sherk, T. E. (1978) Development of the compound eyes of dragonflies (Odonata). III. Adult compound eyes. *J. Exp. Zool.*, **203**, 61–80.

Snyder, A. W. (1979) Physics of vision in compound eyes. In *Handbook of Sensory Physiology* VII/6A, ed. H. Autrum, pp. 225–313. Berlin: Springer.

Snyder, A. W., Stavenga, D. G. & Laughlin, S. B. (1977) Spatial information capacity of compound eyes. *J. Comp. Physiol.*, **116**, 183–207.

Stavenga, D. G. (1979) Pseudopupils of compound eyes. In *Handbook of Sensory Physiology* VII/6A, ed. H. Autrum, pp. 357–439. Berlin: Springer.

de Vries, H. (1956) Physical aspects of the sense organs. *Prog. Biophys. Biophys. Chem.*, **6**, 208–64.

Walls, G. L. (1942) *The Vertebrate Eye and its Adaptive Radiation.* New York: Hafner.

Wehner, R. (1981) Spatial vision in arthropods. In *Handbook of Sensory Physiology* VII/6C, ed. H. Autrum, pp. 287–616. Berlin: Springer.

Zeil, J. (1983) Sexual dimorphism in the visual system of flies: the compound eyes and neural superposition in Bibionidae (Diptera). *J. Comp. Physiol.*, **150**, 379–93.

Zeil, J., Nalbach, G. & Nalbach, H-O. (1986) Eyes, eyestalks and the visual world of semi-terrestrial crabs. *J. Comp. Physiol.*, A. **159**, 801–11.

6
The light response of photoreceptors

P. A. McNaughton

Photoreceptors perform the first step in the analysis of a visual image, namely the conversion of light into an electrical signal. The cellular mechanism of this process of energy transformation or transduction has become much clearer in recent years as a result of advances in the study of the biochemistry and physiology of single photoreceptors, and it is on this aspect that this brief review mainly focuses. It should not be forgotten, though, that photoreceptors perform a more complex task than mere energy conversion and amplification. Photoreceptors *adapt* by altering the gain of transduction to accord with the prevailing level of illumination, and they thereby widen the range of light intensities over which they can respond. The first stage of *temporal analysis* occurs in the photoreceptors: time-dependent conductance mechanisms in the inner segment membrane ensure that the voltage signal which drives the transfer of information to second-order cells reaches a peak earlier than the current change across the outer membrane. Finally, the *synaptic transfer* itself seems to be highly non-linear, so that even a small hyperpolarization caused by steady illumination greatly reduces the gain of signal transfer. All of these features must be considered by those studying higher levels of information processing in the visual system, and it should be borne in mind that the photoreceptors do not present a faithful spatial and temporal map of the external world to second-order neurons in the visual pathway any more than the visual system as a whole presents an unprocessed image to an imaginary homunculus sitting at the seat of consciousness deep within the brain.

The biochemistry of phototransduction

Rhodopsin, the light-absorbing pigment, comprises a protein, opsin, linked covalently to the light-absorb-ing chromophore, 11-*cis* retinal. An incident photon of light interacts with the electrons in the alternating chain of single and double bonds in the backbone of 11-*cis* retinal, causing the promotion of these electrons to an excited state from which relaxation to the all-*trans* form of the backbone can occur. After this initial energy input the rhodopsin decays through a series of states culminating in the release of all-*trans* retinal. The later events in the decay are far too slow to be responsible for the light response, though it is possible that they may play a role in light adaptation. The chain of events leading to the closure of ionic channels in the outer segment membrane seems to branch away at an early stage, probably at the point of formation of metarhodopsin II from metarhodopsin I.

The subsequent events have been the subject of intensive study in recent years (see review by Stryer, 1986). Figure 6.1 summarizes our current view, which may have many more steps to be added but which is probably correct in its essential features. An isomerized rhodopsin molecule, formed by the absorption of a photon of light in step 1, is free to diffuse laterally within the disc membrane and is therefore capable of interacting with a number of molecules of transducin, which it converts from the inactive to the active state by causing a bound molecule of guanosine diphosphate (GDP) to be exchanged for the triphosphate (GTP). The ratio of rhodopsin molecules to transducin molecules in the disc membrane is about 10:1, but each isomerized rhodopsin is capable of activating about 500 transducins in the course of random lateral diffusion. The first two steps thus allow efficient collection of photons, by virtue of the preponderance of rhodopsin molecules, together with a high gain.

In the third step of the pathway an active molecule of transducin switches on a single molecule of phosphodiesterase (PDE), the enzyme responsible for

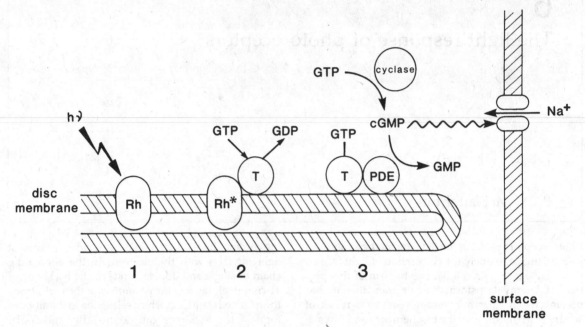

Fig. 6.1. Diagram of the light-sensitive cascade. In step 1 the 11-*cis* retinal chromophore of a rhodopsin molecule, Rh, absorbs a photon of light, converting it into the active form, Rh*. In step 2 an Rh* interacts with a molecule of transducin, T, converting it to the active form by catalyzing the release of a bound GDP and the uptake of GTP. Each Rh* is capable of activating a large number of transducin molecules (probably about 500). In step 3 a single active molecule of transducin switches a single phosphodiesterase into an active state, thus catalyzing the hydrolysis of cGMP to GMP. When the level of cGMP is lowered the light-sensitive channels close. The diagram does not show the inactivation of the various steps in the pathway, nor does it show the possible interactions of intracellular calcium with the pathway.

breaking down 3',5'-cyclic guanosine monophosphate (cGMP) to GMP. As far as we know the interaction of transducin with PDE is one-to-one, so no further gain is introduced at this step, but considerable gain is introduced at the next step: each PDE breaks down about 500 molecules of cGMP during the time course of a single photon response.

This much has been known, at least in outline, for several years. The final step linking cGMP to the change in ionic current flowing across the outer segment membrane was missing, and most researchers imagined either that cGMP controlled ionic channels in the membrane indirectly, perhaps by modulating the activity of a protein kinase which phosphorylated the channels, or that cGMP controlled or modulated the release of calcium ions which were themselves the primary internal transmitter. The answer proved to be simpler than either of these possibilities: cyclic GMP directly modulates the light-sensitive channels without the intervention of any other intermediate or cofactor (Fesenko, Kolesnikov & Lyubarsky, 1985). Two, or perhaps three, molecules of cGMP interact

cooperatively with a channel (Fesenko *et al.*, 1985; Haynes, Kay & Yau, 1986; Zimmerman & Baylor, 1986) to open it and allow the passage of Na ions and, to a lesser extent, of Ca ions (Hodgkin, McNaughton & Nunn, 1985). There is also gain at this step, although less than might be expected: a channel passes 15 to 20 Na ions during its open lifetime (Detwiler, Conner & Bodoia, 1982; Bodoia & Detwiler, 1985; Gray & Attwell, 1985). The low conductance of the channel in normal conditions seems to be due to a blocking action of divalent ions, the function of which is to reduce the contribution to the noisiness of the light response of channel opening and closing (Hodgkin, McNaughton & Nunn, 1985).

The activation of the pathway shown in Fig. 6.1 is reasonably well understood, but what is much less clear are the processes responsible for shutting it off. An isomerized rhodopsin is the target of a rhodopsin kinase which phosphorylates up to eight sites at the C-terminal end; this phosphorylation is the signal for the binding of a second protein (the 48K protein or 'arrestin') which terminates the interaction of rhodopsin with further transducins (Kühn, Hall & Wilden, 1984). The activity of transducin is thought to be terminated by its intrinsic GTP-ase activity, which cleaves the terminal phosphate from GTP to return the enzyme to the inactive GDP-bound form. The problem here is that the measured GTP-ase activity is two orders of magnitude too slow to turn off the light response. Whether the *in vitro* measurements of GTP-ase activity are unreliable or whether some other factor is involved has yet to be determined.

Finally, the return of the cGMP level to the dark value after a flash of light is thought to be speeded by an increase in the activity of the guanylate cyclase responsible for producing cGMP from GTP. The increase in the production rate of cGMP in light means that the flux of cGMP through the pathway shown in Fig. 6.1 is more light sensitive, in the steady-state, than is the level of cGMP itself (Goldberg, Ames, Gander & Walseth, 1983), and suggests the operation of a negative feedback system of the kind required to explain light adaption. Quite how this negative feedback operates has not yet been finally established, but the most plausible suggestion to date is that the drop in internal free calcium concentration which is known to follow the light response (see below, p. 69) increases the activity of the guanylate cyclase (Cohen, Hall & Ferrendelli, 1978; Lolley & Racz, 1982; Hodgkin, McNaughton & Nunn, 1985; Pepe, Panfoli & Cugnoli, 1986; Koch & Stryer, 1988).

The light sensitive pathway shown in Fig. 6.1 has many parallels with the β-adrenergic pathway, and probably with other hormone systems as well. Olfaction, too, operates by a similar mechanism, although here, as in the β-adrenergic system, the final target of the G-protein is an adenylate cyclase rather than a phosphodiesterase (Pace, Hanski, Salomon & Lancet, 1985; Nakamura & Gold, 1987). The analogies between the pathways in the various systems are so close – extending to similar structures of the principal proteins and to similar actions of pertussis and cholera toxins on the pathways (Van Dop *et al.*, 1984) – that there can be no doubt that the cellular mechanisms for photoreception, olfaction and some hormone effects have evolved from a common ancestor mechanism.

Certain features of the pathway shown in Fig. 6.1 make it particularly suitable for detecting photons with high gain and low noise. First, the high overall amplification in the pathway is achieved in a cascade of stages each of lower gain, as in a photomultiplier tube. The gains of one or more of these stages must be regulated to produce the phenomenon of light adaptation. As noted above some at least of this gain regulation appears to occur by an action of calcium on the guanylate cyclase, though additional gain regulation at one or more of the steps in the pathway linking rhodopsin isomerization to PDE activation is also a possibility. Second, the intrinsic noisiness of the pathway is low. The noisiness can be considered under two headings: the dark noise, and the variability in response to a steady light. The activation energy of rhodopsin in high, so thermal isomerizations of rhodopsin in darkness are rare events, although these events appear to constitute the main source of dark noise for the retina as a whole (Barlow, 1957; Baylor, Nunn & Schnapf, 1984). Two further sources of noise contribute to the variability of the outer segment membrane current. A low-frequency noise source has the temporal properties of shot noise filtered by two of the four time constants needed to describe the overall single-photon response, and may therefore be due to a noise source halfway along the transduction chain shown in Fig. 6.1 (Baylor, Matthews & Yau, 1980). A possible site for this noise source is a random variation in the number of phosphodiesterase molecules active in darkness. A second noise source of higher frequency can be attributed to the random opening and closing of light-sensitive channels (Bodoia & Detwiler, 1985; Gray & Attwell, 1985). As noted above, the small value of the unit conductance of a single light-sensitive channel in the normal environment of a photoreceptor outer segment is important in reducing the contribution of this noise source. These last two sources of noise outweigh the contribution of thermal isomerization of rhodopsin to the variability of the membrane current in darkness, but they seem to be removed from the signal, probably by a combination of temporal filtering and a thresholding operation, before it is transmitted from the retina to the brain (Baylor, Nunn & Schnapf, 1984).

The second major source of noise – the variability in response to a steady light – appears to be little greater than the inescapable variability imposed by the quantum nature of light. The single-photon response is remarkably stereotyped, much more so than expected if the lifetime of an isomerized rhodopsin molecule were determined by a single Poisson process (Baylor, Lamb & Yau, 1979). The observation that arrestin, the protein which terminates the activity of an isomerized rhodopsin, binds preferentially to multiply phosphorylated rhodopsin is interesting in this context: if a single first-order process terminated the activity of rhodopsin the variance of the single-photon response would, in the absence of other noise sources, be equal to its amplitude, while if eight independent processes of equal rate are required the variance would be reduced by a factor of 8.

Characteristics of the light-sensitive current

The picture of the circulating light-sensitive current appearing in many elementary textbooks is shown in Fig. 6.2A. This picture is not incorrect in its essential features, but some points need elaboration. First, the idea that the light-sensitive current crossing the outer segment membrane is carried purely by Na^+ ions is now known to be incorrect: a small but significant contribution to the light-sensitive current (probably about 10%) comes from Ca^{2+} ions passing through the light-sensitive channel (Hodgkin, McNaughton & Nunn, 1985). The light-sensitive channel is in fact not highly selective for Na^+ ions, since the currents carried by equimolar concentrations of monovalent cations are in the ratio Li:Na:K:Rb:Cs=1.1:1.0:0.8:0.6:0.15 (Hodgkin, McNaughton & Nunn, 1985), and the light-sensitive current is carried principally by Na^+ for the simple reason that Na^+ is the major external cation.

The second important contribution to the outer segment membrane current comes from the operation of a mechanism responsible for extruding the calcium which enters through the light-sensitive channel (Yau & Nakatani, 1984b; McNaughton, Cervetto & Nunn, 1986; Hodgkin, McNaughton & Nunn, 1987; Hodgkin & Nunn, 1987). The principal – and probably the only – means by which calcium is extruded across the outer segment membrane of the photoreceptor, against the steep inwardly directed electrical and concentration

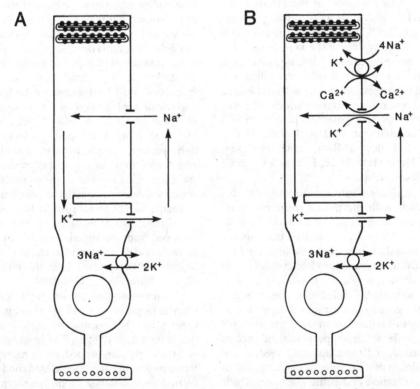

Fig. 6.2. A: the picture of circulating light-sensitive current as presented in many textbooks; B: some necessary modifications to the scheme in A. The light-sensitive channel is imperfectly selective, and about 10% of the light sensitive current is carried by Ca^{2+} ions. The light-sensitive channel discriminates poorly amongst alkali metal cations, and a substantial efflux of K^+ ions through the light-sensitive channel is therefore to be expected, although it has not been directly demonstrated.

    The calcium ions flowing in through the light sensitive channel are extruded by a $4Na^+:1Ca^{2+}$, $1K^+$ exchange which does not depend on energy sources other than that supplied by the transmembrane Na gradient. Since one charge enters the outer segment for every Ca^{2+} extruded, the current carried by the exchange is about 5% of the light-sensitive current, and therefore the Na^+ influx associated with exchange activity is about 20% of the light-sensitive current. The time constant of turnover of the exchangeable fraction of internal Ca^{2+} is about 0.5 s, while the time constant of turnover of Na^+ is of the order of 100 s.

gradients, is a mechanism which depends on external sodium, and which is usually therefore referred to as the Na:Ca exchange. Recent work (Cervetto *et al.*, 1989) has shown that the exchange is more complex than previously thought, and that potassium ions are cotransported with calcium in an electrogenic exchange of stoichiometry $4Na^+:1Ca^{2+},1K^+$, with a substantial contribution to the driving force of the exchange coming from the transmembrane K^+ gradient. With a stoichiometry of $4Na^+:1Ca^{2+},1K^+$ one charge enters the outer segment for every Ca^{2+} ion extruded, and an inflow *j* of calcium ions through the light-sensitive channel therefore contributes an additional inflow of current of *j*/2 in the process of being extruded from the outer segment. The exchange is not directly light-sensitive, although its activity is modulated indirectly by light through changes in the intracellular calcium concentration. For instance, after a bright flash of light the current carried by the exchange declines with a time constant of 0.5 s (in a salamander rod) because the intracellular calcium level declines with this time constant after the calcium influx through the light-sensitive channels has been terminated.

A revised picture of the flow of current in darkness in a rod is shown in Fig. 6.2B. The light-sensitive current and the Na:Ca,K exchange are the only mechanisms contributing in any significant degree to outer segment membrane current, since the resistance of the outer segment membrane when light-sensitive channels are closed and when the exchange is deactivated is found to be in excess of 40 GΩ (Baylor & Nunn, 1986; Lagnado & McNaughton, 1987b). The inner segment membrane contains a variety of conductance mechanisms which shape the response to light of the cell membrane potential, and it contains in addition the Na:K pumps responsible for maintaining the normal gradients of Na and K. The conductance mechanisms in the inner segment have little effect on the circulating dark current flowing between inner and outer segments, since over the normal range of intracellular voltages the light-sensitive current is almost independent of membrane potential (Baylor & Nunn, 1986).

Control of intracellular calcium

Calcium ions are now no longer thought to occupy the central rôle of internal transmitter in the light response for two main reasons: the evidence favouring cGMP as the internal transmitter, reviewed above, is now strong; and, secondly, light is now known to cause a decline in the free concentration of intracellular Ca

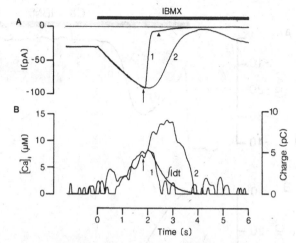

Fig. 6.3. The effect of a flash of light on free $[Ca]_i$. A: the outer segment membrane current from a single rod, recorded with a suction pipette; B: the free intracellular [Ca] measured simultaneously with aequorin. The $[Ca]_i$ was first increased into the range of maximum sensitivity of aequorin by applying the phosphodiesterase inhibitor IBMX, which opens light-sensitive channels by inhibiting the breakdown of cGMP. In the traces labelled 1 a bright flash of light was delivered at the arrow, while the traces labelled 2 were recorded without a flash. The triangle in A marks the Na:Ca exchange current observed after a bright flash has suppressed all the light-sensitive current. The integral of the exchange current is plotted in B (smooth trace). Modified from McNaughton, Cervetto & Nunn, 1986.

instead of the increase required by the calcium hypothesis. The evidence for this second assertion is shown in Fig. 6.3. The free $[Ca]_i$ in a single rod outer segment was monitored using the calcium-sensitive photoprotein aequorin while the light-sensitive current was recorded with a suction pipette. A flash of light can be seen to cause a delayed decline in $[Ca]_i$, with no evidence for a release of Ca coincident with the flash.

Figure 6.3 also shows the Na:Ca,K exchange current (marked with a triangle on the record of membrane current). There is a good correlation between the decline in free $[Ca]_i$, measured with aequorin, and the charge transferred by the Na:Ca,K exchange (shown as the continuous trace in Fig. 6.3B), demonstrating that the Na:Ca,K exchange is the principal mechanism for Ca extrusion from the outer segment.

Further information on the operation of the Na:Ca,K exchange was obtained in the experiment shown in Fig. 6.4. Here the normal external solution

70   *P. A. McNaughton*

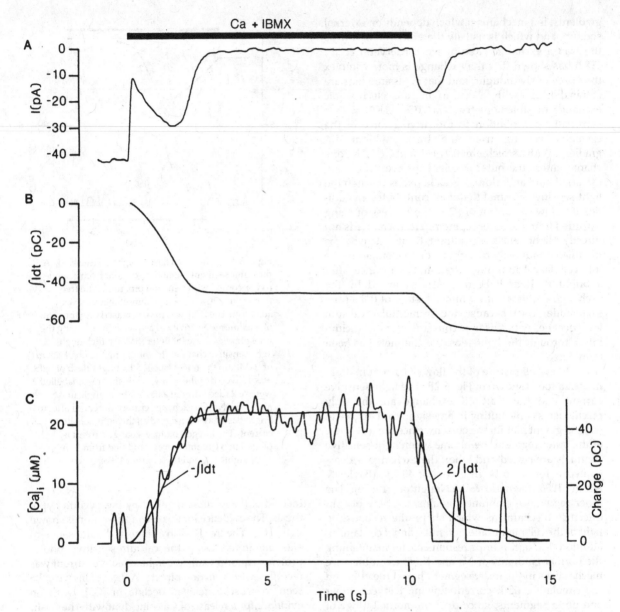

Fig. 6.4. The Na:Ca, K exchange stoichiometry and intracellular buffering power. A: the membrane current recorded during application of a solution in which Ca is the only permeant ion; IBMX has been included in the solution to hold light-sensitive channels open (duration of exposure shown by black bar). Light-sensitive channels were closed after the first few seconds by the strong aequorin light emission, and remained closed until after the end of the trace shown. The light-sensitive inward current observed on return to normal [Na] is due to the operation of the electrogenic Na:Ca exchange. B: the integral of membrane current, starting at the moment of admission of isotonic Ca. The total influx of charge carried by Ca^{2+} was 46 pC, and the charge transferred during the operation of the Na:Ca exchange was 20.6 pC, consistent with an exchange stoichiometry of $4Na^+:1Ca^{2+}$, $1K^+$. C: the free $[Ca]_i$ obtained from the aequorin light emission (irregular trace), compared with the time courses of the integral of calcium influx (first part of smooth trace) and twice the integral of the Na:Ca exchange current (second part of smooth trace). The right-hand ordinate shows the charge flow in pC (1 pC=10^{-12}C); from the known intracellular volume a charge flow of 1 pC changes the total $[Ca]_i$ by 10 μM. The measured maximum increase in free $[Ca]_i$ is 22 μM. Modified from McNaughton, Cervetto & Nunn, 1986.

was replaced at zero time with an isotonic $CaCl_2$ solution. The changes in current on replacing Ringer with isotonic Ca are due partly to the elevation in Ca, which suppresses the light-sensitive current by a direct action on light-sensitive channels (Hodgkin, McNaughton & Nunn, 1985), and partly to the inclusion of the phosphodiesterase inhibitor IBMX, which causes a delayed increase in light-sensitive current by inhibiting the breakdown of cGMP (Cervetto & McNaughton, 1986). Fortunately the origin of the changes in light-sensitive current is not particularly important in this experiment, where the intention was to load the outer segment with a known quantity of Ca which can be calculated from the integral of the light-sensitive current. The influx of Ca was terminated in this experiment by the strong light emission from the aequorin used to measure $[Ca]_i$, and the light-sensitive current remained suppressed until after the end of the trace shown in Fig. 6.4A. The inward current activated transiently on return to normal [Na] is due to the operation of the electrogenic Na:Ca,K exchange. The integral of the light-sensitive current, shown in Fig. 6.4B, can be seen to be approximately double the charge transferred by the Na:Ca exchange on restoration of normal levels of external Na, consistent with an exchange stoichiometry of $4Na^+:1Ca^{2+},1K^+$.

The light emission from the aequorin can be converted to free $[Ca]_i$ using standard methods (Fig. 6.4C; for details see McNaughton, Cervetto & Nunn, 1986). The free $[Ca]_i$ is found to rise with the same time course as the integral of the inward calcium current (smooth curve in the first part of Fig. 6.4C), but the expected concentration change calculated from the calcium influx and from the measured volume of the cell is about twenty times larger than the measured change in free $[Ca]_i$, showing that 95% of the Ca entering the cell is rapidly bound to an internal Ca buffer. A similar result is obtained when calcium is pumped from the cell by the Na:Ca,K exchange: the decline in free $[Ca]_i$ mirrors the integral of the pump current reasonably faithfully, but is about twenty times smaller than the change in total $[Ca]_i$ calculated from the current carried by the exchange. We conclude that the intracellular calcium binding system takes up calcium in a rapid and reversible manner, and from the observation that free $[Ca]_i$ is approximately proportional to total $[Ca]_i$ over the concentration ranges observed in this experiment we conclude that the intracellular buffer system is of large capacity and low affinity. A possible origin of the intracellular buffer observed in these experiments is the headgroups of the phosphatidyl serine components of the lipid bilayer, which are known to take up calcium

(McLaughlin *et al.*, 1981). What is noteworthy about the calcium buffer in the rod outer segment by comparison with that in other cells is how weak the intracellular buffering actually is: in most cells far fewer than one in twenty of the calcium ions entering the cell would be free, and the intracellular buffers in most cells (sarcoplasmic reticulum, mitochondria, etc.) are more complex in their behaviour than the simple and rapidly reversible system observed in the rod outer segment.

The picture of calcium handling in the rod outer segment which emerges from these experiments can be summarized as follows: the outer segment membrane in darkness is quite permeable to calcium, and the rapid influx through the light-sensitive channels is matched by an equally rapid efflux carried by an active $4Na^+:1Ca^{2+},1K^+$ exchange mechanism. Rather little of the calcium entering the cell is bound, at least on a time scale of a few seconds, and consequently the exchangeable calcium in the outer segment turns over with a short time constant, of about 0.5 seconds. A bright light closes the light-sensitive channels, making the outer segment membrane almost totally impermeable to calcium, and consequently the internal Ca declines rapidly after the flash. These observations and others have suggested to a number of workers that calcium might be the internal transmitter for light adaptation, and there is now a considerable amount of evidence to support this view. It has been known for some time that reducing the activity of the Na:Ca exchange by reducing the external concentration of Na, which produces an increase in free $[Ca]_i$, has effects opposite to those of light adaptation: the

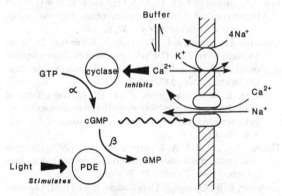

Fig. 6.5. Possible mechanism for the interaction of intracellular calcium ions with the light-sensitive pathway. The rate of formation of cGMP from GTP, α, is increased by a fall in intracellular [Ca] while the rate of hydrolysis of cGMP, β, is increased by light by means of the pathway shown in Fig. 6.1.

response to a weak flash is prolonged and the sensitivity is increased (Yau, McNaughton & Hodgkin, 1981). Similarly, a brief elevation in external Ca prolongs the flash response (Hodgkin, McNaughton & Nunn, 1984). Stabilizing the intracellular Ca by incorporating calcium buffers into the cell should slow changes in free $[Ca]_i$, and the onset of light adaptation in response to a weak step of light is also found to be slowed (Torre, Matthews & Lamb, 1986).

The main open question is: at which point in the light-sensitive pathway does calcium act? There is good evidence for an action of calcium in inhibiting the guanylate cyclase responsible for producing cGMP (see above), and it seems likely that some of the effects

of light adaptation are produced by this means. The mechanism is outlined in Fig. 6.5: switching on a steady light closes light-sensitive channels, thereby blocking part of the calcium influx and causing a decline in free $[Ca]_i$. This decline in free $[Ca]_i$ releases the guanylate cyclase from inhibition, increasing the production of cGMP and thus causing a partial recovery of the lightsensitive current. This kind of negative feedback mechanism is clearly what is required to explain light adaptation, but it may not be the whole story and an interaction of calcium with the light-sensitive pathway at one or more of the stages coupling an isomerized rhodopsin to the phosphodiesterase remains an open possibility.

References

Barlow, H. B. (1957) Increment thresholds at low intensities considered as signal/noise discriminations. *J. Physiol.*, **136**, 469.

Baylor, D. A., Lamb, T. D. & Yau, K-W. (1979) Responses of retinal rods to single photons. *J. Physiol.*, **288**, 613.

Baylor, D. A., Matthews, G. & Yau, K-W. (1980) Two components of electrical dark noise in toad retinal rod outer segments. *J. Physiol.*, **309**, 591.

Baylor, D. A. & Nunn, B. J. (1986) Electrical properties of the light-sensitive conductance of rods of the salamander *Ambystoma tigrinum*. *J. Physiol.*, **371**, 115–45.

Baylor, D. A., Nunn, B. J. & Schnapf, J. L. (1984) The photocurrent, noise and spectral sensitivity of rods of the monkey *Macaca fascicularis*. *J. Physiol.*, **357**, 575.

Bodoia, R. D. & Detwiler, P. B. (1985) Patch-clamp recordings of the light-sensitive dark noise in retinal rods from the lizard and frog. *J. Physiol.*, **367**, 183–216.

Bok, D., quoted in Fain, G. L. & Lisman, J. E. (1981) Membrane conductances of photoreceptors. *Progress in Biophysics and Molecular Biology*, **37**, 91–147.

Cervetto, L., Lagnado, L., Perry, R. J., Robinson, D. W. & McNaughton, P. A. (1989) Extrusion of calcium from rod outer segments is driven by both sodium and potassium gradients. *Nature*, **337**, 740–3.

Cervetto, L. & McNaughton, P. A. (1986) The effects of phosphodiesterase inhibitors and lanthanum ions on the light-sensitive current of toad retinal rods. *J. Physiol.*, **370**, 91–109.

Cohen, A. I., Hall, I. A. & Ferrendelli, J. A. (1978) Calcium and cyclic nucleotide regulation in incubated mouse retinas. *J. Gen. Physiol.*, **71**, 595–612.

Detwiler, P. B., Conner, J. D. & Bodoia, R. D. (1982) Gigaseal patch clamp recording from outer segments of intact retinal rods. *Nature*, **300**, 59–61.

Fesenko, E. E., Kolesnikov, S. S. & Lyubarsky, A. L. (1985) Induction by cyclic GMP of cationic conductance in plasma membrane of retinal rod outer segment. *Nature*, **313**, 310–13.

Goldberg, N. D., Ames, A., Gander, J. E. & Walseth, T. F. (1983) Maganitude of increase in retinal cGMP metabolic flux determined by ^{18}O incorporation into nucleotide L-phosphoryls corresponds with intensity of photic stimulation. *J. Biol. Chem.*, **258**, 9213–19.

Gray, P. & Attwell, D. (1985) Kinetics of light-sensitive channels in vertebrate photoreceptors. *Proc. Roy. Soc.*, **B223**, 379–88.

Haynes, L. W., Kay, A. R. & Yau, K-W. (1986) Single cyclic GMP-activated channel activity in excised patches of rod outer segment membrane. *Nature*, **321**, 66–70.

Hodgkin, A. L., McNaughton, P. A. & Nunn, B. J. (1984) Comparison between the effects of flashes of light and brief pulses of calcium on the current of toad and salamander rods. *J. Physiol.*, **357**, 10P.

Hodgkin, A. L., McNaughton, P. A. & Nunn, B. J. (1985) The ionic selectivity and calcium dependence of the light-sensitive pathway in toad rods. *J. Physiol.*, **358**, 447–68.

Hodgkin, A. L., McNaughton, P. A. & Nunn, B. J. (1987) Measurement of sodium–calcium exchange in salamander rods. *J. Physiol.*, **391**, 347–70.

Hodgkin, A. L. & Nunn, B. J. (1987) The effect of ions on sodium–calcium exchange in salamander rods. *J. Physiol.*, **391**, 371–98.

Koch, K-W. & Stryer, L. (1988) Highly cooperative feedback control of retinal rod guanylate cyclase by calcium ions. *Nature*, **334**, 64–6.

Kühn, H., Hall, S. W. & Wilden, U. (1984) Light-induced binding of 48-kDa protein to photoreceptor membranes is highly enhanced by phosphorylation of rhodopsin. *FEBS Letters*, **176**, 473–8.

Lagnado, L. & McNaughton, P. A. (1987a) Light responses and Na:Ca exchange in isolated salamander rod outer segments. *J. Physiol.*, **390**, 11P.

Lagnado, L. & McNaughton, P. A. (1987b) Voltage dependence of Na:Ca exchange in isolated salamander rod outer segments. *J. Physiol.*, **390**, 162P.

Lolley, R. N. & Racz, E. (1982) Calcium modulation of cyclic GMP synthesis in rat visual cells. *Vision Res.*, **22**, 1481–6.

McLaughlin, S., Mulrine, N., Gresalfi, T., Vaio, G. &

McLaughlin, A. (1981) The adsorption of divalent cations to bilayer membranes containing phosphatidyl-serine. *J. Gen. Physiol.*, **77**, 445–73.

McNaughton, P. A., Cervetto, L. & Nunn, B. J. (1986) Measurement of the intracellular free calcium concentration in salamander rods. *Nature*, **322**, 261–3.

Nakamura, T. & Gold, G. H. (1987) A cyclic nucleotide-gated conductance in olfactory receptor cilia. *Nature*, **325**, 442–4.

Pace, U., Hanski, E., Salomon, Y. & Lancet, D. (1985) Odorant-sensitive adenylate cyclase may mediate olfactory reception. *Nature*, **316**, 255–8.

Pepe, I. M., Panfoli, I. & Cugnoli, C. (1986) Guanylate cyclase in rod outer segments of the toad retina: effect of light and Ca^{2+}. *FEBS Letters*, **203**, 73–6.

Stryer, L. (1986) Cyclic GMP cascade of vision. *Ann. Rev. Neurosci.*, **9**, 87–119.

Torre, V., Matthews, H. R. & Lamb, T. D. (1986) Role of calcium in regulating the cyclic GMP cascade of phototransduction in retinal rods. *Proc. Natl. Acad. Sci. USA*, **83**, 7109–13.

Van Dop, C., Yamanaka, G., Steinberg, F., Sekura, R. D., Mandark, C. R., Stryer, L. & Bourne, H. R. (1984) ADP-ribosylation of transducin by pertussis toxin blocks the light-stimulated hydrolysis of GTP and cGMP in retinal photoreceptors. *J. Biol. Chem.*, **259**, 23–6.

Yau, K-W., McNaughton, P. A. & Hodgkin, A. L. (1981) Effect of ions on the light-sensitive current in retinal rods. *Nature*, **292**, 502–5.

Yau, K-W. & Nakatani, K. (1984a) Cation selectivity of light-sensitive conductance in retinal rods. *Nature*, **309**, 352–4.

Yau, K-W. & Nakatani K. (1984b) Electrogenic Na–Ca exchange in retinal rod outer segment. *Nature*, **311**, 661–3.

Yau, K-W. & Nakatani, K. (1985) Light-induced reduction of cytoplasmic free calcium in retinal rod outer segment. *Nature*, **313**, 579–82.

Zimmerman, A. L. & Baylor, D. A. (1986) Cyclic GMP-sensitive conductance of retinal rods consists of aqueous pores. *Nature*, **321**, 70.

7

Is there more than meets the eye?

D. I. Vaney and A. A. Hughes

In a recent review entitled 'Why can't the eye see better?', Horace Barlow (1986) discussed how optical factors, photoreceptor characteristics and the dynamic range of retinal ganglion cells limit visual performance. Barlow's question, like all good riddles, demands a shift in perspective before it can be tackled. In this essay we pose a complementary puzzle, 'is there more than meets the eye?' Although there is no doubt that much remains to be discovered about the retina, we question whether the apparent simplicity of retinal function critically underestimates the sophistication of early stages of visual processing.

The complexity of visual coding by retinal ganglion cells is often presented in terms of those receptive field characteristics that may provide the neural substrate for psychophysical phenomena. Thus the centre–surround organization of concentric cells is related to the coding of chromatic or luminance contrast; the On and Off pathways underpin the efficient signalling of increased light and darkness; the spatial and temporal properties of X and Y ganglion cells seem matched to the requirements of pattern vision and motion detection. Although this approach has inherent appeal, the sophistication that psychophysicists and central physiologists demand of retinal function is, in fact, rather limited.

Hierarchical concepts of visual processing deny to retinal function those characteristics that are presently perceived to be intrinsic to cortical function. For example, the long-range horizontal interactions between cortical modules are thought to underlie such diverse processes as vernier acuity and figure–ground discrimination. In the retina, however, the many amacrine connections beyond the classic receptive field are credited with little more than producing the periphery effect. The emphasis on vertical integration within the retina ignores the considerable potential for physiological interactions between neurons serving adjacent or isolated retinal fields.

This narrow view of retinal complexity has remained intact because it is braced by convergent physiological and psychophysical ideas. However, if we now ask 'What could the retina do?', our perspective is broadened. If it is accepted that the complexity of neuronal hardware is reflected in the sophistication of visual processing, then demonstration of unexpected diversity in the structure and connectivity of retinal neurons might point to novel coding capabilities.

Neuronal diversity and coding complexity

Twenty years ago, Werblin & Dowling (1969) proposed that simple circuits, involving a handful of interneurons converging on a retinal ganglion cell, could give rise to concentric fields with transient or sustained responses. In the outer retina, luminance coding by the photoreceptors is transformed through signal averaging and multiplicative feedback into contrast coding by the bipolar cells. Although these second-order neurons code relatively simple information, the shift from photopic to scotopic vision is a delicate process, requiring changes in photoreceptor and horizontal cell coupling, as well as the ordered recruitment of bipolar and amacrine cells in the rod-signal pathway. Such adaptive processes may themselves be intricate without increasing the complexity of visual coding.

In the inner retina, bipolar convergence accounts for increased receptive field size, and complementary push–pull inputs may enhance the dynamic range and gain of the signal. Lateral to this direct pathway, amacrine cells probably generate the

Box 1. How many types of retinal neurons?

The five major classes of retinal neurons include many subtypes, each with a characteristic dendritic morphology that receives a stereotyped input from a restricted range of neurons. Consequently, the receptive field properties and visual responses of each retinal type are distinctive and, when transmitted to selective output neurons, lay the foundation for the parallel processing of visual information. The number and diversity of neuronal type thus provide a useful measure of the complexity of retinal processing.

In mammalian retina, simple interactions between three or four types of photoreceptors and two types of horizontal cells shape the response properties of the bipolar cells. Multiple types of bipolars can be distinguished by their receptor contacts, dendritic spread and axonal lamination; they form dichotomies according to whether they serve photopic or scotopic vision, long or short wavelength cones, On- or Off-centre ganglion cells, and perhaps an excitatory or inhibitory function.

Although physiological analysis indicates that there are at least 13 types of ganglion cells in cat retina, the relative density of each is only known for the four brisk-concentric types (On and Off Y-cells, On and Off X-cells). Their morphological correlates, the alpha and beta cells, account for 50% of the 170 000 ganglion cells in cat retina. Are there enough ganglion cells left over to provide continuous coverage of the retina by each of the sluggish-concentric and non-concentric types? Assuming that each ganglion cell type achieves three-fold coverage by the receptive field centre (compared with 2.75 for Off-centre Y-cells), Levick (1986) estimated that only 45 000 additional ganglion cells would be required (Fig. 7.1A). The Y-cells and larger non-concentric types achieve complete retinal coverage with 3000 cells or less, representing only 2% of the ganglion cell total.

Using Golgi methods, Kolb *et al.* (1981) distinguished 22 types of amacrine cells in cat retina on the basis of field size, branching pattern and dendritic stratification. Apart from the problems of identifying a neuronal type from only one or a few stained cells, it is inevitable that many types will not be represented in such samples. Similarly, evaluations of amacrine heterogeneity based on pharmacological diversity are limited by the histochemical probes available. We have sought an objective estimate of the number of amacrine types in rabbit retina, based on the relative incidence of 13 amacrine populations whose cellular distribution, dendritic morphology and transmitter content have been characterized: the sample ranges from the dense AII amacrines to the sparse dopaminergic cells. The 13 types account for about 25% of neurons in the amacrine sublayer, suggesting that there are 40 to 50 amacrine types in total (Fig. 7.1B). It thus appears that there are 70 to 80 neuronal types in mammalian retina, and even a three figure total does not seem implausible.

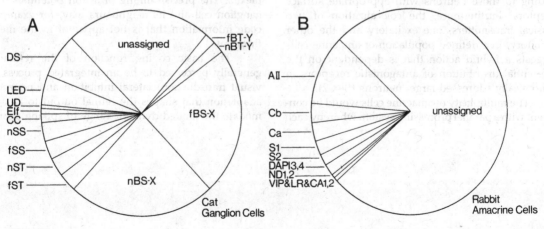

Fig. 7.1.

antagonistic surround, which appears qualitatively different from the multiplicative bipolar surround. In mammalian retina, a well defined amacrine system channels the output from rod bipolars into the On and Off pathways, and the periphery effect must also be amacrine mediated.

It seems, however, that these diverse functions account for only a fraction of the processing capability of amacrine cells. Even allowing for the intricate neural interactions that underlie non-concentric ganglion cells, such as the generation of direction selectivity, there are many more amacrine types and related circuits than are required by present wiring schemes.

The density distribution of 13 diverse types of amacrine cells have been mapped in the rabbit retina: they comprise only 25% of all amacrines, suggesting that there are 40 to 50 amacrine types in total (Box 1). Of these, only the cholinergic, dopaminergic and rod (AII and 'reciprocal') amacrine systems are regarded as well characterized. The limitations of our understanding are starkly underlined, however, by the recent finding that cholinergic amacrine cells in mammalian retinae also contain the inhibitory transmitter GABA and its synthetic enzyme.

Most of the neurotransmitters and neuromodulators found in the brain have been localized in the vertebrate retina, usually in specific populations of amacrine cells. This pharmacological diversity underpins a wide range of neuronal interactions, and allows a subtlety of effect that presently escapes the microelectrode. At one level is the distinction between 'anatomically addressed' transmitters which act directly on the postsynaptic cell, and 'chemically addressed' transmitters which spread diffusely before binding to those neurons with appropriate surface receptors. Furthermore, the colocalization of two classical transmitters, one excitatory and the other inhibitory, in a defined population of amacrine cells suggests a hybrid action that is dependent on the differential distribution of antagonistic receptors in anatomically addressed target neurons (Box 2).

The multiplicity of amacrine cells would be consistent with a parallel processing system whereby each type of ganglion cell receives input from a few specific types of amacrines. However, this does not seem to be the case. Application of selective agonists and antagonists to the retina indicates that, in general, each neurotransmitter has diverse effects on the receptive field properties of a wide range of ganglion cells. While this is not unexpected for ubiquitous transmitters such as GABA or glycine, it is surprising for the cholinergic amacrines, whose narrowly stratified processes are coextensive with only a few types of ganglion cells.

In principle then, a ganglion cell that branches in both the On and Off sublaminae, may receive either a direct or modulatory input from some 60 types of retinal interneurons. It becomes apparent that a comprehensive wiring diagram of the retina, specifying all the components and their synaptic connections, may only be of limited utility in understanding how the retina processes visual information: the dynamic interactions of such a complex system, involving a plethora of receptors, cannot be predicted simply by assessing which inputs are sequentially active.

Text books still emphasize that information flow in the retina is unidirectional, despite increasing evidence to the contrary. Most local circuits in the retina provide facility for neuronal feedback, and a variety of specialized systems, such as the interplexiform network, the superficial plexus and the centrifugal fibres, specifically serve this function. While it is widely accepted that negative feedback at the amacrine level may sharpen the response properties of transient ganglion cells, there is little consensus concerning the function of recurrent synapses from ganglion cell dendrites to amacrine processes, and from ganglion cell axons to processes in the superficial plexus. The precise timing of action potentials in a ganglion cell and its neighbours may, for example, code information that is not apparent in the mean firing rate.

The basic coding function of the retina is generally perceived to be an integrated process of visual transduction, lateral inhibition and neuronal adaptation that shapes the retinal output to accommodate the limited dynamic range of spiking axons.

Box 2. GABA, GABA, everywhere

Barlow & Levick's (1965) hypothesis that horizontal cells provide the asymmetric inhibition necessary for direction selectivity was overturned by the finding that GABAergic antagonists abolish the selectivity of directional ganglion cells in rabbit retina. It was argued that because GABA is an amacrine cell transmitter, direction selectivity must be a property of the inner retina, a conclusion now supported by other studies. GABA is indeed a ubiquitous transmitter in the inner plexiform layer, being synthesized by every third amacrine cell. However, recent studies on rabbit retina indicate that interplexiform cells are also GABA-positive; Barlow's wiring scheme was therefore dismissed prematurely, particularly in the light of DeVoe's novel finding that some bipolar cells in turtle retina show a form of direction selectivity.

Many of the ganglion cells in rabbit retina are also GABA-immunoreactive and, in monkey retina, about 25% of the photoreceptors synthesize GABA. The widespread distribution of GABA in the retina indicates that pharmacological dissection of these pathways must be interpreted with caution, but there is consensus that the temporal processing of complex visual information is largely mediated by amacrine cell inhibition in the inner plexiform layer. We also find varicose GABA-positive processes in the nerve fibre layer of rabbit retina: they arise from the inner plexiform layer, divide repeatedly and are not aligned with the fibre bundles (Fig. 7.2A). These processes are thus distinct from optic axons and may be amacrine dendrites contributing to the superficial plexus.

It seems possible that the morphological diversity of GABAergic amacrine cells may be matched by a pharmacological diversity, such that each type has a unique neurochemical 'signature'. In mammalian retinae, distinct populations of GABA-immunoreactive amacrines have been identified that either accumulate serotonin, show NADPH-diaphorase activity, or contain dopamine, substance P or acetylcholine, as illustrated below. The fluorescent dye DAPI selectively stains the array of displaced cholinergic amacrines in the ganglion cell layer of rabbit retina (Fig. 7.2B); all are strongly labelled following reaction with a GABA antiserum (Fig. 7.2C). The coexistence of acetylcholine and GABA in the interneurons presynaptic to direction selective ganglion cells is of particular interest, because non-linear interactions between these transmitters appear to underlie the mechanism of direction selectivity. With appropriate wiring, the centrifugal segregation of input and output synapses on cholinergic amacrines could provide the asymmetric inhibition necessary for direction selectivity; we propose that ganglion cells which respond to different preferred directions receive synaptic input from different segments of the cholinergic dendritic field.

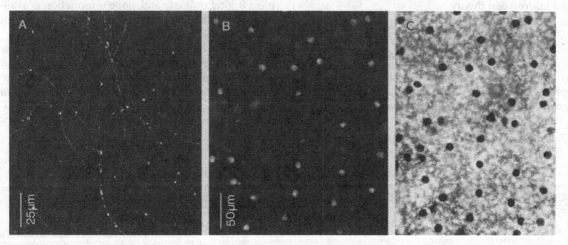

Fig. 7.2.

However, these are essentially outer plexiform functions and the much thicker, inner plexiform layer might seem superfluous, particularly so in the primate fovea, where the midget system preserves the photoreceptor grain in multiple arrays of concentric ganglion cells. If there is much more to retinal coding (complex receptive fields notwithstanding), the mechanisms in question must involve sophisticated processing by the amacrine cells.

The operational unit of amacrine function ranges, according to cell type, from a single dendritic varicosity or branch of the dendritic tree to a local neuronal plexus formed by overlapping dendritic fields (Box 3). The multiple strategies for spatial sampling adopted by amacrine cells contrast with the unitary organization of other retinal neurons, which integrate incoming signals within territorially distinct dendritic fields. Thus, the morphological and pharmacological diversity of retinal amacrine cells provides only a base measure of the complexity of inner retina processing. The extensive dendritic field overlap of many amacrine types provides an added dimension whose consequences for visual processing are unpredictable and not presently amenable to experimental investigation.

Recent advances in retinal research thus serve to reinforce the empirical belief that the complexity of early visual processing can be properly assessed only at the ganglion cell level: all the information available to higher visual centres must be coded in the firing of the optic nerve fibres. However, current research does challenge us to reassess what the eye is telling the brain. Classic methods of receptive field analysis will have a role in this process, but they must be combined with complementary tools from biological cybernetics and information theory.

Visual coding: optimization

In 1959, Barlow summarized the classic approach to optimally encoding information so as to ensure, in accord with the principles of Shannon & Weaver (1949), the efficient transfer of information from one region of the nervous system to another without loss. Such encoding strips away predictability, or redundancy, and effects a more compact representation of information. Throughout his account, Barlow described such a system as having an 'output' in the form of a 'display' without redundancy. This optimization is thus primarily concerned with the transfer of information, not its analysis. At some level the non-redundant display was envisaged to be employed by the nervous system for finding useful sensory associations.

Concentric units have long been regarded as sampling apertures which basically relay an image for such higher level processing. It is generally assumed that beta cells, brisk-sustained X-units, have the ability to provide a substrate for pattern vision by transmitting all the information necessary for a potentially reconstructible neural representation of the optical image. We know enough about the beta cells in the cat to be able to discuss the relationship between receptive field size, spatial cut-off frequency and cell density in some detail, given simple information theory concepts and the assumption that they form a straightforward array of sampling apertures.

The brain may employ two separate maps, one On and one Off, to reconstruct the world from their rectified information. Alternatively, On and Off cells may form a unified sampling array of interdigitated functional pairs with their dendritic and receptive fields displaced relative to one another (Box 4). The latter organization suggests goals additional to neuronal impulse economy. Sophisticated versions of the sampling theorem would permit the attainment of greater resolving power from a given number of samplers if local ordinate and slope information is available about the image brightness over a range of orientations.

Simple cells form a commonly encountered class involved at an early stage of cortical processing and may mimimally obtain the input from one or more pairs of adjacent On and Off beta cells. The output of such cells might be regarded as a band limited deriva-

Box 3. Spatial sampling by retinal amacrine cells

The remarkable diversity in the morphology and pharmacology of retinal amacrine cells is not reflected physiologically in their receptive field properties. However, the visual responses recorded at the cell body may not be representative of the activity in amacrine dendrites: the close apposition of input and output synapses provides scope for local interactions that may be highly non-linear in character and isolated from activity elsewhere in the dendritic field. The diversity of amacrine function can be inferred from the unexpected variety in the coverage patterns of different types. Wässle (1986) has shown that retinal neurons which integrate signals over the whole dendritic field, such as horizontal cells and ganglion cells, form distinct territories with each point on the retina overlapped by only a few cells of each type. The regular distribution of their dendritic fields thus provides efficient sampling of the visual space.

Such territorial organization is shown by AII amacrine cells, which are the interneurons between rod bipolars and retinal ganglion cells. The three-fold overlap of their dendritic fields in cat retina is comparable to that of the beta ganglion cells. Only five AII amacrines converge on each beta cell, and their narrow-field organization thus preserves the receptive-field centre size under scotopic conditions.

The spatial organization of medium and wide-field amacrine cells is quite different. The cholinergic amacrines in rabbit retina, for example, comprise two matching populations whose processes are narrowly stratified in the On and Off sublaminae of the inner plexiform layer. The dendritic overlap of each type is ten times that of integrating neurons, ranging from 25 to 70. Although the 50–80 terminal dendrites of a cholinergic amacrine are closely spaced, a group of distal terminals may be separated from an adjacent group by a thin dendritic path, 200–800 μm long (Fig. 7.3A): a single arborization may thus comprise multiple subunits. The cholinergic plexus has a striking fasciculated topology that appears to match the looping morphology of the post-synaptic, On-Off direction selective ganglion cells.

By contrast, serotonin-accumulating amacrines in rabbit retina blanket the inner margin of the plexiform layer, forming a rich plexus interrupted only by Müller stalks. The two types involved, termed S1 and S2 amacrines, have similar density distributions but the dendritic field size of S1 cells (Fig. 7.3B, left) is four times that of S2 cells (right). Each S1 amacrine gives rise to 19–30 thin radial processes that extend for 600–1700 μm; consequently their dendritic field overlap is extraordinary, ranging from 550 to 900. Each square millimetre of retina thus contains 6–8 metres of S1 dendrites and, woven as a cloth, these fibres would have a spacing of only 0.3 μm. Such a pervasive neuropil may provide an effective substrate for diffuse transmitter release, as proposed for serotonergic fibres elsewhere in the nervous system.

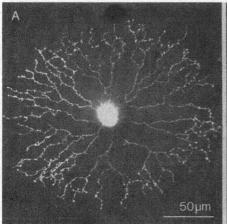
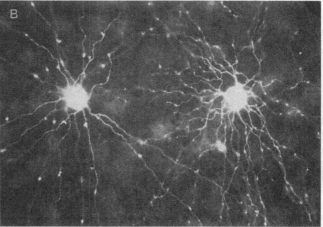

50μm

Fig. 7.3.

Box 4. Beta cells: A dichotomous or unitary system?

The cat's area of best vision contains 1000 cones per square degree. Shannon's sampling theorem thus suggests a potential grating resolution of 16 cycles per degree. This cannot be achieved in a generalized task because the peak density of ganglion cells relaying information to the brain is only 400 cells per square degree, and this population comprises at least 13 functional types of units.

What proportion of the ganglion cells could relay a generalized image to the brain? Indeed, do any of the ganglion cell types function as ideal samplers? The sustained response and linear summation of X ganglion cells make them candidates for such a task. Their morphological correlate, the beta cells, comprise half the ganglion cell population and have the highest density of any type, 264 ganglion cells per square degree in the central area. On this basis they could resolve a grating of some 8 cycles per degree, a value close to that claimed for the cat in psychophysical experiments. The system thus behaves as if the beta cells are independent sampling apertures. However, there is a problem. In this analysis the beta cells are treated as one population, but they actually comprise equal numbers of functionally distinct On (Fig. 7.4A) and Off (Fig. 7.4B) subtypes. Barlow (1986) suggested that the On and Off dichotomy economizes on nerve impulses. A cell signalling both an increase and a decrease in brightness would require a high maintained firing rate to permit appropriate modulation. Two channels would also double the dynamic range of the system.

We might thus expect On and Off beta cells to occur in functional pairs, each forming half of the channel sampling a given region of visual space. The effective sampling density would then be halved, and the beta array would attain a maximum grating resolution of only 5.5 cycles per degree.

Spatial irregularity of the sampling array must reduce the reconstruction quality of the image, although elaborate algorithms can minimize this effect. Wässle *et al.* (1981) argued that, because the array regularity of the On or the Off beta cells is greater than that of the combined population, they do not function cooperatively but rather form separate systems. However, the dendritic trees of each array are distributed more regularly than their cell bodies, so the regularity of the receptive fields of the combined beta population may yet approach that of the subtypes.

Although the On and Off cell bodies are necessarily physically separated in the retinal ganglion cell layer, the dendritic trees ramify respectively in the On and Off sublaminae of the inner plexiform layer. If the On and Off cells do comprise functional halves of one channel, then the dendritic trees and receptive fields of an adjacent beta pair might be expected to overlap completely. However, when the dendritic trees of neighbouring On and Off beta cells are injected with dye they do not occupy the same field. This argues against the single channel concept.

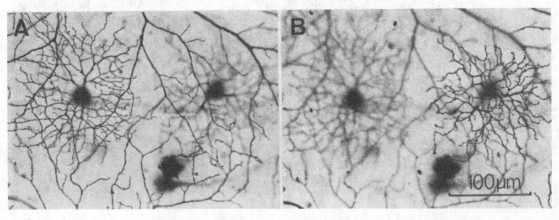

Fig. 7.4.

tive of the retinal image. A given beta cell can be combined with neighbours of the opposite class over a range of retinal sectors, to generate cortical simple cells of differing orientation selectivity. An inhomogeneous array of retinal cells thus potentially contains the information necessary for a grating resolution close to that of a homogeneous population of sampling apertures of the small density if it is analysed appropriately. Thus cortical orientation selectivity might be regarded as a passive outcome of an optimal encoding strategy. Of course, this does not preclude more analytic roles, such as orientation detection, for such cells.

For efficiency, in the absence of noise, an optimal system encodes at each level only that information which will be used at the next; the information will also be coded in a manner which permits functional access by the system at the next stage. The strategy at a given stage reflects those which precede and follow. System design should thus be influenced by bottom-up and top-down factors. If the more complex models of beta cell function are valid, it is apparent that the cortical mechanisms may be linked in such a fashion with the spatial arrays and properties of retinal cells.

To help assess the validity of the models we require knowledge, as yet unavailable, of the cat's psychophysical grating resolution as distinct from its ability to detect gratings. The animal resolves gratings of 5 cycles per degree but acuities of over 10 cycles have been reported. Confirmation of higher resolutions by means of orientation discrimination tasks would minimize the possibility of simple detection and lend support to the more sophisticated models. There are simply not enough beta cells to attain a high grating resolution from independent On and Off sampling arrays.

Since Kuffler's time, our puzzlement as to retinal function has increased with the discovery of so many classes of receptive field. In principle, their specialized information might be reconstructed from the beta cell array by high level analysis, if the fields were ideal sampling apertures. The avoidance of the reconstruction task by introducing non-concentric receptive fields to provide suitable information to brain areas involved in specific tasks is understandable. In cat and rabbit, however, nearly all classes of retinal receptive field project to the visual cortex as well as to specialized midbrain sites. The failure of the beta system to relay certain spatial and temporal information from the photoreceptor array may require other types of receptive field to fill the gap. No theoretical analysis has yet been attempted for such

fields. We do not know if they have an independent representation at the cortical level or function as one system involving the beta cells.

Visual coding: integration

Craik (1967) suggested that the nervous system embodies a model of the environment. Optimal encoding may provide for information transfer without loss but it also incorporates a partial model of the significant habitat. When information is reduced or compacted, optimization introduces information about the world because some of the redundancies eliminated have their origin in the visual environment itself. Photoreceptors may have photopigments matched in sensitivity to the wavelengths of light available at the place and time the animal is active. The presence of uniformity in the visual image permits the use of lateral inhibition and predictive coding for economy of signalling.

However, much additional redundancy may be eliminated by the selective acquisition of only that subset of visual features of importance to the species. Colour-opponent cells may be organized in an optimal manner with respect to the cone pigments present; their number does not appear to be determined by properties of the external world. High retinal cell densities, such as an area or fovea, are selectively located to deal with parts of the visual field important in terms of the animal's lifestyle, rather than with overt features of the visual world. In this sense, the retina may already be regarded as involved in something more than optimal information transfer.

If the lifestyle of the species drives the redundancy elimination of topographic sampling and information processing then its primary determinants are genetically encoded. There will be wide variation in the weighting and analysis of different regions of visual field according to lifestyle.

Is the complexity of the retina relative to its known functions too high? The observed degree of complexity may simply be available to ensure reliable function or provide some degree of context-dependent redundancy in addition to the basic context-free encoding. To tackle such questions we need insight into the manner in which the visual system achieves integrative processing. The information theory approach emphasizes topographic sampling, the location of edges, shapes and colour within real or Fourier space and, perhaps at some higher level, the recognition of objects by pontifical cells uniquely tuned to given inputs. McKay (1986) has described these as systems embodying an *explicit* neural image of the world but the nature of the display and its use remain problematic.

By contrast, McKay suggests a visual system with 'conditional readiness for action' in which the external world is represented *implicitly*. The neural apparatus would be organized to seek covariation in its input, as represented in parallel analysers, separately identifying object components, elements of given distance and regions of colour which move together. Features of the world remain represented only in this most general sense as a state of the system which controls its present motor activity.

Our current understanding is open. The beta system may provide an *explicit*, relatively independent, information source for pattern recognition; other classes of cell being involved in activities as yet undetermined. Alternatively, the retina may comprise a set of parallel channels, the beta system not providing an *explicit* relay of the information required but rather contributing to an *implicit* system.

The psychophysics of vision begin with the 'given' features of cortical organization, orientation selectivity, colour, binocularity etc. and regard the 'ill-posed problem' facing the brain as one of reconstructing as near as possible an accurate representation of the world in which the animal moves, eats, and is eaten, from information so reduced by the ocular apparatus as to permit many, non-unique solutions. The role of the retina is neglected. In this sense little has changed since 1604. In his *Ad Vitellionem Paralipomena*, Kepler left the function of the retina for posterity to solve:

> Here the image or picture is composed by the visual spirits that reside in the retina and the nerve, and whether it is made to appear before the soul or the tribunal of the visual faculty by a spirit in the hollows of the brain, or whether the visual faculty, like a magistrate sent by the soul, goes forth from the administrative chamber of the brain into the optic nerve and retina to meet this image, as though descending to a lower court – I leave to be disputed. . . .

It is apparent that limited cortical facilities for sensory information processing must be competing for space and that selective pressure will ensure retinal encoding provides a minimal demand on central analysis in terms of the balance of requirements in a given lifestyle. Thus the brain, through evolutionary experience, determines retinal structure and processing, perhaps establishing a strategy common across the vertebrates.

Is there any bottom-up determination in the system? In a sense, yes, if the optics are seen as potentially flexible in design and determined by central needs, an ultimate limit is set by the information available from the environment. However, we do not see this as determining retinal design *per se*. Rather, the lifestyle of a species establishes the redundancies employed and the subset of available information accessed as relevant. It remains one of our most challenging problems to determine whether the emerging complexity of retinal architecture will indicate substantially greater variety of adaptation to given lifestyles than are presently apparent.

Acknowledgements

Figure 7.4 was kindly provided by Brian Boycott and Heinz Wässle. The authors acknowledge the support of the National Health and Medical Research Council. NVRI is an affiliate institute of the University of Melbourne.

References

Ariel, M. & Daw, N, W. (1982) Pharmacological analysis of directionally sensitive rabbit retinal ganglion cells. *J. Physiol.*, **324**, 161–85.

Barlow, H. B. (1959) Sensory mechanisms, the reduction of redundancy, and intelligence. In *Mechanisation of Thought Processes*. National Physical Laboratory Symposium No. 10. London: HMSO.

Barlow, H. B. (1986) Why can't the eye see better? In *Visual Neuroscience*, ed. J. D. Pettigrew, K. J. Sanderson & W. R. Levick, pp. 3–18. Cambridge: Cambridge University Press.

Barlow, H. B. & Levick, W. R. (1965) The mechanism of directionally selective units in rabbit's retina. *J. Physiol.*, **178**, 477–504.

Brecha, N. C., Eldred, W., Kuljis, R. O. & Karten, H. J. (1984) Identification and localization of biologically active peptides in the vertebrate retina. *Progr. Retinal Res.*, **3**, 185–226.

Buchsbaum, G. & Gottshalk, A. (1983) Trichromacy, opponent colour coding and optimum information transmission in the retina. *Proc. Roy. Soc. Lond.* B**220**, 89–113.

Cleland, B. G., Harding, T. & Tulunay-Keesey, U. (1979) Visual resolution and receptive field size: examination of two kinds of cat retinal ganglion cell. *Science*, **205**, 1015–17.

Craik, K. J. W. (1967) *The Nature of Explanation*. Cambridge: Cambridge University Press.

French, A. S., Snyder, A. W. & Stavenga, D. G. (1977) Image degradation by an irregular retinal mosaic. *Biol. Cybern.*, **27**, 229–33.

Hughes, A. (1977) The topography of vision in mammals of

contrasting lifestyle: Comparative optics and retinal organisation. In *Handbook of Sensory Physiology*, Vol. VII/5, The Visual System in Vertebrates, ed. F. Crescitelli, pp. 697–756. Berlin: Springer-Verlag.

Hughes, A. (1981) Cat retina and the sampling theorem; the relation of transient and sustained brisk-unit cut-off frequency to α and β-mode cell density. *Exp. Brain Res.*, **42**, 196–202.

Hughes, A. (1985) New perspectives in retinal organisation. *Progr. Retinal Res.*, **4**, 243–313.

Koch, C. & Poggio, T. (1987) Biophysics of computation: neurons, synapses, and membranes. In *Synaptic Function*, ed. G. M. Edelman, W. E. Gall & W. M. Cowan, pp. 637–97. New York: John Wiley.

Kolb, H., Nelson, R. & Mariani, A. (1981) Amacrine cells, bipolar cells and ganglion cells of the cat retina: a Golgi study. *Vision Res.*, **21**, 1081–114.

Lam, D. M.-K., Li, H.-B., Su, Y.-Y. T. & Watt, C. B. (1985) The signature hypothesis: co-localizations of neuroactive substances as anatomical probes for circuitry analyses. *Vision Res.*, **25**, 1353–64.

Levick, W. R. (1986) Sampling of information space by retinal ganglion cells. In *Visual Neuroscience*, ed. J. D. Pettigrew, K. J. Sanderson & W. R. Levick, pp. 33–43. Cambridge: Cambridge University Press.

Masland, R. H. & Tauchi, M. (1986) The cholinergic amacrine cell. *Trends Neurosci.*, **9**, 218–23.

McKay, D. M. (1986) Vision – the capture of optical co-variation. In *Visual Neuroscience*, ed. J. D. Pettigrew, K. J. Sanderson & W. R. Levick, pp. 365–73. Cambridge: Cambridge University Press.

Peichl, L., Ott, H. & Boycott, B. B. (1987) Alpha ganglion cells in mammalian retinae. *Proc. Roy. Soc. Lond.* **B231**, 169–97.

Poggio, T., Torre, V. & Koch, C. (1985) Computational vision and regularisation theory. *Nature*, **317**, 314–19.

Rosenfeld, A. & Kak, A. C. (1981) *Digital Picture Processing*. 2nd edn. New York: Academic Press.

Schall, J. D. & Leventhal, A. G. (1987) Relationships between ganglion cell dendritic structure and retinal topography in the cat. *J. Comp. Neurol.*, **257**, 149–59.

Shannon, C. E. & Weaver, W. (1949) *The Mathematical Theory of Communication*. Urbana Ill: University of Illinois Press.

Soodak, R. E. (1987) The retinal ganglion cell mosaic defines orientation columns in striate cortex. *Proc. Natl. Acad. Sci.*, **84**, 3936–40.

Sterling, P., Freed, M. & Smith, R. G. (1986) Microcircuitry and functional architecture of the cat retina. *Trends Neurosci.*, **9**, 186–92.

Vaney, D. I. (1986) Morphological identification of serotonin-accumulating neurons in the living retina. *Science*, **233**, 444–6.

Vaney, D. I. (1986) Parallel and serial pathways in the inner plexiform layer of the mammalian retina. In *Visual Neuroscience*, ed. J. D. Pettigrew, K. J. Sanderson & W. R. Levick, pp. 44–59. Cambridge: Cambridge University Press.

Vaney, D. I. & Young, H. M. (1988) GABA-like immunoreactivity in cholinergic amacrine cells of the rabbit retina. *Brain Res.*, **438**, 369–73.

Wässle, H., Boycott, B. B. & Illing, R.-B. (1981) Morphology and mosaic of on- and off-beta cells in the cat retina and some functional considerations. *Proc. Roy. Soc. Lond.*, **B212**, 157–75.

Wässle, H. (1986) Sampling of visual space by retinal ganglion cells. In *Visual Neuroscience*, ed. J. D. Pettigrew, K. J. Sanderson & W. R. Levick, pp. 19–32. Cambridge: Cambridge University Press.

Werblin, F. S. & Dowling, J. E. (1969) Organization of the retina of the mudpuppy, *Necturus maculosus*. II. Intracellular recording. *J. Neurophysiol.*, **32**, 339–55.

8

Quantum efficiency and performance of retinal ganglion cells

L. N. Thibos and W. R. Levick

Introduction

What is quantum efficiency? Following Rose's (1946) pioneering work, Horace Barlow provided a clear answer to this question a quarter of a century ago (Barlow, 1962) by defining quantum efficiency as:

$$F = \frac{\text{Least quantity of light theoretically required for performing a task}}{\text{Least quantity required in practice for performing that same task}}$$

Barlow stressed the importance of adhering to a strict definition of what is meant by the overall quantum efficiency of visual performance (Barlow, 1977). The emphasis is appropriate because his equation is more than a mere definition, it is a way of thinking about how real visual detectors behave:

> Now imagine a human subject and an ideal device performing the same task: with no filter in front of it, the ideal device will of course perform better, but by interposing the appropriate filter its performance can be reduced until it matches that achieved by the subject. The fraction of light transmitted by this filter is then equal to the overall quantum efficiency, F, as defined above.
>
> (Barlow, 1962; pp. 155–6).

Barlow's idea was a major step forward for at least three reasons. First, it emphasized the importance of identifying the task. Second, it suggested the use of an absolute standard of comparison, the ideal detector, for assessing the performance of real visual systems. Third, it offered a specific method for making that comparison: handicap the ideal detector until its performance falls to the level of the inferior, real device. In so doing, one obtains a conceptual model of how the real system performs. A real detector acts like an ideal detector looking through a filter that passes only a fraction F of the incoming photons.

Beyond the specification of an absolute figure of merit for real visual detectors, Barlow emphasized that the concept of quantum efficiency is chiefly of interest in leading one to factors *other than* quantum fluctuations that limit performance. In this spirit, we propose to pursue the foregoing ideas by asking: how do we know that it will always be possible to match the performance of a real detector just by placing a neutral filter in front of the hypothetical ideal device? And if it is not possible, what have we learned about those other factors Barlow foresaw?

Performance of an ideal photon detector

To tackle these questions requires that we be more specific about what is meant by 'performance'. Consider the following detection experiment. A steady light source emits P photons per unit time and the signal to be detected is a change of mP photons per unit time, where m is a modulation parameter within the range -1 to $+1$. On some trials just the steady light is present and on other trials the signal occurs. These two conditions are randomly presented with equal probability and the observer's task is to decide after each trial whether or not the stimulus condition had been presented. The observer's performance in this case is given by two numbers:

Y = proportion of trials on which the subject correctly said the signal was present,

X = proportion of trials on which the subject incorrectly said the signal was present.

A simplifying assumption is sometimes made that X, the rate of false-positive responses, is fixed in order that performance may be specified solely by Y, the frequency-of-seeing. In general, however, both X and Y will vary with the detector's decision criterion and so both must be included in a specification of performance. In the context of signal detection theory (Green & Swets, 1966; Egan, 1975), the covariation of Y with X is known as a receiver operating characteristic (ROC) and it is this curve which embodies the various modes in which a given performance is manifested. Assessment of ROC curves is aided by two fiducial lines: the positive diagonal, which indicates chance performance, and the negative diagonal, which is the axis for displaying a special measure of signal detectability called d'.

The design of an ideal detector for an incremental ($m>0$) or for a decremental ($m<0$) change of stimulus luminance is dictated by the statistical nature of light. For low levels of illumination, the arrival of photons may be described by the Poisson random process (Mandel & Wolf, 1965). It is known that the optimal method for detecting an increase in the rate of Poisson events is to count the events (Cox & Lewis, 1966) and decide in favor of the hypothesis of 'stimulus presented' if the number exceeds some criterion. Alternatively, to detect optimally a decrease in mean rate, one should say the stimulus occurred if the number of events is less than some criterion. These decision rules enable the ROC curves for an ideal detector to be determined theoretically from the probability distribution functions for Poisson random variables. It so happens that ideal photon detectors have ROC curves which are very nearly linear when plotted on Gaussian probability cordinates (Thibos, Levick & Cohn, 1979). This simplifies matters considerably because the entire performance curve of the ideal device can be summarized by just two numbers, slope and intercept of the ROC curve with the d' axis. The following approximate formulae for slope and d' in terms of known stimulus parameters P and m were derived:

$$d' \cong |m| P^{1/2}(1+m)^{-1/4} \tag{1}$$

$$\text{slope} \cong (1+m)^{-1/6} \tag{2}$$

Note that these equations reveal two Poisson signatures of quantal fluctuations. First, d' for a decrement stimulus is always greater than d' for an increment stimulus of the same magnitude ($|m|$). Second, ROC slope is greater than unity for decrements and less than unity for increments.

To be a useful model for real visual neurons, the ideal detector must be handicapped in some way so that it performs at the same level. A general way of thinking of this handicap is to envision the stimulus photons traversing a hypothetical 'black box' *en route* to the ideal detector. Inside the box is some mechanism which hampers the detector by changing the mean

rate or modulation of the photon stream. Later on we will be more specific about what might be inside the black box, but for now we need make only one key restriction: that the black box does not alter the essential Poisson nature of quantal fluctuations. Accordingly, we will be considering as a class all those handicap mechanisms for which the stream of output particles emerging from the box remains a Poisson random process. To remind us of this key assumption, we will refer to this kind of handicap as a 'Poisson' box.

Because the output of a Poisson box is a Poisson random process, a simple counter remains the ideal detector of the photic input and its ROC will be a straight line. If P' is the mean rate of events emerging from the Poisson box, and m' is the effective modulation of the output stream caused by the stimulus, then by equations 1, 2, above, the ROC will have intercept and slope:

$$d' \cong |m'| (P')^{1/2}(1+m')^{-1/4} \tag{3}$$

$$\text{slope} \cong (1+m')^{-1/6} \tag{4}$$

Filter handicap

Barlow's proposition was that the black box contains a filter. We conceive of an optical filter as a device which randomly deletes photons and it is known that random deletion of events of a Poisson process preserves the Poisson nature of the process (Parzen, 1962). Therefore, Barlow's handicap qualifies as a Poisson box. Since the filter will reduce the steady light P and the signal mP by the same fraction F, signal modulation is not affected by a filter. Accordingly, the parameters of the ROC curve will be given by equations 3, 4 when we make the substitutions:

$$P' = FP \tag{5}$$

$$m' = m \tag{6}$$

Note that to close approximation, ROC slope for Poisson signals is independent of the mean rate of the steady light and depends only on the amount of signal modulation. Therefore, the handicap imposed by a filter is manifest graphically by a parallel shifting of the ROC curve towards the chance line in accordance with the reduced d'. An example of this behavior is shown in Fig. 8.1A for incremental stimuli and Fig. 8.1B for decremental stimuli of fixed modulation ($|m|=67\%$). In the next section we will compare these theoretical curves against experimental ROCs obtained from retinal neurons.

Performance of cat retinal ganglion cells

In a neurophysiological experiment, detection performance depends not only on the visual neuron being recorded, but also on the fidelity of equipment used to monitor the cell, the measure of neural response extracted by the experimenter and the experimenter's strategy for deciding whether or not the stimulus occurred based solely on the observed response. Since retinal ganglion cells signal visual information to the brain by all-or-none action potentials, the fidelity requirement is met by accurately measuring the time of occurrence of each neural event. What is not so obvious is the best measure of response, which may be different for different types of ganglion cells. The time course of response is perhaps simplest in sustained ganglion cells, which respond to changes in stimulus luminance by a more or less sustained change in their rate of discharge. A natural measure of response for this cell type is the number of nerve impulses occurring during the interval over which the discharge is displaced from that due to the steady light. The decision strategy for an on-type cell (one which increases its discharge rate in response to an incremental stimulus) would then be to say the stimulus occurred if the number of nerve impulses counted is greater than some criterion. Alternatively, if the stimulus to be detected is a decrement, the experimenter should say the stimulus occurred if the number of nerve impulses counted is less than some criterion. If the discharge pattern of a ganglion cell were a Poisson random process, then the foregoing strategy would be the best one. However, this is not a good statistical model for cat retinal ganglion cells (Barlow & Levick, 1969; Barlow, Levick & Yoon, 1971) so it is possible that the above experimental method imposes an additional handicap upon the preparation of which we are not aware.

Many factors can act to reduce ganglion cell performance to a level below the theoretical maximum. The best performance occurs when these biological and experimental factors are minimized and the cell is limited mainly by the quantal fluctuations in the stimulus itself. Such conditions are difficult to achieve experimentally and cells which show evidence of being limited by quantal fluctuations are relatively rare. One such cell provided the data of Fig. 8.1, taken from the study of Levick, Thibos, Cohn, Catanzaro & Barlow (1983). This was a dark adapted, retinal ganglion cell of the on-center, brisk-sustained class. The stimulus configuration was a small spot of light contained within the center component of the receptive field. The spot was on continuously at a level dim

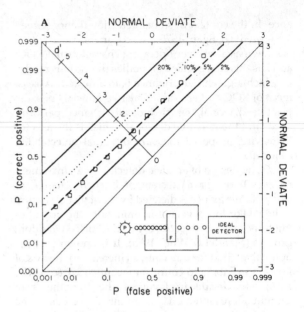

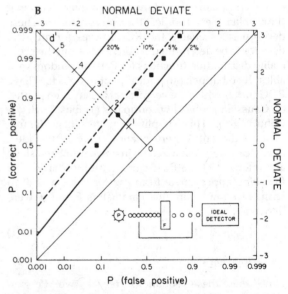

Fig. 8.1. ROC curves for a retinal ganglion cell (symbols) compared to those of an ideal detector handicapped by an attenuating filter (lines). Stimulus was a small spot of light (0.21 deg) centered on the receptive field of a cell (G-9-8) in the dark-adapted cat retina. The signal to be detected was a brief (0.1 s), 67% increment (A) or 67% decrement (B) of a steady light with mean luminance 87.5 photon (507 nm) per stimulus duration (600 trials). Inset shows model of retinal ganglion cell as a Poisson box. Inside the box is a filter of transmission factor F. ROC curves for the model are a family of parallel lines, corresponding to various values of filter factor F, as indicated by number near each line.

enough to avoid light adapting the cell (P=88 photons/ 0.1 s) and the stimulus to be detected was a brief (0.1 s) change ($|m|$=0.67) of the steady level which occurred once every 0.6 s. The cell's ROC curves for the incremental stimulus (Fig. 8.1A) and for the decremental stimulus (Fig. 8.1B) both show the Poisson signature expected when quantal fluctuations are a major factor limiting performance. First, these ROC curves were closely fitted by straight lines when plotted on Gaussian coordinates. Second, least-squares regression of the data indicated that the detectability (d'=1.25) of the increment stimulus was less than the detectability (d'=1.59) of the decrement stimulus of the same modulation magnitude. Third, ROC slope (0.97) for the increment was less than unity and slope (1.19) for the decrement was greater than unity.

We are now in a position to consider the question posed in the introduction: can the ROC curves for a retinal ganglion cell be matched by the ROC curves for an ideal detector handicapped by a filter? The cell of Fig. 8.1 is a good candidate for a match since it shows signs of quantum limited behavior just as the ideal detector does. Comparison of the ganglion cell data with the family of theoretical curves for an increment stimulus (Fig. 8.1A) indicates a reasonable fit for the curve corresponding to the filter value F=5.0%, although the slope is not quite right. The more troublesome result, however, is that the data for the decrement stimulus are not well matched by the corresponding theoretical curve (Fig. 8.1B) but instead are fitted best by a curve for the lower value of F=3.7%. This discrepancy is too large to be ignored.

The difficulties encountered in matching the ROC data for this ganglion cell are indicative of a fundamental limitation of the theoretical model. In principle, the slope of an empirically obtained ROC may not be the same as that of an ideal detector with various levels of neutral filter handicap. In such a case, an empirical ROC is free to cut across the parallel family of theoretical ROC curves so that each point of the empirical ROC corresponds to a different value of F. Consequently, no single choice of filter can produce a match between the full ROC curves of real and filter-handicapped, ideal detectors. The problem becomes acute when the stimulus is a decrement of 100% modulation. If the steady light provides even a few photons per trial, an ideal detector can perform without error by always saying the signal is present when zero photons are caught and saying there is no signal when it catches one or more photons. In this case, signal detectability is indefinitely large, the ROC curve is indeterminate, and introducing a filter poses no handicap. For real ganglion cells, however, removing all of the light does not necessarily remove all of

the variability of the cell's discharge and so the cell cannot attain perfect performance. Thus, the model of an ideal detector handicapped by a filter is certainly inadequate, but through this failure comes the kind of success forecast by Barlow since it shows that real detectors are limited by more than an inability to catch every quantum.

Noise handicap

Since an attenuating filter by itself is insufficient to mimic real detectors, it becomes necessary to model the equivalently handicapped, ideal detector in another way. Barlow solved a similar problem in the analysis of frequency-of-seeing curves for human subjects by suggesting that there exists a source of biological noise which produces neural events indistinguishable from the natural response to light (Barlow, 1956). Since these events occur even in the dark, they have been called 'dark light events' or 'eigengrau'. Unfortunately, the first phrase carries with it an apparent contradiction of terms which can be unsettling for the student, and the second does not convey the essential idea of discrete events. Therefore, we propose to coin a new word to stand for those hypothetical events which are confusable with the absorption of photons but which are due to internal, biological causes and may therefore occur even in complete darkness. As they are complementary to photons, the elementary particles of light, let these particles of darkness be known as 'scotons', from the Greek root Σκοτοσ (*skotos*) meaning darkness.

For present purposes we make the simplifying assumption that these hypothetical scotons have the statistical properties of a Poisson random process. Since the superposition of two independent trains of Poisson events is another Poisson train (Cox & Lewis, 1966), a black box containing an additive source of Poisson noise of mean rate S scotons/unit time qualifies as a Poisson box. Since photons and scotons are assumed to be physiologically indistinguishable, the effective rate of background events is

$$P' = P + S \tag{7}$$

whereas the effective modulation caused by the stimulus decreases to

$$m' = mP/(P+S) \tag{8}$$

Applying these results to the general expressions for d' and slope given by equations 3 and 4, we see that the weakness of the filter model has been averted by the use of the noise model. By increasing S, ROC slope approaches unity and d' approaches 0 as required. Thus it is conceivable that a particular value of S could produce a match of both slope and intercept of ROCs for real and ideal detectors. Further, the noise model avoids the critical weakness of the original filter model because any positive value of S will keep d' finite even for 100% decrements.

A test of the noise model is presented in Fig. 8.2A, which illustrates the performance of another retinal ganglion cell for the detection of 100% decrements of a steady light emitting on average $P=61$ photons/unit time. The ROC curve has slope 1.20 and crosses the d' axis at 2.01. To reduce d' of the ideal detector to that of the ganglion cell requires $S=860$ scotons/unit time, which implies an effective modulation of -6.6%. But the slope of the theoretical ROC curve (solid line) is then 1.01, which is too far from the experimental value to be explained on the basis of experimental variability. A second test of the model also suggests the noise model is inadequate. Since the model assumes that the internal noise is independent of the light stimulus, the amount of noise present should be the same regardless of whether the stimulus is an increment or a decrement. Therefore, by calculating the amount of noise necessary to account for decrement performance, it should be possible to predict ganglion cell performance for an increment. As shown in Fig. 8.2A, however, the prediction (dashed line) clearly fails to match the ganglion cell data (open squares).

The reasons the noise model fails can be understood as follows. In order to reduce the infinite detectability of the 100% decrement stimulus, the ideal detector must be handicapped with a source of noise events which has a mean rate much higher than the steady level of the light stimulus. Consequently, the effective modulation provided by the stimulus is very low. When the modulation is low, increments and decrements are about equally detectable. Thus the two theoretical ROC curves in Fig. 8.2 are nearly identical. For the retinal ganglion cell, however, the Poisson signature of the light source is clearly evident in the ROC curves as signal detectability is significantly higher for the decrement stimulus than for an increment of the same magnitude. This is an indication that the model has the wrong proportions of photons and scotons. Evidently the quantal fluctuations of the stimulus are of much greater importance for the ganglion cell than for the model and this is why the model fails.

Filter plus noise handicap

From the preceding it is clear that our hypothetical Poisson box must contain more than just either a filter

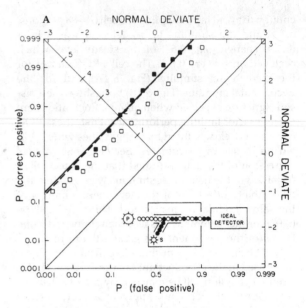

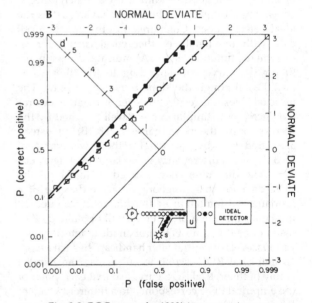

Fig. 8.2. ROC curves for 100% increment (open symbols and dashed lines) and decrement (closed symbols and solid lines) of a spot of light (0.43 deg) supplying 61 photons (507 nm) per stimulus duration (0.5 s). Cell H-1-8, 1000 trials. Theoretical curves in (A) are for the noise-only model (see inset), where the ideal detector is handicapped by an added noise source of rate $S = 860$ scotons per stimulus duration. Curves in (B) are for noise + filter model (see inset), where the ideal detector is handicapped by a noise source of rate $S = 82$ scotons per stimulus duration and by a filter which passes $U = 12\%$ of photons and scotons.

or a source of noise. The obvious next step is to incorporate both components into the model, which is equivalent to an arbitrary sequence of noise and filter stages. It is convenient, but not essential, to suppose the filter acts after the superposition of photons and scotons. The only effect of this order is to measure scotons in the same units as the input photons. Let the transmission factor of the filter be U, which stands for the fraction of quantal events, both photons and scotons, utilized by the ideal detector. The effective, steady rate of events seen by the ideal detector is

$$P' = U(P+S) \qquad (9)$$

and the effective modulation caused by the stimulus is

$$m' = mP/(P+S) \qquad (10)$$

In principle, the two parameters d' and slope are sufficient to determine the two unknowns of the model, U and S. A straightforward approach would be to estimate slope and d' of an empirical ROC by least-squares regression and then use equations 3 and 4, in conjunction with 9 and 10, to determine the model's parameters. This method guarantees that an empirical ROC will be well described by the model since the ROC of the model is in fact the best fitting straight line to the data. To test the model, it could be used to predict the results of other experiments, say with different modulation strengths or different intensity levels.

In practice, the above method of parameter estimation is often unsatisfactory because it yields results which have a large statistical uncertainty. Consider, for instance, the ROC curve for an incremental stimulus. According to equation 2, the range of possible slope values is 1.0 to 0.89, which corresponds to the modulation range of 0 to 100%. Suppose the empirical ROC slope is B and we ask the question, what is the 95% confidence interval for this value? To answer this question, we need to know the statistical properties of ROC slope for Poisson signals. These are not known theoretically, but computer simulation for typical stimulus parameters has indicated that ROC slope has a Gaussian distribution with standard deviation given approximately by $SD = \sqrt{(3/N)}$, where N is the number of stimulus trials used to generate the ROC curve (Thibos *et al.*, 1979). Under the best of conditions, $N=1000$ is about the most that could be expected of a physiological experiment so the 95% confidence interval for slope of an increment ROC would be $B \pm SD \times t_{(.05,k-2)}$, where $t_{(.05,k-2)}$ is Student's t-statistic for $k-2$ degrees of freedom and k is the number of ROC points used to determine slope. The smallest confidence interval occurs when k is large,

and under this assumption the interval is $B-0.1$ to $B+0.1$. Unfortunately, even this minimum range of uncertainty for B completely overlaps the full range of possible slope values expected for a detector of Poisson signals. In other words, it appears that we will learn nothing about the parameters of the model from measurements of ROC slope for an increment. The situation is not quite so hopeless for a decrement stimulus, as the permissible range of slopes is somewhat larger. Nevertheless, these practical problems suggest an alternative approach should be developed.

A better method for estimating the parameters of the model is based on detectability measurements for an increment (d'_+) and a decrement (d'_-) stimulus of the same magnitude m. Applying equation 3, the ratio $r = d'_-/d'_+$ yields an estimate of the effective modulation magnitude m':

$$m' = (r^4-1)/(r^4+1) \qquad (11)$$

from which the model parameters may be estimated:

$$S = P(m/m'-1) \qquad (12)$$

$$U = d'_+ d'_- (1-m'^2)^{1/4}/Pmm' \qquad (13)$$

Applying these equations to the data of retinal ganglion cell of Fig. 8.2A indicates that this cell performs the same as the ideal detector model with $U=12\%$ and $S=82$. The theoretical ROC curves for the model, shown by the lines in Fig. 8.2B, appear to fit the data reasonably well. More searching tests of the model would involve prediction of results for other stimulus conditions based on the model parameters determined from the initial experiment. This requires long periods of stable physiological behavior which has been achieved for only a small number of cells. Nevertheless, on those occasions it was possible to verify that a model with fixed parameters could adequately describe the performance of retinal ganglion cells over the full range of modulations at a fixed background level and over about 1 log unit range of backgrounds above absolute threshold (Levick *et al.*, 1983).

In summary, the performance of the brisk-sustained type of cat retinal ganglion cell can be adequately matched by a theoretical model consisting of an ideal detector handicapped by a source of added noise and an attenuating filter. Simpler models consisting of either one or other of these handicaps can be ruled out, since neither is sufficient to account for ganglion cell performance over a range of stimulus conditions. The proposed model seems irreducible for other reasons as well. It is certain that ganglion cells cannot utilize all incident quanta since some are undoubtedly reflected, scattered and absorbed by the ocular media. Therefore, some kind of attenuating filter seems essential to the model. Similarly, the presence of retinal noise cannot be denied since retinal ganglion cells typically have a variable maintained discharge in the dark. This noise can only come from intrinsic, biological sources. The challenge for the future will be to determine how useful this simple model will be in describing the performance of other cell types in the dark-adapted condition and in accounting for the changes of performance brought on by light adaptation.

Quantum efficiency revisited

Two problems have been identified with Barlow's original formulation of quantum efficiency. First, in general the ROC curve for real detectors of light may cut across the family of theoretical ROC curves for an ideal detector, each curve corresponding to a different value of quantum efficiency, so that no single value of F will produce a match between empirical and theoretical curves. Second, the quantum efficiency cannot be determined when the stimulus is a decrement of 100% modulation. Although there is no satisfactory resolution of the latter problem, it would be possible to resolve the former by adopting a convention which specifies which performance point on the experimental ROC curve is to be matched by the theoretical model. A natural choice is to require the theoretical curve to intersect the empirical ROC at the negative diagonal. In other words, the suggested convention is to say that the real and ideal detectors have equal performance when they have equal d'. For the model, d' is known from equations 3, 5 and 6:

$$d' = |m|(FP)^{1/2}(1+m)^{1/4} \qquad (14)$$

Setting d' of this equation to the experimentally determined value for the real detector, and solving for F, gives a simple formula for the real detector in terms of its own performance and the given signal parameters:

$$F = d'^2(1+m)^{1/2}/Pm^2 \qquad (15)$$

A general expression for the efficiency of an arbitrary Poisson box may be obtained by equating d' for an ideal detector handicapped by a Poisson box (equation 3) with d' for an ideal detector handicapped by a filter (equation 14) and solving for F. This gives the desired result in terms of the signal parameters before and after the box:

$$F = (P'/P)(m'/m)^2[(1+m)/(1+m')]^{1/2} \qquad (16)$$

Explicit formulae for special cases of interest follow immediately from this general solution. When the box contains a filter of transmission U, then $m=m'$ and $P=UP$, so quantum efficiency is just the filter's transmission factor:

$$F_{filter} = U \qquad (17)$$

Unlike the case of a filter handicap, when the box contains a source of added noise, quantum efficiency is not fixed but depends upon stimulus parameters P and m. This is shown by substituting the expressions of equations 7 and 8 into equation 16:

$$F_{noise} = (P/P+S)[(1+m)/(1+mP/(P+S))]^{1/2} \qquad (18)$$

Finally, when the box contains both a filter and a source of added noise, quantum efficiency is found from equations 9, 10 and 16 to be:

$$F_{noise+filter} = (UP/P+S)[(1+m)/(1+mP/(P+S))]^{1/2} \qquad (19)$$

The product rule for a sequence of inefficient stages in the visual system was one of the attractive features of Barlow's original formulation of quantum efficiency. By this rule, the overall quantum efficiency of series of concatenated filters is the product of their individual efficiencies. Given the above development, it is now possible to verify the more general product rule for the quantum efficiency of a series of Poisson boxes. According to the convention suggested above, each box in the sequence will have the same effect on d' as does some filter, the value of which is given by equation 19, and so its efficiency is equal to the filter's transmission factor. By extension, a series of Poisson boxes will have the same overall effect on d' as a series of filters. But a series of filters is equivalent to a single filter which reduces d' by the same amount. The transmission of this single filter is, by definition, equal to the overall quantum efficiency of the series of Poisson boxes. It is also, by computation, equal to the product of the transmission factors of the individual filters and thus the efficiencies of the individual Poisson boxes. It should be kept in mind that in the general case the efficiency of a Poisson box depends upon signal parameters at its own input. Therefore, the order of the boxes is important and changing the order will in general change the overall quantum efficiency.

The foregoing analysis provides a tool for assessing the relative importance of the noise component and filter component of the Poisson box used by Levick *et al.* (1983) to model the behaviour of cat retinal ganglion cells. Factoring out the two components is a specific application of product rule, for it is evident from equations 17, 18 and 19 that:

$$F_{noise+filter} = F_{filter} \times F_{noise} \qquad (20)$$

The quantum efficiency of eight retinal ganglion cells studied by Levick *et al.* (1983) ranged from 2% to 11% and averaged 7%. ROC curves for these cells were matched by ROC curves for the filter+noise model presented above and the parameters of the model were presented in their Table 1. The range of quantum efficiencies for the filter component for the eight cells was 3% to 29% with an average of 14%. The range of efficiencies for the noise component was 35% to 81% and the mean was 55%. This comparison reveals that the inability of the ganglion cell to utilize all of the incident quanta of light had a much greater effect on the cell's overall quantum efficiency than did the internal source of biological noise.

References

Barlow, H. B. (1956) Retinal noise & absolute threshold. *J. Opt. Soc. Am.*, **46**, 634–9.

Barlow, H. B. (1962) A method of determining the overall quantum efficiency of visual discriminations. *J. Physiol.*, **160**, 155–68.

Barlow, H. B. (1977) Retinal and central factors in human vision limited by noise. In *Vertebrate Photoreception*, ed. H. B. Barlow & P. Fatt, London: Academic Press. pp. 337–58.

Barlow, H. B. & Levick, W. R. (1969) Changes in the maintained discharge with adaptation level in the cat retina. *J. Physiol.*, **202**, 699–718.

Barlow, H. B., Levick, W. R. & Yoon, M. (1971) Responses to single quanta of light in retinal ganglion cells of the cat. *Vision Res.*, **3**(suppl), 87–101.

Cox, D. R. & Lewis, P. A. W. (1966) *The Statistical Analysis of Series of Events.* London: Methuen.

Egan, J. P. (1975) *Signal Detection Theory and ROC Analysis.* New York: Academic Press.

Green, D. M. & Swets, J. A. (1966) *Signal Detection Theory and Psychophysics.* New York: John Wiley and Sons.

Levick, W. R., Thibos, L. N., Cohn, T. E., Catanzaro, D. & Barlow, H. B. (1983) Performance of cat retinal ganglion cells at low light levels. *J. Gen. Physiol.*, **82**, 405–26.

Mandel, L. & Wolf, E. (1965) Coherence properties of optical fields. *Review of Modern Physics*, **37**, 231–87.

Parzen, E. (1962) *Stochastic Processes.* San Francisco: Holden-Day.

Rose, A. (1946) A unified approach to the performance of photographic film, television pickup tubes, and the human eye. *Journal of the Society of Motion Picture Engineers*, **47**, 273–94.

Thibos, L. N., Levick, W. R. & Cohn, T. E. (1979) Receiver operating characteristic curves for Poisson signals. *Biol. Cybern.*, **33**, 57–61.

9

Neural interactions underlying direction-selectivity in the rabbit retina

C. W. Oyster

One of Horace Barlow's early ideas about the processing of visual information was the 'password' hypothesis (Barlow, 1961), which has to do with the selection and transmission of information about specific, meaningful (i.e. non-redundant) aspects of the visual world. This notion came, at least in part, from his discovery that some of the frog's retinal ganglion cells had response properties consistent with their being 'detectors of snapworthy objects' – flies, for example (Barlow, 1953). Subsequently, the remarkable study by Lettvin, Maturana, McCulloch & Pitts (1959) provided irresistible impetus to the idea that the encoding and transmission of visual information is a highly selective procedure.

From the work on frog retina, it became obvious that the speed and direction of moving stimuli are of considerable importance to the visual system (Lettvin et al., 1959; Maturana et al., 1960). This result was extended to mammalian retina when Barlow & Hill (1963) demonstrated the presence of direction-selective ganglion cells in the rabbit retina. By now, direction-selective ganglion cells have been found in a wide variety of vertebrate retinas. Although these neurons differ somewhat in their response properties, all respond maximally to an appropriate stimulus moving through the receptive field in a particular, 'preferred', direction and respond minimally, if at all, to the same stimulus moving in the opposite, 'null', direction. Responses to other directions of stimulus movement are less than maximal.

As it happens, the topic of direction-selectivity is a very broad one. Direction-selective neurons are found at a variety of places in both vertebrate and invertebrate visual systems and must be considered in the general context of the analysis of image motion by the visual system (see, for example, Hildreth & Koch, 1987). Among the numerous questions that can be raised is the issue of generating a direction-selective neuron *de novo*, that is, of synthesis by the appropriate combination or interaction of non-directional elements. This process occurs early in the rabbit's visual system, as Barlow & Hill (1963) pointed out, thereby providing an excellent opportunity to understand the neural circuitry that produces this striking example of visual information encoding.

Direction-selectivity in the rabbit retina

There are two classes of direction-selective ganglion cells in rabbit retina, the ON–OFF and ON direction-selective cells (Barlow, Hill & Levick, 1964). ON–OFF direction-selective cells are more frequently encountered and their response properties have been more thoroughly studied; they will be the main subject of the discussion to follow. Before pursuing this topic, however, it is worth noting that the ON direction-selective cells are not simply variants within the ON–OFF cell class. ON direction-selective cells have a unique dendritic morphology (Amthor, Takahashi & Oyster, 1989) and, unlike the ON–OFF cells, project primarily to the pretectal and accessory optic system nuclei (Collewijn, 1975; Simpson, Soodak & Hess, 1979). The ON direction-selective cells also differ in their distribution of preferred directions (Oyster & Barlow, 1967) and in their sensitivity to movement velocity (Oyster, Takahashi & Collewijn, 1972).

One in every four or five ganglion cell recordings in rabbit retina is from an ON–OFF direction-selective cell (Levick, 1967; Oyster, 1968; Caldwell & Daw, 1978; Amthor et al., 1989). The receptive field maps consist of ON and OFF responses to small, stationary stimuli; these cells also respond to either light or dark moving stimuli. The direction-selectivity to a moving stimulus is illustrated in Fig. 9.1, where response magnitude is plotted in polar coordinates as a function of movement direction. For a stimulus moving in the preferred direction, that is, to the right in Fig. 9.1, the cell fired a maximum number of action potentials. Opposite movement (to the left) elicited only a few potentials that correspond to the cell's normally low maintained discharge at that level of ambient illumination. Stimulus movements along an axis perpendicular to the preferred-null axis produced roughly equal responses that are clearly less than maximal. The resulting direction sensitivity function is cardioid-like, with a cusp representing the null direction.

Preferred directions vary from cell to cell, but the range of possible directions is highly restricted. Basi-

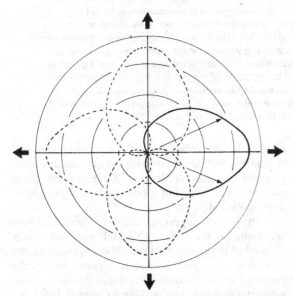

Fig. 9.1. Directional response functions for ON–OFF direction-selective ganglion cells. In this polar coordinate diagram, response magnitude in number of action potentials and direction of stimulus movement are combined as vectors, two of which are illustrated. For a given cell, a response function is created by connecting the ends of all its response vectors as a smooth curve. The resulting functions, like the one shown with a heavy filled line, is cardioid-like in shape; the maximum response (preferred) direction is 180° from the minimum response (null) direction, which creates the cusp of the cardioid. As shown by three other response functions (dashed curves), an ON–OFF direction-selective cell may have only one of four possible preferred directions, which are 90° apart. Adapted from Oyster, 1968.

cally, the cell population includes only four preferred directions (Oyster & Barlow, 1967) which, in Fig. 9.1, are right, left, up, and down. For the rabbit's laterally directed eyes, these directions are approximately anterior, posterior, superior, and inferior in the visual field.

The operational mechanism for direction-selectivity

In an elegant series of studies, Barlow & Levick (1965) developed the evidence and control experiments that led to an operational description of direction-selectivity in the ON–OFF cells. The essential points are, first, that separate stimuli within a cell's receptive field will interact if the stimuli are not too far apart; in other words, the interaction is local, operating within small parts of the total receptive field. Second, the interaction is inhibitory; spatially and temporally separate stimuli may produce inhibition of the second response by its predecessor. Third, the inhibition is not equally effective in all directions around a given point in the receptive field; inhibition is most effective along the null direction.

The scheme Barlow and Levick proposed as consistent with their observations is illustrated in Fig. 9.2A. Vertical pathways connect small clusters of photoreceptors (A, B, C, D, & E) to the ganglion cell via intermediate relays; these connections are all excitatory. A second kind of pathway contains lateral inhibitory connections; in Fig. 9.2A, only the preferred-null axis is represented and the inhibitory connections extend only in the null direction (left). Stimulus movement from E to A will generate excitation at the ganglion cell only through the vertical pathway from the photoreceptors at E; the others will be cancelled by the lateral inhibitory pathways. The sequence A to E, however, will provide excitation at the ganglion cell from all points. The inhibitory pathways still operate, but the excitation in the vertical pathways will reach the ganglion cell before the inhibition can cancel it. Note also that a stimulus at E may cancel excitation arising from D, but will not affect excitation coming from C, B, or A, thus conforming to the requirement that inhibition be local.

Since other directions of movement produce less than maximal responses, inhibition cannot be confined to the null direction, though this is not shown in Fig. 9.2A. This point was made explicitly by Wyatt & Daw (1975), who demonstrated that some inhibitory spread occurs in all directions *except* the preferred direction. Thus, one can think of the mechanism depicted in Fig. 9.2A as being elaborated in other

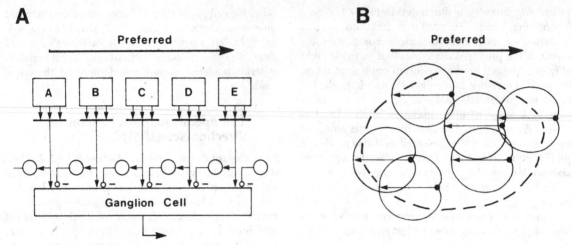

Fig. 9.2. A – The operational mechanism for direction-selectivity in ON–OFF ganglion cells. This diagram, which is a modified version of that shown by Barlow & Levick (1965), illustrates groups of photoreceptors (A to E) connected by bipolar cells to a ganglion cell. Lateral inhibitory connections (here shown as unidirectional) are mediated by amacrine cells. The essential point is that excitation elicited in the bipolars by a stimulus moving from E to A is cancelled by the amacrine-mediated inhibition. Excitation generated by movement from A to E will be effective because it arrives at the ganglion cell prior to the inhibition. Only one of the two sets of cone bipolars is illustrated. B – Hypothetical regions of inhibition generated by stimuli at different points in a direction-selective cell's receptive field. Note that inhibition is thought to spread maximally in the null direction, regardless of receptive field location, and minimally in the preferred direction. Inhibition will be generated by either light (ON) or dark (OFF) stimuli. A different kind of inhibitory spread is illustrated by Wyatt & Daw (1975).

directions around a point in the receptive field, but with less extensive lateral inhibition. The spread of inhibition as a function of movement direction should resemble a cardioid whose axis of symmetry is the preferred-null axis; some of the possible inhibitory cardioids are illustrated in Fig. 9.2B. It is worth emphasizing that these direction-selective 'subunits' are not known to be discrete entities; they are probably best envisioned as continuous, overlapping and, the implications of Fig. 9.2A notwithstanding, not easily countable. (Parenthetically, these inhibitory cardioids have never been measured experimentally – Wyatt & Daw (1975) delimited the area within which inhibition could spread *to* a given point, not the area within which inhibition spreads *from* a point in the receptive field. The two areas need not be the same.)

The retinal location of direction-selective interactions

In its operational form, Barlow and Levick's model for direction-selectivity does not assign the lateral inhibitory connections to any specific neurons. The most obvious choices, however, are horizontal cells or amacrine cells. From information available at the time, Barlow and Levick chose the former, thereby suggest-

ing that bipolar cells would be the basic elements of direction-selectivity. Under this hypothesis, direction-selective ganglion cells would simply be those ganglion cells receiving inputs from direction-selective bipolar cells.

It is now apparent, however, that direction-selectivity for the rabbit's ON–OFF ganglion cells is elaborated in the inner retina, although this may not be true in other species. Recent reports suggest the presence of direction-selective bipolar cells in turtle retina, for example (DeVoe, Guy & Criswell, 1985), but the results presently available are not conclusive.

The principal evidence for direction-selectivity being elaborated in the rabbit's inner plexiform layer (IPL) comes from studies of retinal neurotransmitters and their antagonists. Both GABA (γ-aminobutyric acid) antagonists and anticholinesterases will abolish direction-selectivity in the ON–OFF cells (Wyatt & Daw, 1976; Caldwell, Daw & Wyatt, 1978; Ariel & Daw, 1982). In rabbit retina, GABA and acetylcholine can be localized to amacrine cells by uptake autoradiography or immunohistochemical methods. Very recent studies indicate that the cholinergic amacrine cells also contain GABA and its synthetic enzymes (Vaney & Young, 1988; Brecha, Johnson, Peichl & Wassle, 1988).

There is no convincing evidence that rabbit horizontal cells utilize either GABA or acetylcholine as a neurotransmitter. The rabbit retina does contain interplexiform cells (Oyster & Takahashi, 1977) and because their neurotransmitters are unknown, some are at least potentially GABA-ergic (see, for example, Mosinger & Yazulla, 1987). This is a modest caveat, however, and the available evidence points to direction-selectivity being a consequence of inner plexiform layer interactions among bipolar cells, amacrine cells, and ganglion cells.

Morphology of ON–OFF direction-selective cells

Physiological evidence suggests that ON (depolarizing) and OFF (hyperpolarizing) cone bipolars in rabbit retina, like these in other species, terminate in the inner and outer sublaminae of the inner plexiform layer (Bloomfield & Miller, 1986). Since ON–OFF direction-selective cells respond to both phases of illumination, it has been assumed that these cells have bistratified dendritic arbors, thereby receiving direct inputs from both sets of cone bipolars (see, for example, Ariel & Daw, 1982).

This assumption is correct, although another class of ON–OFF ganglion cell in rabbit retina, the local-edge-detector (Levick, 1967), is *not* bistratified (Amthor *et al.*, 1989). ON–OFF direction-selective cells have most of their dendrites confined to two narrow planes in the inner and outer IPL (Amthor, Oyster & Takahashi, 1984), as shown in the upper part of Fig. 9.3. The exceptions are the few branches that traverse vertically through the IPL to connect the branching planes.

The dendritic branching of an ON–OFF direction-selective cell in a flat-mount view (Fig. 9.3, lower) is quite complex, with considerable crossing of dendrites. This complexity is largely due to superposition of the two branching planes, however, and matters are simplified by illustrating the two planes separately, as in Fig. 9.4. Within each plane, the dendrites can now be seen to form a space-filling network with very few instances of dendrites crossing one another. This illustration, unlike the computer reconstruction in Fig. 9.3, shows small spines and spine-like appendages throughout the dendritic field. Careful inspection will also reveal that small diameter terminal branches are distributed randomly throughout each of the branching areas.

ON–OFF direction-selective cells have three or four main dendrites arising from the soma; each of these main dendrites and all of its higher order bran-

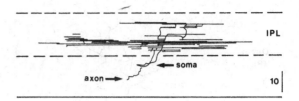

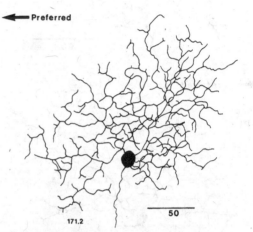

Fig. 9.3. Side or sectioned view (upper) and flatmount view (lower) of an ON–OFF direction-selective ganglion cell. The rather complex branching pattern of the direction-selective cell dendrites seen in the flatmount view is composed of two separate levels of branching in the IPL, whose borders are indicated by dashed lines. Dimension scales are in µm.

ches can be considered anatomically as a separate dendritic system. Most commonly, a dendritic system has lower order branches in the inner IPL with higher order dendrites traversing to the outer IPL where further branching occurs. On occasion, the entire dendritic system is confined to the inner IPL. Alternatively, a main dendrite from the soma may go directly to the outer IPL with all the subsequent branching in this plane.

The effect of this branching scheme is illustrated in Fig. 9.5A, where each dendritic system is indicated with boundaries drawn by connecting the free terminal endings with straight line segments and with different degrees of shading for the three dendritic systems. Generally, each branching plane is filled with branches from at least two dendritic systems; since there are very few crossing branches, it follows that individual dendritic systems are not spatially overlapping. Instead, they fit together, covering the plane like pieces of a jigsaw puzzle.

In some cells, a branching plane may consist of branches from only one dendritic system; it is there-

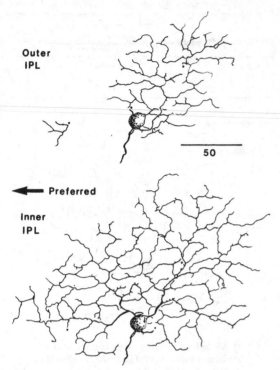

Fig. 9.4 Separate flatmount views of the two IPL branching planes for an ON–OFF direction-selective cell (same cell as in Fig. 9.3). The branching patterns are space-filling in character, but with very few dendrides crossing one another. Dendritic spines and small diameter terminal branches are distributed throughout each branching plane. Dimension scale is in μm. Adapted from Amthor, Oyster & Takahashi, 1984.

fore unlikely that the property of direction-selectivity is in any way related to the anatomical subunits created in the branching planes by different dendritic systems. It is much more likely that direction-selectivity can be elaborated within an individual dendritic system, or a portion thereof, and furthermore, that direction-selectivity is elaborated separately in the inner and outer branching planes. It is also clear that neighboring points in a dendritic field may fall within different dendritic systems and be separated by considerable electrotonic distances; thus, their spatial interaction is likely to be a consequence of the input circuitry and not a result of interaction within the dendritic arbor.

These and other morphological features of the ON–OFF direction-selective cells make the important point that the preferred direction of an ON–OFF cell is not revealed through its dendritic morphology. It is

true that individual cells can be recognized as different – their branching patterns, though basically similar, are sufficiently idiosyncratic that they are easily distinguishable from one another. None of their morphological features, however, show the 90° or 180° rotations that would be expected from the 90° or 180° differences in preferred direction among cells. To a large extent, it appears that the cells are morphologically interchangeable.

Finally, the inner and outer IPL branching planes are often of different size and do not completely overlap. On average, however, the branching areas are about 125 μm in diameter for ON–OFF cells in the visual streak. This value, combined with esimates of ON–OFF direction-selective cell density, results in a coverage factor very close to 4.0 (Amthor et al., 1989). This four-fold coverage factor estimate is consistent with the notion that each point in visual space can activate four ON–OFF direction-selective cells each, one assumes, having a different preferred direction.

Inputs to the ON–OFF direction-selective cells

None of the physiologically identified ON–OFF direction-selective cells has been studied by electron microscopy, but a Golgi-stained ganglion cell with the characteristic bistratified morphology of the ON–OFF cells has been examined (Famiglietti, 1985a). The first conclusion to be drawn from this work is that ON–OFF direction-selective cells receive cone bipolar inputs, apparently in both branching planes. The spatial distribution of the bipolar contacts is not known, but since spines and terminal branches are found throughout the ON–OFF cells' branching planes, the probable spatial array of bipolar inputs is illustrated schematically in Fig. 9.5B (cone bipolar terminals have been assigned a diameter of 20 μm).

Fig. 9.5B illustrates the simple assumptions that bipolar terminals tile both branching planes, that is, cover the areas without gaps or significant overlap, and that all bipolar terminals within reach of ON–OFF cell dendrites make some synaptic contact with them. These dual arrays of excitatory inputs must be selectively and independently cancelled to produce direction-selectivity and the resulting preferred direction must be the same for both the ON and OFF levels of dendritic branching.

The other source of input to the ON–OFF cells is, not surprisingly, from amacrine cells (Famiglietti, 1985a). The crucial question, which the electron microscopy has not answered at this point, concerns the exact type or types of amacrine cells involved.

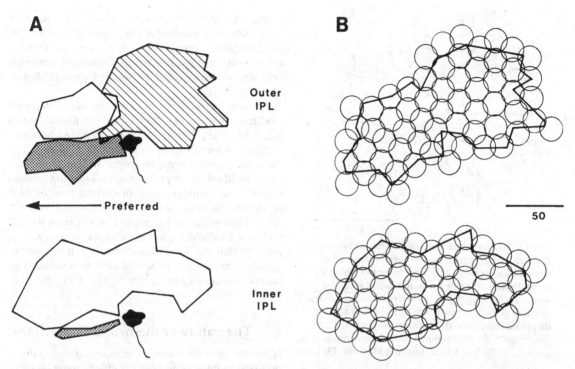

A

Outer
IPL

Preferred

Inner
IPL

B

50

Fig. 9.5. A – Anatomical subunits in the direction-selective cell branching planes. Regions occupied by branches of different dendritic systems are illustrated by different levels of shading. A given system most commonly has branches at both levels, but this is not always true. A dendritic system may ramify exclusively at either of the two IPL levels. Branches from different systems have little or no spatial overlap at the same level. B – Presumed spatial relationship between cone bipolar terminals and the branching planes of a direction-selective cell. Bipolar terminals are illustrated as 20 μm diameter circles that cover the plane with few gaps and little overlap. The dimension scale is in μm and applies to both A and B.

Here, one must rely on the aforementioned pharmaco-logical studies that implicate GABA and cholinergic amacrine cell systems (Wyatt & Daw, 1976; Caldwell, Daw & Wyatt, 1978; Ariel & Daw, 1982). The GABA system in rabbit retina is not well understood in terms of morphology, except in the general sense that some amacrine cells, with somata in the inner nuclear layer and the ganglion cell layer, exhibit GABA and/or GAD-like immunoreactivity (e.g. Mosinger & Yazulla, 1987). It is therefore of considerable interest that much of the GABA-like immunoreactivity can be co-localized with cholinergic amacrines (Vaney & Young, 1988; Brecha *et al.*, 1988) because the cholinergic amacrine cell system has been very thoroughly studied.

The starburst amacrine cells

When stained with Golgi methods, one group of rabbit amacrine cells attract particular attention because of their striking radial symmetry; they have been called

'starburst' amacrine cells, in recognition of their characteristic morphology (Famiglietti, 1983). These beautiful neurons have been shown to be cholinergic; one cell from the rabbit's visual streak, injected with Lucifer yellow by Tauchi & Masland (1984), is shown in Fig. 9.6. The cell illustrated here had its soma in the ganglion cell layer with its branches ramifying in the inner part of the inner plexiform layer. There is a second set of starburst amacrines with somata in the inner nuclear layer and processes ramifying in the outer part of the IPL (Tauchi & Masland, 1984; Famiglietti, 1983). The ramification levels of the two sets of starburst amacrine cells appear to be the same as the planes in which the direction-selective cells' dendrites branch. These cells usually have four major branches radiating from the soma; these major den-drites generally divide once or twice near the soma. Most of the high order branching, however, occurs at some distance from the soma, forming a fairly dense annulus of high order branches. The branches in this annular zone are relatively thick and have numerous

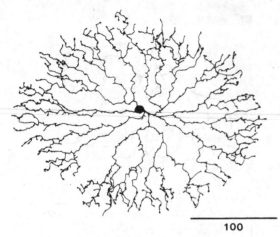

100

Fig. 9.6. Starburst amacrine cell in flatmount view. This cell, characteristically, has considerable radial symmetry with most of the high order branching at some distance from the soma. In this instance, the soma was in the ganglion cell layer and the processes ramified in the inner part of the IPL, i.e. it is a displaced amacrine cell. There are also starburst amacrines of the conventional variety. Dimension scale in μm. Redrawn from Tauchi & Masland, 1984.

varicosities (Fig. 9.6). These terminal branches are certainly coarser than the main processes arising from the soma, a feature that is thought to endow these cells with an unusual property.

Miller & Bloomfield (1983) used dendritic length and diameter measurements from HRP-filled starburst amacrines to model the cells' electrotonic properties. They concluded that, to an unusual degree, each major dendritic system is electrotonically isolated from other systems on the same cell. To put it another way, each dendritic system on a starburst amacrine cell can be thought of as an independent functional unit. Each of these functional units is highly directional in the sense that the preferred path of current flow is somafugal.

Another sense in which these cells are directional is their distribution of inputs and outputs. Starburst amacrine cells receive synaptic inputs throughout their dendritic arbors; some of the inputs are from cone bipolars and the remainder are from other amacrine cells of unknown type (Famiglietti, 1983). Synaptic outputs, however, seem always to be to ganglion cells and are confined to the annular zone of thickened, varicose branches; it is estimated that the output zone occupies some 50 to 60% of the total dendritic area (Famiglietti, 1985b). If it is true that all of the starburst amacrine output goes to ganglion cells, it follows that these neurons are not inter-connected,

directly or indirectly. Only a small percentage of amacrine–amacrine contacts is required to alter this interpretation dramatically, however, and more recent work has established that starburst amacrine cells are interconnected to some degree (Millar & Morgan; 1987).

Some of the essential characteristics of starburst amacrine cells are summarized by the illustration in Fig. 9.7A. The cell from Fig. 9.6 is depicted here as a circular, sectored disc with a thick annular rim. The rim is the region of synaptic output and the sectors are the individual dendritic systems. Radiating arrows indicate the dominant path of current flow in each sector. Inputs to the starburst amacrine cell near the apex of one sector will produce outputs from the cell within a localized region some distance away. It is possible that this kind of asymmetry can be used to generate the asymmetric lateral inhibition required by Barlow and Levick's model for the ON–OFF direction-selective cells.

The nature of the neural interactions

No matter how the lateral inhibition underlying direction-selectivity is generated, its effects must be local, i.e. confined to a small part of the cells receptive (or dendritic) field. This requirement places restrictions on both the location of inhibitory inputs and the way in which the inhibition operates. Several local circuit schemes have been proposed (Miller, 1979; Torre & Poggio, 1978; Koch, Poggio & Torre, 1986) in which the main considerations are the effects of near simultaneous excitation and inhibition at various locations in a direction-selective cell's dendritic arbor.

Inhibitory inputs are extremely effective in cancelling excitatory inputs that are nearby. Moreover, the cancellation can be highly local when the excitatory and inhibitory interactions occur on dendritic spines or fine diameter dendritic branches (Torre & Poggio, 1978). Thus, an essential requirement for direction-selectivity can be satisfied by the appropriate relative location of excitatory and inhibitory inputs. Since ON–OFF direction-selective cells have numerous dendritic spines, and over half of the dendritic branches are small diameter terminals scattered throughout the dendritic field, suitable locations for the requisite excitatory–inhibitory interactions are certainly present. Recent models of current flow show that the localization requirement can be met by the actual dendritic morphology of the ON–OFF cells (Koch *et al.*, 1986).

Inhibition in these neuronal models works by shunting the excitation, that is, without producing a

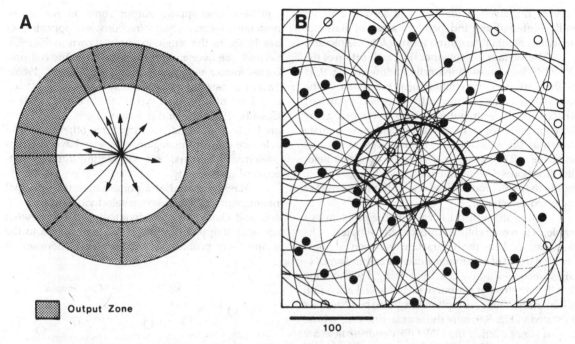

Output Zone

100

Fig. 9.7. A – Schematic view of the starburst amacrine from Fig. 9.6. The shaded annulus is the region in which the amacrine cell has outputs to ganglion cells; inputs *to the amacrine cell* may occur throughout the dendritic field. Sectors were generated by enclosing the regions containing the high order tributary branches of the 0th and 1st order dendrites (order is somafugal). These anatomical subunits may have an unusual degree of electrotonic isolation from one another. Arrows indicate the major direction of current flow in each of the sectors. B – Overlap of dendritic fields of starburst amacrine cells with the dendritic field of an ON–OFF direction-selective cell. Only one branching plane is illustrated. The array of starburst amacrine somata has been taken from Masland, Mills & Hayden, 1984. Cell density is 482 cells/mm^2 and the dendritic fields, shown here as circles, are 250 μm in diameter. The dark irregular contour delimits the dendritic field of a direction-selective cell (mean diameter of 125 μm). Over 40 starburst amacrines have output zones that overlap the ganglion cell's dendritic field. Overlapping amacrine cells have somata shown as filled circles. The dimension scale is in μm and applies to both A and B.

large hyperpolarization of the cell membrane (Torre & Poggio, 1978; Koch *et al.*, 1986). Since the effects are localized, there is no reason to expect the inhibition to produce detectable changes in the membrane potential recorded from the cell soma. Intracellular recordings from ON–OFF direction-selective cells are consistent with this hypothesis; stimuli moving in the null direction do not produce hyperpolarizing potentials (Amthor *et al.*, 1989; but see Miller, 1979).

An implicit assumption in all of the models for direction-selectivity is that a direction-selective cell can in some way select or recognize the appropriate set of inhibitory inputs from all those that are potentially available to it. The assumption is simplified by confining our attention to the starburst amacrine cells, but the specific inputs that are selected, and how they are selected, still remains to be considered.

Spatial organization of direction-selectivity

The problem of input selection is illustrated in Fig. 9.7B. The small circles are the somata of starburst amacrine cells from a patch of retina near the lower edge of the visual streak (from Masland, Mills & Hayden, 1984 – Fig. 7). The somata are in the ganglion cell layer and their processes ramify in the inner IPL. The large circular arcs show the extents of the dendritic fields of the starburst amacrines. At this retinal location, the fields are about 250 μm in diameter (Tauchi & Masland, 1984). Since the cells are close together (density illustrated is 482 cells/mm^2) and their processes spread extensively, there is considerable spatial overlap; each point on the retina falls within the dendritic fields of 40 to 50 starburst amacrines (Tauchi & Masland, 1984). Note that only one of the two relevant IPL levels is illustrated; a second diagram with a different and independent array of starburst amacrines would be required to complete the picture.

The average area of inner IPL ramification of the ON–OFF direction-selective cells is shown in Fig. 9.7B by the dark irregular contour near the center of the amacrine cell array; its mean diameter is 125 µm. The amacrine cells with output zones overlapping the direction-selective cell's dendritic field have somata shown as filled circles. Out of the large number of amacrine cell processes that cross its dendritic field, the direction-selective cell must receive only those inputs that will produce just one of the four possible preferred directions.

Before attempting to deal with the problem as a whole, it is worthwhile to consider the simplest of its elements, namely the interaction between a single functional unit of a starburst amacrine cell and an ON–OFF direction-selective cell. In so doing, I will assume that the *net* effect of starburst amacrine cell activation is inhibitory. This assumption has yet to be tested. As indicated in Fig. 9.8, only those amacrine cells whose output zones overlap the ON–OFF dendritic field are directly relevant; a single dendritic system from one of those amacrines is shown with the correct absolute scale. Two possible sites of synaptic input to *the amacrine cell* are shown by arrows. The large arrow lies outside the ganglion cell's dendritic field. The input, presumably from cone bipolars, will not affect the ganglion cell directly, but activation of the amacrine cell process will produce inhibition in the output zone delineated by the dashed contour line. Simultaneous excitatory inputs to the ganglion cell within the amacrine cell output zone will be suppressed to some extent. Other amacrine cells at different locations (some of which are shown by small circles) will have output zones that overlap, so it appears that the stimuli applied to starburst amacrines outside the ganglion cell's dendritic field can produce the 'silent' inhibitory surround that is characteristic of the ON–OFF direction-selective cells.

An excitatory bipolar input at the site of the small arrow can be expected to have two effects. First, it will provide excitation to the ganglion cell dendrites at that point. Second, by also activating the amacrine cell, it generates a zone of inhibition that spreads predominantly leftward, in this case, but in other directions as well. Simultaneous excitation at point A is subject to cancellation whereas point C will be unaffected. In this simple form, at least, a direction-selective subunit can be generated.

Unfortunately, the difficulties with this simple model are all too obvious. First, other amacrine cells will have overlapping output zones in which the preferential conduction directions are opposite, or nearly so, to the single example shown in Fig. 9.8. Second, the overlapping starburst amacrine cell processes form a very dense plexus (Famiglietti, 1985b; Tauchi & Masland, 1985) that may have to be regarded as a kind of functional syncitium (Masland, Mills & Cassidy, 1984; Masland & Tauchi, 1986). Third, there are likely to be dendrites from three other direction-selective cells in this region; they may have different preferred directions, and will require different patterns of connectivity.

Having arrived at a point where the principal neurons involved in direction-selectivity can be identified and characterized individually, it is somewhat disconcerting to admit that a unique solution to the connectivity problem is not apparent. There are at

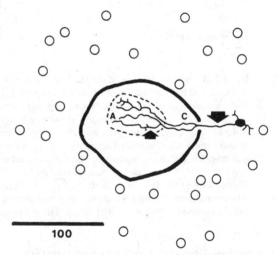

Fig. 9.8. Relationship between a starburst amacrine cell subunit and the dendritic field of a direction-selective ganglion cell. Two of the possible sites of synaptic input to *the amacrine cell* are indicated by arrows. Input at the site of the large arrow activates only the amacrine cell; it will mediate inhibition to the ganglion cell within the region shown by the dashed contour. This will be 'silent' inhibition and may account for the inhibitory surrounds of the direction-selective cell receptive fields. Input at the site of the smaller arrow will also produce inhibition within the zone delimited by the dashed contour; simultaneous excitation to the ganglion cell at point A will be cancelled, but simultaneous excitation at point C will not. This simple model of a direction-selective subunit is difficult to expand to include processes from other starburst amacrines, some of whose somata are shown in the illustration as small circles. Dimension scale in µm.

least two major obstacles remaining, and both are fundamental issues concerning the organization of the retina.

The first problem concerns the specificity of connections among retinal neurons; it can be addressed by the following question. Does a developing neuron, such as a ganglion cell, recognize potential input neurons as individuals or is recognition based on more broadly defined types or classes of neurons? Using direction-selectivity as an example, the question deals with whether or not the direction-selective ganglion cells make connections with all of the starburst amacrine cells within reach. The assumption implicit in most considerations of the direction-selective mechanism is that they do *not*, thereby implying that starburst amacrine cells are recognizable as individuals or as small subsets of individuals.

At present, the hard fact is that we do not know what degree of specificity is involved in the recognition and establishment of connections among retinal neurons. As a result, models for retinal circuitry are unavoidably based on insecure premises, regardless of the degree of specificity that one assumes to exist.

A second difficulty is that a single ganglion cell receives inputs from numerous amacrine and bipolar cells that are unlikely to be functionally isolated from one another. The starburst amacrine cells, for example, may constitute an interconnected array, or network; the properties of this or any other array of real neurons are not known. Direction-selectivity may be a local consequence of the large scale organization of the input array. If so, the mechanism for direction-selectivity is an inherent property of the networks of starburst amacrine cells. Thus the solution to the problem of direction-selectivity may require an understanding of how such a large neuronal network may operate.

What I am suggesting is that the neuronal connectivity underlying direction-selectivity cannot be easily extricated from the larger issues of retinal development and organization. Therein lies much of the importance of the problem. Unlike the operations performed by most other retinal ganglion cells, direction-selectivity is highly asymmetric; it appears that this asymmetry is not a morphological property of the individual neurons that contribute to direction-selectivity. If the task is to understand the retinal circuits that perform specific information processing tasks, and to do this with generalizable principles of retinal organization, the mechanism for direction-selectivity presents a particularly rigorous challenge.

Acknowledgements

It is difficult to express adequately my gratitude to Professor Horace B. Barlow, who was my graduate advisor at Berkeley. Despite the passing of twenty years, I remain indebted for the generous gift of his time, his effort, and his thought in my behalf.

The studies on morphology of rabbit direction-selective cells were done in collaboration with Dr Franklin R. Amthor and Professor Ellen S. Takahashi, with technical assistance from Ms Laura Engstrand and Dr Myong-Suk Lee. Our work was supported by USPHS Grants EY02207, EY03895, EY05070, EY03039 (CORE Grant – UAB) and RR05807 (BRSG).

References

Amthor, F. R., Oyster, C. W. & Takahashi, E. S. (1984) Morphology of on–off direction-selective ganglion cells in the rabbit retina. *Brain Res.*, **298**, 187–90.

Amthor, F. R., Takahashi, E. S. & Oyster, C. W. (1989) Morphologies of rabbit retinal ganglion cells with complex response properties. *J. Comp. Neurol.*, **280**, 97–121.

Ariel, M. & Daw, N. W. (1982) Pharmacological analysis of directionally sensitive rabbit retinal ganglion cells. *J. Physiol.*, **324**, 161–85.

Barlow, H. B. (1953) Summation and inhibition in the frog's retina. *J. Physiol.*, **119**, 69–88.

Barlow, H. B. (1961) Possible principles underlying the transformations of sensory messages. In *Sensory Communication*, ed. W. A. Rosenblith, pp. 217–34. New York: MIT Press and Wiley & Sons.

Barlow, H. B. & Hill, R. M. (1963) Selective sensitivity to direction of movement in ganglion cells of the rabbit retina. *Science*, **139**, 412–14.

Barlow, H. B., Hill, R. M. & Levick, W. R. (1964) Retinal ganglion cells responding selectively to direction and speed of image motion in the rabbit. *J. Physiol.*, **173**, 377–407.

Barlow, H. B. & Levick, W. R. (1965) The mechanism of directionally selective units in rabbit's retina. *J. Physiol.*, **178**, 477–504.

Bloomfield, S. A. & Miller, R. F. (1986) A functional organization of ON and OFF pathways in the rabbit retina. *J. Neurosci.*, **6**, 1–13.

Brecha, N., Johnson, D., Peichl, L. & Wässle, H. (1988) Cholinergic amacrine cells of the rabbit retina contain glutamate decarboxylase and gamma-aminobutyrate *Proc. Natl. Acad. Sci. USA*, **85**, 6187–91.

Caldwell, J. H. & Daw, N. W. (1978) New properties of rabbit retinal ganglion cells. *J. Physiol.*, **276**, 257–76.

Caldwell, J. H., Daw, N. W. & Wyatt, H. J. (1978) Effects of picrotoxin and strychnine on rabbit retinal ganglion cells: lateral interactions for cells with more complex receptive fields. *J. Physiol.*, **276**, 277–98.

Collewijn, H. (1975) Direction-selective units in the rabbit's nucleus of the optic tract. *Brain Res.*, **100**, 489–508.

DeVoe, R. D., Guy, R. G. & Criswell, M. H. (1985) Directionally selective cells of the inner nuclear layer of the turtle retina. *Invest. Ophthal. and Vis. Sci. (Suppl.)*, **26**, 311.

Famiglietti, E. V. (1983) On and off pathways through amacrine cells in mammalian retina: the synaptic connections of 'starburst' amacrine cells. *Vision Res.*, **23**, 1265–79.

Famiglietti, E. V. (1985a) Synaptic organization of ON–OFF directionally selective ganglion cells in rabbit retina. *Soc. Neurosci. Abstr.*, **11**, 337.

Famiglietti, E. V. (1985b) Starburst amacrine cells: morphological constancy and systematic variation in the anisotropic field of rabbit neurons. *J. Neurosci.*, **5**, 562–77.

Hildreth, E. C. & Koch, C. (1987) The analalysis of visual motion: from computational theory to neuronal mechanisms. *Ann. Rev. Neurosci.*, **10**, 477–533.

Koch. C., Poggio, T. & Torre, V. (1986) Computations in the vertebrate retina: gain enhancement, differentiation and motion discrimination. *Trends Neurosci.*, **9**, 204–11.

Lettvin, J. Y., Maturana, H. R., McCulloch, W. S. & Pitts, W. H. (1959) What the frog's eye tells the frog's brain. *Proc. Inst. Rad. Eng.*, **47**, 1940–51.

Levick, W. R. (1967) Receptive fields and trigger features of ganglion cells in the visual streak of the rabbit's retina. *J. Physiol.*, **188**, 285–307.

Masland, R. H. & Tauchi, M. (1986) The cholinergic amacrine cell. *Trends Neurosci.*, **9**, 218–23.

Masland, R. H., Mills, J. W. & Cassidy, C. (1984) The functions of acetylcholine in the rabbit retina. *Proc. Roy. Soc. Lond.*, **B223**, 121–39.

Masland, R. H., Mills, J. W. & Hayden, S. A. (1984) Acetylcholine-synthesizing amacrine cells: identification and selective staining by using radioautography and fluorescent markers. *Proc. Roy. Soc. Lond.*, **B223**, 79–100.

Maturana, H. R., Lettvin, J. Y., McCulloch, W. S. & Pitts, W. H. (1960) Physiology and anatomy of vision in the frog. *J. Gen. Physiol.*, **43**, 129–75.

Millar, T. J. & Morgan, I. G. (1987) Cholinergic amacrine cells in the rabbit retina synapse onto other cholinergic amacrine cells. *J. Neurosci. Lett.*, **74**, 281–5.

Miller, R. F. (1979) The neuronal basis of ganglion cell receptive field organization and the physiology of amacrine cells. In *The Neurosciences, Fourth Study Program*, ed. F. O. Schmitt & F. G. Worden, pp. 227–45. New York: MIT Press.

Miller, R. F. & Bloomfield, S. A. (1983) Electroanatomy of a unique amacrine cell in the rabbit retina. *Proc. Natl. Acad. Sci. USA*, **80**, 3069–73.

Mosinger, J. L. & Yazulla, S. (1987) Double-label analysis of GAD- and GABA-like immunoreactivity in the rabbit retina. *Vision Res.*, **27**, 23–30.

Oyster, C. W. (1968) The analysis of image motion by the rabbit retina. *J. Physiol.*, **199**, 613–35.

Oyster, C. W. & Barlow, H. B. (1967) Direction-selective units in rabbit retina: distribution of preferred directions. *Science*, **155**, 841–2.

Oyster, C. W. & Takahashi, E. S. (1977) Interplexiform cells in rabbit retina. *Proc. Roy. Soc. Lond.*, **B197**, 477–84.

Oyster, C. W., Takahashi, E. S. & Collewijn, H. (1972) Direction-selective retinal ganglion cells and control of optokinetic nystagmus in the rabbit. *Vision Res.*, **13**, 183–93.

Simpson, J. I., Soodak, R. E. & Hess, R. (1979) The accessory optic system and its relation to the vestibulocerebellum. In *Reflex Control of Posture and Movement*, ed. R. Granit & O. Pompeiano. *Prog. Brain Res.*, **50**, 715–24.

Tauchi, M. & Masland, R. H. (1984) The shape and arrangement of the cholinergic neurons in the rabbit retina. *Proc. Roy. Soc. Lond.*, **B223**, 101–19.

Tauchi, M. & Masland, R. H. (1985) Local order among the dendrites of an amacrine cell population. *J. Neurosci.*, **5**, 2494–501.

Torre, V. & Poggio, T. (1978) A synaptic mechanism possibly underlying directional selectivity to motion. *Proc. Roy. Soc. Lond.*, **B202**, 409–16.

Vaney, D. I. & Young, H. M. (1988) GABA-like immunoreactivity in cholinergic amacrine cells of the rabbit retina. *Brain Res.*, **438**, 369–73.

Wyatt, H. J. & Daw, N. W. (1975) Directionally sensitive ganglion cells in the rabbit retina: specificity for stimulus direction, size, and speed. *J. Neurophysiol.*, **38**, 613–26.

Wyatt, H. J. & Daw, N. W. (1976) Specific effects of neurotransmitter anatagonists on ganglion cells in rabbit retina. *Science*, **191**, 204–5.

10

Detection and discrimination mechanisms in the striate cortex of the Old-World monkey

M. J. Hawken and A. J. Parker

Introduction

The sensory systems of man measured at absolute threshold are extraordinarily sensitive. Under favourable conditions, the behavioural performance is close to perfect and the most significant limitations on the human observer are the physical limitations imposed by the nature of the detection task, such as the random fluctuations in the number of quanta arriving at the cornea from a flash of light of very weak intensity (Hecht *et al.*, 1942), or limitations imposed at the transduction stages, such as random, thermally-induced decomposition of photopigment molecules (Barlow, 1956). These demonstrations force one to consider a mechanistic question: namely, how is psychophysical performance of this quality supported by the individual elements of the nervous system, and, in particular, if the essential limitations on performance, even under a restricted set of conditions, can be shown to be either external to the organism or within the primary sense organs, how can information transmission be so reliable throughout the remainder of the system? In this work, we have examined the performance of neurons in the first visual cortical area of Old-World Primates (V1 or striate cortex) on a number of tasks that have identifiable counterparts in perceptual behaviour.

There are a number of psychophysical tasks that are theoretically important in studying perceptual behaviour because they offer a 'systems analysis' of the visual system and its individual components. The study of these tasks has led to the steady evolution of a number of relatively sophisticated, quantitative models of early visual processing, which all incorporate the concept of a set of 'receptive fields' of different sizes or scales that are bandpass in the spatial frequency domain and orientation selective (Campbell & Robson, 1968). These developments in models of spatial vision have resulted from information gathered from a number of different approaches to the same problem – mostly psychophysical and neurophysiological, and more recently computational. In their most highly developed form, these models can predict the threshold visibility of patterned targets of arbitrary spatial organization (Watson, 1983). Therefore, if we wish to attempt to formulate an account of how the operation of neural elements of the striate cortex could support psychophysical performance, this framework provides a sound basis for further progress.

Analysis of thresholds

Before the comparison of neural and psychophysical performance is actually approached, we need to consider what measure or measures of the impulse activity of nerve cells are appropriate for comparison with psychophysical measures of threshold, which are typically defined in terms of the stimulus intensity required to support a certain probability of response by the subject. Techniques of analysing the discharge of nerve cells to extract thresholds have been explored in detail, particularly for vertebrate retinal ganglion cells (Barlow & Levick, 1969; Cohn *et al.*, 1975). Fundamental to these techniques is the recognition that the variability in a neuron's discharge pattern will limit its ability to signal the detection of a weak stimulus or the discrimination of two stimuli closely-spaced on some dimension.

Since psychophysical techniques analyse the probability of detection for a single presentation of the stimulus target (or in the case of discrimination for a pair of targets), it is the response variability of a single neuron to a single stimulus presentation that is most relevant for comparison with psychophysics. In the case of detection, the variability of the resting discharge itself together with the intrinsic sensitivity of the cell for the stimulus in question sets a lower limit on the threshold. In order to analyse the variability of the responses of the cell, we have made use of different techniques as appropriate – construction of a full receiver operating characteristic (ROC) curve (Cohn et al., 1975; Tolhurst et al., 1983; Bradley et al., 1987), construction of a neurometric function for a particular criterion response (Barlow & Levick, 1969; Tolhurst et al., 1983) and threshold tracking techniques (Derrington & Lennie, 1982; Hawken & Parker, 1987). Here, we describe in more detail only one of these, namely the construction of a neurometric function.

With this technique, the response of the neuron to a set of stimuli is measured over a number of trials. Typically, the total number of impulses within the stimulus duration is used as an index of the cell's response, but other possibilities can be considered, such as the modulation of the spike train in synchrony with the drift of bars of the grating or more complex measures based on the occurrence of particular temporal sequences of spikes within the discharge of the cell (Dayhoff & Gerstein, 1983a,b; Richmond et al., 1987). In the case of a simple count of spikes, a criterion number is selected in such a way that the probability of exceeding the criterion in the 'no-stimulus' condition is 0.02–0.05, which is close to the probability in a psychophysical experiment often exhibited by human observers reporting the detection of a stimulus when none was presented (i.e. false alarm rate). The probability of the neuron's output exceeding this criterion is plotted as a function of stimulus intensity and both for cells and observers this curve has a sigmoid shape, well described by a cumulative Gaussian function or a Weibull or Quick function (see Fig. 10.4). The value of intensity supporting a particular detection rate (say 0.5) can be taken as an estimate of the threshold of the cell.

Of the other methods for extracting thresholds, constructing an ROC curve involves the simultaneous application of several criteria to the cell's discharge pattern, much in the way that rating-scale data are treated in psychophysics, while the tracking techniques find a single point on the neurometric function that supports a given detection rate in combination with a fixed false alarm rate. The tracking techniques involve a sacrifice of some of the detailed information about a cell's behaviour, but are faster and more useful when a large number of measures is required. The point of all these techniques, both in neurophysiology and psychophysics, is to allow the threshold of the

system, which is determined by the location of the sigmoid curve relative to the abscissa, to be segregated from the statistical reliability of the response of the system, which is given by the slope of the sigmoid curve. Once this has been done it is more reasonable to compare thresholds of cells and observers.

This preamble to examining thresholds in V1 neurons would be incomplete without appreciating that a single V1 cell is only a component of the complete visual system and, relative to the complete visual system, it has a restricted range of sensitivities. This point must also be taken into account in comparing single cell thresholds with psychophysical thresholds. To take an extreme case, it is unreasonable to expect a V1 neuron with a spatially-restricted receptive field to have a measurable threshold for stimuli presented *outside* the receptive field. This would be equivalent to expecting a light-meter to register a signal for light that was not actually falling on its sensor array. A more practically relevant case is that when a spatially-extended target, such as a sinusoidal grating, is presented, the cell must necessarily behave as if it were viewing this grating target through a spatially-restricted 'window of visibility' (Watson, 1983). This window of visibility is of course the cell's receptive field. The shape of this window is important in determining the sensitivity of any device to a spatial target. A light-meter with an elongated row of sensors will register a lower threshold for a bar of light aligned with the row rather than orthogonal to the row. Therefore, in selecting a psychophysical stimulus configuration for measurement of a threshold, it is important to place the psychophysical observer at the same relative disadvantage as the neuron, which can be achieved by presenting psychophysical stimuli matched carefully in profile and visual eccentricity to the neurophysiologically-measured properties of V1 receptive fields.

Hence, a quantitative model or description of the cell's receptive field profile is needed. One method of acquiring this is to combine the techniques developed for the analysis of visual receptive fields using sinusoidal grating stimuli (Enroth-Cugell & Robson, 1984) with the threshold tracking techniques (Derrington & Lennie, 1982). The advantages of sinusoidal gratings for the characterization of receptive field properties and the extent to which it is valid to apply a linear model of the receptive field have been delimited carefully (Enroth-Cugell & Robson, 1966; Movshon et al., 1978; Shapley & Lennie, 1984). In this work, the threshold contrast sensitivity of cells as a function of spatial frequency was measured and the resulting data were described with a model based on the sum of up to three difference-of-Gaussian functions (Hawken & Parker, 1987). The orientation selectivity of the neuron was also measured and, in combination with the other spatial parameters of the receptive field, was used to estimate the length summation behaviour of the receptive field (Parker & Hawken, 1988). Together these measures estimate a full two-dimensional profile of the receptive field and thus allow an evaluation of the 'window of visibility' for the V1 neuron in question. Of course, the shapes of receptive field profiles of individual V1 neurons differ widely and it is necessary to carry out this procedure on an individual basis for each cell.

In summary, the actual measurements of threshold for detection or discrimination in any device will be controlled by at least two important parameters. First, there is the statistical reliability of the generation of signals when a stimulus is applied and this is generally controlled by the intrinsic noise of the device. Second, there are factors such as the spatial size of the sensor that would affect the sensitivity of almost any device for the stimulus in question. To deal with the first problem, techniques developed for analysing threshold sensitivity of retinal ganglion cells can be applied to the cortex. To deal with the second, quantitative models of the two-dimensional shapes of receptive field profiles of V1 neurons can be obtained and used as a set of 'probe' stimuli in psychophysical experiments.

Acuity limit and detection of fine spatial detail

One of the classic descriptors of pattern vision is acuity or spatial resolution measured with grating targets. The spatial modulation transfer function of the optics of the eye is one of the physical limits to spatial resolution; in humans, this is about 60 cycles/degree in photopic conditions with an optimal pupil size (Campbell & Green, 1965). Psychophysical measurements of the spatial resolution in humans indicate that they have acuities close to this value, 55–60 cycles/degree.

The spatial frequency tuning and acuity for two neurons are shown in Fig. 10.1. Figure 10.1A (top) shows the response as a function of spatial frequency in the conventional style of averaged response. This cell was recorded from V1 of the savannah dwelling vervet monkey (*Cercopithecus aethiops*) and had essentially zero background activity, so that in principle a single spike could be taken as a reliable index of the presence of a signal. The neurometric function in Fig. 10.1A (bottom) is derived simply on the basis of

whether or not the cell fired at all during a stimulus presentation. The estimated grating resolution is 55 cycles/degree. In Fig. 10.1B the spatial frequency tuning is shown for a cell whose acuity is amongst the highest we have recorded in V1 of the tree dwelling cynomologus monkey (*Macaca fascicularis*). Here, reliable detection occurs with a response rate of three spikes or more and the acuity derived from the neurometric function is 25 cycles/degree (Fig. 10.1B, bottom).

Unfortunately, there are no behavioural estimates of acuity in vervet monkeys, but the performance of the cell in Fig. 10.1A is better than that measured behaviourally in other species of Old-World monkeys. The acuity difference between the vervet and the cynomologus cells in Fig. 10.1 is probably explained partly in terms of a small difference in eccentricity of the two receptive fields. There is a very sharp reduction in resolution with small movements away from the fovea in humans (Wertheim, 1895). Another factor that may contribute to the acuity difference is the difference in the foveal cone density between these two species of Old-World monkeys. Perry & Cowey's (1985) measurements on vervet retinae indicate a foveal cone density of about twice that of cynomologus retinae. It seems reasonable to conjecture that individual V1 neurons in primates can provide a signal reliable enough to support the behaviourally-measured foveal acuity.

Contrast detection and discrimination

One of the most informative features of the behaviourally-determined spatial contrast sensitivity function within the context of the multiple channel model of early visual processing is the provision of an estimate of the sensitivity of the system at different spatial frequencies or spatial scales. Based on results from psychophysical experiments, the sensitivity for achromatic gratings is dependent on the spatial frequency, the number of grating cycles, the eccentricity, the duration of the stimulus presentation and the mean luminance of the display (Campbell & Robson, 1968; Graham *et al.*, 1978; Howell & Hess, 1978; Legge, 1978; Watson, 1979; Robson & Graham, 1981). Therefore, it is of some importance to take all these variables into consideration when attempting a comparison between the performance of single neurons and the performance of a psychophysical observer.

Our approach has been to apply a two-dimensional model to the receptive fields of V1 neurons and to estimate the spatial dimensions of the receptive

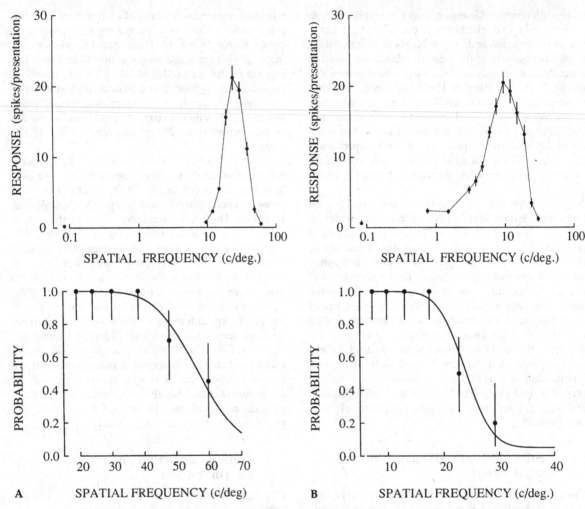

Fig. 10.1. A: the response (mean ± sem) as a function of spatial frequency for a layer 4cβ complex cell from a vervet monkey (*Cercopithecus aethiops*). The receptive field centre was within 0.2° of the fovea. The lower graph plots the neurometric function for the high-frequency portion of the spatial frequency tuning. The solid curve is the best-fitting Weibull function, estimating the grating resolution as 55 cycles/degree. B: spatial frequency response (mean ± sem) function for a layer 4cβ simple cell from a cynomologus monkey (*Macaca fascicularis*). The receptive field centre was between 0.25° and 0.5° eccentric. As in A the lower graph gives the neurometric function, based on exceeding a criterion of 3 spikes (5% false alarm rate). The acuity for this neuron is 25 cycles/degree. Each response in A & B is based on 20 trials of 2 cycles of a drifting grating (temporal frequency: A, 2 Hz; B, 2.6 Hz).

field by applying the model to the spatial contrast sensitivity functions and orientation tuning functions of each cell. This procedure provides a quantitative estimate of the spatial profile of sensitivity over the receptive field and, although these estimates are somewhat indirect, they are arguably more accurate than anything that could be achieved by direct measurement of the point-weighting functions of foveal V1 cells. Subsequently we measured the contrast sensitivity of human observers to a range of stimuli, whose spatial parameters spanned the whole

range of receptive field sizes estimated for the V1 population and whose duration of presentation, temporal frequency of modulation and eccentricity of presentation were all matched as closely as possible to the conditions under which the V1 neurons were tested.

An example of the contrast sensitivity and orientation tuning measurements for a single cell are shown in Fig. 10.2A, with the solid curves being derived from the model. The contrast sensitivity for this cell was obtained from a staircase procedure (Derrington &

Lennie, 1982; Hawken & Parker, 1987) that maintained the false alarm rate for the cell at 5% or less. For this cell, application of the model implies a spatial profile such as that shown in Fig. 10.2B; on the left is the spatial weighting in the direction orthogonal to the preferred orientation, on the right is shown the weighting along the direction of the preferred orientation. This neuron's receptive field was centred at an

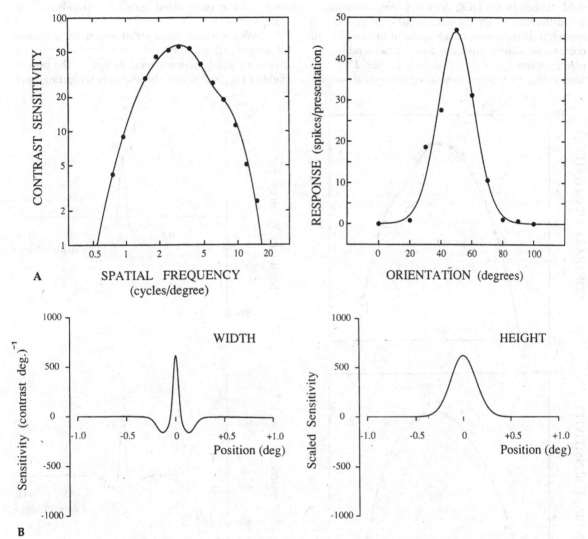

Fig. 10.2. A, left: a plot of contrast sensitivity as a function of spatial frequency for a layer 6 simple cell. The solid circles show the measured contrast sensitivity values, while the solid curve is the best-fitting even symmetric version of a d-DOG-s function used to model the receptive field profile. In the right-hand graph, the solid circles show the response of the same cell to a 6.0 cycle/degree moving grating for a range of orientations. Orientations between 0° (vertical grating moving rightward) and 100° (10° from horizontal moving up and to the left) define the range of orientations and therefore the orientation tuning curve. The solid curve is the predicted orientation tuning derived from the estimated 2-D organization of the cell's receptive field. B, left: the spatial weighting function of the receptive field orthogonal to the preferred orientation (width), for the cell whose contrast sensitivity and orientation tuning are shown in A. The spatial weighting is the even symmetric version of the d-DOG-s function and is the inverse transform of the solid curve in the spatial frequency domain shown in A (left); right: the predicted spatial weighting along the length of the receptive field, parallel to the preferred orientation (height). The convolution of these two spatial weighting functions produces a receptive field with a long relatively narrow central region flanked by two wider antagonistic regions.

eccentricity of 1 degree from the fovea. We have approximated the range of receptive field shapes with a model that is simply a difference-of-Gaussians (DOG) function orthogonal to the preferred orientation and a Gaussian along the length of the receptive field. Although the DOG does not completely mimic the difference of DOGs with separation (d-DOG-s) model, it does provide an adequate fit to most V1 cell contrast sensitivity functions and is considerably simpler than the d-DOG-s (Hawken & Parker, 1987). As seen in Fig. 10.3, when comparing the spatial weight-

ing functions, the central excitatory region is almost identical between d-DOG-s and DOG functions and the largest discrepancy is the shape and spatial extent of the flanking regions. A set of stimuli was constructed so that their normalized luminance profiles matched the normalized sensitivity profiles of the receptive fields.

We measured the contrast sensitivity of human observers to these stimuli over the range of eccentricities from which neurons were sampled. The bottom right of Fig. 10.3 shows the stimulus weighting func-

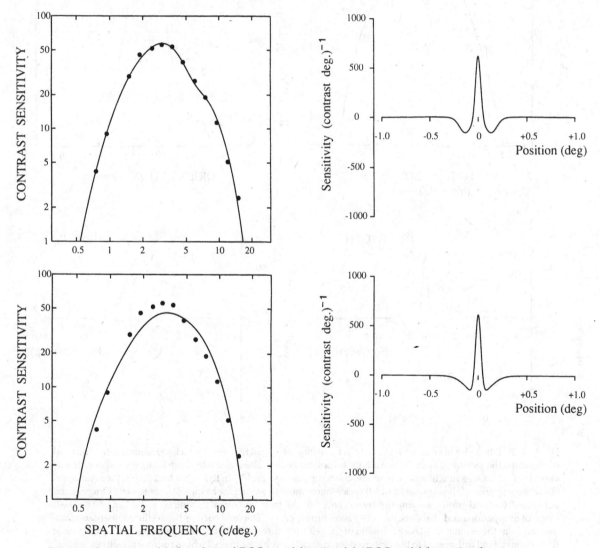

Fig. 10.3. Comparison of the best-fitting d-DOG-s model (top) and the DOG model (bottom) to the contrast sensitivity measurements of the simple cell described in Fig. 10.2. At the top right is the even symmetric spatial weighting of the d-DOG-s function with the bottom right showing the spatial weighting of the DOG for comparison.

tion used to measure the psychophysical threshold to compare with the neural threshold of the cell whose contrast sensitivity function is shown in Figs. 10.2 and 10.3. The contrast threshold obtained from a human observer to the stimulus in this bottom right figure was 32.2 dB while the contrast threshold of the cell was 31.7 dB, a negligible difference. The concept of choosing a stimulus target matched in shape to the receptive field profile can be given clearer justification in terms of the theory of ideal observers. If an observer's performance is noise limited and the spatial and temporal characteristics are known exactly, then the optimal linear filter is a cross-correlation device. Thus if the observer is equipped with a neuron similar in characteristics to the one recorded in the monkey, the optimal strategy for the human observer is to 'use' that neuron when the stimulus target is presented.

For each cell, the response as a function of contrast was measured at one spatial frequency close to the optimal to cross-check the measurements of

sensitivity using a method closely comparable to the psychophysical method (see p. 104). The neurometric functions in Fig. 10.4 were constructed with a criterion chosen to maintain the false alarm rate at less than 5%. The sensitivity for this cell ranges from 2.8 to 3.1% contrast, with the slope of the neurometric function ranging from 2.4 to 3.1. The slopes of the psychometric functions for human observers were mostly in the range 1.5–5.0, with a geometric mean of 2.7. When the threshold is adjusted for a grating stimulus rather than the DOG, then the thresholds for the cell and the observer could be interchanged without any loss of performance of the cell or the observer.

To compare the peak contrast sensitivity of V1 neurons with the thresholds of human observers, the spatial dimensions of the psychophysical target were matched to the two-dimensional receptive field profile of each cell. Analysis of a sample of 75 V1 neurons treated in this way indicates that many have sensitivities which are close to those of the human observer

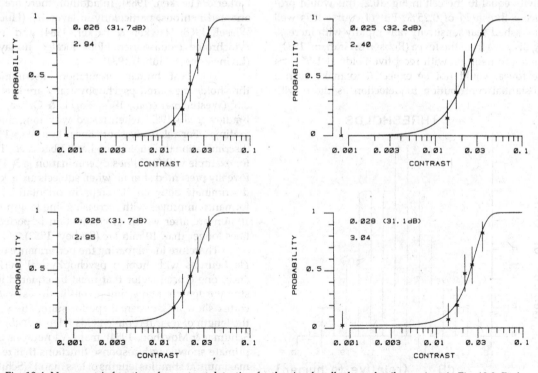

Fig. 10.4. Neurometric functions for contrast detection for the simple cell whose details are given in Fig. 10.2. Each graph shows an independent estimate of the neurometric function for this cell, based on analysis of two sequential cycles of an eight cycle presentation. The grating spatial frequency was 3.75 cycle/degree moving at 2.6 Hz. The star symbols are the measured probabilities of exceeding a criterion based on 40 trials at each contrast, while the solid curve in each graph is the best-fitting Weibull function from which the values of threshold (α) and slope (β) are obtained. In each of the four graphs the threshold contrast is given by the top value (i.e. for the top left graph 0.026 & 31.7 dB) while the slope is given below (i.e. 2.94).

(Fig. 10.5). On the basis of this analysis, many neurons can reliably detect spatially discrete stimuli with a sensitivity sufficient to match psychophysical behaviour.

Of course, with a spatially-extended target much of the stimulus would be outside the limits of a single neuron's receptive field, but neighbouring cells could contribute to detection. If the summation across a large number of neurons can be described by probability summation (an assumption for which there is admittedly little conclusive evidence either way), then there would be a pronounced reduction in threshold. Consider the detection of a 3 cycle/degree grating that covers the whole screen in our experiments, about 18 by 18 cm at a distance of 342 cm. If, purely by way of illustration, one considered only a set of neurons with even-symmetric receptive fields whose peaks were centred at the peaks and troughs of the grating target, about 300 neurons would contribute to the detection if their field centres were located at the peaks and troughs of each cycle. If all 300 neurons had a sensitivity equal to the cell in Fig. 10.2, this would produce a threshold of 0.25%. But of course it is well established that sensitivity falls rapidly with increasing distance from the fovea (Robson & Graham, 1981). Therefore neurons with receptive fields at 1.5° from the fovea would not be expected to make such a substantial contribution to detection as those with

receptive fields right in the foveal representation. Weighting the sensitivity according to the eccentricity gives a threshold of 0.53%, close to the measured values of threshold sensitivity. Of course, this analysis only suggests in principle what could be achieved and the real situation must be very different, but it appears that the independent actions of single neurons, each covering their own discrete portion of visual space through their own 'window of visibility', might be sufficient to support the detection even of spatially-extended stimuli at threshold.

Orientation

One of the most remarkable features of cortical receptive fields of both cat and monkey found by Hubel & Wiesel (1962; 1968) is orientation selectivity. In monkey V1, orientation bandwidth (full width at half height) ranges from around 10° for the most narrowly tuned cells to full widths in excess of 100° (Schiller *et al.*, 1976b; Poggio *et al.*, 1977; De Valois *et al.*, 1982a; Parker & Hawken, 1988). In addition there are non-oriented neurons, particularly in layer 4cβ (Hubel & Wiesel, 1968; Hawken & Parker, 1984) and in the cytochrome oxidase rich blobs located in layer 3 (Livingstone & Hubel, 1984).

The best human orientation discrimination thresholds measured psychophysically are less than 0.5° (Westheimer *et al.*, 1976; Vogels & Orban, 1986; Bradley *et al.*, 1987) when tested with long lines or gratings. For relatively short lines, less than 1°, the discrimination threshold is higher (Orban *et al.*, 1984), for example with 0.5° lines discrimination is 3–4°. For foveally presented stimuli, when subjects are asked to discriminate between 10° steps in orientation, performance improves with increasing line length up to 10 min arc after which discrimination is perfect for lines longer than 10 min arc (Scobey, 1982).

Therefore in comparing the performance of single neurons with human psychophysical performance, one crucial factor that must be equated is the stimulus length. Many simple cells in the cat's striate cortex show a Gaussian shape for summation along the length of their receptive fields (Henry *et al.*, 1978; Schumer & Movshon, 1984); many V1 neurons in the primate show length-response functions that reach a maximum at stimulus lengths of less than 1° (Schiller *et al.*, 1976a). Recently we have attempted to estimate the length of foveal V1 receptive fields, based on measurements of orientation selectivity and an assumption of a Gaussian weighting of sensitivity along the receptive field (Parker & Hawken, 1988). While a few cells had height space constants of greater than 0.5°, the median

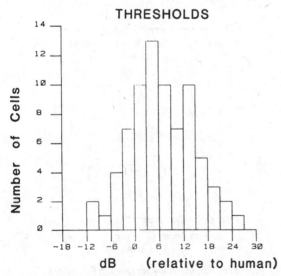

THRESHOLDS

Fig. 10.5. Histogram of the distribution of a sample of 75 V1 neurons where each threshold is given relative to the psychophysical threshold of human observers. It can be seen that a substantial number of neurons have thresholds quite close to the human contrast thresholds.

value was about 15 min arc. In conventional receptive field plots with bars, the estimated values might be 2–4 times these two numbers, depending on the brightness of the bar. Therefore it is probably most reasonable to compare psychophysical thresholds for relatively short stimuli with those of V1 cells.

Recent work in cat V1 shows cells whose orientation discrimination is close to the limits required to support behavioural performance (Bradley *et al.*, 1987; Skottun *et al.*, 1987). For cat V1 neurons, orientation discrimination thresholds are, on average, 20% of the full width of the orientation tuning function (Bradley *et al.*, 1987), so for the most narrowly tuned cells (10° or so) the discrimination thresholds are 2°–3° at best. In the monkey, there are a few cells with orientation bandwidths in the 10° range, which therefore might be

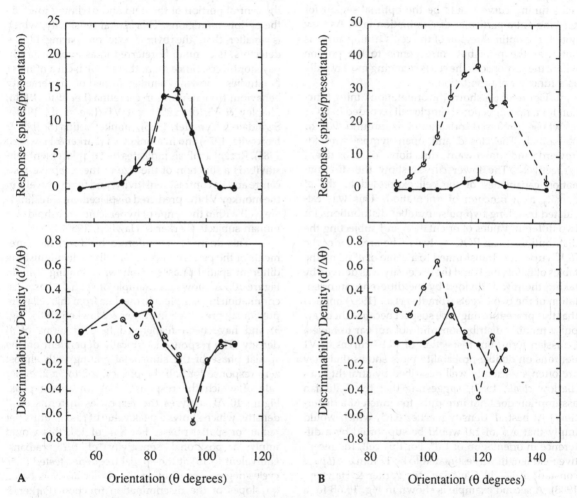

Fig. 10.6. A: the upper graph shows the orientation tuning response function for a layer 3 simple cell. The solid curve shows the response to upward movement, with the peak response being at 90° (horizontal grating). The dashed curve give the tuning for downward movement over the same range of orientations. The solid symbols are the mean response for upward movement with the vertical bars indicating +1 sd. Open circles are for downward movement. The lower graph shows discrimination density as a function of orientation derived from pairs of ROC curves and shows that the best discrimination occurs where the rate of change of response is steepest and not at the peak of the function. B: the orientation tuning function for a direction selective layer 6 simple cell is shown in the upper graph, measured at orientations 5° apart. The preferred orientation (120°) is an oblique stimulus moving rightward and downward (dashed curve). The response to upward leftward moving gratings of the same orientation (solid curve) is much reduced. The lower graph shows the discrimination density as a function of orientation where it can be seen that the peaks of $d'/\Delta\phi$ occur either side of the peak response.

expected to produce discrimination thresholds of about 2°, if the signal to noise characteristics of primate neurons are similar to those of the cat. Measurements of discrimination in the primate are shown in Fig. 10.6. The data, from our own experiments, are from monkey V1 neurons analysed with the ROC techniques similar to those used by Bradley *et al.* (1987). A particular advantage of their technique is that it allows an objective determination of which portion of the cell's tuning curve would be the optimal region for carrying out a particular discrimination task. As they noted, the optimal region of the cell's tuning curve is not near the peak but corresponds to the portion where the response of the cell is changing most rapidly as a function of orientation.

Figure 10.6A shows the orientation tuning function for a non-directional simple cell recorded in layer 3, whose preferred orientation is around 90° or horizontal. The closed and open symbols are for upward and downward directions of movement respectively. The lower curves show the discrimination capabilities of the cell expressed as the d' density as a function of orientation. This was calculated by taking two pulse number distributions for two different values of orientation and subjecting the distributions to an ROC analysis. The area under the ROC curve was transformed to a value of d' using the tables of Elliot (1964) and the d' density was derived by taking the raw d' divided by the difference in orientation of the two targets. [Bradley *et al.* (1987) implied that this procedure might be suspect because their raw pulse number distributions did not appear to have a Gaussian form, but inspection of ROC curves of V1 neurons on double-probability plots shows that they are often sufficiently well described by straight lines (Barlow *et al.*, 1987), suggesting that the Gaussian assumption does not introduce too much of a distortion.] At best, d' density reaches 0.65, which would imply that a d' of 1.0 would be supported by a difference in orientation of 1.8°. For this cell, the receptive field length was estimated to be 17 min arc (space constant of height Gaussian, see Parker & Hawken, 1988). A second example is shown in Fig. 10.6B for a cell that was highly selective for direction as well as orientation. For the preferred direction, d' density reaches a peak value of 0.65 suggesting a d' of 1.0 would be supported by an orientation difference of just less than 2.0°. It is interesting to note that, even though there is a ten-fold difference in peak response at the preferred orientation for the two directions of movement, there is only about a factor of 2 to 3 difference in d' density for orientation discrimination.

Hyperacuity and pattern discrimination

Scobey & Horowitz (1972) showed that cat retinal ganglion cells are capable of signaling stimulus displacements much smaller than the dimensions of the receptive field centre. Furthermore they showed that displacement sensitivity was a function of the distance from the receptive field centre, being most sensitive in the central portion of the field and declining towards the peripheral regions. This spatial sensitivity, which is smaller than the overall size or spacing of the detectors, is commonly referred to as hyperacuity in psychophysics. Since then, there have been a number of studies showing similar forms of hyperacuity behaviour from neurons in cat retina (Lee *et al.*, 1981a; Shapley & Victor, 1986), cat V1 (Lee *et al.*, 1981b; Swindale & Cynader, 1986), monkey retina (Scobey & Horowitz, 1976) and in monkey V1 (Parker & Hawken, 1985). Recent analysis indicates that displacement sensitivity is a function of the size of the receptive field centre and its contrast sensitivity, and for many cells in the monkey V1 the predicted displacement thresholds are well within the range of hyperacuity thresholds for human subjects (Parker & Hawken, 1985).

This analysis is reinforced by direct measurements of the performance of V1 cells in distinguishing different spatial phases of sinewave grating stimuli. Figure 10.7A shows an example of spatial phase discrimination in a simple cell; the data from this cell were previously presented in Parker & Hawken (1985, Fig. 3) and have been reanalysed here in terms of d' density. The response is critically dependent on the spatial phase of the sinusoidal grating with almost zero response for half the phases, $\pi/2$ to $3\pi/2$, either side of which the response rises towards a peak. Figure 10.7B analyses the responses in terms of d' density, which shows a peak value of four d' units per radian of spatial phase. For a d' of 1.0, this would imply a positional sensitivity of 0.25 radians, equivalent to 15″ at the spatial frequency tested (9.56 cycles/degree), confirming the earlier analysis based on slopes of the discrimination function (Parker & Hawken, 1985). The spatial acuity of this cell was 15.4 cycles/degree, i.e. each cycle of the sinewave subtends approximately 4 min arc, so the positional sensitivity is 16 times better than the conventional resolution acuity.

Another form of pattern discrimination task, which also involves the registration of small differences in the spatial distribution of luminance over the target, is spatial frequency discrimination. Psychophysical

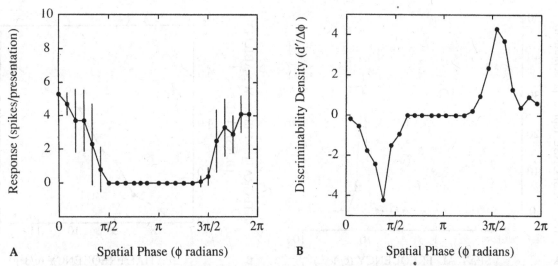

Fig. 10.7. A: the response to 380 ms presentations of a grating stimulus at 24 different spatial phases throughout 2π radians for a layer 6 simple cell. The spatial frequency of the grating was 9.56 cycles/degree therefore distance between successive spatial positions is 15.6" arc. The solid symbols represent the mean response while the vertical bars are ±1 sd. B: the discrimination density per radian plotted as a function of relative spatial phase. There are two very clear peaks corresponding to the rapid transition from a reliable response to zero response in A. This indicates a positional threshold of about 15" of arc for this neuron.

observers have difference thresholds for the discrimination of different spatial frequencies of around 4% of the standard spatial frequency (Campbell *et al.*, 1970), but with targets restricted in vertical and horizontal extent the difference threshold can be as large as 10% (Heeley, 1985). When the standard frequency is relatively high, say 10 cycles/degree, a difference threshold of 4% implies a difference of 9" between the separation of successive pairs of peaks of the sinusoid, well within the hyperacuity range. Some V1 neurons have very narrow spatial frequency tuning functions when tested with high contrast gratings suggesting they may be candidates to support this level of performance (Parker & Hawken, 1985; Bradley *et al.*, 1987). Figure 10.8A shows the spatial frequency tuning of a layer 3 complex cell that had a peak response at 12 cycles/degree. Analysis of the low frequency portion of the tuning function in terms of cumulative *d'* density (Barlow *et al.*, 1987) gives a discrimination threshold of 4.7%.

Conclusion

From these results, it seems reasonable to conclude that for a number of psychophysical tasks, it is possible to find neurons whose threshold performance is, in an objective, statistical sense, close to that of a psychophysical observer. The existence of this correspondence has been found for somatosensory primary afferent fibres with receptive fields on the volar aspects of the fingers (Vallbo & Johansson, 1976). However, it would be more speculative to conclude that psychophysical thresholds actually bear a direct relationship to the individual sensitivities of single cortical neurons under normal conditions. Unfortunately, it is possible to give plausible arguments both for the view that psychophysical thresholds should be lower than neural thresholds and the converse. In the first case, it may be argued that statistical averaging over a population of neurons will lower the psychophysical thresholds relative to the neural. On the other hand, the efficacy of any such statistical averaging must be limited to some degree by the fact that cortical cells in V1 appear to have a threshold nonlinearity in their *d'* vs contrast functions (Barlow *et al.*, 1987). In the second case, it may be argued that the chief problem for the psychophysical observer is that he is equipped with a large number of neurons, only a fraction of which are relevant for the current task; if the observer's nervous system cannot reliably identify the relevant neurons, then the background activity of the irrelevant neurons may contribute a significant amount of noise, and so it would be necessary for the thresholds of the relevant neurons to be considerably lower than the psychophysical threshold. This second case is a modified version of

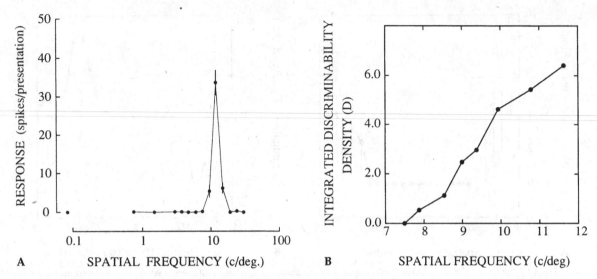

Fig. 10.8. A: the response tuning function of a layer 3 complex cell to a range of spatial frequencies from 0.75 to 24.0 cycles/degree with the cell responding at only three spatial frequencies, 9.56, 12.0 and 15.0 cycles/degree. B: for a range of spatial frequencies on the low frequency limb of the response tuning function the integrated discriminability density is plotted against spatial frequency. Interpolation between the middle four points of the function gives a spatial frequency difference threshold at 4.7% for a d' of 1 at 9.0 cycles/degree. Also of interest is the fact that performance is reasonably good over a range as large as 6 d' units.

the stimulus uncertainty argument presented in the signal detection theory literature.

Both of these possibilities are difficult to test rigorously, but perhaps the best test would come from experiments of the style already carried out using axonal recording from the tactile sensory nerves in awake human subjects (Vallbo & Johannson, 1976). In this case, it is possible to observe the trial-by-trial correlations in the behaviour of the neuron and the psychophysical observer. A similar kind of experiment can be conceived for the visual cortex using the techniques of recording from awake behaving primates, but such an experiment would have to meet the criteria for neural thresholds discussed above and, in addition, arrange for simultaneous measurement of a psychophysical threshold in the animal, accurate control for the effects of eye movements and a lengthy search for the most sensitive neurons in the cortex. Although this would be difficult, other possible approaches would be somewhat indirect at best.

Whatever the outcome of such an experiment, it is clear that single neurons do carry highly reliable signals about events in the outside world – at least the reliability is no worse than that experienced as a consequence of fluctuations in behavioural thresholds. But equally it is clear that for some of the psychophysical tasks studied here, relying on the

activity of just one cortical cell would be wholly inadequate. The activity of the cortical cell is easily altered by changes in the stimulus other than those manipulated in the physiology experiment. For example, in the case of spatial frequency discrimination, changes in the contrast of the test and comparison gratings from trial to trial do not greatly upset human discrimination performance, but presumably such changes would significantly degrade the performance of cells in V1. To deal with this kind of variation in the stimuli, the visual system needs to construct a signal about spatial frequency that is invariant with changes in stimulus contrast. Demonstrating the existence of cells that are highly sensitive to changes in spatial frequency is an important first step in offering an explanation for human discrimination performance, but such demonstrations do not show how the visual system constructs a measure that could be used directly for controlling responses in the discrimination task.

Acknowledgements

This research was supported by grant 7900491 to C. Blakemore from the MRC, NATO grant 85/0167, Wellcome Trust major equipment grant and USAF grant AFOSR-85-0296.

References

Barlow, H. B. (1956) Retinal noise and absolute threshold. *J. Opt. Soc. Am.*, **46**, 634–9.

Barlow, H. B. & Levick, W. R. (1969) Three factors limiting the reliable detection of light by retinal ganglion cells of the cat. *J. Physiol.*, **200**, 1–24.

Barlow, H. B., Hawken, M. J., Kaushal, T. P. & Parker, A. J. (1987) Human contrast discrimination and the threshold of cortical neurons. *J. Opt. Soc. Am.*, **A4**, 2366–71.

Bradley, A., Skottun, B. C., Ohzawa, I., Sclar, G. & Freeman, R. D. (1987) Visual orientation and spatial frequency discrimination: a comparison of single neurons and behaviour. *J. Neurophysiol.*, **57**, 755–72.

Campbell, F. W. & Green, D. G. (1965) Optical and retinal factors affecting visual resolution. *J. Physiol.*, **181**, 576–93.

Campbell, F. W. & Robson, J. G. (1968) Application of Fourier analysis to the visibility of gratings. *J. Physiol.*, **197**, 551–6.

Campbell, F. W., Nachmias, J. & Jukes, J. (1970) Spatial frequency discrimination in human vision. *J. Opt. Soc. Am.*, **60**, 555–9.

Cohn, T. E., Green, D. G. & Tanner, W. P. (1975) Receiver operating characteristic analysis. Application to the study of quantum fluctuation effects in optic nerve of *Rana pipiens*. *J. Gen. Physiol.*, **66**, 583–616.

Dayhoff, J. E. & Gerstein, G. L. (1983a) Favored patterns in spike trains. I detection. *J. Neurophysiol.*, **49**, 1334–48.

Dayhoff, J. E. & Gerstein, G. L. (1983b) Favored patterns in spike trains. II application. *J. Neurophysiol.*, **49**, 1349–63.

Derrington, A. M. & Lennie, P. (1982) The influence of temporal frequency and adaptation level on receptive field organization of retinal ganglion cells in the cat. *J. Physiol.*, **333**, 343–66.

DeValois, R. L., Yund, E. W. & Hepler, N. (1982a) The orientation and direction selectivity of cells in the macaque visual cortex. *Vision Res.*, **22**, 531–44.

Elliot, P. B. (1964) Tables of d'. In *Signal Detection and Recognition by Human Observers*, ed. J. A. Swets, Appendix 1, pp. 651–84, New York: J. Wiley and Son Inc.

Enroth-Cugell, C. & Robson, J. G. (1966) The contrast sensitivity of the retinal ganglion cells of the cat. *J. Physiol.*, **187**, 517–52.

Enroth-Cugell, C. & Robson, J. G. (1984) Functional characteristics and diversity of cat retinal ganglion cells. *Invest. Ophthal. and Vis. Sci.*, **25**, 250–67.

Graham, N., Robson, J. G. & Nachmias, J. (1978) Grating summation in fovea and periphery. *Vision Res.*, **18**, 815–25.

Hawken, M. J. & Parker, A. J. (1984) Contrast sensitivity and orientation selectivity in laminar IV of the striate cortex of Old World monkeys. *Exp. Brain Res.*, **54**, 367–72.

Hawken, M. J. & Parker, A. J. (1987) Spatial properties of neurons in the monkey striate cortex. *Proc. Roy. Soc. Lond.*, B**231**, 251–88.

Hecht, S., Shlaer, S. & Pirenne, M. (1942) Energy, quanta, and vision. *J. Gen. Physiol.*, **25**, 819–40.

Heeley, D. W. (1985) Retinal image sampling as a limiting process in the visual discrimination of sine wave gratings in man. *J. Physiol.*, **367**, 17P.

Henry, G. H., Goodwin, A. W. & Bishop, P. O. (1978) Spatial summation of responses in receptive fields of simple cells in cat striate cortex. *Exp. Brain Res.*, **32**, 245–66.

Howell, E. R. & Hess, R. F. (1978) The functional area for summation to threshold for sinusoidal gratings. *Vision Res.*, **18**, 369–74.

Hubel, D. H. & Wiesel, T. N. (1962) Receptive fields, binocular interaction and functional architecture in the cat's visual cortex. *J. Physiol.*, **160**, 106–54.

Hubel, D. H. & Wiesel, T. N. (1968) Receptive fields and functional architecture of monkey striate cortex. *J. Physiol.*, **195**, 215–43.

Lee, B. B., Elepfandt, A. & Virsu, V. (1981a) Phase of responses to moving sinusoidal gratings in cells of cat retina and lateral geniculate nucleus. *J. Neurophysiol.*, **45**, 807–17.

Lee, B. B., Elepfandt, A. & Virsu, V. (1981b) Phase of response to sinusoidal gratings of simple cells in cat striate cortex. *J. Neurophysiol.*, **45**, 818–28.

Legge, G. (1978) Space domain properties of a spatial frequency channel in human vision. *Vision Res.*, **18**, 959–69.

Livingstone, M. S. & Hubel, D. H. (1984) Anatomy and physiology of a color system in the primate visual cortex. *J. Neurosci.*, **4**, 309–56.

Movshon, J. A., Thompson, I. D. & Tolhurst, D. J. (1978) Spatial summation in the receptive fields of simple cells in the cat's striate cortex. *J. Physiol.*, **283**, 79–99.

Orban, G. A., Vandenbussche, E. & Vogels, R. (1984) Human orientation discrimination tested with long stimuli. *Vision Res.*, **24**, 121–8.

Parker, A. J. & Hawken, M. J. (1985) The capabilities of cortical cells in spatial-resolution tasks. *J. Opt. Soc. Am.*, A**2**, 1101–14.

Parker, A. J. & Hawken, M. J. (1988) 2-dimensional spatial structure of receptive fields in the monkey striate cortex. *J. Opt. Soc. Am.* A**5**, 598–605.

Perry, V. H. & Cowey, A. (1985) The ganglion cell and cone distributions in the monkey's retina: implications for central magnification factors. *Vision Res.*, **25**, 1795–1810.

Poggio, G. D., Doty, R. W. & Talbot, W. H. (1977) Foveal striate cortex of behaving monkey: single neuron responses to square-wave gratings during fixation of gaze. *J. Neurophysiol.*, **40**, 1369–91.

Richmond, B. J., Optican, L., Podell, M. & Spitzer, H. (1987) Temporal encoding of two-dimensional patterns by single units in the primate inferior temporal cortex. I. Response characteristics. *J. Neurophysiol.*, **57**, 132–46.

Robson, J. G. & Graham, N. (1981) Probability summation and regional variation in contrast sensitivity across the visual field. *Vision Res.*, **21**, 409–18.

Schiller, P. H., Finlay, B. L. & Volman, S. F. (1976a) Quantitative studies of single-cell properties in monkey striate cortex: I. Spatiotemporal organization of receptive fields. *J. Neurophysiol.*, **39**, 1288–319.

Schiller, P. H., Finlay, B. L. & Volman, S. F. (1976b) Quantitative studies of single-cell properties in monkey striate cortex: II. Orientation specificity and ocular dominance. *J. Neurophysiol.*, **39**, 1320–33.

Schumer, R. A. & Movshon, J. A. (1984) Length summation in simple cells of cat striate cortex. *Vision Res.*, **24**, 565–71.

Scobey, R. P. (1982) Human visual orientation discrimination. *J. Neurophysiol.*, **48**, 18–26.

Scobey, R. P. & Horowitz, J. M. (1972) The detection of small image displacements by cat retinal ganglion cells. *Vision Res.*, **12**, 2133–43.

Scobey, R. P. & Horowitz, J. M. (1976) Detection of image displacement by phasic cells in peripheral visual fields of the monkey. *Vision Res.*, **16**, 15–24.

Shapley, R. M. & Lennie, P. (1984) Spatial frequency analysis in the visual system. *Ann. Rev. Neurosci.*, **8**, 547–83.

Shapley, R. M. & Victor, R. (1986) Hyperacuity in cat retinal ganglion cells. *Science*, **231**, 999–1002.

Skottun, B., Bradley, A., Sclar, G., Ohzawa, I. & Freeman, R. D. (1987) The effects of contrast on visual orientation and spatial frequency discrimination: a comparison of single cells and behavior. *J. Neurophysiol.*, **75**, 773–86.

Swindale, N. S. & Cynader, M. S. (1986) Vernier acuity of neurons in cat visual cortex. *Nature*, **319**, 591–3.

Tolhurst, D. J., Moshon, J. A. & Dean, A. F. (1983) The statistical reliability of signals in single neurons in cat and monkey visual cortex. *Vision Res.*, **23**, 775–86.

Vallbo, A. B. & Johansson, R. (1976) Skin mechanoreceptors in the human hand: neural and psychophysical thresholds. In *Sensory Functions of the Skin in Primates: with Special Reference to Man*, ed. Y. Zotterman, pp. 185–98. Oxford: Pergamon Press.

Vogels, R. & Orban, G. A. (1986) Decision processes in visual discrimination and line orientation. *J. Exp. Psychol. Human Perception and Performance*, **12**, 115–32.

Watson, A. B. (1979) Probability summation over time. *Vision Res.*, **19**, 515–22.

Watson, A. B. (1983) Detection and recognition of simple spatial forms. In *Physical and Biological Processing of Images*. ed. O. J. Braddick & A. C. Sleigh, pp. 100–14. Berlin: Springer-Verlag.

Wertheim, T. (1895) Uber die indirekte Sehscharfe. *Zeitschrift fur Psychol, und Physiol, Sinnesorg*, **BVII**, s185, 173–87.

Westheimer, G., Shimamura, K. & McKee, S. P. (1976) Interference with line orientation sensitivity. *J. Opt. Soc. Am.*, **66**, 332–8.

Colour

11
The two subsystems of colour vision and their rôles in wavelength discrimination

J. D. Mollon, O. Estévez and C. R. Cavonius

Introduction

Horace Barlow makes only occasional forays into the field of colour vision (Barlow, 1958, 1982), but when he does, he always leaves us with much to think about. In his 1982 paper 'What causes trichromacy?', he gave us a novel way of considering the information content of a coloured spectrum: he expressed the detailed structure of the colour spectrum in terms of its Fourier components and he treated the three photopigments (Fig. 11.1) as low-pass filters that would differentially attenuate the different Fourier components. Owing to the broad bandwidth of the filters, the visual system is insensitive to the fine structure of the colour spectrum; that is to say, if the amplitude of a stimulus varies periodically with wavelength and if the period of this modulation is small, then the response of the visual system will show little variation as the phase of the modulation is changed (Barlow, 1982).

In considering his main question – that of why our colour vision is three-dimensional – Barlow was led also to ask several secondary questions: 'Why do the photopigments have such broad bandwidths?', 'Are broad bandwidths deleterious to hue discrimination?' and 'Why are the peak sensitivities of the pigments so asymmetrically placed in the spectrum?' We hope that the present paper may say something in answer to these secondary questions. We first put forward a general view of the early stages of colour vision, the view that it consists of two subsystems, one recently overlaid on a much earlier one; and then we review some experimental work on wavelength discrimination, work that bears on the two subsystems of colour vision.

The emerging view of colour vision is one that has long been suggested by the distribution of colour discrimination among the mammals (Jacobs, 1982); by the relative incidences of different forms of colour blindness in man (Ladd-Franklin, 1892); and by a number of asymmetric features of our colour vision, such as the relative paucity of the short-wave receptors (compared with the middle- and long-wave receptors) and indeed the asymmetric arrangement of the absorbance curves of the photopigments (Gouras, 1984; Mollon, 1986; Mollon & Jordan, 1988). It is a view consistent with Derrington, Krauskopf & Lennie's electrophysiological analysis of the parvocellular layers of the lateral geniculate nucleus (Derrington et al., 1984). But, above all, it is a view prompted by the molecular biology of the visual pigments published by Nathans and his collaborators (Nathans et al., 1986a,b). The most salient findings of Nathans et al. are: first, that the genes for the long- and middle-wave pigments lie very close together on the q-arm of the X-chromosome, and second, that the amino-acid sequences for the two pigments are 96% identical. It appears that visual pigments all consist of seven helices, which span the membrane and form a palisade surrounding the retinal, the prosthetic group that gives the pigment its spectral sensitivity (Fig. 11.2). The solid circles in the diagram to the bottom right of Fig. 11.2 show the small number of amino acids that Nathans et al. identify as different between the long- and middle-wave pigments. The strong implication is that these two pigments were differentiated only very recently,[1] by duplication of an ancestral gene. On the

[1] 'Very recently' would here mean 'within the last 30 to 40 million years' (see Nathans et al., 1986a). That the duplication event occurred after the divergence of platyrrhine and catyrrhine monkeys is also suggested by the fact that New-World primates appear to have only one X-chromosome locus for a visual pigment (Mollon, Bowmaker & Jacobs, 1984; Bowmaker, Jacobs & Mollon, 1987)

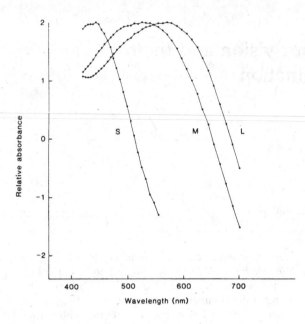

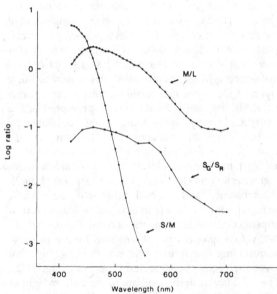

other hand, the gene for the short-wave pigment is located on chromosome 7 and the amino-acid sequence for that pigment differs as much from the sequences for the long- and middle-wave pigments as it does from that for the rod pigment, rhodopsin: the implication is that the short-wave pigment has long enjoyed an independent existence.

The two subsystems of colour vision

These considerations suggest the nature of the two subsystems that underlie human colour vision.

Widespread among mammals is a primordial, dichromatic, system of colour vision that compares the rates at which photons are absorbed in the short-wave cones, on the one hand, and, on the other, in a second class of cone with a peak sensitivity that varies across species but lies always in the green to yellow region of the spectrum (Jacobs, 1982). This ratio is extracted by a minority class of ganglion cells that exhibit little sensitivity to spatial contrast: such cells (and their counterparts in the parvocellular laminae of the lateral geniculate nucleus) behave as if they draw antagonistic inputs from coextensive or nearly coextensive regions of the receptor array, and thus this subsystem comes close to being a pure colour system (Gouras, 1984; Derrington & Lennie, 1984). There is some evidence that a morphologically distinct channel subserves the extraction of this primordial colour information: Mariani (1984) has described an uncommon type of primate bipolar cell that resembles the usual midget invaginating bipolar, except that the cell body gives rise to several dendrites and may make contact with two, well-separated, cone pedicles (which Mariani takes to be short-wave cones). The short-wave cones, and the higher-order cells that carry their signals, can be sparsely distributed, because they are given little part to play in the analysis of spatial detail (Tansley & Boynton, 1976; Thoma & Scheibner, 1980); and this in turn is likely to be because the short-wave component of the retinal image is chronically degraded, since non-

Fig. 11.1. The upper panel shows the spectral sensitivities of the short-wave (S), middle-wave (M) and long-wave (L) cones. These 'König fundamentals' are those derived by Estévez from the Stiles–Burch 2-deg colour-matching data. In the lower panel are plotted the log ratio of middle-wave to long-wave cone sensitivity (M/L) and the log ratio of short-wave to middle-wave sensitivity (S/M). Also plotted in the lower panel is the log ratio of middle-wave to long-wave cone sensitivity (S_G/S_R), as obtained by electrophysiological recording from individual cones of *Macaca fascicularis* by Nunn,

Schnapf & Baylor (1985) (this function is arbitrarily placed on the ordinate). In order to allow direct comparison with the electrophysiological results, which were obtained by transverse illumination of receptors, the sensitivities of the 'König fundamentals' are given as absorptances for a pigment solution of low concentration. There is only a very small shift in the position of the maximum of M/L when allowance is made for self-screening of the pigment *in vivo*; and pre-receptoral absorption cannot change the position of the maximum.

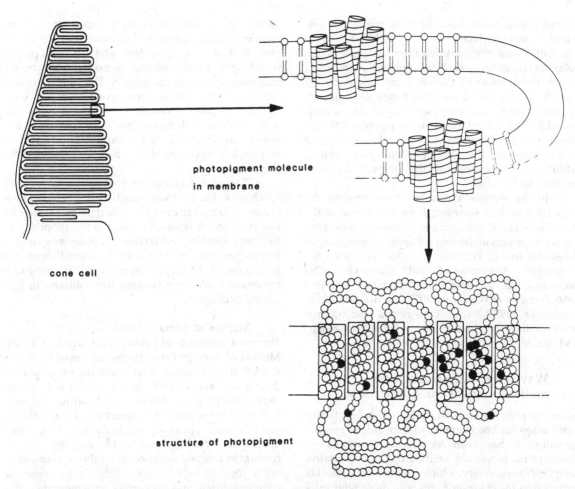

photopigment molecule in membrane

cone cell

structure of photopigment

Fig. 11.2. The structure of visual pigments. The upper panels illustrate the arrangement of the pigment molecules in the infolded membranes of the outer segment of a cone: each molecule consists of seven transmembrane helices, which cluster around the chromophore. At the bottom right is represented (after Nathans) the sequence of amino acids in the protein part of the photopigment: the filled circles indicate those amino acids that differ between the long- and middle-wave pigments of the human retina.

directional skylight dilutes the shadows of the natural world and since the eye itself is subject to chromatic aberration.

In the Old World monkeys and in man, the ancestral subsystem is overlaid by a second colour vision system that compares the rates at which quanta are caught in the long- and middle-wave cones. This recently evolved system is parasitic, we suggest, on a channel that still has as its chief purpose the analysis of spatial detail. The substrates for this channel are the midget bipolars, the midget (or 'Pβ') retinal ganglion cells, and the predominant type of parvocellular unit in the lateral geniculate nucleus. Such cells draw their antagonistic inputs not only from distinct classes of cone but also from distinct regions of the field; and

thus they respond both to colour and to spatial contrast.[2]

In summary then, the three cone pigments of

[2] It is not uncontroversial to claim that this channel still has for its main business the analysis of spatial detail. On the basis of the higher contrast sensitivity and higher gain of the magnocellular system, Shapley & Perry (1986) have suggested that the *principal* function of the parvocellular laminae is colour vision. And there have been several reports that maximal spatial resolution is similar for units in the magnocellular and parvocellular streams of the visual system (e.g. Blakemore & Vital-Durand, 1986; Crook, Lange-Malecki, Lee & Valberg, 1988). For a detailed discussion of the position adopted here, see Mollon & Jordan (1988).

normal human vision have different origins and different evolutionary rôles. The ancestral middle-wave pigment, maximally sensitive near the peak of the solar spectrum, subserved the primary purposes of vision, the analyses of motion, form, and depth. A long time ago, the short-wave cones were added, sparingly, for the sole purpose of colour vision. Most recently, the ancestral middle-wave pigment differentiated to give a second dimension of colour vision; but in this case, both the daughter pigments developed within the constraints of the original function, namely, spatial vision.

In the sections that follow, we consider the respective rôles in wavelength discrimination of the two subsystems of colour vision. In treating separately the contributions of the two subsystems, our analysis resembles that of Walraven and Bouman, who distinguished 'deuteranopic' and 'tritanopic' components of hue discrimination (Walraven & Bouman, 1966; Bouman & Walraven, 1972), or that of Judd & Yonemura (1970), who constructed the normal wavelength-discrimination curve from 'protanopic' and 'tritanopic' components.

Wavelength discrimination: methodological considerations

In one respect, the modern study of wavelength discrimination has been curiously backward. In psychoacoustics, it has been for twenty years almost unacceptable to use any method but two-alternative temporal forced-choice, which minimizes the effect of variation in the observer's criterion; those who work on spatial frequency have nearly as honourable a record; and even in colour vision it is commonplace to use such performance measures when chromaticity is modulated on displays with fixed phosphors. But, to the shame of our sub-branch of visual science, the discrimination of wavelength is still commonly measured by a time-honoured method of adjustment (Wright & Pitt, 1935): the subject increases the difference in wavelength until the standard and variable fields look different and then sees if he can eliminate the perceptual differences by adjusting the luminance of the variable. If he can, he increases the wavelength difference and repeats the process until the two half-fields look different at all luminance settings. It is easy to imagine that the criterion used by the observer might differ according to the spectral region being examined, and in particular, according to which subsystem of colour vision (i.e. which ratio of cone signals) was mediating discrimination.

Two obstacles may excuse the psychophysical

backwardness that has characterised studies of wavelength discrimination. The first is the mechanical one, that it has been less easy to manipulate wavelength in real time than to manipulate acoustic frequency or spatial frequency. This difficulty has passed with the introduction of monochromators with integral stepping motors: the experiments we describe were all done with monochromators that allow the centre wavelength of the passband to be adjusted in steps of 0.05 nm (Type M300E, Bentham Instruments, Reading, UK).

The second difficulty is that in some parts of the spectrum a change of wavelength can be detected by a change in luminosity more readily than by a change in hue (Laurens & Hamilton, 1923). If we adopt a performance measure and eschew the observer's subjective judgements, then we need to ensure that we are testing colour discrimination and not luminosity discrimination. We have adopted two solutions to this second problem:

Method of Average Error
The most venerable of performance measures is the Method of Average Error, the method used by König & Dieterici to measure wavelength discrimination in their great paper of 1884. In our version of this procedure, the observer views a 2-deg bipartite field, one half of which is fixed in luminance and wavelength. The computer repeatedly offsets the wavelength and luminance of the other half field by amounts that are random in size and direction; the subject, manipulating a joystick in two dimensions, must restore a complete match; and the performance measure is the standard deviation of 50 settings (Mollon & Estévez, 1988). The subject cannot use luminosity as a guide to wavelength: he must himself make a match on both dimensions.

Forced-choice
We have allowed the psychoacousticians to teach us how to measure frequency discrimination by two-alternative forced-choice. When modern measurements of acoustic frequency discrimination were first attempted, the resolution at high frequencies appeared much better than in the classical study of Stücker (1908), who, using Galton whistles, tested Mahler and other musicians of the Vienna Court Opera. Henning (1966), however, introduced small random variations of amplitude into the tones to be discriminated and found that his results agreed with those of Stücker. The implication is that Stücker was not able to blow his Galton whistles absolutely steadily and so was able to secure true measurements of

frequency discrimination. We have translated Henning's paradigm to vision (Mollon & Cavonius, 1987). On each trial, there are two presentations of a bipartite field. The lower, standard, half-field is fixed in wavelength and luminance. On one of the two presentations the wavelength of the upper half-field is the same as that of the standard; and on the other presentation the upper field has a wavelength that is greater by a value $\Delta\lambda$. To prevent the use of luminosity cues, small random variations in the luminance of the upper half-field are introduced within and between trials, the range of variation being ± 0.1 log unit. The subject must indicate on which of two presentations the fields differ in wavelength, and $\Delta\lambda$ is adjusted by a staircase procedure to track the 71% correct point. The value of $\Delta\lambda$ is initially 3 nm; this value is increased by a factor 1.25 after each incorrect response and decreased by a factor 0.8 after two correct responses (Moore, Glasberg & Shailer, 1984). Feedback is given by tone signals after each trial.

The reader may wonder why we did not use a simpler form of the forced-choice paradigm, in which the observer was asked to say whether the longer wavelength was in the upper or lower half of a single bipartite field. A spatial forced choice of this kind was used in the strikingly modern study of Laurens & Hamilton (1923). For our present purposes, a specific difficulty is that 'longer' corresponds to different appearances in different spectral regions; and in particular, when the stimuli are bright, there is a wavelength near 460 nm where excursions in longer and shorter directions give a similar change in appearance (Mollon & Estévez, 1988). The particular forced-choice method we adopted (see above) requires the subject to make only the simplest discrimination: on which of the two presentations is a physical difference in wavelength more likely to have been present. He is not asked to report the direction of the difference.

The short-wave pessimum

Figure 11.3 offers an overall view of wavelength discrimination as examined by the two-alternative temporal forced-choice method (see above). The troland value of the lower, standard, half-field was always 50, with Judd's correction (Wyszecki & Stiles, 1982, Table 5.2.2) being applied below 460 nm; and the duration of each presentation was 800 ms (these turn out to be significant parameters). The bandwidths of the monochromators were set at 1 nm, and broadband gelatin blocking filters, appropriate to the standard wavelength, were placed in the final com-

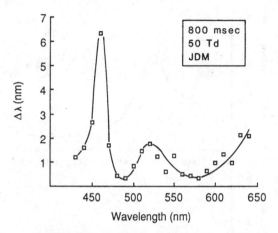

Fig. 11.3. Wavelength discrimination measured by two-alternative temporal forced-choice. For details of methods, see text. Observer: JDM.

mon beam. Thresholds were estimated from the last 16 of 20 reversals of the staircase. Wavelengths were sampled every ten nanometers in two different randomised sequences; the plotted thresholds represent the means of the two separate estimates for each wavelength.

As in the classical data (König & Dieterici, 1884; Wright & Pitt, 1935), there are two clear minima in the function of Fig. 11.3, near 490 nm and 580 nm. Owing to the forced-choice method, the absolute values of the thresholds in these regions are lower than those found with adjustment methods (Wright & Pitt, 1935), dropping to as little as 0.25 nm. It is noteworthy that the visual system achieves this impressive resolution with photodetectors that have a bandwidth of the order of 100 nm (Fig. 11.1). But perhaps the most salient feature of the present results is the size of the peak at 460 nm, where the threshold rises to 7 nm. We shall refer to this peak as the 'short-wave pessimum'. The useful term 'pessimum' was introduced by Robert Weale (Weale, 1951) and it avoids the ambiguity of speaking of a maximum in the wavelength-discrimination function. In the rest of this paper, we concentrate on an analysis of the short-wave region of the spectrum, since it serves well to illustrate the rôle in wavelength discrimination of the two subsystems of human colour vision and the factors that limit their performance.

Figure 11.4 gives a magnified view of discrimination in the short-wave region. Measurements were made by the method of average error (Mollon & Estévez, 1988) and standard wavelengths were sampled every 5 nm). The thresholds are typically lower than those obtained by forced-choice, since here they

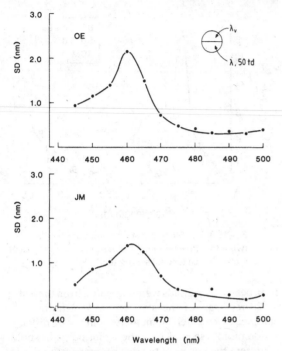

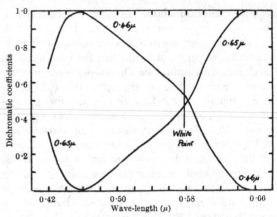

Fig. 11.5. Dichromatic coefficient curves for a centrally fixated colour-matching field that subtended 20' of arc (from Willmer & Wright, 1945). The primaries were 460 and 650 nm; the units of these two stimuli were chosen to be equal in a match to a yellow of 582.5 nm, and the values for the 460-nm (b) and 650-nm (r) coefficients in any match were adjusted to bring $b + r = 1$. All wavelengths between 420 and 650 nm could be matched by positive mixtures of the two primaries, and this is the basis for our argument that the ratio of middle- to long-wave cone sensitivity must peak near 460 nm (see text). Reproduced by permission of Professors E. N. Willmer and W. D. Wright.

Fig. 11.4. Wavelength discrimination in the short-wave region, measured by the method of average error. The ordinate represents the precision (standard deviation) of settings of the variable wavelength (λ_v) when matching standard wavelengths (λ) in the range 445 to 500 nm. Each data point represents the r.m.s. value for two independent sets of 25 matches. Results are shown separately for two of the present authors. Note the well-defined peak in the function at 460 nm, the 'short-wave pessimum'.

represent the standard deviation of matches, but again a sharply defined peak occurs at 460 nm.

So, at this point in the spectrum, neither of the two subsystems of colour vision seems to be doing us much good. But the reasons are different, we suggest, for the two subsystems. Consider first the subsystem that compares the quantum catches in the middle- and long-wave cones. The most obvious factor that must limit wavelength discrimination (and the factor considered in traditional analyses) is the rate of change with wavelength of the ratio of quantum catches. Near 460 nm the ratio of middle-wave to long-wave sensitivity ($M:L$) goes through a shallow maximum (see Fig. 11.1, lower panel) and the rate of change must slow down to zero. That this is so is implied by the colour-matching functions for tritanopes, who lack short-wave cones, and by the corresponding functions for normal observers viewing under tritan conditions (Fischer, Bouman & Ten Doesschate, 1952; Wright,

1952; Willmer & Wright, 1945; Alpern, Kitahara & Krantz, 1983). Figure 11.5 shows colour matching results for W. D. Wright when the bipartite stimulus field was confined to the central 20' of the foveola, conditions under which the eye is dichromatic and matches are thought to depend only on the long- and middle-wave cones (Willmer & Wright, 1945). The ordinate of Fig. 11.5 shows the proportion of each primary in the match and the important result is that all wavelengths between 420 and 650 nm can be matched by positive mixtures of the 460-nm and 650-nm primaries. Provided that we allow the minimal assumption that the ratio $M:L$ is higher at 460 nm than at 650 nm, these tritanopic colour-matching results oblige us to conclude that the ratio $M:L$ is maximal at 460 nm. For suppose the maximum occurred at some other wavelength λ_x, then *ex hypothesi* monochromatic light of 460 nm would give a smaller ratio of middle- to long-wave signals than did λ_x. Adding the 650-nm primary could only reduce the ratio further. There would be no positive mixture of the 460-nm and 650-nm primaries that gave the high ratio of cone signals produced by λ_x, and thus a colour match would not be possible. So, there cannot be another wavelength, λ_x, that represents the maximum.[3] Of course, it is tritan colour-matching data, along with protan and deutan data, that constrain the König fundamentals to be what they are.

We should like to labour this point a little. The understanding of colour vision was historically held back by the application of colour names to the receptors. König was among the first securely to grasp that a red light is not a light that maximally stimulates the long-wave cones but a light that produces a high ratio of long- to middle-wave cone excitation. 'Red', 'green' and 'blue' cones have today been expelled from almost all but ophthalmological textbooks; yet respectable visual scientists still use the terms 'red–green' and 'blue–yellow' for the second-order channels of the visual system. This is not an innocuous practice: it misleads students and their betters alike. In fact, the so-called 'red–green' channel is maximally polarised by red light on the one hand, and on the other by a wavelength (460 nm) close to unique blue; while the so-called 'blue–yellow' channel is maximally polarised by violet light and red or yellow light. It remains an open question whether there exist, at a more central stage, red–green and yellow–blue processes that correspond to those postulated by Opponent Colours Theory (Mollon & Cavonius, 1987).

That the ratio M:L passes through a shallow maximum in the blue spectral region is independently suggested by results obtained from a modification of Stiles' two-colour increment-threshold method (Estévez & Cavonius, 1977). And if further confirmation be needed, it is given by the M and L cone sensitivities recorded electrophysiologically from macaque cones by Nunn *et al.* (1985): the log ratio of these sensitivities is shown in the lower panel of Fig. 11.1.

So, this is the explanation – a traditional one – why the M vs. L subsystem is of little help to wavelength discrimination at 460 nm: the rate of change of the ratio slows down to zero. But the ratio of short-wave to middle- or long-wave sensitivity (S:M or S:L), extracted by the more ancient subsystem, is seen to be changing rapidly in the region of 460 nm (Fig. 11.1, lower panel). Why cannot our ancient subsystem

[3] An objection occasionally put to us, from those who know something of colour theory, is that it is well known that colour-matching results are compatible with an infinite number of sets of fundamental sensitivities; and that one cannot therefore deduce the position of the maximal value of M:L from tritan colour mixing results. But an objection of this kind cannot counter the specific conclusion being drawn here from dichromatic data.

help us here? The answer is suggested by three experimental operations that paradoxically improve wavelength discrimination at 460 nm.

Three paradoxes of wavelength discrimination

Reduction of intensity: the König–Dieterici Anomaly

In the region of 460 nm, wavelength discrimination can be paradoxically improved by reducing the luminance of the stimuli. Such an effect is visible in the classical curves of König & Dieterici (1884), and Mollon & Estévez (1988) have proposed that it should be known as the 'König–Dieterici Anomaly'. The anomaly was rediscovered by McCree (1960). It is also apparent in the wavelength-discrimination curves given for normal observers by Haase (1934), and those for a deuteranope given by Walraven & Bouman (1966). The latter data (obtained at 1 and 10 trolands) are especially instructive, since the deuteranope's discrimination may be thought to depend only on the comparison of short- and long-wave cone signals; and the improvement near 460 nm is seen to be a consequence of a leftward shift of the deuteranope's U-shaped function as luminance is reduced (see Fig. 11.9).

Figure 11.6 shows direct measurements of the König–Dieterici Anomaly at 460 nm, using the method of average error. Each data point represents the root-mean-square value for three independent sets

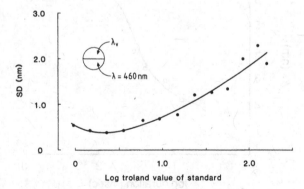

Fig. 11.6. The König–Dieterici Anomaly, measured by the method of average error. The figure shows the precision (standard deviation) of wavelength matches for monochromatic standard lights of 460 nm plotted as a function of their luminance. Each data point represents the r.m.s. value for three independent sets of 25 matches. Note that discrimination is best at low luminance.

of 25 matches. In this experiment the standard deviation of wavelength matches falls from around 2.0 at 100 td to well under half a nanometer at 5 td.

Reduction of duration

The second operation that paradoxically improves wavelength discrimination at 460 nm is a shortening of stimulus duration. Figure 11.7 shows results obtained by two-alternative temporal forced-choice for durations between 8 and 800 ms. Different durations were sampled in random order in two separate sequences. The standard and variable fields formed the lower and upper halves of a 2-deg bipartite field, the standard field had a troland value of 50, and the bandwidth of the monochromators was 1 nm. Other details of the procedure were as described for the experiment of Fig. 11.3.

It can be seen from Fig. 11.7 that discrimination at 460 nm improves systematically as duration is reduced below 50 ms. Under the conditions of the present experiments, reduction of duration and reduction of intensity thus produce effects in the same direction; but it is interesting to note that we have here an instance – perhaps unique – where reducing duration has an effect that is opposite in direction from the effect of reducing *area*: a reduction of field-size usually *impairs* wavelength discrimination in the region of 460 nm (Willmer & Wright, 1945), whereas we find

here that the threshold falls when duration is reduced.[4]

The König–Dieterici Anomaly and the effect of reducing stimulus duration both point to a saturating signal as the explanation why the older subsystem cannot sustain good discrimination for 50-td lights near 460 nm: when the quantum flux presented to the short-wave cones is reduced, by lowering the stimulus luminance or by shortening duration, we suppose that there is a shift to shorter wavelengths of the spectral region where the older subsystem begins to be saturated (and that there is an concomitant shift of the region of optimum discrimination, since the middle wavelengths now give too small a quantum catch in the short-wave cones[5]). But what is the site of the saturation? Do the short-wavelength cones themselves saturate, as in the model of Vos & Walraven (1972), or does the saturation occur in a post-receptoral colour-differencing system? There is also the (less plausible) possibility that rods, initially saturated, come to play a rôle in the discrimination of 2-deg centrally-fixated fields when stimulus energy is reduced.

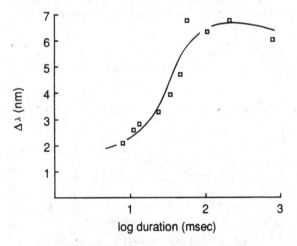

Fig. 11.7. Wavelength discrimination at 460 nm as a function of the duration of the flash. Measurements were made by a two-alternative temporal forced-choice procedure and the observer was JDM. Notice that performance improves as stimulus energy is reduced.

[4] Farnsworth (1958) suggested that discrimination was relatively better for the tritan direction of colour space at short durations. It is not clear whether his result is related to the one shown in Fig. 11.7, since (a) the range of durations over which his improvement occurred (2000 vs 200 ms) is of a different order from the critical range found here and (b) the improvement was only relative to discrimination on a red–green dimension and the absolute values of the thresholds were higher at 200 ms. Farnsworth does not give the luminance of his stimuli.

[5] A hypothesis of this kind will readily explain the results of Foster, Scase & Taylor (1987), who found that wavelength discrimination near 500 nm was severely impaired when the duration of a 100-td stimulus was reduced from 1 s to 3 ms. The short-wave cone system has a particularly large critical duration: for a 100-td 500-nm stimulus the value is of the order of 130 ms (Krauskopf & Mollon, 1971, Figure 3). Thus, for the ancient, 'deutan', subsystem of colour vision, a change in duration from 1000 to 3 ms represents a reduction of, say, 1.65 log units in the effective stimulus energy. This attenuation of the stimulus will shift the minimum of the deutan discrimination to shorter wavelengths (Walraven & Bouman, 1966). Wavelength discrimination at 500 nm will deteriorate, owing to an inadequate quantum catch in the short-wave cones. The sharp cusp near 500 nm in the 3-ms data of Foster *et al.* can be interpreted as the intersection of separate 'deutan' and 'tritan' functions (see Fig. 11.9).

Cancellation by added fields

There is a third experimental operation that counter-intuitively lowers wavelength-discrimination thresholds at 460 nm; and this effect shows that at least some of the saturation occurs in a post-receptoral channel which draws inputs from the short-wave cones on the one hand and from the long- or middle-wave cones on the other. In this experiment (Mollon & Estévez, 1988), we held constant at 40 td the luminance of the standard half-field. To both halves of the bipartite field we added yellow-green light (560 nm) of increasing intensity, the added light forming a uniform, steady, circular field. In this case then, the quantum catch of the short-wave cones themselves cannot fall; it effectively remains constant as the yellow-green field is increased. If the short-wave cone signal is already saturated, then adding yellow-green light will not make it less so. Thresholds were measured by the method of average error.

The abscissa of Fig. 11.8 shows the troland value of the added yellow-green field (note that the 460-nm field is fixed). For each observer the standard deviation of the matches is halved at a point between 2.0 and 3.0 log units of added yellow-green light. In this case, the recovery cannot be explained by a release

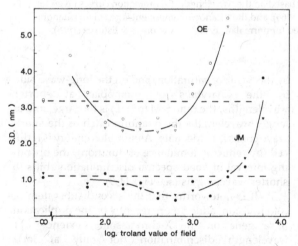

Fig. 11.8. The precision (standard deviation) of wavelength matches at 460 nm as a function of the log troland value of a 560-nm 'desaturating' field. The 460-nm standard field was fixed at 40 td. Data are shown for two independent runs for two of the authors. The results for OE have been displaced vertically by 2 nm. The horizontal broken line indicates the precision of matches when no desaturant was used.

from saturation of the signals of the short-wave cones themselves (nor of rod signals); rather we may suppose that the saturation occurs in a post-receptoral colour-differencing channel that draws signals of opposite sign from the short-wave cones, on the one hand, and some combination of the middle- and long-wave cones, on the other. 460-nm light of 50 td places this channel in a saturating region of its response characteristic; and adding an opposing middle-wave field brings the channel back to a sensitive part of its operating range. The 560-nm light is a desaturant in both the phenomenological and the mechanistic sense. By this account, the present result is essentially the same as the 'combinative euchromatopsia' (the facilitation of increment sensitivity) observed for violet targets when a long-wave auxiliary field is added to a primary blue field (Mollon & Polden, 1977; Polden & Mollon, 1980).

In conclusion, then, an analysis of wavelength discrimination at short wavelengths suggests that our hue discrimination is limited by two factors, first, by the rate of change with wavelength of the ratios of quantum catches and, second, by the limited dynamic range of post-receptoral channels. In the case of the younger subsystem (the middle-wave/long-wave system), of course, both factors may operate at 460 nm, since the ratio of quantum catches there reaches its extreme value.

The rôles of the two subsystems

So, if a full answer is one day to be given to the questions raised by Horace Barlow in his 1982 paper (see Introduction, above), we think it will be inappropriate to treat human colour vision as a single system, designed all at once and for the sole purpose of hue discrimination. Rather, it will be necessary to consider the evolutionary history of colour vision, and the constraints imposed by the eye's other functions.

Initially, we suppose, there was a single cone pigment in the mid-spectral region. It was designed to subserve the chief tasks of vision, the discrimination of movement, flicker and form. To ensure high sensitivity, its bandwidth was broad and its peak wavelength was close to the peak of the daylight spectrum. Later, a second class of cones were (very frugally) added. These cones, with their peak sensitivity at short wavelengths, far removed from that of the middle-wave cones, served only for colour vision. By comparing their quantum catch with that of the middle-wave cones, the visual system achieved the most basic form of colour discrimination, the discrimi-

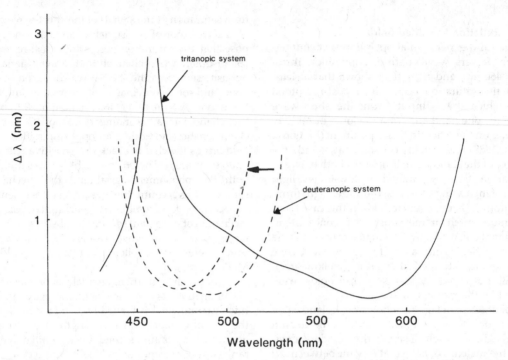

Fig. 11.9. The 'deuteranopic' and 'tritanopic' component functions that underlie normal hue discrimination. The rightmost of the broken lines represents the deuteranopic component when the troland value of the field is of the order of 100; when the troland value is reduced the deuteranopic function shifts leftwards as shown. The functions shown are schematic, but the deuteranopic component is based on the wavelength-discrimination curves given for deuteranopes by Pitt (1944) and by Walraven & Bouman (1966); and the tritanopic component is based on tritanope 'A' in the study of Wright (1952) and the functions obtained for normal observers by Cavonius & Estévez (1978) under tritan conditions of viewing.

nation of the sign and the gradient with which an object's reflectance changed from one end of the spectrum to the other. Subjectively, this ancient discrimination is the discrimination of warm colours from cool, the discrimination of reds, browns, yellows and olives from blues and blue-greens – and both of these from neutral greys and whites. If we adopt Barlow's Fourier approach to colour mechanisms, but consider the *subsystem* (rather than the individual photopigment) as a channel, then the job of the ancient subsystem is to extract the lowest Fourier component of colour information, i.e. the phase and amplitude of the variation between one end of the visible spectrum and the other. At the level of 50 td, the ancient subsystem does not support the discrimination of monochromatic or near-monochromatic lights, except in a small spectral interval near 500 nm; this is the interval where monochromatic lights yield ratios of short- to middle-wave excitation that resemble the ratios produced by daylight. The interval is limited on the short-wave side

by the Scylla of saturation, and on the long-wave side by the Charybdis of tritanopia: at shorter wavelengths, the ratio $S:M$ (or $S:L$) is too large, and at longer wavelengths the quantum catch of the short-wave cones is inadequate. As stimulus energy is reduced (by reducing luminance or duration), the operating interval of good spectral discrimination shifts to shorter wavelengths (see Fig. 11.9).

It is noteworthy that the second subsystem of colour vision, added more recently by the duplication of a gene on the X-chromosome, extends our wavelength discrimination not only at long wavelengths, but also at short (Fig. 11.9). It has always been of interest that tritanopes (who depend on the second subsystem alone) enjoy good hue discrimination throughout the spectrum, except in the vicinity of 460 nm (Wright, 1952; Fischer *et al.*, 1952; see Fig. 11.9); and in normal vision, at least for stimuli of 50 td or more, it is the ratio $L:M$ that sustains the discrimination of wavelengths below 460 nm. This may be one consequence of the substantial overlap of the middle- and long-wave cone sensitivities:[6] there is no wavelength that produces a very large or very small value of the ratio M:L. If the peak sensitivities of the middle- and long-wave cones were more separated (or of their bandwidths were narrow), we should expect the spectral discrimination of the second subsystem to be limited in the same way as the first: as soon as we left the narrow spectral window where the antagonistic cone signals were in balance, one of the two inputs would quickly become very large while the other would be limited by a failing quantum catch.[7]

So, the second subsystem extends discrimination in the wavelength domain. But there is another way of looking at its job: perhaps its true function is to extend discrimination in the Fourier domain. This is the domain to which we were introduced by Barlow (1982), although here it is the subsystem, rather than the photopigment, that is taken as the filter. Because the absorbance spectra of the long- and middle-wave pigments overlap so substantially, the second subsystem will be insensitive to the low Fourier components that well stimulate the ancient subsystem; its

maximal response will be to intermediate components, although, as Barlow (1982) showed us, it must always be limited by the bandwidths of its two underlying photopigments.

It is often claimed that higher Fourier components are rare in the reflectances of the natural world (e.g. Lennie & D'Zmura, 1988), but this is the case only when spectroradiometric samples are taken from large surfaces. If the measurement is confined to part of an individual leaf or individual fruit, then fine detail is readily apparent in the spectra of the world of plants (Goodwin, 1965). Perhaps it was for discrimination among the carotenoids, the chlorophyls, and the flavins that the second subsystem of colour vision was given to us.

Acknowledgements

We are grateful to L. Winn for instrument making, to S. Astell and G. Jordan for experimental assistance, and to H. B. Barlow and S. Shevell for comments on the text. The experiments described above were supported by MRC Grant G8417519N.

References

Alpern, M., Kitahara, K. & Krantz, D. H. (1983) Classical tritanopia, *J. Physiol. (Lond.)*, **335**, 655–81.

Barlow, H. B. (1958) Intrinsic noises of cones. In *Visual Problems of Colour*, National Physical Laboratory Symposium No. 8, vol. 2. London: HMSO.

Barlow, H. B. (1982) What causes trichromacy? A theoretical analysis using comb-filtered spectra. *Vision Res.*, **22**, 635–43.

Blakemore, C. & Vital-Durand, F. (1986) Organization and post-natal development of the monkey's lateral geniculate nucleus. *J. Physiol. (Lond.)*, **380**, 453–91.

Bouman, M. A. & Walraven, P. L. (1972) Color discrimination data. In *Handbook of Sensory Physiology*, vol. VII/4, ed. D. Jameson & L. M. Hurvich, pp. 484–516. Berlin: Springer.

Bowmaker, J. K., Jacobs, G. H. & Mollon, J. D. (1987) Polymorphism of photopigments in the squirrel monkey: a sixth phenotype. *Proc. Roy. Soc. Lond.*, **B231**, 383–90.

Cavonius, C. R. & Estévez, O. (1978) π Mechanisms and cone fundamentals. In *Visual Psychophysics and Physiology*, ed. J. C. Armington, J. Krauskopf & B. R. Wooten, pp. 221–31. New York: Academic Press.

Crook, J. M., Lange-Malecki, B., Lee, B. B. & Valberg, A. (1988) Visual resolution of macaque retinal ganglion cells. *J. Physiol. (Lond.)*, **396**, 205–24.

Derrington, A. M. & Lennie, P. (1984) Spatial and temporal contrast sensitivities of neurones in lateral geniculate nucleus of macaque. *J. Physiol. (Lond.)*, **357**, 219–40.

---

[6] Two other possible explanations can be distinguished. (a) Since the eye exhibits chromatic aberration and since the long- and middle-wave cones both continue to be used for form vision, spatial resolution would be impaired if the peak sensitivities became too separated in the spectrum (Barlow, 1982). (b) There may be no rapid evolutionary route from the ancestral middle-wave opsin to an opsin with an amino-acid sequence that gives a peak sensitivity lying below 530 nm. These explanations, and the one given in the text, are not, of course, exclusive.

[7] Despite the relatively limited range of values of the ratio M:L, it may still be the case that no individual Pβ ganglion cell accommodates the full range. Whereas the retinal ganglion cells that draw inputs from short-wave cones form a very homogeneous group, a wide variation has been reported in the relative weightings of long- and middle-wave cone inputs to those colour-opponent units that collectively comprise the second subsystem (Zrenner & Gouras, 1983). This variation is conventionally expressed as a variation in spectral neutral points. The response function of any individual cell may exhibit maximal sensitivity over only a limited range of values of M:L, while the subsystem as a whole, comprising a population of cells, accommodates the full range.

Derrington, A. M., Krauskopf, J. & Lennie, P. (1984) Chromatic mechanisms in lateral geniculate nucleus of macaque. *J. Physiol. (Lond.)*, **357**, 241–65.

Estévez, O. & Cavonius, C. R. (1977) Human color perception and Stiles' π mechanisms. *Vision Res.*, **17**, 417–22.

Farnsworth, D. (1958) A temporal factor in colour discrimination. In *Visual problems of colour*, National Physical Laboratory Symposium No. 8, London: HMSO.

Fischer, F. P., Bouman, M. A. & Ten Doesschate, J. (1952) A case of tritanopy, *Documenta Ophthal.*, **5**, 55–87.

Foster, D. H., Scase, M. O. & Taylor, S. P. (1987) Anomalous loss in blue–green hue discrimination in very brief monochromatic stimuli presented to the normal human eye. *J. Physiol. (Lond.)*, **381**, 64P.

Goodwin, T. W. (1965) *Chemistry of Plant Pigments*. New York: Academic Press.

Gouras, P. (1984) Color vision. In *Progress in Retinal Research*, vol. 3, ed. N. N. Osbourne & G. J. Chader. New York: Pergamon.

Haase, G. von (1934) Bestimmung der Farbtonempfindlichkeit des menschlichen Auges bei verschiedenen Helligkeiten und Sättingungen. Bau eines empfindlichen Farbpyrometers. *Annalen der Physik*, **20**, 75–105.

Henning, G. B. (1966) Frequency discrimination of random-amplitude tones. *J. Acoust. Soc. Amer.*, **39**, 336–9.

Jacobs, G. H. (1982) *Comparative Color Vision*. New York: Academic Press.

Judd, D. B. & Yonemura, G. T. (1970) CIE 1960 UCS diagram and the Müller theory of color vision. *Proceedings of the International Color Association, Stockholm, Sweden, 1969*, pp. 266–74. Göttingen: Munsterschmidt.

König, A. & Dieterici, C. (1884) Über die Empfindlichkeit des normalen Auges für Wellenlängenunterschiede des Lichtes. *Annalen der Physik*, **22**, 579–89.

Krauskopf, J. & Mollon, J. D. (1971) The independence of the temporal integration properties of individual chromatic mechanisms in the human eye. *J. Physiol. (Lond.)*, **219**, 611–23.

Ladd-Franklin, C. (1892) A new theory of light sensation. In *International Congress of Psychology, 2nd Congress*. London. (Kraus reprint, 1974).

Laurens, H. & Hamilton, W. F. (1923) The sensibility of the eye to differences in wave-length. *Amer. J. Physiol.*, **65**, 547–68.

Lennie, P. & D'Zmura, M. (1988) Mechanisms of color vision. *CRC Critical Reviews*. **3**, 333–400.

Mariani, A. P. (1984) Bipolar cells in monkey retina selective for the cones likely to be blue-sensitive. *Nature*, **308**, 184–6.

McCree, K. J. (1960) Small-field tritanopia and the effects of voluntary fixation, *Optica Acta*, **7**, 317–23.

Mollon, J. D. (1986) Molecular genetics: understanding colour vision. *Nature*, **321**, 12–13.

Mollon, J. D., Bowmaker, J. K. & Jacobs, G. H. (1984) Variations of colour vision in a New World primate can be explained by polymorphism of retinal photopigments. *Proc. Roy. Soc., Lond.*, **B222**, 373–99.

Mollon, J. D. & Cavonius, C. R. (1987) The chromatic antagonisms of opponent process theory are not the same as those revealed in studies of detection and discrimination. In *Colour Deficiencies VIII*, ed. G. Verriest (Documenta Ophthalmologica Proceedings Series 46). The Hague: Martinus Nijhoff.

Mollon, J. D. & Estévez, O. (1988) Tyndall's paradox of hue discrimination. *J. Opt. Soc. Am. A*, **5**, 151–9.

Mollon, J. D. & Jordan, G. (1988) Eine evolutionäre Interpretation des menschlichen Farbensehens *Die Farbe*, **35136**, 139–70.

Mollon, J. D. & Polden, P. G. (1977) Further anomalies of the blue mechanism. *Invest. Ophthal. and Vis. Sci. (Suppl.)*, **1b**, 140.

Moore, B. C. J., Glasberg, B. R. & Shailer, M. J. (1984) Frequency and intensity difference limens for harmonics within complex tones. *J. Acoust. Soc. Amer.*, **75**, 550–61.

Nathans, J., Thomas, D. & Hogness, D. S. (1986a) Molecular genetics of human color vision: the genes encoding blue, green and red pigments. *Science*, **232**, 192–202.

Nathans, J., Piantanida, T. P., Eddy, R. L., Shows, T. B. & Hogness, D. S. (1986b) Molecular genetics of inherited variation in human color vision. *Science*, **232**, 203–10.

Nunn, B. J., Schnapf, J. L. & Baylor, D. A. (1985) The action spectra of rods and red- and green-sensitive cones of the monkey *Macaca fascicularis*. In *Central and Peripheral Mechanisms of Colour Vision*, ed. D. Ottoson & S. Zeki. London: Macmillan.

Pitt, F. H. G. (1944) The nature of normal trichromatic and dichromatic vision. *Proc. Roy. Soc. Lond.*, **B132**, 101–17.

Polden, P. G. & Mollon, J. D. (1980) Reversed effect of adapting stimuli on visual sensitivity. *Proc. Roy. Soc. Lond.*, **B210**, 235–72.

Shapley, R. & Perry, V. H. (1986) Cat and monkey retinal ganglion cells and their visual functional roles. *Trends Neurosci.*, **9**, 229–35.

Stücker, N. (1908) Über die Unterschiedsempfindlichkeit für Tonhöher in verschiedenen Tonregionen. *Z. f. Sinnesphysiologie*, **42**, 392–408.

Tansley, B. W. & Boynton, R. M. (1976) A line, not a space, represents visual distinctness of borders formed by different colors. *Science*, **191**, 954–7.

Thoma, W. & Scheibner, H. (1980) Die spektrale tritanopische Sättigungsfunktion beschreibt die spektrale Distinktibilität. *Farbe und Design*, **17**, 49–52.

Vos, J. J. & Walraven, P. L. (1972) An analytical description of the line element in the zone-fluctuation model of colour vision – I. Basic concepts. *Vision Res.*, **12**, 1327–43.

Walraven, P. L. & Bouman, M. A. (1966) Fluctuation theory of colour discrimination of normal trichromats. *Vision Res.*, **6**, 567–86.

Weale, R. A. (1951) Hue discrimination in para-central parts of the human retina measured at different luminance levels. *J. Physiol. (Lond.)*, **113**, 115–22.

Willmer, E. N. & Wright, W. D. (1945) Colour sensitivity of the fovea centralis. *Nature*, **156**, 119.

Wright, W. D. (1952) The characteristics of tritanopia. *J. Opt. Soc. Am.*, **42**, 509.

Wright, W. D. & Pitt, F. H. G. (1935) Hue-discrimination in normal colour-vision. *Proc. Physical. Soc.*, **46**, 459–73.

Wyszecki, G. & Stiles, W. S. (1982) *Color Science.* New York: Wiley.

Zrenner, E. & Gouras, P. (1983) Cone opponency in tonic ganglion cells and its variation with eccentricity in rhesus monkey retina. In *Color Vision: Physiology and Psychophysics*, ed. J. D. Mollon & L. T. Sharpe, pp. 211–23. London: Academic Press.

12

The effect of the angle of retinal incidence on the color of monochromatic light

M. Alpern

Introduction

An almost unknown spin-off of the elegant, but inapt, pupillometer used by Stiles & Crawford (1933) to measure pupil area* was the discovery that lights going through different regions of the pupil do not have the same effect on the color sense (Stiles, 1937). This was named the Stiles–Crawford Effect of the second kind (SCII) by Hansen (1943) to distinguish it from that widely known spin-off: the discovery that lights going through different parts of the pupil do not have the same effect on the brightness sense (Hansen's Stiles–Crawford Effect of the first kind or SCI). The literature on this subject has been reviewed elsewhere (Alpern, 1986).

The first SCI experiments were with white light. Would the effect for monochromatic light of different wavelengths all be the same? When Stiles (1937) asked this question, he found that two fields of monochromatic light of the same wavelength but different angles of incidence on the retina could not be matched, no matter how the radiance of one was varied. As a first step, subjects ignored the hue and saturation differences and made the fields equally bright. These results were well quantified by the equation for a parabola,

$$\log I_o/I = \varrho(\lambda)[r-r_o]^2. \tag{1}$$

In this equation r is the position of pupil entry, I is the radiance for a match, and the subscript o represents

*A subject equated the brightness of two photometric fields. One was seen in Maxwellian view; the light from this field reaching the subject's retina was independent of the area of his pupil. The other was seen in normal view, and the amount of light from it reaching his pupil depended on the pupil area.

these values at r where I is a minimum. $\varrho(\lambda)$, a parameter quantifying the magnitude of SCI, was indeed found to be wavelength dependent, smallest near the middle of the spectrum, large at either end.

As a second step, Stiles tried to measure the color effect. To do this, subjects matched two photometric fields, one formed by rays of light striking the retina obliquely from the margin of the exit pupil, the other formed by rays striking the retina as foveal chief rays. Subjects adjusted the wavelength and the radiance of the 'off-axis' set of rays to match the field illuminating the retina with chief rays and quantified the result by the difference in wavelength of the two monochromatic beams at the match. The results are known as the 'Stiles–Crawford hue shift'. These initial measurements of Stiles provide rare examples in which Stiles resorted to Class B psychophysical experiments under apparatus exigencies, although a Class A experiment was clearly indicated. Still, for a quarter of a century this initial 'hue shift' experiment was the paradigm of all attempts to quantify SCII. Though even today many confuse the hue shift with a full quantification of SCII, a sharp distinction is needed because there are clear saturation changes as well.

A reasonably complete quantitative description of SCII has been realized only on one eye – the left eye of J. M. Enoch (Enoch & Stiles, 1961). Three normally incident primaries were matched to a monochromatic test, the angle of incidence on the retina of which was varied parametrically. Enoch & Stiles also reported results of a few experiments on a second subject comparing the chromaticities of only two test lights, one incident on the retina as a chief ray, the other incident obliquely from the exit pupil margin. Further data using this 'two point method' have been obtained by Alpern, Kitahara & Tamaki (1983) and Alpern &

Tamaki (1983) on two other normal trichromats. Since then, three others have been studied here, but their results are not yet published.

Some individual differences exist among these seven normal trichromats, but the general pattern is clear. An obliquely incident monochromatic beam of light in spectral range $m<18\ 350\ \text{cm}^{-1}$ ($\lambda>545$ nm) appears of longer wavelength and less saturated than light of the same wavelength incident as a chief ray. For $18\ 350\ \text{cm}^{-1}<m<19\ 750\ \text{cm}^{-1}$ or so, the obliquely incident beam appears more saturated and of shorter wavelength than chief rays, while as m increases beyond $19\ 750\ \text{cm}^{-1}$ (506.3 nm), the wavelength of the obliquely incident ray again appears to be longer than that of its chief ray counterpart, while the test gradually becomes less saturated.

Stiles's original theory dismissed the possibility that the effect might be due to differential prereceptor differences in the two beams. Instead, it developed from calculations suggesting that the three species of receptors exhibited the effect to different degrees; and that the SCI effect would be smallest in the part of the spectrum where absorption of light was highest. Stiles noted that this might be achieved by differential screening of the two different beams by the visual pigment in the outer and inner segments. It remained for Brindley (1953) to bring Stiles's concept into line with the more recently discovered fact that effective absorption is confined to the photoreceptor outer segment (OS). In Brindley's version, the visual pigment is in the OS in substantial concentration. Lights striking the retina as foveal chief rays are absorbed by the pigment throughout the full OS length, while oblique rays incident from the margin of the exit pupil are absorbed in a much smaller OS traverse. Hence the density of visual pigment which absorbs oblique rays – and defines the action spectra of cones for them – is much more dilute. Brindley introduced the term 'self-screening' for this mechanism. He calculated the quantitative difference using the Beer–Lambert law of absorption and applied his calculations to the change in color-matching behavior he found when all the colorimeter beams were moved from the center to the margin of the pupil. Brindley found that only the long-wave cone visual pigment needed to be in sufficiently high concentration for 'self-screening' to occur in order to explain his results.

But in explaining the 'hue shift' data of four subjects, Walraven & Bouman (1960) and Walraven (1962) expanded the theory of 'self-screening' in two ways, first by supposing the concentration of the visual pigments in all three species of foveal cones to

be high, and secondly by assuming two other sources of light loss, namely by leakage in the outer and inner segments. These were zero for normal incidence and wavelength independent. Light leakage in the inner segment was mainly responsible for SCI. Enoch & Stiles (1961) applied Walraven's theory to their data on J.M.E. (assuming reasonable estimates of absorbancy index spectra of the three kinds of pigment) and required peak densities of 1.0 and 0.7 for the visual pigments in the middle- and long-wave sensitive cones respectively. These high densities were reached without recourse to leakage in the inner segment; when they were added, the density estimates were still higher. Their results were inconsistent with short-wave sensitive cones showing 'self-screening'.

About the time that Enoch & Stiles's results were published, Toraldo di Francia's (1949a,b) analogue of cones as 'dielectric rod antennae' to explain SCI began to catch hold, and by 1973 a quantitative waveguide theory had been developed by Snyder & Pask (1973) to account for SCI by quantifying the wavelength dependency of $\varrho(\lambda)$. The inevitable extension of such considerations to the full SCII has yet to be undertaken, but Pask & Snyder (1975) provide a fit to hue shift results by such a formulation. In its original version, the Snyder–Pask photoreceptor model has five curve-fitting parameters: the diameters d_i, d_o of the inner and outer segments respectively, and the indices of refraction n_i, n_o, n_s of the inner and outer segments and of the surrounding space respectively where $n_s<n_i<n_o$.

In all this, the view in Stiles's original paper that the color – as distinct from the color matching functions (CMFs) – of a monochromatic light remains free of any prereceptor distortions prevailed. Theorists generally supposed that the action spectrum of the three species of cones providing the physical basis of foveal trichromacy depended upon the angle of incidence of light striking the retina in a way which differed for each cone species and was in addition to, and independent of, any prereceptor distortions which may or may not occur. In contrast to this general line of theory, Weale's recent (1981a,b) theory of the hue shift requires the assumption that the action spectrum of each one of the three species of foveal cones was independent of the angle of incidence of light on the retina. Weale accounted for the hue shift by three prereceptor factors: (i) losses by reflection at the cornea, (ii) absorption in the lens, and (iii) attenuation of the high spatial frequencies by the obliquely incident rays.

This essay summarizes recent work in my

laboratory as it relates to all three of these explanations for SCII. That work suggests that each is inadequate to account for the facts uncovered.

Results

In order that all theories could be applied to measurements of variation in color matching with angle of retinal incidence, Alpern & Kitahara (1983) undertook to measure directly the wavelength dependency of the directional sensitivity of each one of the three foveal cone mechanisms. It is a constraint on the strength of the inferences from their results that there is no generally accepted psychophysical way in which this can be done. They elected the field sensitivity mechanisms of the three Stiles foveal $\Pi_j(\mu)$ mechanisms ($j=3,4,5$). Although there is no room here to describe the details of the method, which may be found in the original paper, it is necessary to emphasize that the method uses foveal fixation, and that the 5°-in-diameter circular background field traverses the pupil while the 1° test always traverses the eye as a foveal chief ray. The consequence of these circumstances is that two of the three factors in Weale's theory (F_1 and F_3) are so small that they can be safely ignored. Furthermore, losses in the lens (F_2) which bears, according to Weale's hypothesis, the brunt of the changes with wavelength, have for the data presented below been corrected by the results of *ad hoc* measurements of the transmissivity of the subject's own lens (as well as of his macular pigment). The results shown in Fig. 12.1 represent the wavelength directional sensitivity of each mechanism at the retinal level.

Each point in this figure represents the value of $\varrho_j(\mu)$ emerging from a computer fit of eqn 1 to empirical estimates of the radiances of a monochromatic background of a given wavenumber (m) required for the elevation of the Π_j threshold by a factor of ten, for backgrounds entering the observer's pupil at 9–11 different positions scanning its horizontal diameter. The computer algorithm also provides an estimate of the variance from which the standard errors (sem) of the estimate can be calculated; the line drawn through each datum in the figure is limited by ±1 sem.

The curves in Fig. 12.1 are derived from theory; the dashed line shows the best fits (as judged by eye) to the 'self-screening' theory of Walraven & Bouman (1960) as modified by Enoch & Stiles (1961); the thin solid lines show results of the best fits (also judged by eye) of the waveguide theory of Snyder & Pask (1973) to the wavelength variation of the directional sensitivity parameter rho for Π_3 (above), Π_4 (in the middle) and Π_5 (below). The dashed-dot line [fitted to $\varrho_5(\mu)$

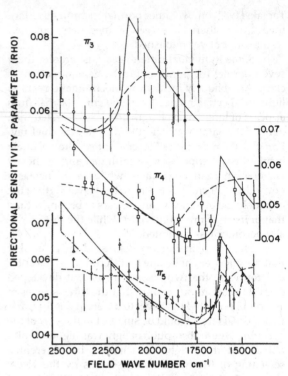

Fig. 12.1. The field wave frequency dependency of the directional sensitivity parameter $\varrho_j(\mu)$ of eqn 1a determined by the field sensitivities of the W. S. Stiles foveal cone mechanisms $\Pi_j(\mu)$ for $j = 3, 4, 5$. The symbols represent the mean values ±1 sem of the results of Alpern & Kitahara (1983) corrected for losses in the lens, macular pigment, and remaining eye media: circles for $\varrho_3(\mu)$, squares for $\varrho_4(\mu)$, and triangles for $\varrho_5(\mu)$. The dashed line describes the result of the best fitting 'self-screening' predictions; the solid line shows the expectation of the simple Snyder–Pask waveguide theory. The procedures for fitting these curves and determining relevant parameters of each model are described by Zwas (1979) and the explicit values used for these results listed by Alpern (1983). The dashed-dot line fitted to $\varrho_5(\mu)$ data is the best fit of a modified Snyder–Pask model in which responses from four Π_5 subsets were pooled as described by Alpern (1983). The graph showing the Π_5 result is modified only slightly from Fig. 2A of Alpern (1983).

data only] shows predictions of an elaboration of the simple Snyder–Pask theory in which the population of long-wave sensitive cones whose responses are modelled, is supposed comprised of four subsets each of which has slightly different inner segment diameters and indices of refraction from the others. The details of this calculation are previously described (Zwas, 1979;

Alpern, 1983). Indeed, the specifications of the curve-fitting parameters for the curves in this figure are given in Alpern (1983).

That the directional sensitivity parameter rho for each of the three cone mechanisms is substantially (i.e. 4–7×) larger than the directional sensitivity parameter of the rods (Alpern, Ching & Kitahara, 1983) is inconsistent with Weale's theory. The testing of each of the other models, if it is to be anything more than curve-fitting the data in Fig. 12.1, requires independent measurements of change in color with change in the angle of retinal incidence free from distortions in the lens, as Weale (1961, 1981a,b) emphasized. His theory of the hue shift mainly depends upon the facts that the lens is colored and that in order to reach the same part of the retina with different angles of obliquity, the light must pass through different regions of the lens. In order to avoid this complexity, Enoch & Stiles (1961) and Alpern, Kitahara & Tamaki (1983) have plotted the chromaticity of monochromatic lights incident on the retina at different angles of incidence in the WDW* chromaticity diagram where all preretinal distortions in the chromaticities of monochromatic lights are factored out. For this purpose, they used three normally incident primaries to match the test, whether normally or obliquely incident. However, a fundamental assumption of this method of describing such results is that the effects of oblique incidence operate at a level of organization in the visual system where the effects of radiation of different wavelengths are still compounded by the simple linear laws. Alpern & Tamaki (1983) found evidence for doubting the generality, if not the validity, of this assumption.

To obviate this difficulty in the present context, Alpern, Kitahara & Fielder (1987) have resorted to Brindley's (1953) strategy of studying the effect of angle of retinal incidence on matching, i.e. comparing the trichromatic color matches made when all four beams of the colorimeter were incident on the retina

---

*WDW are the initials of Professor W. D. Wright the colorimetrist pioneer who introduced the system of plotting results of color matching of spectrally pure test lights with a color triangle in which the chromaticity coordinates are normalized at *five* different loci in the spectrum rather than just at the wavelengths of the three reference primaries, as was then the invariable practice. It has the great advantage that for such test lights (but *no others*) chromaticities are independent of any spectral losses in the eye prior to absorption in the visual pigments. The details of the system are explicit in eqn 4. It has become general practice since, when using this system, to honor Prof. Wright by referring to such a triangle with his initials.

from the margin of the exit pupil to those made when all four beams were incident as foveal chief rays. [Alpern & Tamaki (1983) found no reason to doubt the linear laws of color matching under these conditions.] Unlike Brindley, however, Alpern, Kitahara & Fielder studied the entire visible spectrum instead of just the red–green range. This had the advantage of facilitating the comparison of WDW chromaticities (u, v, w) to obviate the pernicious influence of differences in the three prereceptor factors of Weale's theory (most importantly, the lens) and of testing Brindley's idea of 'self-screening' under more demanding circumstances than he required. [It may be recalled that plots in a chromaticity diagram are normalized so that $u+v+w=1.0$. They found it more convenient to plot the *change* in WDW chromaticity on shifting from the foveal chief rays (angle of incidence=0°) to an angle of incidence of 7.5° from the temporal exit pupil margin.]

The results for the same subject, whose data are given in Fig. 12.1, are plotted as $\triangle u=u'-u$ (triangles above), $\triangle v=v'-v$ (squares in the middle), and $\triangle w=w'-w$ (circles below) (where primed values represent oliquely, unprimed values normally, incident matches) in Fig. 12.2. Each symbol in Fig. 12.2 represents a mean chromaticity difference between three repetitions of the experiment through the pupil center and three through its edge, while the ends of the line through the symbol represent the 95% confidence limits of that chromaticity difference. (Where no lines are found, the plots of those limits are closer together than the extremes of the symbol.)

The lines show predictions of various theories to be described shortly. Consider, first, Weale's assumption that the action spectra of the three species of foveal cones are independent of the angle of incidence of the monochromatic light striking the retina. If it were true, there should be no differences between the WDW chromaticities of chief rays and obliquely incident monochromatic rays of the same wavelength because the WDW normalization factors out the prereceptor factors upon which, according to Weale's hypothesis, the Stiles–Crawford hue shift depends. That almost one-third of the lines specifying the 95% limit of chromaticities of the color changes in Fig. 12.2 do not include zero is therefore taken as strong evidence against Weale's original theory. In confronting his original theory with hue shift data, Weale (1981a) found a rather unsatisfactory fit in the short-wave region of the spectrum which he dealt with by the *ad hoc* hypothesis that the short-wave sensitive cones are not subject to cut-off of high spatial frequencies of obliquely incident rays because they (like the rods) are

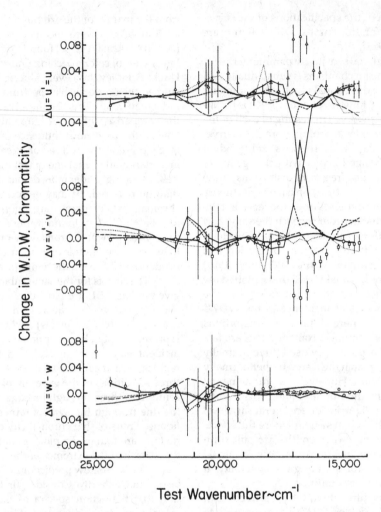

Fig. 12.2. Changes in the WDW chromaticity when all beams of the colorimeter are moved from incident on the retina as a chief ray to an angle of incidence of 7.5° from near the temporal margin of the exit pupil. Symbols are means enclosed by lines whose extremes define the 95% confidence limits of the results of three repetitions of the experiment (in each experimental session the individual measurements being repeated two or three times) on the same observer whose results are shown in Fig. 12.1: triangles, $\Delta u = u' - u$, the change in the chromaticity measured with the long-wave sensitive primary; squares, $\Delta v = v' - v$, the change in chromaticity measured with the middle-wave sensitive primary; circles, $\Delta w = w' - w$, the change in chromaticity measured with the short-wave sensitive primary. The lines are theoretical; thin solid lines are the simple waveguide hypothesis. It was calculated using the theoretical (i.e. solid) lines of Fig. 12.1 (Snyder–Pask model) to infer the $\Pi_i(\mu')$ spectra. Short dashed lines were calculated with the aid of those same solid lines to infer $\Pi_3(\mu')$ and $\Pi_4(\mu')$, but the dashed-dot line in Fig. 12.1 to infer $\Pi_5(\mu')$ (i.e. modified Snyder–Pask model). The dotted lines were obtained with the help of the dashed lines in Fig. 12.1 ('self-screening' model) to infer the $\Pi_i(\mu')$ spectra. The long dashes show the lines found by using the symbols to calculate empirical spectra. To infer $\Pi_i(\mu')$ from these irregular points, the data were then smoothed by fitting them with sixth or seventh order polynomials. They are not based on a priori theoretical constructs. The heavy solid lines are the results of Alpern et al. (1987) based on 'self-screening' by optimizing the fit with a computer search routine. A variety of the most recent experimental estimates of absorbancy index spectra (or spectral distribution of absorption coefficients) were tried in this curve fitting. The heavy solid lines represent the best fitting of these which depended upon the absorption coefficients derived from the Wyszecki & Stiles (1980) study. Where two (or more) curves run together, only the most conspicuous is shown. (For details, see text.) None of these theoretical or *ad hoc* fits is satisfactory.

not diffraction limited. In this modified form one does not generally expect WDW chromaticities to be free of prereceptor factors which are by hypothesis different for one cone species at a given wavelength than for the other two. However, for the observer whose results are shown in Fig. 12.2, it was found for all wavenumbers smaller than the green primary ($m=19\ 000$ cm^{-1}) that no short-wavelength primary was ever required for 'off-axis' color matches. The only reasonable explanation is that the short-wave sensitive foveal cones make no contribution to the perception of obliquely incident monochromatic light in this part of the spectrum.

If that is the explanation, then the attenuation of obliquely incident monochromatic rays by the three prereceptor factors of Weale's theory applies equally well to the species of cones whose excitation *does* contribute to those perceptions, and the predictions of the modified theory is then no different from Weale's unmodified theory in this part of the spectrum. When the results in Fig. 12.2 are examined in this light, it is clear that substantial changes in frequency of non-zero chromaticity do occur for $m<19\ 000$ cm^{-1}. Indeed, the frequency in which the 95% confidence limits of the changes in WDW chromaticity do not include zero increases from almost one-third to almost two-thirds of the instances where this consideration applies. Hence, these results exclude both of Weale's (1981a) hypotheses as explanations for the changes in color matching found for this observer and offer further evidence for the view that the action spectra of foveal long- and medium-wave sensitive cones are closely dependent upon the angle of incidence of light on the retina.

But what do the results tell us about current explanations for that dependency? Consider the dotted lines fitted to the data in Fig. 12.2 in the following way. First, a sixth or seventh order polynomial was fitted to the $\Pi_3(\mu)$, $\Pi_4(\mu)$ and $\Pi_5(\mu)$ field sensitivity action spectra respectively of Alpern & Kitahara (1983) for normal angle of incidence on the retina. Designating these spectra as f_r, f_g, f_b respectively, one calculates the color matching functions $\bar{r}$, $\bar{g}$, $\bar{b}$:

$$\left| \begin{array}{c} \bar{r} \\ \bar{g} \\ \bar{b} \end{array} \right| = A^{-1} \left| \begin{array}{c} f_r \\ f_g \\ f_b \end{array} \right| \tag{2}$$

where

$$A = \left| \begin{array}{ccc} f_r(1) & f_r(2) & f_r(3) \\ f_g(1) & f_g(2) & f_g(3) \\ f_b(1) & f_b(2) & f_b(3) \end{array} \right| \tag{3}$$

has a non-zero determinant.

$$u = \frac{\bar{r}[\bar{g}(4)/\bar{r}(4)]}{\bar{r}[\bar{g}(4)/\bar{r}(4)] + \bar{g} + \bar{b}[\bar{g}(5)/\bar{b}(5)]}$$

$$v = \frac{\bar{g}}{\bar{r}[\bar{g}(4)/\bar{r}(4)] + \bar{g} + \bar{b}[\bar{g}(5)/\bar{b}(5)]} \tag{4}$$

and

$$w = 1 - (u+v).$$

In these equations $f_r(i)$, $\bar{r}(i)$, etc. refer to the values at the wave-numbers i, and $i=(1,2,3)$ represent the wavenumbers of the reference primaries, while $i=(4,5)$ represent the wavenumbers of the two WDW normalization values.

Next, the field sensitivity action spectra for oblique incidence was obtained using the dashed smooth curves in Fig. 12.1 ('self-screening') in conjunction with eqn 1a and the 'on-axis' $\Pi_j(\mu)$ action spectra to calculate the 'off-axis' [$\Pi_j(\mu')$] values for 3.0 mm temporal pupil entry of the colorimeter beams:

$$\log \Pi_j(\mu')/\log \Pi_j(\mu) = \varrho_j(\mu)\ (r-r_o)^2 = 9.0\varrho_j(\mu). \tag{1a}$$

These 'off-axis' values were then substituted for f_r,f_g,f_b in eqns 2 and 3, and eqn 4 solved for the 'off-axis' chromaticities u',v' and w'.

It is clear that the dotted lines drawn in Fig. 12.2 from this theoretical frame fail to intersect the 95% confidence limits of the chromaticity changes much more often than 5% of the time. This suggests that either 'self-screening' is not capable of explaining the changes in WDW chromaticity with change in angle of obliquity measured on this observer, or the $\Pi_j(\mu)$ field sensitivity spectra do not provide a valid operational definition of the action spectra of the cone mechanisms subserving his foveal color matches.

If the $\Pi_j(\mu)$ spectra do not validly represent the action spectra for color matching, then some more appropriate set should do the job. One can, with 'self-screening' theory, calculate the spectra appropriate for oblique incidence, given the parameters in the model (e.g. peak densities for normal and oblique incidence) and the characteristics (e.g. λ_{max}, shape of absorbancy index spectra) of the action spectra for normal incidence. Alpern *et al.* (1987) have used a variety of different modern estimates of these foveal chief ray spectra, including electrophysiological estimates from photocurrent of monkey cone outer segments by Nunn, Schnapf & Baylor (1984), the microspectro-photometric estimates from 58 long-wave, 45 middle-wave and 5 short-wave sensitive cones of seven human eyes by Dartnall, Bowmaker & Mollon (1983), and the estimates of Estévez (1979) from the psychophysically measured CMFs of Stiles & Burch

(1955) in a search routine to optimize the fit of 'self-screening' theory to the changes in WDW chromaticity with change in the angle of incidence of the color-imeter beams, such as are illustrated by the symbols in Fig. 12.2.

The most successful of all these fits is shown in the figure as the heavy solid line. The action spectra used in this instance were found by Wyszecki & Stiles (1980) to optimize the fit of 'self-screening' theory to the changes in WDW chromaticity with increase of test radiance from 10^3 to 10^5 td (chief ray color matching). Though of all the efforts to fit these WDW chromaticity changes with change in angle of retinal incidence this fit is the most successful, it is nevertheless the case that 29% of the lines defining the 95% confidence limit of the chromaticity differences shown in this figure fail to intersect the lines predicted by this theoretical formulation. These and similar results on three other normal trichromats do not augur a favourable future for 'self-screening' as an explanation for SCII, no matter how the action spectra of human foveal cones which underly color matching of normally and obliquely incident lights are ultimately defined. Of course, the catalog of possibilities tested by Alpern et al. (1987) was by no means exhaustive, but within the examples studied were a broad diversity of results from experiments spanning the gamut of the best modern techniques for inferring the action spectra of human cones, and Alpern et al. (1987) found that the discrepancies between theory and data remaining after using any one of them, were both large and more similar than the differences between the various fits.

If neither prereceptor factors nor 'self-screening' is to account for the change in color with change in the angle of incidence, the most probable alternative is waveguides. To evaluate this alternative, the simple Snyder–Pask model (solid line) fitted to the $\varrho_j(\mu)$ results in Fig. 12.1 were applied to the $\Pi_j(\mu)$ field sensitivity action spectra (normal incidence) and substituted in eqn 1a to calculate $\Pi_j(\mu')$ spectra and hence another set of theoretical predictions of u',v',w'. The changes in WDW $\triangle u, \triangle v, \triangle w$ predicted in this way are plotted in Fig. 12.2 as a thin solid line. The result is a disappointingly poor quantitative description of the measured changes. Can this be improved by modifying the Snyder–Pask model? Perhaps, but our efforts so far in this regard still yield disappointing predictions. The calculation yielding the thin solid line in Fig. 12.2 was repeated with only one modification, the substitution of the dashed-dot line fitted to $\varrho_5(\mu)$ data in Fig. 12.1 for the solid line to obtain the $\Pi_5(\mu')$ spectrum. (The dashed-dot line in Fig. 12.1 fits the

triangles in this figure more closely than the solid line. It allows for variability in the index of refraction and diameter of the inner segment of long-wave sensitive cones.) The results of this calculation are shown in Fig. 12.2 by short dashes, and they do not appreciably improve the ability of waveguide theory to predict these changes in WDW chromaticity with change in angle of obliquity.

Discussion

Since not one of the theoretical curves fitted to the $\Pi_j(\mu), \Pi_j(\mu')$ spectra provided a reasonable fit to the measured chromaticity changes, it is appropriate to return to the question as to the validity of these spectra for matching. One way of dealing with this question is to predict the WDW chromaticity changes of Fig. 12.2 relying on the empirical $\Pi_j(\mu), \Pi_j(\mu')$ spectra alone. To this end, the $\Pi_j(\mu')$ spectrum was computed from the circles, squares and triangles in Fig. 12.1 (rather than from the smooth theoretical curves fitted to them, as has been done heretofore), using eqn 1a and sixth (or seventh) order polynomials fitted to the results. These smoothed spectra were substituted in eqns 2, 3 and 4 to calculate u',v' and w' once more. The predicted values of $\triangle u, \triangle v$ and $\triangle w$ are shown in Fig. 12.2 as longer dashed lines. They provide convincing evidence that the operations which define the $\Pi_j(\mu), \Pi_j(\mu')$ field sensitivity action spectrum are not a valid way of specifying the action spectra of foveal cones which contain the visual pigments absorbing normally and obliquely incident photons underlying the color-matching behavior studied here.

This conclusion is reinforced by Alpern, Kitahara & Tamaki's (1983) discovery that this same $\Pi_j(\mu), \Pi_j(\mu')$ set provides a quite unsatisfactory fit to this observer's 'off-axis' WDW chromaticity changes as measured by three normally incident primaries. Emphasizing this interpretation of their result at that time was mitigated by Alpern & Tamaki's (1983) nearly simultaneous discovery that Grassmann's laws of additivity of color matches did not hold for three normally incident primaries matched to an obliquely incident test. Since they also found these additivity laws held for the conditions of the color comparisons yielding the data in Fig. 12.2, and since the longer dashed lines in that figure are a quite unsatisfactory fit to those data, those circumstances cannot mitigate that conclusion for comparison of WDW chromaticities obtained at different angles of retinal incidence when all beams traverse the eye together. It therefore seems unreasonable any longer to suppose that the similar discrepancies noted earlier by matching three chief ray primaries to an obliquely incident test do not have the identical fundamental cause.

The strongest inference to be made from these results is that the action spectra of foveal cones are clearly dependent upon the angle of incidence of light on the retina [contrary to the assumptions of Weale's (1981a) theory].

The results do not provide support for either 'self-screening' or waveguide. The evidence here is clearly more damaging to the former. However, the difficulties of providing a more valid test of waveguide theory need to be pointed out. Because of the large number of curve-fitting parameters and the sensitivity of the model to small details of the oblique action spectra, (unlike 'self-screening' theories) adequate test of the model requires valid empirical action spectra for for obliquely, as well as normally, incident light. Hence, before an accurate model of this kind can be tested, a more valid experimental way of measuring the foveal cone action spectra throughout the spectrum must be found.

This problem, which vexed the physiology of color vision for about a century, had until now been regarded as solved. The solution was the very operation – defining Stiles's $\Pi_j(\mu)$ foveal cone mechanism – the present results prove to be invalid. It is difficult to know where to turn next. The recently developed method of Stockman (Stockman & Mollon, 1986) is one possibility, but it has difficulties – not only because it deals only with the long- and medium-wave sensitive mechanisms, whereas Alpern, Kitahara & Tamaki (1983) show that the major problem may well be with the short-wave sensitive cones, but also because the extremely small dimensions of the test and field make it difficult, if not impossible, to correct for Weale's (1981a) third factor in order to obtain accurate spectra for oblique incidence at the level photons are absorbed. Another recent possibility (Eisner & MacLeod, 1981), like earlier ones (Wald, 1964), does not promise isolation of a single mechanism with the same probability everywhere in the visible spectrum. One otherwise standard approach, i.e. working backward from the CMFs (Enoch & Stiles, 1961) cannot be used because they are derived from the phenomena to be explained. The most pressing need emerging from these studies is a time-honored one in the history of color vision: a better way of validly measuring the action spectra of human foveal cones to normally and obliquely incident light non-invasively, independent of color matching.

Conclusions

(1) The action spectra (at the level of photon absorption) of foveal cones upon which color matching depends are strongly dependent upon the angle of incidence of the light.

(2) This dependency (contrary to a fundamental assumption in Weale theory) must be a major, if it is not the only, consideration in any viable explanation for the change in color of monochromatic lights with change in the angle of incidence on the retina (or SCII).

(3) Theorectical accounts of this dependency which depend upon 'self-screening' by the visual pigments in cone outer segments, are inconsistent with results of color matching of monochromatic lights at different angles of incidence of the color-imeter beams.

(4) Theoretical accounts attempted so far of this dependency based on photoreceptors modelled as waveguides are also inconsistent with these color matching results. However, this work also suggests that the operations which define the action spectra of the foveal cone mechanisms for normally and obliquely incident rays, upon which the parameters of the waveguide model depend, are invalid.

(5) A more rigorous test of waveguide models awaits the development of a more valid way of measuring the dependency of the action spectra of foveal cones upon angle of retinal incidence non-invasively.

Afterword

Horace Barlow (1961) once began a paper with this sentence: 'A wing would be a most mystifying structure if one did not know that birds flew.'

I picked up what little I know about philosophy of science from early contacts with a disciple of the Vienna Circle and from Hans Reichenbach's (1951) book, so it is perhaps excusable that discussions of Horace's teleological fantasies are prominent in our correspondence over the years. On 21 September 1964, he wrote:

If I understand myself, what I said about bird's wings was that it would be unenlightened, not to say stupid, to study their anatomy and physiology without taking into account that they were used by the bird for flying. If you did not know that the bird flew, you would be unlikely to make much sense of their wings. The idea is just the same with dark adaptation, but I am using the argument the other way around: arguing *from* the fact that we cannot make sense of a certain feature to the probability that there is some unknown factor involved analogous to the use of wings for flying.

I came across this letter while writing this paper and (though I have never yet been able to find a way to provide any teleological question with any experimental answer) must admit that what Horace says about how long it takes to recover sensitivity in the dark after a full bleach strikes a responsive chord as I ponder the differing dependency of individual action spectra of the three species of photoreceptors of color vision on the angle of retinal incidence. It makes sense for cone (and not rod) receptors to give less emphasis to the aberration-prone rays reaching it from the margin of the exit pupil than to aberration-free chief rays. But has nature gone through a complex evolutionary process to develop cone (and not rod) receptors with visual pigments with different absorption spectra for light incident on the retina obliquely than those appropriate for chief rays, for the sole purpose of making the longitudinal chromatic aberration of the eye less obvious by reducing the visibility of out-of-focus blur circles produced by the violet and red spectral extremes? Is the production of this wavelength variation in the magnitude of SCI the whole *raison d'être* for an angle of incidence dependency of the absorption spectra of retinal cones (and not rods) which differs for each one of the three species? On the surface this seems like cracking nuts with a road grader, considering that the chief ray absorption spectra of the long-and middle-wave sensitive cones already serve this end, as does the failure of the short-wave sensitive cones to contribute to heterochromatic brightness and to the resolution of high spatial frequencies. Or is there some unknown factor analogous to 'the use of wings to fly' that future work must elucidate before we can make sense of the anatomy and physiology of the change in color with change in the angle of retinal incidence of monochromatic light? It is not the first time in my experience that Horace has had the last word. He ends that same letter thus: 'It is simply an observational fact that biological mechanisms become adapted through natural selection to a high degree of efficiency, in many cases. When we cannot understand this aspect of the mechanism we are studying, our knowledge is incomplete; knowing where your knowledge is incomplete is often the first step toward new knowledge.'

Acknowledgement

Assisted by Grant EY00197-32 from the National Eye Institute. The generous assistance of Kenji Kitahara, MD, Hiroshi Kitahara, MD, Dan Kirk and Austra Liepa is gratefully acknowledged.

References

Alpern, M. (1983) A note on theory of the Stiles–Crawford effects. In *Colour Vision: Physiology and Psychophysics*, ed. J. D. Mollon & L. T. Sharpe, pp. 117–29. London: Academic Press.

Alpern, M. (1986) The Stiles–Crawford effect of the second kind (SCII): a review. *Perception*, **15**, 785–99.

Alpern, M., Ching, C. C. & Kitahara, K. (1983) The directional sensitivity of retinal rods. *J. Physiol.*, **343**, 577–92.

Alpern, M., Kitahara, H. & Fielder, G. H. (1987) The change in color matches with retinal angle of incidence of the colorimeter beams. *Vision Res.*, **27**, 1763–78.

Alpern, M. & Kitahara, K. (1983) The directional sensitivities of the Stiles' colour mechanisms. *J. Physiol.*, **338**, 627–49.

Alpern, M., Kitahara, K. & Tamaki, R. (1983) The dependence of the colour and brightness of a monochromatic light upon its angle of incidence on the retina. *J. Physiol.*, **338**, 651–68.

Alpern, M. & Tamaki, R. (1983) The saturation of monochromatic lights obliquely incident on the retina. *J. Physiol.*, **338**, 669–91.

Barlow, H. B. (1961) Possible principles underlying the transformations of sensory messages. In *Sensory Communication*, ed. W. A. Rosenblith, pp. 217–34. New York: MIT Press and Wiley.

Brindley, G. S. (1953) The effects on colour vision of adaptation to very bright lights. *J. Physiol.*, **122**, 322–50.

Dartnall, H. J. A., Bowmaker, J. K. & Mollon, J. D. (1983) Human visual pigments microspectrophotometric results from the eyes of seven people. *Proc. Roy. Soc. Lond.*, **B220**, 115–30.

Eisner, A. & MacLeod, D. I. A. (1981) Flicker photometric study of chromatic adaptation: selective suppression of cone inputs by colored backgrounds. *J. Opt. Soc. Am.*, **71**, 705–18.

Enoch, J. M. & Stiles, W. S. (1961) The colour change of monochromatic light with retinal angle of incidence. *Optica Acta*, **8**, 329–58.

Estévez, O. (1979) On the fundamental data base of normal and dichromatic color vision, pp. 138–9. Thesis, University of Amsterdam. Amsterdam: Krips Repro Mepro.

Hansen, G. (1943) Zur Kenntnis des physiologischen Apertur-Farbeffektes (Stiles–Crawford Effect II Art). *Die Naturwissenschaften*, **31**, 416–17.

Nunn, B. J., Schnapf, J. L. & Baylor, D. A. (1984) Spectral sensitivity of single cones in the retina of *Macaca fascicularis*. *Nature*, **309**, 264–6.

Pask, C. & Snyder, A. W. (1975) Theory of the Stiles–Crawford effect of the second kind. In *Photoreceptor Optics*, ed. A. W. Snyder & R. Menzel, pp. 145–58. Berlin: Springer.

Reichenbach, H. (1951) *The Rise of Scientific Philosophy*. Berkeley: University of California Press.

Snyder, A. W. & Pask, C. (1973) The Stiles–Crawford Effect – explanation and consequences. *Vision Res.*, **13**, 1115–17.

Stiles, W. S. (1937) The luminous efficiency of monochromatic rays entering the eye pupil at different points and a new colour effect. *Proc. Roy. Soc. Lond.*, **B123**, 90–118.

Stiles, W. S. & Burch, J. M. (1955) NPL colour-matching investigations (1955). Mean results for pilot group of ten subjects. Appendix to Stiles, W. S. (1955). Interim report to the Commission Internationale de l'Eclairage Zurich 1955 on the National Physical Laboratory's investigations of colour matching. *Optica Acta*, **2**, 176–81.

Stiles, W. S. & Crawford, B. H. (1933) The luminous efficiency of rays entering the eye pupil at different points. *Proc. Roy. Soc. Lond.*, **B112**, 428–50.

Stockman, A. & Mollon, J. (1986) The spectral sensitivities of the middle- and long-wavelength cones: an extension of the two-colour threshold technique of W. S. Stiles. *Perception*, **15**, 729–54.

Toraldo di Francia, G. (1949a) The radiation pattern of retinal receptors. *Proc. Physical Soc. Lond.*, **B62**, 461–2.

Toraldo di Francia, G. (1949b) Retinal cones as dielectric antennas. *J. Opt. Soc. Am.*, **39**, 324.

Wald, G. (1964) The receptors of human color vision. *Science*, **145**, 1007–16.

Walraven, P. L. (1962) *On the Mechanisms of Colour Vision*. Institute for Perception RVO-TNO. Soesterberg, The Netherlands.

Walraven, P. L. & Bouman, M. A. (1960) Relation between directional sensitivity and spectral response curves in human cone vision. *J. Opt. Soc. Am.*, **50**, 780–4.

Weale, R. A. (1961) Notes on the photometric significance of the human crystalline lens. *Vision Res.*, **1**, 183–91.

Weale, R. A. (1981a) On the problem of retinal directional sensitivity. *Proc. Roy. Soc. Lond.*, **B212**, 113–30.

Weale, R. A. (1981b) On matching colours. *Vision Res.*, **21**, 1431–2.

Wyszecki, G. & Stiles, W. S. (1980) High-level trichromatic color matching and the pigment bleaching hypothesis. *Vision Res.*, **20**, 23–37.

Zwas, F. (1979) Wavelength variation in directional sensitivity of the long- and medium-wave sensitive foveal cones of red–green dichromats. *Vision Res.*, **19**, 1067–76.

13
Fourier Interferometric Stimulation (FIS): the method and its applications

R. Gemperlein, R. Paul and A. Steiner

History and basics

In order to describe the efficiency of a physiological system it is important to know its transfer characteristics for complex stimuli. It is not necessary to measure the reaction of the system for stimuli of every possible time-course. If a system can be linearly approximated, one can restrict oneself to the transfer characteristics for sinusoidal stimuli. All other stimulus time-courses can be represented as a sum of sine shaped components of varying amplitude and phase. Hearing can be tested with pure tones, and the spatial resolution of the eye is examined with spatial gratings that are modulated sinusoidally in brightness.

In principle, colour vision could be analogously examined with spectral lights that have sine shaped spectral energy distribution. Newton used rectangular 'comb spectra', and Barlow (1982) explained how comb spectra with a sinusoidal modulation of energy with wavelength can be used for the analysis of colour vision.

In 1969 R. Gemperlein came across a paper about a Fourier interferometer working in the infrared region of the spectrum, and he had the idea of using an interferometer for the visible and ultraviolet spectral region as a spectral modulator for a light source for the examination of the visual system. After preliminary experiments and discussions with various commercial firms in 1974, the realization of this idea started in 1976 based on a doctoral thesis in the physics department of the *Technische Universität* in Munich. Here Heinz Parsche had constructed a Fourier spectrometer for the visible and UV spectral region. With this instrument Rüdiger Paul, while working on his diploma, proved the possibility of realizing this idea, with Parsche's support. These experiments showed the need for a special set-up, since a high input energy to the interferometer demands a design entirely different from that of Parsche's instrument, which was constructed for experiments in Raman spectroscopy using very weak light sources. We therefore developed our own instrument with the support of the *Deutsche Forschungsgemeinschaft*.

The development of this instrument was vindicated by the unexpected discovery of fine structure in the ultraviolet region of the action spectrum of the photoreceptor in the blowfly *Calliphora erythrocephala* (see the section on spectral sensitivity in insects below). The short measurement time led to applications in ophthalmology (see the section on analysis on the human eye) and the technique has also been used to measure human contrast sensitivity functions for comb filtered spectra (see the section on psychophysical measurements). This article emphasizes the potential advantages of Fourier Interferometric Stimulation (FIS) and shows a range of preliminary results on a variety of topics.

Methods

The experimental set-up for investigations using FIS consists of a classical Michelson interferometer where one mirror is moved back and forth at constant velocity through the white light (zero path-difference) position to vary the path-difference.

The principle is explained in Fig. 13.1. A beamsplitter divides the light source into two equivalent light sources, which are recombined after reflexion from two mirrors and interfere at the beamsplitter. If one visualizes light as an electromagnetic wave the output will be weakened periodically, if the path difference equals half that wavelength times an odd number, and will add up to maximal intensity at

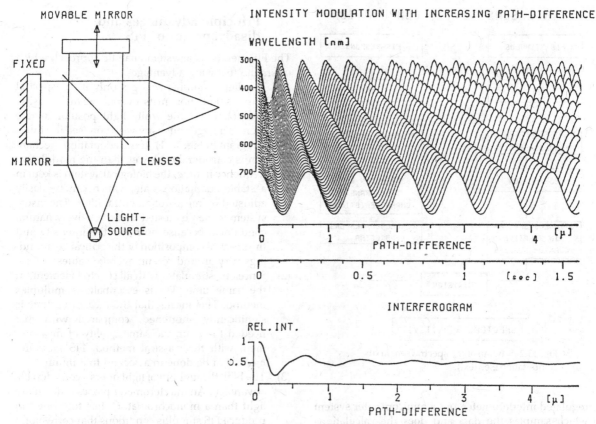

Fig. 13.1. Scheme of a Michelson interferometer with one movable mirror (top left). The resulting intensity modulation for each wavelength from 300 to 700 nm is sketched in relation to the optical path difference, where zero is the adjusted position of both mirrors causing no path difference (top right). Because the mirror moves with a constant speed of 1.45 μm/s, a time scale is also given. All modulated wavelengths are summed up to show the intensity variation of the FIS stimulus with path difference or time.

multiples of that wavelength. The intensity variation for each wavelength is plotted in Fig. 13.1 as a function of wavelength, depending on the path-difference. If the mirror is moving with a constant speed of $V = 1.45$ μm/s the same picture gives us the time modulation of each frequency. In our case the He–Ne laser line is modulated by $f = 2 \times V/\lambda = 2.9/0.632 = 4.59$ Hz. From this formula it follows that each wavelength is coded with a typical modulation frequency in time. From blue to red these frequencies are, in the experiments reported here, 4.14–7.25 Hz for 700–400 nm. The modulation degree of the interferometer output is 60–80%, but of course this can be reduced by dilution if the influence of non-linearities is feared (see the section on psychophysical measurements).

In addition, light from a He–Ne laser passes through the instrument to act as a reference beam, which serves as an absolute wavelength reference and is used for dynamic path regulation. In this way accurate linear mirror movement is guaranteed. The regulating electronics provides sampling pulses at intervals of λ/8 of the He–Ne wavelength of 632.8 nm. The sampling pulses trigger the data acquisition of the computer. The mirror is moved linearly back and forth through the white light (zero path-difference) position. The path-difference is measured in wavelengths of the He–Ne reference laser. This allows averaging of stimuli and responses, since the sampling points always lie at the same positions in relation to the interferogram. The whole instrument is stabilized above room temperature at approximately 36°C by means of an electronically regulated heater. Additional filtering of the lamp spectrum in the infrared helps to stabilize the instrument.

The entire apparatus for carrying out optical experiments consists of a 150 W Xenon arc-lamp, the

SPECTRAL SENSITIVITY COMPUTATION

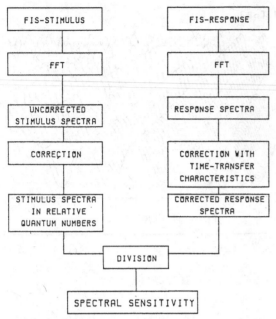

Fig. 13.2. Scheme of the spectral sensitivity computation (see text).

regulated interferometer and a minicomputer system which samples the data and does the calculations (Gemperlein, 1980). The light stimulus can be brought to the eye in different forms by the usual optical means, for example with the help of a light guide or by irradiation of an Ulbricht sphere to provide a Ganzfeld stimulus.

For the calculation of spectral sensitivity, Fourier transformations of stimulus and response interferograms are carried out. The calculation of spectral sensitivity is summarized in Fig. 13.2. Fourier transformation of the stimulus and response interferogram gives the spectra. The stimulus spectrum is corrected for the spectral characteristics of the photomultiplier to get the real lamp spectrum as transmitted through the interferometer. The reaction spectrum is corrected, if necessary, for the time transfer characteristics of the system examined. If one divides the response spectrum by the stimulus spectrum and scales on 100%, one derives the spectral sensitivity, since the FIS-method is a linear analysis. Steiner (1984) fully analysed the influence of nonlinearities, and showed that these interfere less than might be feared (see also the section on spectral sensitivity in insects).

Principle advantages and disadvantages of FIS

The FIS-method is a system-analytic approach which offers the following advantages:

(1) The light stimulus changes only in its spectral composition, not in its overall mean intensity, except around the white light position where there is a larger intensity variation (see the interferogram in Fig. 13.1). If the adaptation mechanism is considerably slower than the modulation frequency in time, the biological system is kept in a stable adaptation state, which can be easily adjusted by means of a neutral filter. The visual system is thereby tested under relatively natural conditions, because normally the intensity and the spectral composition of the optical surroundings vary around certain average values.

(2) Since one stimulates with all spectral elements at the same time, FIS is essentially a multiplex method. This means that the measuring time is significantly shortened, compared with that needed to obtain the same quality of measurement with the classical method. FIS measurements can be done in a second to a minute.

(3) The high throughput of light offers a considerable advantage. An interferometer passes much more light than a monochromator, therefore one can produce FIS stimulus conditions that correspond to a sunny day.

(4) FIS has high spectral resolution. The spectral resolution is a function of the greatest path difference used in stimulation and can be chosen arbitrarily.

(5) An absolute wavelength scale is obtained, because of the use of the He–Ne laser as a reference.

(6) FIS offers a large time frequency range for the measurement, because the mirror velocity can be adjusted to the measurement task within wide limits.

(7) Simultaneous measurements of the stimulus and the response eliminates errors from temporal changes in the lamp spectrum.

(8) Since the range of stimulus frequencies comprises only one octave, one can band-filter the responses. This improves the signal-to-noise ratio and eliminates DC-drift.

(9) FIS is principally a linear procedure. Therefore the spectral sensitivity, calculated by simple division (Fig. 13.2), is subject to a very small error compared to the classical method using a

logarithmic response curve. Because of the limited frequency range, non-linear effects can however be studied. The kind of non-linearity is revealed by the subharmonics and harmonics produced (see the section on analysis of the electroretinogram in butterflies and Fig. 13.5).

(10) As well as the spectral sensitivity, FIS provides information about spectral phase, which describes the delay of the single spectral components in the system.

(11) Fixed adaptational lights can be superimposed on the dynamic FIS stimulus without difficulty.

(12) Consecutive measurements can easily be averaged to increase the quality of the measurement.

(13) Different parameters can be measured in a system simultaneously, for example transmission, reflexion and photo-reaction.

Disadvantages and limitations

The main disadvantage we see is the unfamiliarity of most physiologists with Fourier methods and multiplexing techniques. One measures a complex response, which is the sum of the simultaneous responses to all spectral elements in the stimulus. From this complex response the sensitivity is derived by division and not measured directly as by a constant response criterion. The interpretation and influence of non-linearities seems to be very critical at first glance (see below). A very severe disadvantage is that this instrument, consisting of the inteferometer with control electronics and a computer system for data acquisition and analysis, is currently not commercially available, and therefore has to be constructed.

Spectral sensitivity in insects

Discovery of the fine structure of the absorption of the photopigment in the ultraviolet (UV) range in *Calliphora erythrocephala*

More than 25 years ago, measurements of the spectral sensitivity of the visual cells R1–R6 of the blowfly *Calliphora erythrocephala* had shown that they contain a visual pigment with two sensitivity maxima (Burkhardt, 1962). The first maximum lies in the green spectral range at 500 nm and the second in the ultraviolet range at 360 nm. Different hypotheses were proposed, including the existence of two visual pigments that lie close to each other in the same receptor (Horridge & Mimura, 1975, Rosner, 1975), light-guide effects (Snyder & Pask, 1973), a single pigment with a raised β-absorption band compared with rhodopsin

(Paulsen & Schwemmer, 1979), or the presence of an accessory sensitizing pigment that absorbs additional quanta (Kirschfeld, Francheschini & Minke, 1977).

Through highly resolved FIS measurements, Gemperlein *et al.* (1980) found a surprising fine structure of the absorption spectrum in the UV range (Fig. 13.3). Comparison with published spectra showed that the kind of spectrum we had found could originate from a five-chained polyene. A spectrum comparison allowed Paul (1981) to conclude that the pigment could be retroretinol or retinol, with a planar configuration possibly due to binding to opsin, since only then does such a fine structure show up in the spectrum. Kirschfeld *et al.* (1983) and Vogt & Kirschfeld (1983) tested our results in the classical way and confirmed our findings. Biochemically they identified 3-hydroxyretinol as the sensitizing pigment.

Analysis of the electroretinogram in butterflies; selective adaptation for isolation of receptors

Steiner (1984) examined the spectral sensitivity of the butterflies *Pieris brassicae* (cabbage white), *Parargae aegeria* (speckled wood butterfly) and *Aglais urticae* (small tortoiseshell). Since in butterflies it is very difficult to penetrate single receptor cells, he used the FIS method, together with selective adaptation, and measured the amplitude of the electroretinogram (ERG) in different parts of the compound eye. The interpretation of the spectral sensitivity of the eye was aided by the phase-response and the non-linear reaction.

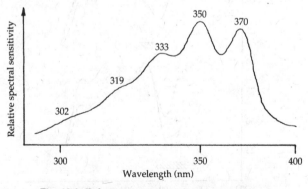

Fig. 13.3. Relative spectral sensitivity of the blowfly *Calliphora erythrocephala chalky* to an ultraviolet FIS stimulus as it can be measured intra- or extracellulary (path difference 72 μm, 1.34 nm resolution at 350 nm.) 100 ERG responses are averaged because of the very low signal-to-noise ratio.

It is a common assumption, that the overall multi-peaked spectral sensitivity of the ERG is caused by separate receptors with maxima at different wavelengths. Fig. 13.4 demonstrates how well the number of receptors existing in an eye can be shown with FIS through selective adaptation. These measurements were carried out in the ventral part of the eye in *Pieris brassicae*. A fixed adaptation light consisting of a particular wavelength band, which is hatched in the illustration, was shifted from red to blue (from top to bottom in Fig. 13.4). The spectral sensitivity without

an adapting light is represented by a dashed line. It is obvious that the receptor absorbing best in the area of the adapting light is saturated in its response and therefore depressed in relation to the others. This result, together with further analysis of the non-linearity and phase, led to the conclusion that there are separate receptors with maxima at 620 nm, 540 nm, 450 nm and 360 nm. The complete analysis can be found in Steiner, Paul & Gemperlein (1987).

Measurements on *Parargae aegeria* serve as an example for the interpretation of phase and non-linearity. Figure 13.5 shows the spectrum of the ERG response from the compound eye of *Parargae aegeria*. The stimulus itself contained only temporal frequencies in the range of 4–8 Hz, each temporal frequency corresponding to a different spectral wavelength (see Methods) indicated by the inserted scale. Normally the components in this range are used for deriving the spectral sensitivity by dividing the corrected stimulus spectrum (not shown here), but in this case the direct response components are also plotted out for higher and lower temporal frequencies with their corresponding phases.

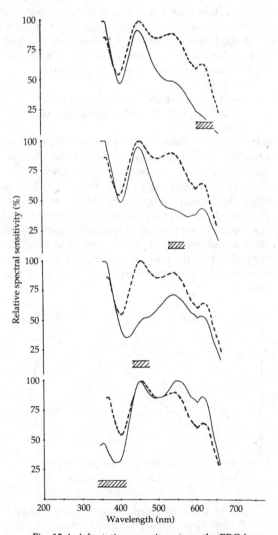

Fig. 13.4. Adaptation experiments on the ERG from the ventral part of the eye of *Pieris brassicae*. Relative spectral sensitivity under 'white light' is plotted as a dashed line. The hatched area shows the adaptation light, varying from red to blue (top to bottom).

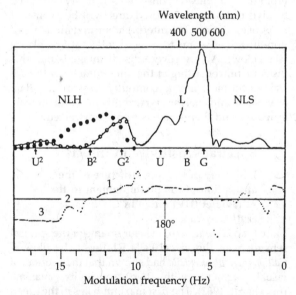

Fig. 13.5. Relative ERG response spectrum of *Parargae aegeria* on a frequency scale, with phase plotted below. NLS: non-linear subharmonics. L: linear response. NLH: non-linear harmonic response. Ultraviolet (U), blue (B) and green (G) and their harmonic responses (U^2, B^2, G^2) are indicated. Open circles: measured non-linear response. Filled circles: predicted non-linear response from one common characteristic.

If all reaction components came from the same receptor, one would expect no great phase differences, since the stimulus frequency range covers only one octave (4–8 Hz, where all reported time transfer functions of insect receptors are flat). But if one stimulates several receptor types simultaneously, they might react with different latencies on the basis of the different amounts of light that they receive and their differing sensitivities. This would lead to phase differences. Let us first concentrate on the linear section of the response spectrum (L in Fig. 13.5). Time frequencies are plotted leftwards to have the corresponding wavelength scale running rightwards as usual: the maxima in the amplitude suggest three receptor types. The phase shows a small increase of U (ultraviolet) over B (blue) after G (green). Since the response (time-frequency) is plotted leftwards in a linear scale on the abscissa, we can find the regions where we have to look for the quadratic distortion of the reaction: U^2, B^2, C^2 by doubling the path that goes from the right margin to U, B, G. Here the phases show clear differences and so reinforce the conclusion that there are three separate receptor systems.

The frequencies above and below the linear response are caused, we believe, by non-linearities of the response. Steiner (1984) has computed the predictions on the basis of non-linearities of single and multicomponent models. Thus non-linearities of the response certainly occur, but it is possible to make use of them in analysing response components. The prediction of the non-linear reaction from the linear reaction component under the assumption of a common response characteristic is plotted with filled circles in Fig. 13.5. Since these do not correspond to the measured reaction, the hypothesis of a common response characteristic can be rejected. Instead one can assume that various separated receptors with differing spectral maxima are involved and predict the open circles, which agree with the measured amplitude and therefore support the hypothesis of separate receptors. Further examples of the results obtained from various insect species can be found in Paul, Steiner & Gemperlein (1986).

Spectral sensitivity in man

Analysis of the human eye by means of ERG and Visual Evoked Cortical Potential (VECP)

The FIS method could be a good method to carry out fast, objective and precise measurements on humans. In cooperation with the eye clinic of the University in Munich we have tried to determine the spectral sensitivity in humans without injury by employing the usual ERG and the evoked potentials recorded over the occipital cortex (VECP) (Adamczyk *et al.*, 1983). The first experiments involving the ERG revealed only the scotopic sensitivity, but in excellent agreement with previously published data (Gemperlein, 1980). In these experiments a visual field of approximately 30 degrees in diameter was irradiated by Maxwellian view, hence stimulating peripheral zones of the retina consisting mainly of rods (together with even more eccentric ones exposed to scattered light). Using Ganzfeld stimulation from an Ulbricht sphere we found suitable conditions for determining the photopic as well as the scotopic spectral sensitivity. For this, an intensity variation of 1:100 was sufficient.

In Fig. 13.6 we see an example of the spectral sensitivity derived from the ERG of a person with normal colour vision. Curve 1 is measured with a stimulus light of 10^3 cd/m². As others have found, even at this high luminance the ERG is still dominated by the rod signal and therefore the spectral response corresponds to scotopic sensitivity with a maximum at 500 nm, even though the luminance is well above psychophysical scotopic levels. With an increase of intensity by a factor of 10 we found that the maximum shifted into the blue range: as far as we know this is the first time such a blue shift has been reported and clearly it needs further investigation. At full light intensity (10^5 cd/m²), the expected Purkinje shift occurs towards yellow (around 550 nm). The exact location of the peak varies slightly with subject and intensity. Note that these unusual results were obtained with the eye adapted to very high luminance

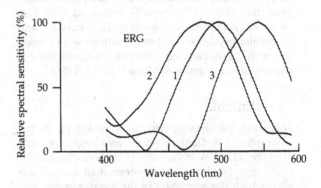

Fig. 13.6. Spectral sensitivity from the ERG of the eye of a person with normal colour vision under Ganzfeld FIS-stimulation with white light. Relative intensity $1 = 10^{-2}$, $2 = 10^{-1}$, $3 = 1$ times maximal luminance, equivalent to 10^5 cd/m². 1: reveals the scotopic sensitivity. 2: maximum shifted to blue 3: photopic Purkinje shift.

levels and the use of Ganzfeld illumination was also found to be essential.

In order to determine such a spectral sensitivity curve, a single experimental run lasting only 17 seconds was sufficient in a relaxed subject. Since the amplitude of the FIS signal lies in the range of 20–50 µV it can be entirely obscured by muscle potentials and therefore 25–49 measurements are averaged for inexperienced patients from the clinic taking 10 to 15 minutes. An analysis of non-linearity and phase similar to that of Fig. 13.5 is being performed and we hope it will enable us to separate the responses from different receptors and/or neurons.

Psychophysical measurements for a spectral contrast sensitivity function

Following a suggestion from J. D. Mollon, Horace Barlow came to Munich with the idea of doing psychophysical measurements in the summer of 1982. The regulation of the interferometer was changed by a new computer program so that the instrument was set at a certain comb frequency, jumping back and forth with a defined path difference, causing a changing colour sensation. This then provided the possibility of a threshold measurement. FIS light was mixed with 'white light' until the subject could no longer detect colour changes with variations of the comb frequency. From these values a sensitivity function, dependent on the comb frequency, was determined. There were several unsatisfactory features of these preliminary measurements but they provided the first psychophysical colour transfer function determined with comb spectra (Barlow et al., 1983). A subject with defective colour vision clearly showed a poorer colour resolution (Fig. 13.7, curve 3) compared with two observers with normal vision (Fig. 13.7, curves 1 and 2). Similar psychophysical examinations were carried out with a modified experimental set-up in the eye clinic of the university of Munich (Pohl, 1985).

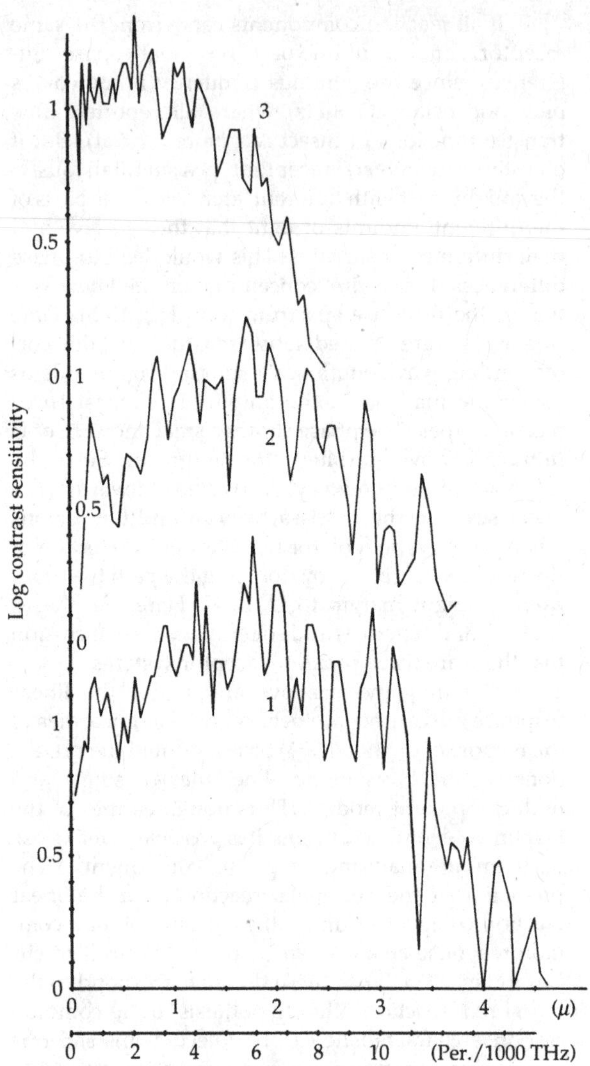

Outlook

Following the development of a prototype in the laboratory of R. Gemperlein, Steiner began the construction of a new instrument in the eye clinic at the University of Munich. A modern digital computer allows both the regulation of the interferometer and the succeeding calculations to be carried out rapidly.

Fig. 13.7. Colour contrast sensitivity function of one deuteranopic (3) and two colour normal observers (1, 2). The psychophysical threshold measurements are described in the text.

With the application of a digital signal processor it should be possible to measure on-line spectral sensitivities and to search for neurons with specific spectral qualities. We hope that these developments will provide a new impulse to the field of colour vision.

References

Adamczyk, R., Gemperlein, R., Paul, R. & Steiner, A. (1983) Objektive elektrophysiologische Bestimmung der skotopischen und photopischen spektralen Empfindlichkeiten des menschlichen Auges mit Hilfe fourierinterferometrischer Stimulation (FIS). *Fortschr. Ophthalmol.*, **80**, 488–91.

Barlow, H. B. (1982) What causes trichromacy? A theoretical analysis using comb-filtered spectra. *Vision Res.*, **221**, 635–43.

Barlow, H. B., Gemperlein, R., Paul, R. & Steiner, A. (1983) Human contrast sensitivity for comb-filtered spectra. *J. Physiol.*, **340**, 50P.

Burkhardt, D. (1962) Spectral sensitivity and other response characteristics of single visual cells in the arthropod eye. *Symp. Soc. Exp. Biol.*, **16**, 86–109.

Gemperlein, R. (1980) Fourier Interferometric Stimulation (FIS). A new method for the analysis of spectral processing in visual systems. In *MEDINFO* 80, ed. D. A. B. Lindberg & S. Kaihara, pp. 372–6. Amsterdam: North Holland Publishing Company.

Gemperlein, R., Paul, R., Lindauer, E. & Steiner, A. (1980) UV fine structure of the spectral sensitivity of flies' visual cells. Revealed by FIS (Fourier Interferometric Stimulation). *Naturwissenschaften*, **67**, 665.

Horridge, G. A. & Mimura, K. (1975) Fly photoreceptors I. Physical separation of two visual pigments in *Calliphora* retinula cells 1–6. *Proc. Roy. Soc. Lond.*, **B216**, 71–85.

Kirschfeld, K., Feiler, R., Hardie, R., Vogt, K. & Franceschini, N. (1983) The sensitizing pigment in fly photoreceptors. Properties and candidates. *Biophys. Struct. Mech.*, **10**, 81–92.

Kirschfeld, K., Franceschini, N. & Minke, B. (1977) Evidence for a sensitising pigment in fly photoreceptors. *Nature (Lond.)*, **269**, 386–90.

Paul R. (1981) Neue Aspekte der spektralen Empfindlichkeit von *Calliphora erythrocephala* gewonnen durch fourierin-terferometrische Stimulation (FIS). Thesis, Munich University (unpublished).

Paul, R., Steiner, A. & Gemperlein R. (1986) Spectral sensitivity of *Calliphora erythrocephala* and other insect species studied with Fourier Interferometric Stimulation (FIS). *J. Comp. Physiol.*, **A158**, 669–80.

Paulsen, R. & Schwemmer, J. (1979) Vitamin A deficiency reduces the concentration of visual pigment protein within blowfly photoreceptor membranes. *Biochim. Biophys. Acta*, **557**, 385–90.

Pohl, W. J. (1985) Untersuchungen von kongenital Farbsinngestörten mittels eines speziell zusammengesetzten polychromatischen Reizlichts. Thesis, Munich University (Unpublished).

Rosner, G. (1975) Adaption and photoregeneration in fly eyes. *J. Comp. Physiol.*, **102**, 269–95.

Snyder, A. W. & Pask, C. (1973) Spectral sensitivity of dipteran retinula cells. *J. Comp. Physiol.*, **84**, 59–76.

Steiner, A. (1984) Die lineare und nichtlineare Analyse biologischer Sehsysteme mit einfachen Sinusreizen und Fourier-Interferometrischer Stimulation (FIS). Thesis, Munich University (unpublished).

Steiner, A., Paul, R. & Gemperlein, R. (1987) Retinal receptor types in *Aglais urticae* and *Pieris brassicae* (Lepidoptera), revealed by analysis of the electroretinogram obtained with Fourier interferometric stimulation (FIS). *J. Comp. Physiol.*, **A160**, 247–58. •

Vogt, K. & Kirschfeld, K. (1983) Sensitizing pigment in the fly. *Biophys. Struct. Mech.*, **9**, 319–28.

14

The chromatic coding of space

K. T. Mullen

Introduction

Colour vision is a means of encoding the spectral reflectance of a surface. Thus the contours, edges or patterns which allow us to distinguish an object against its background may be seen both by virtue of their intensity variation and on the basis of their colour variation. Over the past three decades a relatively new approach to the investigation of colour vision has been emerging. This involves creating a stimulus from which the variations in intensity have been removed and so allowing it to be distinguished solely on the basis of its colour differences. Such stimuli are often termed 'isoluminant'. In this chapter I aim to examine some of the difficulties associated with the use of colour-only stimuli and to assess their contribution to the understanding of the spatial coding of colour vision.

The problems of colour-only stimuli

Chromatic aberrations

There are considerable optical difficulties inherent in the use of chromatic stimuli, which have to be overcome in order to remove all luminance artifacts and ensure that the stimulus can be detected only on the basis of its colour variation. These arise largely from the two types of chromatic aberration of the eye. The chromatic difference of focus, the increasing power of the eye for shorter wavelengths of light, affects the relative contrasts of the sinusoidal component colours in a chromatic grating. (A chromatic grating can be considered as the sum of two luminance modulated gratings added in antiphase.) This is often corrected by using an achromatizing lens, a small pupil or by correcting the relative amplitudes of the component wavelengths. The second aberration is the chromatic difference of magnification. This arises since the longer wavelength components of the image are magnified relative to the shorter wavelengths which alters the relative spatial frequencies of the component gratings in the chromatic stimulus. The result of this aberration is to produce a wavelength dependent difference of position on the retina which increases as a function of eccentricity. Since the fovea is displaced from the optic axis of the eye by approximately 5 degrees towards the temporal retina, a chromatic difference of position may be detectable even for foveal stimuli (see Le Grand, 1967).

The results of experiments, done with Roger Watt, to test whether a chromatic difference of position could be measured in the fovea are shown in Fig. 14.1. A vernier task was arranged with the top and bottom vernier bars of different wavelengths. (See figure legend for details.) Using the method of Watt & Campbell (1985) the bars were set to appear colinear. The figure shows the vernier settings for foveal fixation as a function of the wavelength difference between the bars. Subjective colinearity although variable appears to be affected by the wavelength difference which suggests that there is a wavelength dependent displacement of the two bars on the retina of this subject. The results indicate that the chromatic difference of displacement at the fovea for this subject from 438 nm to 624 nm is approximately 1.3 minutes of arc. The effects of these two aberrations become more troublesome at high spatial frequencies when, in addition, wavelength dependent diffraction effects will occur at the pupil. These have been calculated to be detectable for a 2 mm pupil above the 10 cpd (Van der Horst, de Weert & Bouman, 1967). Overall, these optical problems have hampered the use of high spatial frequency chromatic stimuli in, for example, measuring colour acuity.

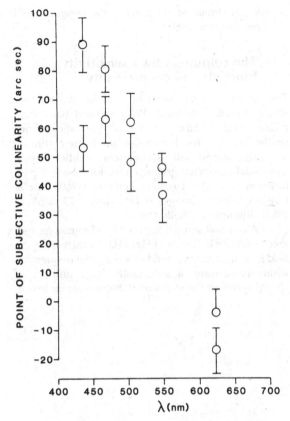

Fig. 14.1. The point of subjective colinearity, in arc seconds, is shown for a vernier task with the two vernier bars of different wavelengths. The wavelength of the fixed bar is 643 nm and the wavelength of the variable bar is given on the abscissa. ±one standard error is shown. A linear regression fitted to the data was used to calculate a vernier displacement of 80 seconds of arc for the wavelength range 438 nm to 624 nm.

example for stimuli of low spatial or temporal frequency, the luminance of colours does not simply predict their brightness. For these reasons a brightness match may be temporal frequency or spatial frequency dependent. Variations in the intensity match may occur with both spatial and temporal frequency (Kelly, 1983; Mullen, 1985; Cavanagh, MacLeod & Anstis, 1987). Thus it is important to equate the intensities of the colours under the appropriate spatial and temporal conditions. The most direct method is simply to measure performance at the task for a range of different relative intensities of the component colours.

Figures 14.2A and B show the results of such a method used to produce a colour-only red/green grating. The ratio of the mean luminances of the com-

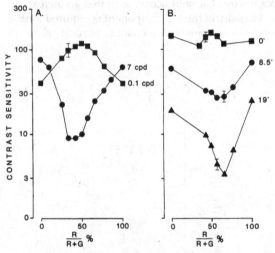

Fig. 14.2. The stimulus is a monochromatic (602 nm) red luminance grating added in antiphase with a green (526 nm) luminance grating. These two component gratings are equal in contrast. The ordinate shows contrast sensitivity (the reciprocal contrast at threshold of either component grating). The abscissa shows the proportion of red to green mean luminances of the component gratings in the composite stimulus, expressed as the percentage of red (R) in the red/green mixture. The summed red and green mean luminances (R + G) are constant. Stimuli are sinusoidally phase reversed at 0.4 Hz. A. The two curves show results for two spatial frequencies (■, 0.1 cpd; ●, 7 cpd) both viewed foveally. The spatial frequency determines whether a maximum or minimum is obtained. B. The curves show results for a grating of 0.8 cpd viewed at three different eccentricities in the nasal visual field (■, 0°; ●, 8.5°; ▲, 19°). A shift in the position of the minimum occurs.

Setting the intensity match

The second difficulty associated with the use of chromatic gratings is how to set the intensities of the two colours in the stimulus so that it can be detected only on the basis of its colour differences. It is essential to establish a quantitative method for finding the intensity match and one of the difficulties is that only under certain conditions will equating the luminance of the colours in the stimuli also result in their brightness being equal. For tasks involving flicker, spatial acuity or making a minimally distinct border the brightness of colours directly depends upon their luminance (eg. Boynton & Kaiser, 1968). Under other conditions, for

ponent colours is varied and contrast sensitivity to the composite stimulus is measured at various points in the complete red to green range. Removing the luminance contrast from the stimulus and adding colour differences causes contrast sensitivity to change, but the direction in which it changes depends on the spatial frequency of the stimulus (Fig. 14.2A). At medium or high spatial frequencies a minimum in sensitivity occurs whereas at low spatial frequencies a maximum is reached. The position of these maxima or minima can be used to indicate the red/green luminance ratio required for a colour-only stimulus.

The luminance ratio required to produce a colour-only grating changes across the visual field, reflecting change in spectral sensitivity with eccentricity. The results in Fig. 14.2B show the change which occurs across the nasal field in the first 19 degrees of eccentricity. The shift occurs such that an increase in the intensity of the red component is required for the match as eccentricity increases beyond about 8

degrees. A similar shift occurs in the temporal field (Mullen, forthcoming).

The colour contrast sensitivity function and colour acuity

The earliest measurements of a colour contrast sensitivity function (Schade, 1958) showed band pass characteristics and a high acuity for chromatic gratings similar to that for luminance modulated stimuli, however almost all subsequent studies using sinusoidal chromatic gratings have found a low pass function (Van der Horst & Bouman, 1969; Hilz & Cavonius, 1970; Granger & Heurtley, 1973; Mullen, 1985) although see Kelly (1983).

A contrast sensitivity function obtained for red/green gratings is shown in Fig. 14.3. By increasing the field size, the results extend to low spatial frequencies while maintaining a sufficiently large number of spatial cycles in the stimulus to minimize any loss in

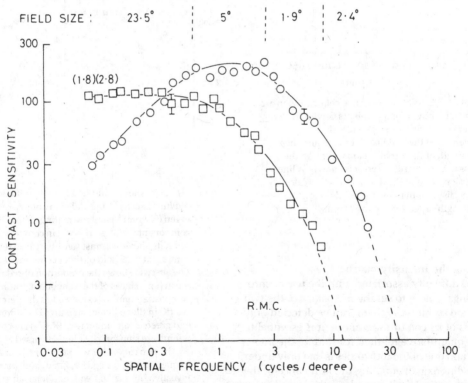

Fig. 14.3. The contrast sensitivity to a red/green chromatic grating (□) compared to a monochromatic luminance grating (○). The red/green intensity match in the chromatic grating is determined using the maxima and minima of Fig. 14.2A. The luminance grating is the green component grating (0% red) of Fig. 14.2A. Figures in brackets indicate the number of spatial cycles displayed in the stimulus at the lowest spatial frequencies. Chromatic aberrations have been corrected (from Mullen, 1985).

sensitivity from the effects of probability summation (Howell & Hess, 1978; Robson & Graham, 1981).

Acuity for these red/green gratings in the figure is relatively low at 10–12 cpd, which is approximately three times lower than the acuity for luminance gratings measured under comparable conditions. Previous studies have found considerably higher acuities for chromatic gratings, although these higher values are probably not based on the detection of their colour differences. For example, Granger & Heurtley (1973) noticed that although their red/green grating lost its colour differences around 12 cpd it could still be detected as an achromatic (yellow/black) grating up to 30 cpd.

Two 'cardinal directions' in colour space can be identified on the basis that temporal modulation between colours at isoluminance in one direction fails to have any adaptive effect on the direction of modulations in the other direction, and vice versa (Krauskopf, Williams & Heeley, 1982). One of these directions is a tritanopic confusion line; all colours along this line produce the same quantum catches in long (L) and medium (M) wavelength cone types and so their discrimination depends on the contribution of short wavelength (S) cones. The second direction is independent of S cone activity; colour modulation at isoluminance along this line produces a constant quantum catch in S cones and so can be discriminated solely by comparing M and L cone quantum catches. These results suggest the presence of separable post receptoral mechanisms subserving colour detection and arising from combinations of these different cone types. Two groups of parvocellular neuron in the primate lateral geniculate nucleus (LGN) have been found which are maximally responsive along the two axes of colour space similar to the cardinal directions (Derrington, Krauskopf & Lennie, 1984). However, the failure of these subcortical neurons to adapt or habituate suggests that the psychophysically defined cardinal directions are determined by groups of neurons located more centrally than the LGN.

One question which arises concerns the spatial properties of these chromatic sub-systems. The red/green grating of Fig. 14.3 barely modulates S cones, and so this contrast sensitivity function is likely to arise from a mechanism (or mechanisms) combining the outputs of L and M cones, such as the one identified by Krauskopf *et al.* (1982). The spatial contrast sensitivity of the chromatic sub-systems which receive S cone modulation have not been measured directly. The contrast sensitivity functions arising from 'isolated' S cone responses, obtained from stimuli on yellow adapting backgrounds, are spatially low pass at low temporal frequencies (Kelly, 1974; Green, 1968) suggesting that in the normal visual system S cone mechanisms have low pass spatial contrast sensitivity.

Identifying the acuity of the S cone chromatic mechanism is hampered by technical difficulties; chromatic stimuli must modulate S cones at isoluminance along a tritanopic confusion line, while being corrected for chromatic aberrations and maintaining an adequate mean luminance. Acuity measured with a pair of chromatic bars (along a tritanopic confusion line) has been estimated to be 5–8 cpd (Eskew & Boynton, 1987). This is likely to be a lower estimate, because only a single spatial cycle of a square wave was used and the stimulus was centrally fixated and so fell largely within the region of foveal tritanopia (Williams, MacLeod & Hayhoe, 1981). An upper bound of the acuity of this chromatic mechanism is presumably given by the acuity of the 'isolated' S cone mechanism. Estimates of S cone acuity range from 5 cpd (Brindley, 1954) to 10–12 cpd (Williams, Collier & Thompson, 1983). Thus, overall it appears that the acuity of the S cone chromatic mechanism at between 5 and 10 cpd is rather lower than that of a chromatic mechanism combining L and M cone outputs.

From our knowledge of luminance vision it would be expected that the overall colour contrast sensitivity function arises from the outputs of a range of spatially selective submechanisms and recent attempts have been made to identify their characteristics. Spatial frequency selective masking between chromatic gratings occurs with a wide spread of masking across spatial frequency, suggesting that the adapted submechanisms are broadly tuned and band pass (De Valois & Switkes, 1983). Thus while psychophysical results indicate the presence of chromatic spatial submechanisms their characteristics and distribution are still illusive.

The early stage of colour processing is by the colour opponent cells of the retino-striate pathway, and the evidence suggests that these act as spatial low pass filters for chromatic modulation, while retaining their band pass selectivity for luminance modulation (Ingling & Martinez, 1983, 1985). It is interesting that such low pass spatial characteristics have not been revealed psychophysically. One consequence of the low pass, low acuity filtering of colour vision is likely to be a reduction in the accuracy with which colour differences can be localized in space. There is evidence to suggest that this is the case, since vernier acuity which requires a high degree of spatial precision is reported to be significantly reduced, by approximately a factor of 1.3 to 3, for isoluminant stimuli (Morgan & Aiba, 1985).

Comparing colour and luminance vision

In Fig. 14.3, the low pass contrast sensitivity function for colour vision is compared to the band pass function of luminance vision on the same contrast scale. (The contrast of the two component gratings is taken as a working measure of the contrast of the composite chromatic grating.) These results show that for low spatial frequencies the combination of the two component gratings in antiphase *can* be seen when neither can be detected on its own, whereas at higher spatial frequencies contrast sensitivity is greater to the individual component gratings. This indicates an advantage of colour vision over luminance vision at low spatial frequencies.

One difficulty which impedes comparisons between colour and luminance vision is that it is like comparing apples with oranges; the qualitative differences making it difficult to find a quantitative comparison. A way around this problem can be found since the cones are a common pathway in the coding of both colour and luminance contrast and so provide a common metric for the comparison. Thus it is possible ible to compare sensitivities to colour and luminance contrast in terms of the receptoral activities produced by each.

A comparison between colour and luminance contrast sensitivity in terms of cone contrasts is given in Fig. 14.4. Sensitivities to the red/green chromatic grating and the green monochromatic grating (from Fig. 14.3) have been calculated in terms of the contrasts of each to a long wavelength and a medium wavelength cone type. Comparisons show that at low spatial frequencies cone contrast sensitivity is considerably higher to chromatic than to luminance grat-

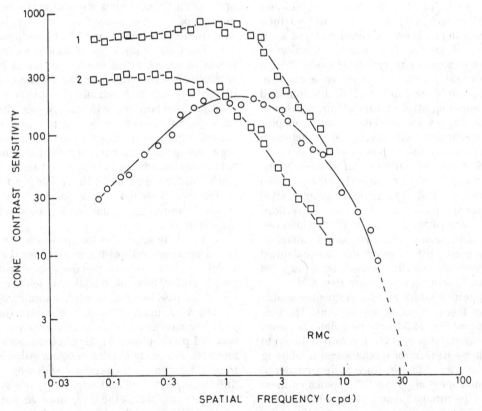

Fig. 14.4. The data of Fig. 14.3 have been replotted in terms of cone contrasts, the contrast of the stimulus to a mechanism with the spectral sensitivity of M or L cones. Top curve (1): contrast sensitivity of L cones to the chromatic grating. Middle curve (2): contrast sensitivity of M cones to the chromatic grating. Lower curve: contrast sensitivity of M and L cones to the luminance grating (the two are identical).

ings. In other words, the chromatic stimulus is detected on the basis of smaller cone modulations than is the luminance stimulus. Since individual classes of cone can signal only the intensity of a stimulus and not its wavelength, it must be the post receptoral combinations of the cone outputs which produces this advantage of colour vision.

In summary, colour vision has emerged as a spatially low pass, low acuity system. We cannot use colour vision to detect the sharp edges or fine detail in the image or to precisely localize edges or borders, all this requires the presence of luminance contrast. Colour vision however provides an additional means of detecting a figure against its background by 'filling-in' the colour of objects or forms, and is particularly sensitive to low spatial frequency colour variation. In view of this dichotomy of spatial function it is interesting that the colour of objects never appears to 'spill-over' the edges or contours which define them. The presence of luminance contrast appears to be able to segregate the chromatic borders to the luminance borders. The effect of border segregation is to 'overlay' the colour and luminance attributes of the image. The absence of border segregation at isoluminance might account for the characteristic 'shimmery' appearance of these colour-only patterns.

Colour vision as a specialization of the central visual field

It is a simple observation that there is a loss of colour sensation in the more peripheral regions of the visual field (see Moreland 1972 for a review, Noorlander *et al.*, 1983; Johnson & Massof, 1982). This should not necessarily be taken to mean that colour vision is a particular specialization of central vision since various forms of colour contrast sensitivity loss across the visual field could account for this effect. For example, one possibility is that there is a discrete specialization for colour localized to the central visual field, which might be characterized by a central region of uniform sensitivity followed by a rapid decline. A contrasting view is that there is no particular central field specialization for colour, in which case colour and luminance contrast sensitivity would decline in parallel across the visual field. A lower foveal contrast sensitivity to chromatic gratings compared with luminance gratings would produce an early 'bottoming out' of colour vision in the periphery with luminance vision remaining.

The results of an experiment to compare how contrast sensitivity to chromatic (red/green) and luminance gratings varies across the visual field are shown in Fig. 14.5. The intensity match between colours was obtained using the method of Fig. 14.2. Colour contrast sensitivity declines systematically across the visual field and this decline is steeper at all spatial frequencies than the decline in luminance contrast sensitivity (Mullen, forthcoming). There is no evidence for any sparing of colour vision relative to luminance vision within the central visual field. Thus while it is true that colour vision may be considered to be a specialization of central vision, it is not one which is discretely localized to one part of the visual field.

The processing of colour independently from other visual attributes?

It has become clear from theoretical discussions that the single colour-opponent neurons of the primate retino-striate pathway are able to act both as low pass filters for isoluminant chromatic modulation and band pass filters for luminance modulations (Ingling & Martinez, 1983, 1985). The idea of neurons doing a 'double duty' by the simultaneous processing of both colour and luminance contrast also receives firm neurophysiological support (Wiesel & Hubel, 1966; Derrington, Krauskopf & Lennie, 1984). The method by which these signals can subsequently be separated remains unclear, however at the level of the striate cortex a segregation of chromatically and achromatically sensitive neurons appears to have begun (Livingstone & Hubel, 1984). Within the prestriate cortex, the colour sensitive neurons cluster in one region (V4) and so are to some extent separated from the processing of other visual attributes such as stereopsis and motion (Zeki, 1978, 1980; Maunsell & Newsome, 1987; Zeki, chapter 30, and see Barlow, 1986).

To what extent is the neurophysiological separation of the processing of colour from that of other visual attributes evident at the psychophysical level? A number of psychophysical observations appear at face value to be compatible with the parallel processing of colour vision from other visual attributes. Adaptation to chromatic temporal modulation fails to affect the detection of luminance modulation and vice versa (Krauskopf, Williams & Heeley, 1982). This is compatible with a separation of the processing of luminance and colour contrast at a cortical level. However, complex spatial frequency specific masking and facilitatory interactions occur between colour and luminance gratings which suggest that at other levels there is no such separation of colour and luminance processing (De Valois & Switkes, 1983).

There is evidence to suggest a distinction

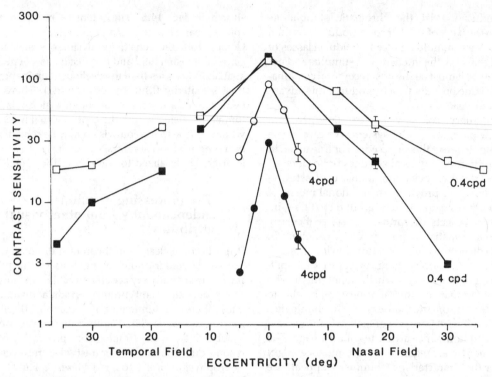

Fig. 14.5. The contrast sensitivity to red/green gratings compared to luminance gratings across the nasal and temporal visual field for two spatial frequencies. Details of stimuli are given in the legend of Fig. 14.2. Stimuli were presented horizontally with four spatial cycles displayed ■, □; 0.4 cpd chromatic and luminance gratings respectively. ●, ○; 4 cpd chromatic and luminance gratings respectively. (From Mullen and O'Sullivan, 1988).

between the contribution of colour and luminance contrast to the perception of motion. Chromatic gratings at isoluminance appear to drift much more slowly than luminance gratings (Moreland, 1982; Cavanagh, Tyler & Favreau, 1984), although this observation in itself is not sufficient to suggest a separation of colour from motion processing. The absence of apparent motion at isoluminance suggests more directly that motion processing cannot utilize chromatic contrasts (Ramachandran & Gregory, 1978). However, the observation that the motion after-effect is not diminished for isoluminant stimuli shows that this conclusion requires qualification (Mullen & Baker, 1985; Derrington & Badcock, 1985; Cavanagh & Favreau, 1985). Overall, interesting differences between the processing of motion from luminance and colour contrast are suggested but any separation of motion processing from colour processing is unlikely to be complete. Quantitative differences between the processing of motion from colour or luminance contrast might also be accounted for, for example, by

differences between the spatio-temporal properties of the colour and luminance filters sub-serving motion processing.

We have seen that despite the differences in spatial resolution and the precision of spatial localization between colour and luminance vision, the colours of objects do not appear to spill-over their luminance edges indicating that mechanisms of border segregation are available which bind colour to luminance borders. Recent demonstrations have also shown that the movement of illusory contours or random dot patterns can 'capture' a stationary chromatic border at isoluminance (Ramachandran, 1987, and see Ramachandran, chapter 31). This observation implies that there are mechanisms which can segregate the colour to moving luminance contours or borders. Thus despite the different perceptual velocities of isoluminant colour and luminance images, the different parts of an object do not appear to separate when it is in motion. The availability of mechanisms to segregate colour to luminance motion would mean that the inability to process motion from colour contrast is no great disadvantage. Only in the rare event of a stimulus being isoluminant would a separation of the colour and luminance attributes of an object occur. Thus an outstanding psychophysical question is to ask about the interactions between colour and luminance processing which serve to bind together these different attributes of the visual image, since without

these mechanisms colour vision would provide us with a perceptually chaotic world.

Acknowledgements

I am grateful for the collaboration of Roger Watt in the experiments for Fig. 14.1, and for the collaboration of Eoin O'Sullivan in the experiments for Fig. 14.5. This article was prepared in August 1987.

References

Barlow, H. B. (1986) Why have multiple cortical areas? *Vision Res.*, **26**, 81–90.

Boynton, R. M. & Kaiser, P. K. (1968) Vision: the additivity law made to work for heterochromatic photometry. *Science*, **161**, 366–8.

Brindley, G. S. (1954) The summation areas of human colour receptive mechanisms at incremental thresholds. *J. Physiol.*, **24**, 400–8.

Cavanagh, P. & Favreau (1985) Color and luminance share a common motion pathway. *Vision Res.*, **25**, 1595–601.

Cavanagh, P., MacLeod, D. I. A. & Anstis, S. M. (1987) Equiluminance: spatial and temporal factors and the contribution of blue-sensitive cones. *J. Opt. Soc. Am.*, **4**, 1428–38.

Cavanagh, P., Tyler, C. W. & Favreau, O. E. (1984) Perceived velocity of moving chromatic gratings. *J. Opt. Soc. Am. A1*, 893–9.

Derrington, A. M. & Badcock, D. R. (1985) The low level motion system has both chromatic and luminance inputs. *Vision Res.*, **25**, 1879–84.

Derrington, A. M., Krauskopf, J. & Lennie, P. (1984) Chromatic mechanisms in lateral geniculate nucleus of macaque. *J. Physiol.*, **357**, 241–65.

DeValois, K. K. & Switkes, E. (1983) Simultaneous masking interactions between chromatic and luminance gratings. *J. Opt. Soc. Am.*, **73**, 11–18.

Eskew, R. T. & Boynton, R. M. (1987) Effects of field area and configuration on chromatic and border discriminations. *Vision Res.*, **27**, 1835–44.

Granger, E. M. & Heurtley, J. C. (1973) Visual chromaticity-modulation transfer function. *J. Opt. Soc. Am.*, **63**, 1173–4.

Green, D. (1968) Contrast sensitivity of the colour mechanisms of the human eye. *J. Physiol.*, **196**, 415–29.

Hilz, R. & Cavonius, C. R. (1970) Wavelength discrimination measured with square wave gratings. *J. Opt. Soc. Am.*, **60**, no 2, 273–7.

Howell, E. R. & Hess, R. F. (1978) The functional area for summation to threshold for sinusoidal gratings. *Vision Res.*, **18**, 369–74.

Ingling, C. R. & Martinez, E. (1983) The spatio-chromatic signal of the r–g channel. In *Colour Vision*, ed. J. D. Mollon & L. T. Sharpe, pp. 433–44. London: Academic Press.

Ingling, C. R. & Martinez, E. (1985) The spatiotemporal properties of the r–g X-cell channel. *Vision Res.*, **25**, 33–8.

Johnson, M. A. & Massof, R. W. (1982) The effect of stimulus size on chromatic thresholds in the peripheral retina. In *Colour Vision Deficiencies VI*, ed. G. Verriest, pp. 15–18. The Hague: Junk.

Kelly, D. H. (1974) Spatio-temporal frequency characteristics of colour vision mechanisms. *J. Opt. Soc. Am.*, **64**, 983–90.

Kelly, D. H. (1983) Spatiotemporal variation of chromatic and achromatic contrast thresholds. *J. Opt. Soc. Am.*, **73**, 742–50.

Krauskopf, J., Williams, D. R. & Heeley, D. W. (1982) Cardinal direction of colour space. *Vision Res.*, **22**, 1123–31.

Le Grand, Y. (1967) Form and space vision. Translated by: M. Millidot & G. G. Heath, revised edition, pp. 5–23. Bloomington: Indiana University Press.

Livingstone, M. S. & Hubel, D. H. (1984) Anatomy and physiology of a colour system in the primate visual cortex. *J. Neurosci.*, **4**, 309–56.

Maunsell, J. H. R. & Newsome, W. T. (1987) Visual processing in monkey extrastriate cortex. *Ann. Rev. Neurosci.*, **10**, 363–401.

Moreland, J. D. (1972) Peripheral colour vision. In *Handbook of Sensory Physiology*, VII/4, ed. D. Jameson & L. M. Hurvich, pp. 517–36. Berlin: Springer-Verlag.

Moreland, J. D. (1982) Spectral sensitivity measured by motion photometry. *Docum. Ophthal. Proc. Series*, Vol. 33, 61–6.

Morgan, M. J. & Aiba, T. S. (1985) Positional acuity with chromatic stimuli. *Vision Res.*, **25**, 689–96.

Mullen, K. T. & Baker, C. L. (1985) A motion aftereffect from an isoluminant stimulus. *Vision Res.*, **25**, 685–8.

Mullen, K. T. & O'Sullivan, E. (1988) Colour contrast sensitivity across the human visual field. *J. Physiol.*, **386**, 66.

Mullen, K. T. (1985) The contrast sensitivity of human colour vision to red–green and blue–yellow chromatic gratings. *J. Physiol.*, **359**, 381–409.

Noorlander, C., Koenderink, J. J., den Ouden, R. J. & Edens, B. W. (1983) Sensitivity to spatiotemporal colour contrast in the peripheral visual field. *Vision Res.*, **33**, 1–11.

Ramachandran, V. S. (1987) Interactions between colour and motion in human vision. *Nature*, **328**, 645–7.

Ramachandran, V. S. & Gregory, R. L. (1978) Does colour provide an input to human motion perception? *Nature*, **275**, 55–7.

Robson, J. G. & Graham, N. (1981) Probability summation and regional variation in contrast sensitivity across the visual field. *Vision Res.*, **21**, 409–18.

Schade, O. H. (1958) On the quality of colour-television images and the perception of colour detail. *Journal of the Society of Motion Picture and Television Engineers*, **67**, 801–19.

Van der Horst, G. J. C. & Bouman, M. A. (1969) Spatio temporal chromaticity discrimination. *J. Opt. Soc. Am.*, **59**, 1482–8.

Van der Horst, G. J. C., de Weert, C. M. M. & Bouman, M. A. (1967) Transfer of spatial chromaticity contrast at threshold in the human eye. *J. Opt. Soc. Am.*, **57**, 1260–6.

Watt, R. J. & Campbell, F. W. (1985) Vernier acuity: interactions between length effects and gaps when orientation cures are eliminated. *Spatial Vision*, **1**, 31–8.

Wiesel, T. N. & Hubel, D. H. (1966) Spatial and chromatic interactions in the lateral geniculate body of the rhesus monkey. *J. Neurophysiol.*, **29**, 1115–6.

Williams, D. R., Collier, R. J. & Thompson, B. J. (1983) Spatial resolution of the short-wavelength mechanism. In *Colour Vision: Physiology and Psychophysics*, ed. J. D. Mollon & L. T. Sharpe, pp. 487–504. London: Academic Press.

Williams, D. R., MacLeod, I. A. & Hayhoe, M. M. (1981) Foveal tritanopia. *Vision Res.*, **21**, 1341–56.

Zeki, S. (1978) Functional specialization in the visual cortex of rhesus monkey. *Nature*, **274**, 423–8.

Zeki, S. (1980) The representation of colours in the cerebral cortex. *Nature*, **284**, 412–8.

Brightness, adaptation and contrast

15

The role of photoreceptors in light-adaptation and dark-adaptation of the visual system

T. D. Lamb

Introduction

The aim of this chapter is to review the contribution of the rod and cone photoreceptors to the adaptational behaviour of the overall visual system. Before doing so it is helpful first to distinguish two rather different phenomena which are both referred to as adaptation, and which may be confused.

Light-adaptation (synonymous with *background adaptation* or *field adaptation*) refers to the ability of the visual system quickly to establish a new steady state of visual performance when the incident level of illumination changes. Such intensity changes may either be increases or decreases in illumination; in both cases a new operating point is reached within several hundred milliseconds, provided the intensity change is restricted to a few log units (e.g. Crawford, 1947).

Dark-adaptation (synonymous with *bleaching adaptation*) refers not simply to the behaviour observed after a reduction in light level, but is instead reserved for the special case of recovery following the cessation of extremely intense illumination, which has 'bleached' a substantial fraction (say more than 0.1%) of the photopigment in the receptors. This recovery may be extremely slow. For example, following exposure to a very intense light bleaching 90% of the rhodopsin, one's visual sensitivity is initially enormously depressed and only recovers to its final dark-adapted level after some 40 minutes.

Shapley & Enroth-Cugell (1984) have set out very clearly the importance of light-adaptation for the visual system. A major purpose of light-adaptation is to provide effective vision over the enormously wide range of intensity which is experienced by the eye. Obviously there must exist mechanisms which permit the visual system to attain extreme sensitivity at the dimmest levels of lighting, yet which avoid saturation and work effectively at very high light levels. But according to Shapley & Enroth-Cugell (1984), a related and probably equally important purpose of light-adaptation is to provide a signal in the visual pathway which is more-or-less independent of the ambient lighting level, and which represents the *contrast* in the visual image. Most of the visual scenes which we normally encounter involve *reflecting* objects, and in a reflected scene the contrast is independent of the mean level of illumination. Extraction of contrast information means that, for scenes comprising reflecting objects, the signals sent from the retina to the brain are invariant with the ambient level of illumination. In this way the brain is presented primarily with information about the scene, rather than with information about the light level.

In order to achieve broadly similar ends a television set incorporates an *automatic gain control* (AGC) circuit which automatically adjusts the receiver's sensitivity very rapidly in approximately inverse proportion to the signal strength, so that a picture of similar contrast is obtained for stations of very different signal strengths. In this way the output of the television set, the picture, is given by the *modulation* of the transmitted signal rather than by the absolute strength of the signal received. For a weak station the gain of the amplifiers in the television set is high and the picture may appear noisy, while for a strong station the gain is greatly reduced and relatively noise-free reception is obtained.

In much the same way, light-adaptation acts automatically and fairly rapidly to adjust visual sensitivity approximately in inverse proportion to the mean light intensity. In cones, and in the rods of lower vertebrates, a substantial part of the control of gain occurs within the photoreceptors themselves. The primate rod system, on the other hand, appears to achieve its automatic gain control primarily through post-receptoral mechanisms.

In contrast to light-adaptation, dark-adaptation serves no useful purpose, and can only represent a disadvantage (Barlow, 1972). In terms of the television receiver analogy, dark-adaptation would correspond to the situation of tuning from an extremely powerful local station to a very weak distant station and finding (to one's surprise) that it was necessary to wait a long time for the receiver to resensitize so that a picture could be obtained. Obviously, the manufacturer of a television receiver with this kind of performance would be likely to have some trouble selling it, and one is left wondering why such an undesirable property should be built into the visual system. One attractive possibility is to suppose that the slowness of dark-adaptation represents an unavoidable consequence of some important property of visual transduction; perhaps it is a consequence of the particular bio-chemistry needed to obtain the enormously high sen-sitivity of the rod photoreceptors.

Light-adaptation and the role of photoreceptors

The performance of the overall visual system when light-adapted to different steady intensities has been studied extensively. Generally speaking, as the back-ground intensity increases, the threshold for the detection of a superimposed test stimulus increases, and the time response of the system improves. Over a wide range of intensities it is often found that the threshold, ΔI, for the detection of a test stimulus is related to the background intensity, I, by an equation of the form:

$$\frac{\Delta I}{\Delta I_0} = \left(1 + \frac{I}{I_D}\right)^n, \tag{1}$$

where ΔI_0 is the absolute threshold, I_D is a constant often referred to as the 'dark light', and the exponent n has a value typically between 0.5 and 1.

Under appropriate circumstances (e.g. large area, long duration test stimulus) the exponent n may approach unity and the increment-threshold relation is then referred to as Weber-law behaviour. Under these conditions the threshold ΔI rises in direct pro-portion to the background intensity I (provided that I is fairly large), and threshold occurs at a constant value of contrast $\Delta I/I$, given by

$$\frac{\Delta I}{I} = \frac{\Delta I_0}{I_D}. \tag{2}$$

It must be noted, however, that Weber-law behaviour such as this is a special case, and that normally n is not exactly equal to unity.

In attempting to relate these psychophysical findings to the results of photoreceptor electrophysio-logy, there are some important gaps in our under-standing. We do not, for example, know to what extent a given desensitization of the photoreceptors will affect the sensitivity of the overall visual system. Since desensitization will decrease not only the signal but also any noise in the receptor (or indeed in whatever cell we are considering), then we cannot make any accurate prediction of the overall result without a much more detailed knowledge of the system.

Despite this problem it is useful to compare the psychophysics with the electrophysiology. In doing so there are certain similarities between the behaviour of cones and the behaviour of the rods of lower vertebrates, which distinguish them from primate rods, and so they will be taken together to begin with. Nevertheless, as will be discussed, there are major differences between rods and cones. For a review of the basic electrophysiology of photoreceptors the reader is referred to Lamb (1984a) and Pugh & Cobbs (1986).

Cones and lower rods

Electrical recordings from cones and from the rods of lower vertebrates have shown that the transduction process in these photoreceptors becomes desensitized in the presence of background illumination, as illustrated in Fig. 15.1 for a toad rod (Lamb, 1984b). The upper-most trace was obtained for flashes presen-ted in darkness, and the peak height of the trace represents the dark-adapted flash sensitivity, S_D. The lower traces were obtained with test flashes presented on steady backgrounds of increasing intensity, and show that in the toad rod the effect of background illumination is both to desensitize the rod and to accelerate its response. That is, the peak of the response not only decreases in size but also moves to earlier times, as the background intensity increases.

The relationship between sensitivity and back-ground intensity for toad rods is plotted in Fig. 15.2 (from Fain, 1976). In order to aid comparison with psychophysical measurements the ordinate plots $1/S$, the reciprocal of the flash intensity. This parameter represents the quantity of light required to elicit a criterion response amplitude, and is therefore com-parable to the threshold, ΔI, in eqns (1) and (2). The straight-line behaviour (with slope of unity) in the

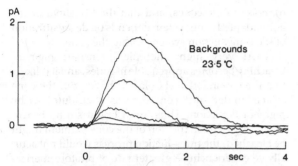

Fig. 15.1. Desensitization of a toad rod by background illumination. Traces plot photocurrent responses to brief dim flashes presented at time zero. Uppermost curve was obtained for flashes presented in darkness, while the remaining curves were for flashes presented on backgrounds of progressively greater intensity. With the brighter backgrounds the test flash intensity was increased in order to obtain a measurable response and the plotted traces have been scaled down accordingly; i.e. the traces are equivalent to sensitivity. Reproduced with permission from Lamb (1984b).

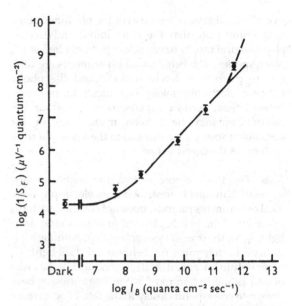

Fig. 15.2. Desensitization of toad rods by background illumination, determined from intracellular voltage responses to dim test flashes. Log reciprocal sensitivity (1/S) is plotted against log background intensity (I), and over a considerable range the results are fitted by a straight line with slope of unity (Weber-law behaviour). Reproduced with permission from Fain (1976).

double logarithmic coordinates of Fig. 15.2 indicates that, over a considerable range of backgrounds, $1/S$ is directly proportional to background intensity I. Hence

$$\frac{S_D}{S} = 1 + \frac{I}{I_0}, \qquad (3)$$

indicating Weber-law behaviour at the level of the photoreceptor, analogous to eqn (1) with $n=1$ in the psychophysical case.

Photoreceptor desensitization of this kind is observed in cones and in the rods of lower vertebrates. The desensitization is known to occur primarily in the light-sensitive outer segment, and is presumably intimately associated with the biochemical cascade of transduction (see for example, Pugh & Cobbs, 1986). From consideration of the very low intensities at which rod desensitization occurs, Donner & Hemilä (1978) and Bastian & Fain (1979) concluded that the desensitization resulting from absorption of a single photon spreads to affect many disks, and therefore that it involves a diffusible messenger substance. The degree of spread of desensitization was investigated by Lamb, McNaughton & Yau (1981), who concluded that the diffusion of a small molecule could account for the observed results. It has recently been shown that a major part of the desensitization is caused by a light-induced decline in cytoplasmic free calcium concentration (Torre, Matthews & Lamb, 1986; Matthews, Murphy, Fain & Lamb, 1988; Nakatani & Yau, 1988; Fain,

Lamb, Matthews & Murphy, 1989; Matthews, Fain, Murphy & Lamb, 1990).

The acceleration of the flash response kinetics which is observed during background illumination is presumably critical in determining the temporal response of the overall visual system. The electrophysiological results indicate that even in the presence of desensitizing backgrounds the early rising phase of the flash response is unaltered, as illustrated in Fig. 15.1 (Baylor & Hodgkin, 1974; Lamb, 1984b). This has the important consequence that although the low-frequency gain of the photoreceptor is decreased during light-adaptation, the high-frequency gain is unaltered (see Tranchina, Gordon & Shapley, 1984; Shapley & Enroth-Cugell, 1984). In psychophysical experiments examining the absolute modulation sensitivity of the visual system as a function of temporal frequency, exactly this behaviour is obtained (Kelly, 1971). An important test of any model of photoreceptor desensitization will be to see whether it correctly predicts the invariant rising phase of the receptor response at the earliest times.

In attempting to compare the response of the

overall visual system with that of the photoreceptors, it is unfortunate that the behavioural and electrophysiological results have seldom been studied in the same species. The behavioural experiments are difficult to perform in lower animals, and the photoreceptor electrophysiology is difficult in primates. Nevertheless, useful comparisons of behaviour and electrophysiology have been made both in the amphibian scotopic system and in the turtle photopic system, as described below.

Rods For the scotopic system the half-saturating intensity I_0 in eqn (3), measured from electrophysiological experiments on rods, does not coincide with the intensity of the psychophysical or behavioural dark-light, I_D, of the overall system (eqn (1)). Although it is difficult to determine the behavioural dark-light, I_D, accurately in lower vertebrates, its value is of the order of 0.01 isomerization $rod^{-1} s^{-1}$ in frogs and has been shown to correspond closely to the rate of occurrence of thermal isomerizations in the rods (Aho, Donner, Hyden, Orlov & Reuter, 1987). The half-desensitizing intensity, I_0, on the other hand, is of the order of 5 isomerizations $rod^{-1} s^{-1}$ in toads (Baylor, Matthews & Yau, 1980), a factor of at least 100 times higher.

Thus, although both the rod electrophysiology and the scotopic behavioural results (in these lower vertebrates) indicate Weber-law behaviour under appropriate conditions, the latter phenomenon is apparently not directly dependent on the former. As in the primate system (discussed below) the behavioural threshold of the rod system is likely to depend to a substantial extent on post-receptoral mechanisms.

Cones In the turtle cone (photopic) system, on the other hand, the half-desensitizing intensity, I_0, for the cones (Baylor & Hodgkin, 1974) appears to correspond quite closely with the behavioural dark-light, I_D, of the photopic system (Fain, Granda & Maxwell, 1977). Hence it is interesting to speculate that in the cone system the psychophysical or behavioural increment-threshold results may be determined directly by the cone electrophysiology. It is also interesting to note that in turtle cones the half-desensitizing intensity, I_0, has been shown to correspond closely to the 'noise equivalent photon rate' of the cone's intrinsic dark noise (Lamb & Simon, 1977).

Taken together these results could indicate that the photopic behavioural results stem directly from desensitization of the cones, and that the photopic 'dark-light' is set by a source of noise intrinsic to the cone photoreceptors. This would mean that the threshold of the dark-adapted cone system depends on noise in the cones, and that the threshold of the light-adapted cone system depends on desensitization of the transduction system within the cone.

At very high photopic intensities pigment bleaching becomes appreciable in cones, and it is likely that the continued Weber-law behaviour of the cone system under such conditions is contributed to by pigment depletion. Thus, on a bright sunny beach, when a substantial fraction of the cone pigment might be bleached, the transduction process would not actually be experiencing a greater rate of photoisomerizations than at a rather lower intensity, since the amount of available photopigment would be reduced. Such a photopigment contribution to Weber-law desensitization can only occur in the cone system. The rods are totally incapacitated at much lower intensities, and are quite unable to respond when even a tiny fraction of pigment (say 1%) is bleached, as is described later.

Primate Rods

The desensitization described above is presumably of very great importance to the functioning of the photopic system and to the scotopic system of lower vertebrates, but it appears to be much less important to the behaviour of the primate scotopic system. Baylor, Nunn & Schnapf (1984) reported that, in contrast to cones and lower rods, the rods of primates do not exhibit Weber-law desensitization. Instead, with background illumination, the size of the primate rod response simply increases with intensity until a compressive saturation sets in as the photocurrent approaches its maximum level (i.e. as the outer segment 'dark current' approaches zero). Other cases in which this type of behaviour is observed have been reviewed by Shapley & Enroth-Cugell (1984). Very recently, Tamura, Nakatani & Yau (1989) have reported that, at relatively high intensities, rods in several mammalian species do in fact adapt to some degree, prior to saturation.

Hence, over much of the psychophysical Weber-law region, individual primate rods continue to operate with essentially full sensitivity. This indicates that the desensitization observed for the overall system is contributed mainly by post-receptoral mechanisms.

An interesting question, then, is why the rods of lower vertebrates should desensitize in a Weber-law manner, beginning at moderately low intensities, whereas primate rods show little such desensitization and instead retain most of their sensitivity until saturation. The answer may lie simply in the prevention of saturation in the larger and slower rods of the lower vertebrates (Fain, 1976; Lamb, 1986). Because of their much larger size and correspondingly larger rhodopsin content (*ca* 20×), together with their lower operating temperature and much slower responses (*ca* 10×), a given light intensity will, in amphibian rods, lead to a state of activation several hundred times greater than in primate rods. In other words, at some arbitrary intensity the number of simultaneous 'photon effects' in a toad rod will be vastly greater than in a monkey rod. But apparently, in order to permit visual detection at extremely low light levels, all rods have evolved a large single-photon response amplitude of several per cent of the standing dark current. Therefore, at a moderate scotopic intensity, where a primate rod would still be able to register single-photon hits, a lower rod would, in the absence of desensitization, be totally saturated and unable to respond. Hence in this way the automatic gain control (AGC) in the cones and lower rods serves to prevent saturation, and thereby to improve the sensitivity of the visual system (Shapley & Enroth-Cugell, 1984). At the higher absolute intensities at which primate rods saturate, the cone photoreceptors are able to respond adequately, so that the near-absence of rod adaptation represents no disadvantage.

Dark-adaptation in rods

Dark-adaptation, or bleaching adaptation, is a term used to describe the recovery both of sensitivity and of other properties of the visual system following exposure of the retina to intense illumination which 'bleaches' a substantial fraction of the pigment in the photoreceptors. It has been known for many years that, following such exposures, recovery of visual sensitivity in the human is composed of two components, a rapid cone-dominated phase followed by a slower rod-dominated phase; only the latter rod phase will be considered here. The original results of Hecht, Haig & Chase (1937) are presented in Fig. 15.3, and illustrate the recovery of sensitivity following exposures of different magnitude. It is important to note that in experiments of this kind the desensitization which is induced by a bleach is vastly greater than would be expected simply from pigment depletion, and a bleach of as little as 1% of the rhodopsin can elevate the visual threshold initially by as much as two log units.

Rushton's theory The 'textbook' theory of dark-adaptation was given by Rushton (1965). The fundamental relation in this work is the 'Dowling–Rushton equation' relating threshold elevation to bleached pigment:

$$\frac{\Delta I}{\Delta I_0} = 10^{aB},$$ (4)

at any time and, *a* is a constant. Subsequent experi-

where *B* is the fraction of pigment remaining bleached ments, however, have shown that this equation is not at all accurate.

Equivalent background intensity In considering any alternative description of dark-adaptation behaviour, it seems important to take full account of the classical observations of Stiles & Crawford (1932) and Crawford (1937). They showed that during the course of dark-adaptation the elevation of threshold could accurately be described in terms of an 'equivalent background intensity'. That is, following an intense bleaching exposure the visual system behaves as if it is viewing the world through a veiling light and, during the course of dark-adaptation, the intensity of this equivalent background slowly fades away.

This 'equivalent background hypothesis' has the great attraction that it removes the need to invoke special mechanisms of desensitization in explaining dark-adaptation. All that is necessary to postulate is that by some unknown mechanisms the after-effects of a bleach give rise to events which the visual system is unable to distinguish from real photon hits. Thus, dark-adaptation simply becomes a special case of light-adaptation, in which the adapting field is stabilized on the retina.

Barlow's hypothesis A description of dark-adaptation, as an alternative to that of Rushton's, was put forward by Barlow (1964). He proposed that, both in fully dark-adapted conditions and during recovery from bleaches, the visual system was limited by *noise* inter-

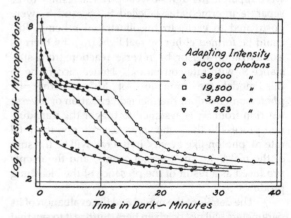

Fig. 15.3. Dark-adaptation curves for a normal observer. Classical results obtained for a series of bleaching intensities, showing distinct rod- and cone-dominated regions. Reproduced with permission from Hecht, Haig & Chase (1937). (Note: the unit of retinal illuminance, the troland, was then called the 'photon').

nal to the photoreceptors. He further proposed that the photoreceptors became noisier during the after-effect of a bleach, thereby raising the visual threshold, as a result of the same signal-to-noise considerations that apply during steady illumination (Barlow, 1956, 1957).

This idea was not developed quantitatively and appears to have received relatively little support over the years. However, as described in the following two sections, electrophysiological recordings from rod photoreceptors suggest that it may be correct, and the idea has been extended to provide a quantitative model of human dark-adaptation behaviour.

A model of dark-adaptation

Using the equivalent background hypothesis of Stiles & Crawford as a basis, I analysed the detailed psychophysical data of Pugh (1975) and formulated a model of dark-adaptation which represents an extension of Barlow's ideas. In this model (Lamb, 1981) the equivalent background hypothesis was taken as literally correct, in that the after-effects of bleaching were assumed to give rise to the generation, within the rod transduction machinery and as a direct consequence of the presence of the bleaching products, of events indistinguishable from photoisomerizations.

These photon-like events were postulated to occur as the result of a tiny degree of reversibility in the chain of inactivation reactions that remove the activated form of rhodopsin, Rh*, from the rod, and the scheme chosen is shown in Fig. 15.4. In order to describe three separate components of recovery which were apparent in Pugh's psychophysical results, three separate intermediates labelled S_1, S_2 and S_3 were postulated to exist. In the illustrated scheme, Rh* could be formed either by real light (r_{hv}), by thermal isomerization (r_0) or by reverse reaction from substance S_1 with rate constant k_{10}. Hence, according to this model the formation of Rh*, whether by photoisomerization, thermal isomerization or reverse reaction from S_1, is assumed to trigger the transduction process in the same way. Accordingly, the total rate of 'photon-like events' in the rod will be the sum of the real light, the thermal events, and the events produced as a result of the presence of the bleaching products.

The details of the model and the evaluation of its parameters will not be given here. Suffice it to say that reconstruction of the behaviour of the model with bleaches ranging from 0.5% to 98% provided an excellent fit to Pugh's psychophysical data (see Lamb, 1981, Figs. 6 and 7).

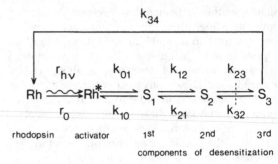

Fig. 15.4. Model indicating origin of 'photon-like events', used to fit dark-adaptation results. Rhodopsin, Rh, is isomerized to the active form Rh* either by light at rate r_{hv}, or thermally at rate r_0. Rh* is inactivated to S_1, which is converted to S_2, and in turn to S_3 before being resynthesized to native rhodopsin. S_1, S_2 and S_3 give rise to the three distinct components observed during recovery, through the reverse reactions with rate constants k_{10}, k_{21} and k_{32}. The time constants of the three components of decay are given by the reciprocals of the respective rate constants of removal, k_{12}, k_{23} and k_{34}; the interconversion of S_2 and S_3 is assumed to be rate-limited. Reproduced with permission from Lamb (1981).

Bleach-induced fluctuations in rods

A clear prediction of this model is the existence in any electrical recordings from rods of photon-like fluctuations following the presentation of bleaches. Such fluctuations have indeed been detected. A recording of toad rod current following a bleach of about 0.7% of the rhodopsin is shown in Fig. 15.5, from Lamb (1980). Prior to the bleach, in the fully dark-adapted state, the baseline was relatively quiet. When the bleaching light was delivered, the current was at first totally suppressed, and as it slowly recovered it was accompanied by greatly increased noise. This noise gradually faded away (after the end of the record illustrated) over a period of 10–20 min.

Although it is difficult to analyse non-stationary records such as these in a quantitative way, it appeared from power spectral analysis that the bleach-induced fluctuations were indistinguishable from the effects of background light (Lamb, 1980). In other words, the rod was behaving as if it was experiencing an enormously increased rate of spontaneous photon-like events, and during the course of dark-adaptation the intensity of this 'equivalent background illumination' gradually declined. Initially the rate of equivalent photon-like events in toad rods was raised to around 1–10 isomerizations s^{-1} by a bleach of about

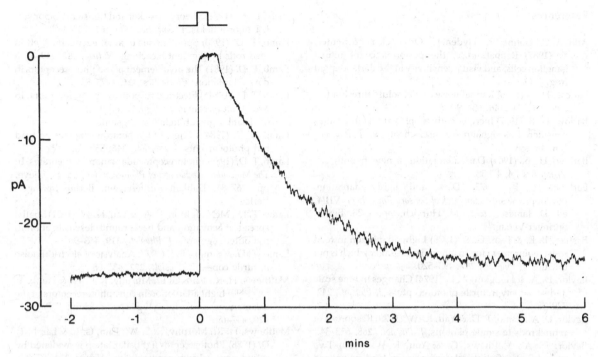

Fig. 15.5. Spontaneous photon-like fluctuations in a toad rod photoreceptor, following exposure of the rod to an intense light bleaching nearly 1% of the pigment. Initially the circulating dark current was completely suppressed, but as the current recovered it was accompanied by pronounced fluctuations. Power spectral analysis showed these fluctuations to be indistinguishable from the noise produced by the random bombardment of photons during illumination with dim light. Reproduced with permission from Lamb (1980).

1%, and the rate of events declined exponentially with a time constant of around 15 min at room temperature.

Hence these results are consistent with the idea that, following a small bleach, the toad rod outer segment experiences a greatly elevated rate of events indistinguishable from photon-events, and that slowly this event rate declines. Similar results to these have been observed in all rods in the toad retina which have been tested with bleaches in the range 0.1% to 2.5%. At higher bleach intensities the rod is, unfortunately, permanently desensitized (presumably as a result of the absence of 11-*cis* retinal) and the lowered sensitivity renders the fluctuations much smaller. This latter result seems consistent with the report that in this species (*Bufo marinus*) not more than 3% of the pigment can be regenerated in the isolated retina (Cocozza & Ostroy, 1987).

Hence, although dark-adaptation is far from being fully understood, it appears possible that it may be explained in terms of photon-like events within the rod transduction machinery, perhaps caused by reverse chemical reactions in the chain of steps which inactivate rhodopsin.

Summary

In summary, it may be said that consideration of the properties of photoreceptors is likely to be of great importance in obtaining a full explanation for the adaptational properties of the visual system. At present it seems that the desensitization of the cones by background light may play a direct role in the desensitization of the photopic system, and that although similar desensitization is observed in the large rods of lower vertebrates, this is unlikely to provide a direct explanation of scotopic light-adaptation. On the other hand dark-adaptation of the scotopic system may well be accounted for simply in terms of unavoidable photon-like events within the transduction machinery which are induced by the presence of bleaching products.

Acknowledgement

Supported by grants from the MRC, the NIH (EY-06154) and the Wellcome Trust.

References

Aho, A. C., Donner, K., Hyden, C., Orlov, O. Yu. & Reuter, T. (1987) Retinal noise, the performance of retinal ganglion cells, and visual sensitivity in the dark-adapted frog. *J. Opt. Soc. Am. A*, **4**, 2321–9.

Barlow, H. B. (1956) Retinal noise and absolute threshold. *J. Opt. Soc. Am.*, **46**, 634–9.

Barlow, H. B. (1957) Increment thresholds at low intensities considered as signal/noise discriminations. *J. Physiol.*, **136**, 469–88.

Barlow, H. B. (1964) Dark-adaptation: a new hypothesis. *Vision Res.*, **4**, 47–58.

Barlow, H. B. (1972) Dark and light adaptation: psychophysics. In *Handbook of Sensory Physiology*, **VII/4**, ed. D. Jameson & L. M. Hurvich, pp. 1–28. Berlin: Springer-Verlag.

Bastian, B. L. & Fain, G. L. (1979) Light adaptation in toad rods: requirement for an internal messenger which is not calcium. *J. Physiol.*, **297**, 493–520.

Baylor, D. A. & Hodgkin, A. L. (1974) Changes in time scale and sensitivity in turtle photoreceptors. *J. Physiol.*, **242**, 729–58.

Baylor, D. A., Lamb, T. D. & Yau, K.-W. (1979) Responses of retinal rods to single photons. *J. Physiol.*, **288**, 613–34.

Baylor, D. A., Matthews, G. & Yau, K.-W. (1980) Two components of electrical dark noise in toad retinal rod outer segments. *J. Physiol.*, **309**, 591–61.

Baylor, D. A., Nunn, B. J. & Schnapf, J. L. (1984) The photocurrent, noise and spectral sensitivity of rods of the monkey, *Macaca fascicularis*. *J. Physiol.*, **357**, 575–607.

Cocozza, J. D. & Ostroy, S. E. (1987) Factors affecting the regeneration of rhodopsin in the isolated amphibian retina. *Vision Res.*, **27**, 1085–91.

Crawford, B. H. (1937) The change of visual sensitivity with time. *Proc. Roy. Soc. Lond.*, **B123**, 68–89.

Crawford, B. H. (1947) Visual adaptation in relation to brief conditioning stimuli. *Proc. Roy. Soc. Lond.*, **B134**, 283–302.

Donner, K. O. & Hemilä, S. (1978) Excitation and adaptation in the vertebrate rod photoreceptor. *Medical Biology*, **56**, 52–63.

Fain, G. L. (1976) Sensitivity of toad rods: dependence on wavelength and background. *J. Physiol.*, **261**, 71–101.

Fain, G. L., Granda, A. M. & Maxwell, J. H. (1977) Voltage signal of photoreceptors at visual threshold. *Nature*, **265**, 181–3.

Fain, G. L., Lamb, T. D., Matthews, H. R. & Murphy, R. L. W. (1989) Cytoplasmic calcium as the messenger for light adaptation in salamander rods. *J. Physiol.*, **416**, 215–243.

Hecht, S., Haig, C. & Chase, A. M. (1937) The influence of light adaptation on the subsequent dark adaptation of the eye. *J. Gen. Physiol.*, **20**, 831–50.

Kelly, D. H. (1971) Theory of flicker and transient responses. I. Uniform fields. *J. Opt. Soc. Am.*, **61**, 537–46.

Lamb, T. D. (1980) Spontaneous quantal events induced in toad rods by pigment bleaching. *Nature*, **287**, 349–51.

Lamb, T. D. (1981) The involvement of rod photoreceptors in dark adaptation. *Vision Res.*, **21**, 1773–82.

Lamb, T. D. (1984a) Electrical response of photoreceptors. In *Recent Advances in Physiology*, **10**, ed. P. F. Baker, pp. 29–65. Edinburgh: Churchill Livingstone.

Lamb, T. D. (1984b) Effect of temperature changes on toad rod photocurrents. *J. Physiol.*, **346**, 557–78.

Lamb, T. D. (1986) Photoreceptor adaptation – vertebrates. In *The Molecular Mechanism of Photoreception*, ed. H. Stieve, pp. 267–86. Dahlem Konferenzen. Berlin: Springer-Verlag.

Lamb, T. D., McNaughton, P. A. & Yau, K.-W. (1981) Spatial spread of activation and background desensitization in rod outer segments. *J. Physiol.*, **319**, 463–96.

Lamb, T. D. & Simon, E. J. (1977) Analysis of electrical noise in turtle cones. *J. Physiol.*, **272**, 435–68.

Matthews, H. R., Fain, G. L., Murphy, R. L. W. & Lamb, T. D. (1990) Light adaptation in cone photoreceptors of the salamander: a role for cytoplasmic calcium. *J. Physiol.*, **420**, 447–69.

Matthews, H. R., Murphy, R. L. W., Fain, G. L. & Lamb, T. D. (1988) Photoreceptor light adaptation is mediated by cytoplasmic calcium concentration. *Nature*, **334**, 67–9.

Nakatani, K. & Yau, K.-W. (1988) Calcium and light adaptation in retinal rods and cones. *Nature*, **334**, 69–71.

Pugh, E. N. Jr (1975) Rushton's paradox: rod dark adaptation after flash photolysis. *J. Physiol.*, **248**, 413–31.

Pugh, E. N. Jr & Cobbs, W. H. (1986) Visual transduction in vertebrate rods and cones: a tale of two transmitters, calcium and cyclic GMP. *Vision Res.*, **26**, 1613–43.

Rushton, W. A. H. (1965) The Ferrier Lecture, 1962. Visual adaptation. *Proc. Roy. Soc. Lond.*, **B162**, 20–46.

Shapley, R. & Enroth-Cugell, C. (1984) Visual adaptation and retinal gain controls. In *Progress in Retinal Research*, **3**, ed. N. N. Osborne & G. J. Chader, pp. 263–346. Oxford: Pergamon Press.

Stiles, W. S. & Crawford, B. H. (1932) Equivalent adaptation levels in localized retinal areas. In *Report of a Joint Discussion on Vision*, pp. 194–211. Physical Society of London, Cambridge: Cambridge University Press. [Reprinted in Stiles, W. S. (1978) *Mechanisms of Colour Vision*. London: Academic Press.]

Tamura, T., Nakatani, K. & Yau, K.-W. (1989) Light adaptation in cat retinal rods. *Science*, **245**, 755–8.

Torre, V., Matthews, H. R. & Lamb, T. D. (1986) Role of calcium in regulating the cyclic GMP cascade of phototransduction in retinal rods. *Proc. Natl. Acad. Sci. USA*, **83**, 7109–13.

Trachina, D., Gordon, J. & Shapley, R. M. (1984) Retinal light-adaptation – evidence for a feedback mechanism. *Nature*, **310**, 314–16.

16

Why do we see better in bright light?

D. I. A. MacLeod, B. Chen and A. Stockman

We have recently been doing some experiments inspired by Horace Barlow's ideas about adaptation and spatial integration. But instead of looking for support for Horace's point of view, we have been hoping to displace one of his ideas by one of our own. This revisionist attitude can be justified by an argument from information theory. Barlow is almost always right, so further demonstrations of his correctness are largely redundant; to catch him out is more difficult but also in a quite objective and technical sense more informative.

It is obvious that at high levels we see textures and details that we miss when the illumination is dim: more light means better sight. This improvement could be due to any of a number of factors, but here we wish to examine one suggestion in particular: that the improvement in vision occurs because light adaptation changes the spatial organization of the retina. That some such change occurs is well documented physiologically. Neurons in the vertebrate visual system typically receive antagonistic influences from the centre and surrounding regions of their receptive fields (Barlow, 1953). Barlow, Fitzhugh & Kuffler (1957) found in cat retinal ganglion cells that light adaptation increases the prominence of the antagonistic surround relative to the centre, thereby reducing the effective size of the central summing area (or, roughly speaking, of the spatial integration region) of each cell. As Barlow (1972) has noted, the effect is rather like reducing the grain size in a photographic film. Like the photographic analog, it could provide an efficient way of regulating sensitivity, because the system would gain a useful improvement in resolution by sacrificing sensitivity that is no longer needed or even desirable. According to this scheme, then, visual sensitivity would be regulated in part through changes in spatial integration.

The psychophysical evidence for a change in spatial integration with light adaptation seems plentiful. Unlike the physiological evidence, it has tended to suggest that the adaptation dependence of spatial integration is pronounced enough to be an important factor in sensitivity regulation. We now wish to reexamine some of that evidence, and to suggest that it can and should be interpreted differently: the psychophysical evidence, we suggest, does not imply a substantial change in spatial integration with light adaptation. Psychophysically, spatial integration is measured by comparing the detection threshold intensities for large and small stimuli, for instance flashed uniform discs of large and small diameters. The state of adaptation can be varied by presenting these test flashes against backgrounds of various intensities. For both small and large test flashes, the threshold intensity increases as background intensity increases, but the rate of increase depends strongly on test flash size. This is illustrated by the two idealized continuous curves in Fig. 16.1 (where test flash intensity is plotted against background intensity in logarithmic coordinates). In this figure, the curve for a large test field reaches unity slope, reflecting the proportional relationship between test flash threshold intensity and background intensity embodied in Weber's Law ($\Delta I/I = constant$); but the slope for the small field is shallower, implying a shortfall from Weber's Law. At low background levels the threshold for seeing the large test flash is much lower than for the small one. This difference is a result of spatial integration: instead of treating local responses from nearby retinal points independently, the visual system adds them together within the central summing area or integration area of each retinal ganglion cell. Roughly speaking, detection requires that the total effect of the responses summed within that area must exceed some criterion.

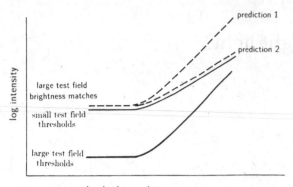

Fig. 16.1. Brightness matches predicted by the spatial integration hypothesis (prediction 1) and the adaptation-dependent nonlinearity hypothesis (prediction 2) (see text for details).

Consequently, as the size of the test flash increases and covers more of the integration area, the threshold intensity falls, until the test flash becomes large enough to cover fully (or extend beyond) the integration area. For large test flashes that completely cover the integration area, decreasing the integration area will make the threshold higher; but for small flashes that fall well inside the integration area, decreasing the area will have little or no effect on threshold. The size of the spatial integration area is accordingly related to the ratio of the threshold intensities for very small and very large flashes, and thus to the vertical separation between the two continuous curves in the log–log plot of Fig. 16.1. For higher background levels (the light adapted case) these curves converge (Barlow, 1958a,b). This increase in relative threshold for the large test flash is usually taken to mean that the area of spatial integration has become smaller in the light adapted case.

We now want to question that interpretation, and to suggest that the converging threshold-versus-background intensity curves (t.v.i. curves) may arise in a quite different way, without any change of spatial integration.

The alternative interpretation is as follows. Consider a single point on the retina, positioned within the boundaries of both the small and the large test flash. At threshold, that point will receive a much greater intensity (or more technically, a much higher retinal irradiance, or radiant flux per unit retinal area) from the small test flash than from the large one. This constitutes a purely local difference between the small and large test flash situations. The local response to the test flash will be greater in the case of the small

flash, simply because of its greater intensity. We can explain the converging t.v.i. curves in terms of purely local processes if we postulate that strong local responses are less affected by background adaptation than weak ones. To put it more precisely, we might suppose that when background illumination drives up the test intensity to evoke a criterion local response, it does so by a smaller factor when the criterion local response is strong (as at small flash threshold) than when it is weak (as at large flash threshold). This would lead to convergence of the t.v.i. curves even if there is no change in spatial integration at all. The postulate is supported by some experiments of Whittle & Challands (1969), who measured the effect of background illumination on sensitivity to *large* test flashes of a range of intensities. They measured the large flash t.v.i. curve, finding it to have the same steeply rising form as shown in Fig. 16.1, but in addition to this they measured the effect of backgrounds on the visual effectiveness of more intense (suprathreshold) test flashes. Instead of setting these flashes to threshold, their subjects adjusted the flash intensity to achieve a criterion subjective brightness. Whittle & Challands determined the test flash intensities required to match a suprathreshold standard flash, when the standard was presented to one eye under fixed adaptation conditions and the variable test flash was presented against a range of background intensities in the other eye. The resulting 'constant brightness curve', representing the test flash intensity required to match the standard as a function of the background intensity, looks (for sufficiently high test intensities) very much like the t.v.i. curve for a small test flash, even though Whittle & Challands used large test stimuli. Yet the constant brightness curve for near-threshold test intensities has a steep slope like the t.v.i. curve for a large test flash. In short, the constant brightness curves for bright and for dim large flashes converge in much the same way as the t.v.i. curves for small and large diameter flashes – just what would be expected if the effects of adaptation depend on the magnitude of the local response to the test flash and not on its size.

If backgrounds do reduce sensitivity by a smaller factor for bright tests than for dim, it follows that the function relating local response to the log of test intensity must be steeper in the light adapted case. There is some evidence for this from physiological experiments, for instance in photoreceptor recordings from insects (Matic & Laughlin, 1981) and primates (Boynton & Whitten, 1970). In our experiments we ask whether the adaptation-dependent nonlinearity suggested by these results and by those of Whittle &

Challands can account for the converging t.v.i. curves without any change of spatial integration.

To test this hypothesis, we compare small and large test field threshold-versus-intensity curves and large test field constant brightness curves. The brightness-matching standard was chosen so that at low background intensities the intensity of the large field required to match it was the same as the threshold intensity of the small field. Thus at low background intensities the local response elicited by the two fields should be the same in both the small flash threshold and the large flash brightness-matching experiments. Now if there is a reduction in spatial integration with increasing background intensity, the large field brightness matching intensities should rise more steeply than the small field threshold intensities. In fact, a pure spatial integration hypothesis predicts that the brightness matching function and the large test field t.v.i. function should be similar in shape, since the test fields used in the two types of measurements are of the same size. This is prediction 1 in Fig. 16.1. However, the response-intensity nonlinearity hypothesis predicts that on increasing the background intensity the small field threshold intensities and the brightness matching intensities should both increase but remain the same as each other (prediction 2, Fig. 16.1).

To make the brightness matches we followed Whittle & Challands in using a display as shown in Fig. 16.2B where the left eye and right eye are stimulated by independently controlled large circular steady backgrounds. These backgrounds were geometrically similar, and they were subjectively in register in the fused binocular field. The stimuli appeared to the subject as shown on the right of the figure: the two flashes to be compared were both seen against a single binocularly fused background. The test flash was made up of two half fields: the intensity of the upper half field – presented to the right eye – could be varied by the subject, while the intensity of the left field – presented to the left eye – was fixed as a standard for brightness matching. The intensity of the upper half field was chosen by the observer to make the fused half circles appear uniform in brightness. The square in Fig. 16.2B is just a finely outlined frame to help maintain binocular fusion and accommodation. All this was done for a range of different background intensities in the right eye, to generate a constant brightness curve in the manner of Whittle & Challands.

For the threshold measurements we presented small or large flashes to the right eye alone, varying the background intensity as before and having the

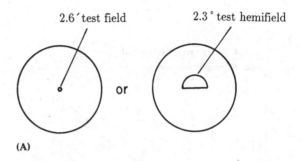

(A)

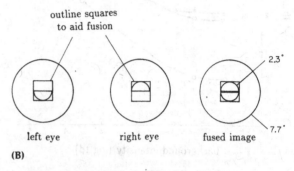

(B)

Fig. 16.2. (A) Subject's field of view in the incremental threshold experiments (right eye). (B) Subject's field of view in the brightness matching experiments (dichoptic).

observer set a threshold by varying the test flash intensity. The large flash was simply the upper half of the test field used for brightness matching. The small flash was a small circular field (see Fig. 16.2A).

We ran these experiments in two different ways with different choices of the colour of the test flashes and background. We used either red flashes on a green background to confine the test response to a single cone type, or else white flashes on a white background. Test durations were 20 ms or 150 ms, too short for major eye movements during the test exposure. Only the 20 ms red on green results are reported here but the white on white results and the 150 ms results are similar (Chen, MacLeod & Stockman, 1987).

In Figs. 16.3A and B the incremental thresholds and equal brightness matches are plotted as a function of background intensity. The large open circles are large (2.3°) test field incremental thresholds, the filled small circles are small (2.6′) test field incremental thresholds and the open and filled triangles are 2.3° brightness matches. For the brightness matches, the standard test field presented to the observer's left eye had an intensity approximately equal to that of the test

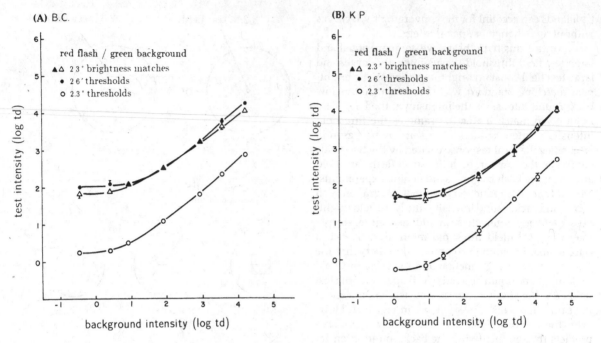

Fig. 16.3. Incremental thresholds and brightness matches plotted as a function of background intensity. The intensities are plotted in log trolands (log td). The test stimulus was a red flash (Wratten no. 25), which was superimposed on a green background (541 nm interference filter). Error bars are ±one S.E.M. based on intersession variation, from at least three sessions, and when not shown they are smaller than the heights of the symbols. (A) Subject B.C. (B) Subject K.P.

field corresponding to the left-most data point of the brightness matching curve. Each data point is the mean of three or four experimental sessions representing a total of 150–200 judgements. The error bars indicate ±1 standard deviation between sessions. Figures 16.3A and B show results for subjects B.C. and K.P. obtained for a 20 ms red test field superimposed on a green background.

Clearly the large field constant brightness curves are similar in shape to the small test flash t.v.i. curves, both being noticeably shallower than the large test flash t.v.i. curves. This agrees with the predictions of the adaptation-dependent nonlinearity hypothesis; the agreement suggests that all or almost all of the difference in shape between the t.v.i. curves can be accounted for on this basis, leaving little or nothing left over to be explained by adaptive changes in spatial integration. As we point out elsewhere (Chen, MacLeod & Stockman, 1987), the small and large test t.v.i. curves of Fig. 16.3 are closer to parallelism than classical idealizations of such data had led us to expect. Instead of an asymptotic slope of 0.5 (thresholds proportional to the square root of the background intensity) our small flash thresholds fall only a little

short of the proportional relationship asserted by Weber's Law, with asymptotic slopes of about 0.8. Nevertheless the convergence of the small and large flash threshold curves is enough to imply a roughly fourfold reduction of integration area, if adaptation-dependent nonlinearity were not considered. But once this nonlinearity is taken into account, the reduction implied by our data is between 0 and at most 29% in area, or 15% in diameter (Chen, MacLeod & Stockman, 1987).

Now there is, as we have noted, good physiological evidence that centre–surround antagonism increases with increasing light adaptation, and this must to some extent decrease the size of the central summing area for the cell. However, analysis reveals that if we define an integration area for the cell by the ratio of its sensitivity for a field of optimal size to its sensitivity for a very small centred field, the change in this area resulting from the loss of the antagonistic surround would be much too small to account for the observed differences between small and large test field t.v.i. functions. Assuming: (i) that the ratio of centre and surround diameters is 1:3 (Hayhoe, 1979; Spillmann, Ransom-Hogg & Oehler, 1987); (ii) that the sensitivity profiles of the centre and surround are Gaussian functions; and (iii) that the sensitivity of the surround for a uniform stimulus is negligible in the dark adapted eye, but becomes as great as that of the centre under light adaptation, so that the integrated sensitivities are equal, we calculate that the change in integration area, in this sense, is no more than 19% and the change in diameter is less than 10% (Chen, MacLeod & Stockman, 1987). Such a small change could be functionally important in some contexts but is insufficient either to account for the converging t.v.i. curves or to generate a clear violation of prediction 2 in Fig. 16.1.

These results lead to a view of the adaptation process in which the enhanced visibility of small test objects or fine detail in bright light is almost entirely due to strictly local processes. The jurisdiction of Weber's Law is limited to cases where the test stimulus is sufficiently weak in its local effects. To the extent that Weber's Law does hold, better vision in bright light is not to be expected: changes in illumination are exactly compensated by a reciprocal adjustment in sensitivity, making the signals independent of illumination[1]. But with small or finely detailed test objects,

Weber's Law fails, because the threshold is high enough for adaptation-dependent nonlinearity to become relevant. Then the change of sensitivity with adaptation is less than given by Weber's Law, and less than would be needed to compensate for a change in light level. In this way, more light can lead to enhanced visibility, even without any change of spatial organization. In short, we see better in bright light not because the grain of the neural response is finer, but because the signals are bigger.

Acknowledgements

This work was supported by NIH Grant EY01711 and by a NATO Postdoctoral Fellowship awarded to A. Stockman. We thank Drs J. B. Mulligan, L. T. Sharpe, H. B. Barlow, C. Enroth-Cugell and P. Whittle for help and advice on an earlier manuscript about this work.

[1] The noise or variability contaminating the signal may also be roughly independent of illumination (Barlow & Levick, 1969). This is our justification for discussing visibility as if it depended on signal strength, rather than signal/noise ratio: with constant noise the two formulations are indistinguishable.

References

Barlow, H. B. (1953) Summation and inhibition in the frog's retina. *J. Physiol.*, **119**, 69–88.

Barlow, H. B. (1958a) Temporal and spatial summation in human vision at different background intensities. *J. Physiol.*, **141**, 337–50.

Barlow, H. B. (1958b) Intrinsic noise of cones. In *Visual Problems of Colour*, Volume 2, pp. 617–30. London: HMSO.

Barlow, H. B. (1972) Dark and light adaptation: psychophysics. In *Handbook of Sensory Physiology*, vol. VII/4, pp. 1–28. Berlin: Springer-Verlag.

Barlow, H. B., Fitzhugh, R. & Kuffler, S. W. (1957) Change of organization in the receptive fields of the cat's retina during dark adaptation. *J. Physiol.*, **137**, 338–54.

Barlow, H. B. & Levick, W. R. (1969) Coding of light intensity by the cat retina. *Rendiconti della Scuola Internazionale di Fisica 'Enrico Fermi'*. XLIII Corso, pp. 385–96. London: Academic Press.

Boynton, R. M. & Whitten, D. N. (1970) Visual adaptation in monkey cones: recordings of late receptor potentials. *Science*, **170**, 1423–6.

Chen, B., MacLeod, D. I. A. & Stockman, A. (1987) Improvement in human vision under bright light: grain or gain? *J. Physiol.*, **394**, 41–66.

Hayhoe, M. M. (1979) After-effects of small adapting fields. *J. Physiol.*, **296**, 141–58.

Matic, T. & Laughlin, S. B. (1981) Changes in the intensity-response function of an insect's photoreceptors due to light adaptation. *J. Comp. Physiol.*, **145**, 169–77.

Spillmann, L., Ransom-Hogg, A. & Oehler, R. (1987) A comparison of perceptive and receptive fields in man and monkey. *Human Neurobiol.*, **6**, 51–62.

Whittle, D. & Challands, P. D. C. (1969) The effect of background luminance on the brightness of flashes. *Vision Res.*, **9**, 1095–110.

Postscript by H. B. Barlow

This chapter elegantly demonstrates that decrease of grain size is a poor analogy of the changes that occur in light adaptation and I retract it without reservation. Nonetheless, changes in spatial organisation at the retinal level may still be responsible for the improvements in vision, and specifically this reorganisation may steepen the incremental luminance/response function in the way that their results require.

At low luminance levels good summation occurs beyond the Ricco limit of complete summation measured at high backgrounds. This probably reflects the fact that, because they lack an inhibitory surround, retinal ganglion cells are efficient transducers of uniformly distributed luminance changes, so at higher levels in the visual pathway good summation of information from many ganglion cells is possible. When the inhibitory surround becomes effective at high backgrounds the ganglion cells no longer respond well to large spots, so such summation is no longer possible, and the summation area, defined by the ratio of large spot to small spot threshold, is decreased. But as Levick and I suggested (*J. Physiol.*, **259**, 737–57, 1976), the main benefit of increased lateral inhibition may be to steepen the response to increments of light at the centre of the receptive field. Brightness matching at high luminance (but not at low) must depend upon the responses of the ganglion cells lying at the border between the two hemifields, and their response functions will benefit from this steepening because an increment applied to one half field will not cover the whole surround.

It would be interesting to see if brightness matching of two separated Gaussian patches followed prediction 1 or prediction 2 in Fig. 16.1.

17

Mechanisms for coding luminance patterns: are they really linear?

A. M. Derrington

Overview

One of the most powerful ideas in vision research in the last two decades has been the notion that luminance patterns are detected by independent linear mechanisms, which are selective for spatial frequency and orientation. This idea is consistent with psychophysical results from masking, sub-threshold summation, and adaptation studies. Moreover, physiological work on the striate cortex shows that simple cells are both linear, and selective for spatial frequency (Movshon *et al.*, 1978) and orientation, making them a potential neural substrate for the detection mechanisms.

There are however some masking results which suggest that, even at modest contrasts, non-linearities may affect the mechanisms detecting luminance patterns.

The aim of this chapter is to present some physiological work which shows that non-linearities do indeed occur early in the visual pathway. A second aim is to show how it might be possible to remove the effects of these early non-linearities by cortical processing.

The chapter falls into four parts. The first part covers the background, describing some of the relevant psychophysical results. The second part describes the non-linear responses of X-cells in the lateral geniculate nucleus of the cat. The third part shows how the non-linear responses could be removed, to make linear receptive fields, like those of cortical simple cells. The final part discusses the implications and raises some unresolved issues.

Evidence for linear, spatial frequency-selective mechanisms

General

One key property of a linear mechanism is that it responds to a sinusoidal input with a sinusoidal output of the same frequency. Its response may differ in amplitude and phase from the input, but it will still be a sinusoid of the same frequency. Moreover, the response to the sum of any number of inputs will be equal to the sum of the responses obtained when each input is presented individually. These two properties have made it possible to investigate the mechanisms of the visual system by simple psychophysical tests which measure interactions between different stimuli. It is the absence of interactions between patterns of different spatial frequencies which leads to the conclusion that the mechanisms which detect spatial patterns are linear and selective for spatial frequency.

There are three kinds of observation on which our current concept of spatial frequency-selective pattern-detection mechanisms is based: adaptation, sub-threshold summation, and masking (see Braddick *et al.*, 1978 for a review). They are all of the same general type: they show that two one-dimensional patterns of the same orientation do not interact with one another inside the visual system unless they have similar spatial frequency.

Adaptation

Perhaps the easiest form of interaction to understand is adaptation or habituation. A subject is first made to view a high contrast pattern, such as a sinusoidal grating, for several seconds (or even minutes), and then his sensitivity to other similar patterns is measured. Blakemore & Campbell (1969) used this technique to show that after adaptation to a sinusoidal grating of one spatial frequency, sensitivity to gratings of similar spatial frequency was depressed, but sensitivity to gratings of very different spatial frequency was unimpaired. This result suggests two things. First, the reduction in sensitivity suggests that the mechanisms which detect sinusoidal gratings are made less sensitive by exposure to a high contrast grating. Second, and much more exciting, the fact that the sensitivity reduction is selective, and only affects spatial frequencies close to that used for adaptation, suggests that each such mechanism is only sensitive to a narrow range of spatial frequencies. However although this experiment provides one of the clearest demonstrations of the existence of spatial frequency selective detection mechanisms, the adaptation technique is so time consuming that it is rarely, if ever, used in conjunction with objective measurements of sensitivity.

Sub-threshold summation

Sub-threshold summation occurs if two patterns, each of which is undetectable, are detectable when added together. The existence of sub-threshold summation between two patterns indicates that they are detected by the same mechanism. If two sinusoidal gratings have similar spatial frequency then sub-threshold summation occurs (Sachs, Nachmias & Robson, 1971), if their spatial frequencies are well separated it does not. Unfortunately the magnitude of sub-threshold summation effects is limited, and great care is necessary to distinguish between changes in sensitivity, and probability effects, which occur when two independently detectable stimuli are presented together.

Masking

In adaptation the reduction in sensitivity is measured after the adaptation stimulus has been removed. In masking the approach is similar except that the high contrast pattern, which causes the reduction in sensitivity, is presented simultaneously with the pattern to which sensitivity is being measured. Masking has two advantages over adaptation. First, it is much quicker, because no pre-exposure to the masking pattern is given, this means that it can conveniently be used in conjunction with objective measurement of sensitivity. Secondly, larger reductions in sensitivity can be obtained. This allows the use of noise masks to measure the spatial frequency tuning of detectors (Henning, Hertz & Hinton, 1981). However it is a masking experiment which raises the possibility that a significant non-linearity may precede the linear spatial frequency-selective mechanisms whose existence is implied by masking, adaptation and sub-threshold summation experiments.

Evidence for non-linearity

Psychophysical evidence

The possibility that even relatively low contrast stimuli might be summed non-linearly was raised by an experiment using a pattern like that illustrated in Fig. 17.1B, an amplitude-modulated (AM) grating. This pattern consists of a high spatial frequency grating whose contrast varies as a sinusoidal function of position. Thus its luminance profile (L_x) can be represented descriptively, as the product of a modulating waveform, of low spatial frequency, and a high frequency carrier,

$$L_x = L_a[1 + C\sin(2\pi f_c x) \{1 + M\cos(2\pi f_m x)\}]. \quad (1)$$

L_a is the space-average mean luminance, C is the contrast, M is the modulation depth (M has a value of 1 in Fig. 17.1B), f_c is the carrier frequency, and f_m is the modulation frequency.

The interesting property of this waveform is that although it is periodic at the modulation frequency, all its components are close to the carrier frequency. This is easier to see if we express equation 1 so that it represents the pattern in terms of its frequency components:

$$L_x = L_a[1 + 0.5CM\sin(2\pi\{f_c - f_m\}x) + C\sin(2\pi f_c x) + 0.5CM\sin(2\pi\{f_c + f_m\}x)]. \quad (2)$$

There are three components, the carrier, which has frequency f_c, and two sidebands which have spatial frequencies $f_c + f_m$ and $f_c - f_m$. When, as in Fig. 17.1, the carrier frequency is high, and the modulation frequency is low, the three frequency components are all much higher than the modulation frequency. Thus a pattern like this should not mask a grating of the modulation frequency. However Henning et al. (1975) observed substantial masking between a high spatial frequency grating, amplitude-modulated at a low spatial frequency, and a grating of the modulation frequency.

The results of a similar experiment, which simply repeats one of Henning et al.'s observations using moving instead of stationary gratings, are shown in Fig. 17.2. Each curve shows detection performance as a function of contrast, in a task where the pattern to be detected (the signal) was a low spatial frequency grating presented either alone (open circles), or added to a high frequency mask whose amplitude was either uniform (filled circles), or modulated at the spatial frequency of the signal

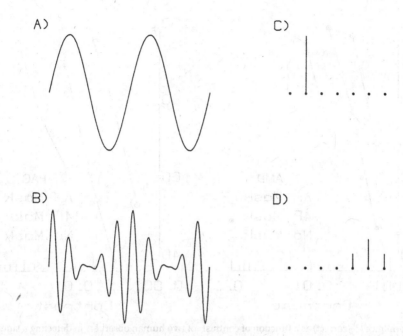

Fig. 17.1. Luminance profiles (A & B) and spatial frequency spectra (C & D) of two stimuli which have the same period, but which have no spatial-frequency components in common. The luminance profiles show luminance (on an arbitrary scale) as a function of spatial position over two periods of each pattern. Each dot in the spatial frequency spectrum represents the position of one spatial frequency component, ranging from zero to the 6th harmonic (F_6) in steps of F_1. The length and the direction of the line at each frequency position represent the amplitude and the phase of the corresponding frequency component. (A) shows the luminance profile of a single sinusoid; (C) shows its spectrum, which contains only a single spatial frequency component. (B) shows the profile of a high frequency sinusoid which is sinusoidally modulated in amplitude at a low frequency; (D) shows the spectrum of (B), which contains components at F_4, F_5 and F_6.

(diamonds). The uniform high-frequency grating produces a modest masking effect, but the amplitude-modulated 10 c/deg grating produces a much larger effect: somewhere between four and eight times as much contrast is needed to detect the signal when this pattern is also present. This is a puzzling observation, because the mechanism most sensitive to the stimulus being detected should be very insensitive to the components of the amplitude modulated mask, as they are of much higher spatial frequency.

However, if some stage of the visual system *preceding* the spatial frequency selective mechanisms, whose existence (and linearity) is suggested by the results described in the preceding section, were non-linear, then we might expect extra frequency components to be generated. These would then form part of the stimulus reaching the array of detection mechanisms, and might conceivably cause the AM grating to stimulate the detectors which are most sensitive to the modulation frequency. One commonly considered form of non-linearity is a stimulus

intensity/response function which, instead of being represented by a linear equation

$$R_i = Ki, \tag{3}$$

is represented by a polynomial

$$R_i = K_1 i + K_2 i^2 + K_3 i^3 \ldots \tag{4}$$

This covers a wide range of non-linearities, including a logarithmic transformation (a logarithmic transformation is often put forward as an explanation of other sensory effects). The effect of the non-linearity can be demonstrated by substituting the equation for the amplitude-modulated grating into equation 4. All of the terms in equation 4 after the first will generate extra components (distortion products), however, as n increases the value of K_n tends to decrease (as also does i^n for our stimuli), so we shall only consider the first non-linear (quadratic) term. We get three new spatial frequency components from the quadratic term; these are at frequencies 0, $2f_m$, and f_m. The component at f_m might well account for the masking,

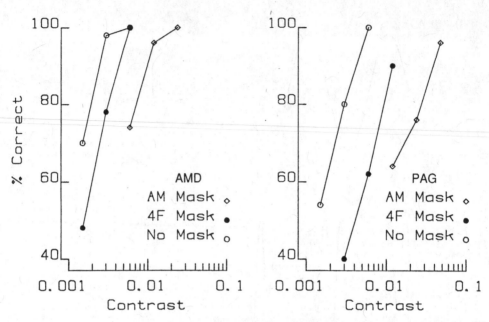

Fig. 17.2. Performance (% correct) as a function of contrast, of two human observers in detecting a sinusoidal grating of spatial frequency 2 c/deg, in a 2 temporal alternative forced choice task. The pattern was presented either alone (open circles), added to a 10 c/deg grating of 25% contrast, which was amplitude-modulated (modulation depth 100%) at 2 c/deg (open diamonds), or added to an 8 c/deg grating of 12.5% contrast (filled circles). All patterns were presented moving at 0.5 deg/s.

since it has the same spatial frequency as the signal, and will therefore activate the same set of spatial frequency-selective detectors.

Physiological distortion products

If the finding that an amplitude-modulated grating masks a grating of its modulation frequency is to be explained by distortion products, as outlined above, then we should expect to observe distortion products in the responses of X-cells in the lateral geniculate nucleus (LGN) of the cat. These are the cells which provide the input for the simple cells in striate cortex, which are the best candidate for a physiological counterpart to the spatial frequency-selective detectors inferred from psychophysical work.

Distortion products, whose amplitudes and phases vary in a way consistent with their being generated by a quadratic non-linearity have been observed in the responses of X-cells (Derrington, 1987). Figure 17.3 shows histograms of the average responses (firing frequency in Spikes/s as a function of time) of an off-centre X-cell to a sinusoidal grating of 0.14 c/deg (A) and to a grating of 0.71 c/deg whose amplitude was sinusoidally modulated at 0.14 c/deg (B). Both patterns were moved across the receptive field at the same velocity, 6.9 deg/s, which meant that 0.98 periods of the pattern crossed the receptive field

every second. Panels C and D show the amplitudes and phases of the modulation components in histograms A and B respectively.

If the mechanisms generating the response of the cell were linear, the histograms should contain modulation components only at those frequencies which correspond to components in the stimulus (illustrated in Fig. 17.1). Although it is true that the largest modulation components in the two responses (F_1 in C and F_4, F_5, and F_6 in D) do in fact correspond to the components in the stimulus, it is clear that there are other components of comparable size. In particular D shows a large component at the modulation frequency F_1; the AM grating contains no component at this frequency.

The simplest possible way of generating a distortion product would be to suppose that the summation processes of the cell act linearly, as in equation 1, and that the non-linearity occurs in the process of generating the response. Thus the actual response R is given by

$$R = K_1 R_i + K_2 R_i^2. \qquad (5)$$

Equation 5 allows us to predict the phase of the F_1 distortion product from the amplitudes and phases of the linear components of the response. Figure 17.4A shows the accuracy of such predictions for the respon-

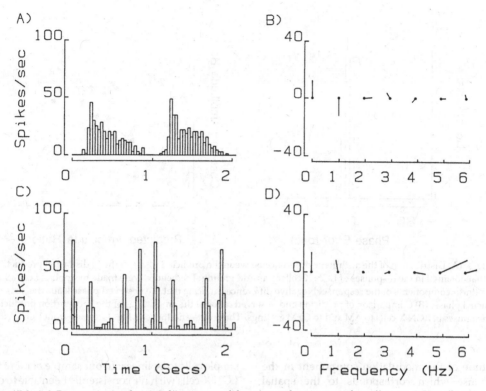

Fig. 17.3. A & B are peri-stimulus time histograms of the averaged responses of an off-centre LGN cell to 20 presentations of a grating moving at 6.9 deg/s. The luminance profiles were: (A) a sinusoid of contrast 0.25, and spatial frequency 0.14 c/deg; (B) an amplitude-modulated (modulation depth 100%; modulation frequency 0.14 c/deg) sinusoid of mean contrast 0.25 and spatial frequency 0.71 c/deg. The binwidth is 32 ms.

C & D show the amplitudes and relative phases of the modulation components in the histograms; C shows those of A, and D shows those of B. The components shown in C and D are zero frequency, 0.98 Hz (the temporal frequency of the grating of 0.14 c/deg), and each of its harmonics up to the 6th. The phases have been normalised by setting the response to the fundamental in C to be 180 degrees away from its phase in the pattern, and shifting all other phases by a corresponding amount (i.e. by scaling the phase shift in proportion to frequency). The length of the line representing each component gives its magnitude (according to the y axis scale), and the direction gives its phase. Note that C contains some amplitude at most harmonics, and that D contains significant responses at the 4th, 5th and 6th harmonics, and also at the fundamental.

ses of 20 LGN X-cells to an amplitude-modulated grating. It shows a frequency distribution histogram of the difference between the observed phase of the F_1 distortion product and the phase predicted from equation 5. In all cases the error in the prediction is less than 20 degrees. The distribution is somewhat skewed, indicating a slight tendency for the observed phase to lead the predicted phase.

The magnitude of the distortion product at F_1 cannot be predicted from the response to a single stimulus, because we need to know the value of K_2/K_1 in equation 5. However we can predict the ratios of the amplitudes of the F_1 distortion products in the responses to two different stimuli, which contain the same spatial frequency components with different phases.

Figure 17.4B shows such a comparison of observed and predicted ratios. The two stimuli were an amplitude-modulated grating, like that shown in Fig. 17.1, and a quasi-frequency modulated grating, which contains the same components but with different relative phases. The agreement between observed and predicted ratios is extremely good, all points fall close to the dashed line which indicates perfect agreement.

Masking by physiological distortion products
Having found that the response of an X-cell to an amplitude-modulated grating contains a component at the modulation frequency, it becomes interesting to look for masking between these stimuli. We can do this easily by using moving gratings, and measuring

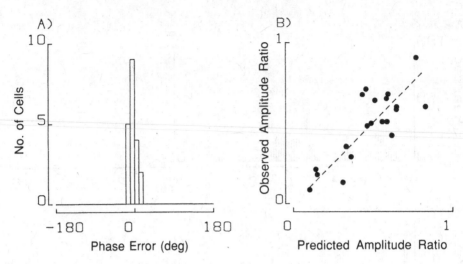

Fig. 17.4. (A) Distribution of the arithmetic difference between the predicted phase of the F_1 distortion product, and that obtained in the responses of LGN X-cells to an AM grating. Predictions were made by applying equation 5 to the linear components of the response. Negative differences indicate that the observed phase leads the predicted phase. (B) Comparison of predicted and observed ratios of the amplitudes of the F_1 distortion products in the responses of LGN X-cells to AM and to QFM gratings. These data and those of Fig. 17.4A are from Derrington, 1987.

the amplitude of the modulation component in the cell's response which corresponds to the spatial frequency component we are trying to detect.

Figure 17.5 shows the results of a detection experiment in which we used the amplitude of the 0.98 Hz modulation-component in an X-cell's response, to detect the presence of a moving sinusoidal grating of frequency 0.14 c/deg, moving at 6.9 deg/s (i.e. so that it generated a modulation in the cell's firing rate at 0.98 Hz). The test pattern was presented either alone (open circles), added to a 0.71 c/deg masking grating (filled circles), or added to a 0.71 c/deg masking grating whose amplitude was modulated at 0.14 c/deg. In each case, performance improves with the contrast of the 0.14 c/deg grating. However, in the presence of either mask, a higher contrast is required to support a given level of performance. As in the psychophysical experiment, the results of which were shown in Fig. 17.2, the modulated masking grating has a much larger effect. This extra masking is presumably attributable to the distortion product (the cell is the same one that provided data for Fig. 17.3).

Can we restore linearity?

Do we need to?
Our results imply that the X-cell input to the striate cortex is non-linear, yet work on striate cortex shows

simple cells to be linear. In our sample of more than 30 LGN X-cells we have consistently been able to observe distortion products in the responses to amplitude-modulated gratings. The few cases where we have failed are almost certainly attributable to our having inadvertently made the wrong choice of stimulus parameters, and then having lost the cell before we could try more appropriate parameters. Thus we can, with a fair degree of confidence, exclude the possibility that there is a sub-set of linear neurons providing input to the striate cortex. This may tempt us to wonder how it might be possible to generate linear psychophysical mechanisms, or to account for the observed linearity of cortical receptive fields.

We cannot simply dismiss the possibility that linear cortical mechanisms might exist: Albrecht & DeValois (1981) recorded the responses of cortical neurons to AM gratings and to gratings of the modulation frequency. They failed to find any examples of neurons which responded both to an amplitude-modulated grating (in which, as in our experiment, the modulation frequency was $\frac{1}{5}$ of the carrier frequency) and also to a grating of the modulation frequency. Thus it seems that the distortion products which we observe in the LGN have somehow been removed, without affecting the (apparently indistinguishable) response to a grating of the modulation frequency.

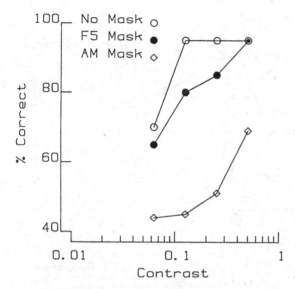

Fig. 17.5. Performance as a function of contrast in an experiment using the responses of a single cell (that which provided the data for Fig. 17.3) to detect a grating of 0.14 c/deg moving at 6.9 deg/s. The grating was presented either alone (open circles), or added to a grating of spatial frequency 0.71 c/deg and 25% contrast which was either uniform (filled circles) or sinusoidally modulated in amplitude (diamonds). Modulation frequency was 0.14 c/deg, modulation depth was 100%. Performance was calculated by measuring the area of ROC curves constructed using the amplitude of the modulation in firing rate at 0.98 Hz as decision variable. Circles are based on 20 presentations; diamonds are the means of four sets of 20 presentations at each of four phases (F_1 phase = 0, 90, 180 or 270 degrees).

A possible mathematical solution

Careful analysis of equation 5 suggests that combining the responses of on-centre and off-centre neurons might provide a relatively simple method for distinguishing between responses that arise as distortion products and those that arise through linear mechanisms. It should be possible to remove the distortion products simply by subtracting the responses of on-centre and off-centre neurons which have superimposed receptive fields. This is possible because the linear part of the response of an on-centre neuron is identical to that of an off-centre neuron except for the sign. Thus

$$R_{on} = -R_{off}, \qquad (6)$$

so if we arrange that our hypothetical cortical neuron receives excitatory input from an on-centre neuron and inhibitory input from an off-centre neuron with a superimposed receptive field, equation 5 gives the response

$$R_{ctx} = W_{on}(K_{1on}R_{on} + K_{2on}R^2_{on}) - W_{off}(K_{1off}R_{off} + K_{2off}R^2_{off}), \qquad (7)$$

where R_{ctx} is the response of our hypothetical cortical subunit, and W_{on} and W_{off} are simply the weights given by the cortical cell to the inputs from the on- and off-centre neurons. We can simplify this by setting the ratio of the weights to give

$$W_{off} K_{2off} = W_{on} K_{2on}, \qquad (8)$$

and by substituting from equation 6 to get

$$R_{ctx} = W_{on} K_{1on} R_{on} + W_{off} K_{1off} R_{on}. \qquad (9)$$

Thus, by the simple process of matching the excitatory input from each on-centre cell with an inhibitory input from an off-centre cell with its receptive field in the same place, the distortion products can be made to cancel, while the linear parts of the responses reinforce each other. Of course this process will not remove cubic distortion products (those generated by a possible R_i^3 term added to equation 5), but these are likely to be much smaller.

A simulation

For those readers who are not completely convinced by this simple mathematical argument, we can simulate the process using real data from LGN cells. We were fortunate enough to record successively the responses of an on-centre X-cell and an off-centre X-cell in the same LGN lamina to the same pair of patterns, a grating of high spatial frequency, amplitude-modulated at a low spatial frequency, and a grating of the modulation frequency. The left-hand column of Fig. 17.6 illustrates the spatial frequency spectra of these patterns: the AM grating has three components, at F_4, F_5 and F_6, the low frequency grating has a single component at F_1.

The middle column of Fig. 17.6 shows the first six modulation components in the responses of the two geniculate neurons to these patterns. For both cells, the response to the AM grating contains a substantial component at the modulation frequency F_1, in addition to the components which correspond to the stimulus, at F_4, F_5 and F_6. The responses to the low frequency grating contain a larger component at F_1, which is of course the frequency which corresponds to the single component in this stimulus. It is the aim of our hypothetical processing scheme to preserve the linear F_1 response in E and F, while removing the one which occurs as a distortion product in C and D.

For clarity, we have altered the phases of all the

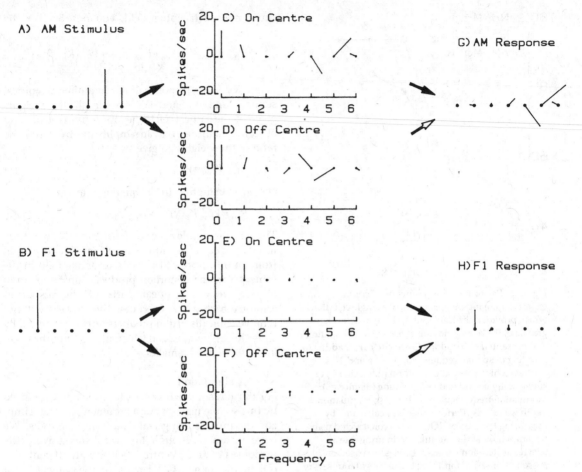

Fig. 17.6. Combining the responses of an on-centre and an off-centre neuron to remove the distortion product in the response to an AM grating. A and B show the spectra of the stimuli, an AM grating (A) and a single sinusoid (B), displayed using the same conventions as Fig. 17.1. C and D show the first six harmonic components in the responses of an on-centre (C) and an off-centre (D) LGN cell, to the AM grating; both responses show a prominent component at F_1. E and F show on-centre (E) and off-centre (F) cells' responses to the single sinusoid. G shows the response of our hypothetical linear cortical input subunit to the AM grating; it was generated by subtracting D from C. Note that the linear components of the response have reinforced one another whereas the F_1 distortion products have almost completely cancelled. H shows the response to a simple sinusoid, generated by subtracting F from E; the linear responses at F_1 have reinforced one another.

responses of each neuron in a manner equivalent to sliding the receptive fields in space so that they are *exactly* superimposed. As a result of this manipulation the linear responses to F_1 are in opposite phase, the on-centre neuron's response being positive, the off-centre neuron's response being negative. Note that this manipulation also causes the on-centre and off-centre neurons' responses to each of the higher frequency components in the AM grating to be in opposite phases.

The right-hand column of Fig. 17.6 shows the

responses of our hypothetical cortical input sub-unit, generated by subtracting the off-centre cell's response to each stimulus from the on-centre cell's response to the same stimulus. Thus G is generated by subtracting D from C, and H is generated by subtracting F from E.

The F_1 distortion product in the response to the AM grating has almost completely vanished, whereas the linear components of the responses to both stimuli have summed almost perfectly. It is important to stress that this dramatic restoration of linearity was produced simply by subtracting the response of the off-centre LGN cell from those of the on-centre LGN cell, and that attempting the same trick with a pair of cells with receptive fields of the same polarity would reduce both the distortion product and the linear response to F_1. This indicates a significant advantage of having separate on-centre and off-centre systems transmitting information about the same pattern.

Discussion

It seems clear that the X-cells, which are generally assumed to be the main input to the cortex for signals about spatial patterns, are non-linear in their responses. This non-linear behaviour of LGN cells provides us with a potential explanation of the masking interactions between AM gratings and gratings of the modulation frequency. There are however several outstanding points, particularly in three areas: firstly there are some psychophysical observations which have seemed hard to reconcile with an explanation of masking by quadratic distortion products, secondly there might be some difficulties in implementing the scheme we have suggested for removing distortion products, and finally there is a possibility that distortion may not be all bad, and in fact it may be very useful in detecting some types of pattern.

Psychophysical questions

Psychophysical experiments on the non-linear responses to AM gratings suggest that the distortion-product grows more slowly with contrast than might be expected of a quadratic distortion product, and fails to show phase-dependent sub-threshold summation effects (Nachmias & Rogowitz, 1983). The slowness of growth with contrast might be caused by changes in gain or phase with contrast, such changes have been described in both geniculate and retinal X-cells (Sclar, 1987; Shapley & Victor, 1978). The failure of sub-threshold summation could well reflect the involvement of both on-centre and off-centre neurons, in which distortion products have different phases relative to linear responses at the same frequency (see Fig. 17.6).

A second question is whether removing the distortion product, in the way suggested above, should prevent AM gratings from masking gratings of the modulation frequency. If the masking is caused by an increase in variance of the F_1 component, which would lead to a reduction in the signal to noise ratio, then we would expect it to persist, even if any change in the amplitude of the F_1 component is cancelled by subtraction as suggested above. On the other hand, if the masking represents response compression, we would expect it to be removed if the distortion were removed before the stage where compression occurs. Two facts suggest that the masking would persist. Firstly, the masking is greatest when the signal is 90 degrees out of phase with the expected distortion product (Henning *et al.*, 1975), which suggests that it is not caused by response compression. Secondly, my unpublished physiological observations show that, at least in some neurons, the variance of the F_1 distortion product does depend on its amplitude, so we would expect some masking to persist even if the mean distortion product is cancelled. One way of addressing this question would be to see whether masking occurs in the responses of cortical neurons which show no overt distortion product.

Removing distortion products

The scheme suggested is to pair each excitatory input from an on-centre cell with an inhibitory input from an off-centre cell with its receptive field in the same place, to form a linear sub-unit. Although this will work best, it might not always be possible to arrange for the two cells to have perfectly superimposed receptive fields. There is a variety of alternative connection schemes which will work for some stimuli but not others.

The simplest alternative is to allow the two receptive fields to be offset along the 'long' axis of the cortical receptive field. In this case the cancellation will work for all stimuli which are uniform along that axis, such as an optimally oriented grating. One consequence of such a scheme would be that linearity would depend on the orientation of the stimulus; there is some evidence for extreme masking interactions between stimuli of differing orientation (Derrington & Henning, 1989).

Another possibility is to have on-centre cells providing the input in 'on' areas of the receptive field, and vice versa; in this case we would add, instead of subtracting, the responses of the two types of cell. This kind of arrangement would only cancel distortion products of certain spatial frequencies. However, even with a modest number of input neurons, it should be possible to arrange that cancellation occurs over the full range of spatial frequencies to which the neuron is sensitive.

How bad is non-linearity?

It is obvious that we can tolerate a degree of non-linearity, since we have no great difficulty in recognising images produced by a number of non-linear processes, such as photography, and television. However there are also aspects of vision for which non-linear distortion products would be positively helpful. One such is the detection of amplitude-modulation, or of beats between two gratings of similar spatial frequency (Badcock & Derrington, 1985), or of complex motion displays (Adelson & Movshon, 1982). Such tasks may be an important component of texture discrimination, and the existence of a distortion product would allow them to be performed at a low level. Thus even though the available evidence suggests that we do not use distortion products for the performance of such tasks (Derrington & Badcock, 1986), it is worth bearing in mind that our scheme for removing distortion products could equally well be used in reverse to extract distortion products for use in such complex tasks.

Conclusions

There are two obvious conclusions to be drawn from the work described here. The first is that significant non-linearities occur early in the visual pathway, and that they affect X-cells. This means that any linear mechanisms which exist in the striate cortex must use special measures to remove the non-linear components of the signals they receive from the lateral geniculate nucleus. The second point is that the dual representation of the visual image in on-centre and off-centre neurons provides one possible means of filtering out the distortion products introduced by the non-linearity. Further work is needed to show whether such filtering does in fact occur.

References

Adelson, E. H. & Movshon, J. A. (1982) Phenomenal coherence of moving visual patterns. *Nature*, **300**, 523–5.

Albrecht, D. G. & DeValois, R. L. (1981) Striate cortex responses to periodic patterns with and without the fundamental harmonics. *J. Physiol.*, **319**, 497–514.

Badcock, D. R. & Derrington, A. M. (1985) Detecting the displacement of periodic patterns. *Vision Res.*, **25**, 1253–8.

Blakemore, C. & Campbell, F. W. (1969) On the existence of neurones in the visual system selectively sensitive to the orientation and size of retinal images. *J. Physiol.*, **203**, 237–60.

Braddick, O. J., Campbell, F. W. & Atkinson, J. A. (1978) Channels in vision: basic aspects. In *Handbook of Sensory Physiology, Vol. 7*, ed. R. Held, H. W. Leibowitz & H.-L. Teuber, pp. 3–38. Berlin, Heidelberg, New York: Springer-Verlag.

Burton, G. J. (1973) Evidence for non-linear response process in the visual system from measurements on the thresholds of spatial beat frequencies. *Vision Res.*, **13**, 1211–55.

Derrington, A. M. (1987) Distortion products in geniculate X-cells: a physiological basis for masking by spatially modulated gratings. *Vision Res.*, **27**, 1377–86.

Derrington, A. M. & Badcock, D. R. (1986) Detecting spatial beats: non-linearity or contrast increment detection? *Vision Res.*, **27**, 343–8.

Derrington, A. M. & Henning, E. B. (1989) Some observations on the masking effects of two-dimensional stimuli. *Vision Res.*, **29**, 241–6.

Henning, G. B., Hertz, G. B. & Broadbent, D. E. (1975) Some experiments bearing on the hypothesis that the visual system analyses patterns in independent bands of spatial frequency. *Vision Res.*, **15**, 887–97.

Henning, G. B., Hertz, B. G. & Hinton, J. L. (1981) Effects of different hypothetical detection mechanisms on the shape of spatial frequency filters inferred from masking experiments. *J. Opt. Soc. Am.*, **71**, 574–81.

Movshon, J. A., Thompson, I. D. & Tolhurst, D. J. (1978) Spatial summation in the receptive fields of simple cells in the cats striate cortex. *J. Physiol.*, **283**, 53–78.

Nachmias, J. N. & Rogowitz, B. E. (1983) Masking by spatially modulated gratings. *Vision Res.*, **23**, 1621–9.

Sachs, M. B., Nachmias, J. N. & Robson, J. G. (1971) Spatial frequency channels in human vision. *J. Opt. Soc. Am.* **61**, 1176–86.

Sclar, G. S. (1987) Expression of 'retinal' contrast gain control by neurons of the cat's lateral geniculate nucleus. *Exp. Brain Res.*, **66**, 589–96.

Shapley, R. M. & Victor, J. D. (1978) The effect of contrast on the transfer characteristics of cat retinal ganglion cells. *J. Physiol.*, **285**, 275–98.

18

Feature detection in biological and artificial visual systems

D. C. Burr and M. C. Morrone

To function efficiently within reasonable information limits, any visual system, biological or artificial, must simplify the image and record it in some economical form (e.g. Barlow, 1957). Image features, such as lines and edges, are rich sources of information. In this chapter we review a simple, efficient and biologically plausible model of how the human visual system may detect, locate and identify edges and lines in any arbitrary image. The model predicts successfully the appearance of many stimuli (including visual illusions), makes accurate quantitative predictions about thresholds and apparent position, and has been applied successfully to artificial visual systems.

Mach bands

Our research started by considering the conspicuous but paradoxical features, the dark and light lines, that appear on waveforms where luminance ramps meet a plateau, or a ramp of different slope. They are usually referred to as 'Mach bands', after the German physicist Ernst Mach, who first observed and studied them more than 100 years ago (Mach, 1865).

Figure 18.1A shows a clear example of Mach bands, on a trapezoidal waveform. The brightness of the pattern does not follow the luminance distribution, but produces sharp black and white bands, separated by a relatively homogeneous region. The stripes are even more apparent in two dimensions. Figure 18.1B is the product of a vertical and horizontal triangle-wave (from Morrone, Ross, Burr & Owens, 1986). Again brightness does not follow luminance, but clear black and white stars appear at the apexes of the waveform.

The standard textbook explanation for the bands (e.g. Ratliff, 1965; Cornsweet, 1970; Fiorentini, 1972) was first advanced by Mach himself: that mutual inhibitory interactions in the retina and visual cortex filter or differentiate the input waveform, producing a waveform with overshoot or undershoot. Mach (1906) suggested that the filter was like a Laplacian–Gaussian operation, which later became the cornerstone to Marr's theories on vision (Marr, 1982, Marr & Hildreth, 1980). This explanation received firm support in the early fifties as Hartline (1949), Barlow (1953) and Kuffler (1953) discovered direct physiological evidence for the lateral inhibition suggested by Mach. Indeed lateral inhibition, or high-pass or band-pass filtering is the basis of most modern theories of vision (e.g. Robson, 1980; Marr, 1982; Watt & Morgan, 1985).

Despite the wide acceptance of lateral inhibition as the complete explanation for Mach bands and other phenomena, it does encounter difficulties. One problem is that it predicts that as the ramp dividing two plateaux is decreased, the bands will become stronger and sharper, reaching a maximum at a step edge. Yet step edges produce no Mach bands (Fiorentini, 1972; Ross, Holt & Johnstone, 1981; Morrone et al., 1986): if they did, every object we see would be surrounded by sharp black and white stripes, which would be most disturbing. Mach bands are unique to situations where a ramp meets a plateau or a ramp of different slope.

The approach of Morrone et al. (1986) to Mach bands was different. They studied the physical properties of stimuli that produce Mach bands, and of those that do not, taking advantage of that useful tool, Fourier analysis, introduced to vision research by Campbell & Robson (1968). The analysis indicated that spatial phase may be important.

Figure 18.2 illustrates schematically the phase relationships of the first four Fourier harmonics of a square-wave, a triangle-wave and a trapezoidal-wave (of equal ramp-width and plateaux). For clarity, all

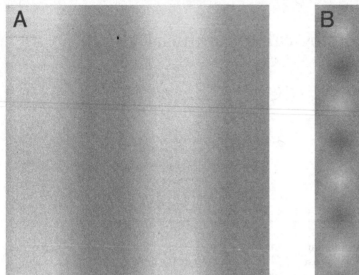

Fig. 18.1. Examples of Mach bands in one and two dimensions. On the left, sharp bands are seen at the knees of the waveform, although there are no corresponding luminance ridges. Stars are seen in the pattern on the right, although the luminance distribution is pyramidal (product of vertical and horizontal triangle-waves).

harmonics have been drawn with equal amplitude (although the amplitude actually decreases with frequency). For the square-wave, the phases of all cosine harmonics are identical at two points in each period, where they cross mean luminance: the phases are all 90° at the positive going edge, and −90° at the negative going edge. For the triangle-wave, harmonics are not in phase at those points, but alternate between 90 and −90° phase. However, arrival-phases are all equal at the apexes of the waveform, where they have 0° or 180° phase. It is at these points that Mach bands appear. For the trapezoid, the first two harmonics are in phase at the mean-luminance crossing point, but the next two are in counterphase. There are no points of perfect phase congruence, but arrival-phases are maximally similar at the knee points of the trapezoid, where they are near 0° or 180° phase.

This led us to suspect that the stimulus for Mach bands is local phase organization at phases at or near 0° or 180°. In a series of experiments reported in detail elsewhere (Morrone *et al.*, 1986; Ross, Morrone & Burr, 1989) the idea was tested and shown to be valid. Mach bands appear on trapezoidal waveforms only when the higher harmonics of the trapezoid, those that break the phase congruence at the mean-luminance cross and cause congruence at the kneepoints, can be resolved by the visual system. When these harmonics were physically removed by smooth digital filtering or by phase inversion, or when the harmonics were undetectable because the spatial

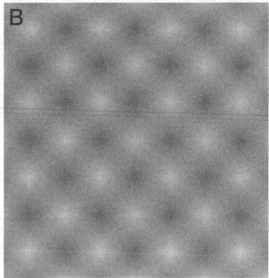

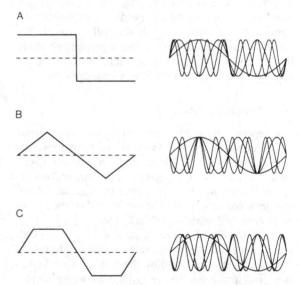

Fig. 18.2. An illustration of how the harmonic components of square-waves, triangle-waves and trapezoids align themselves in phase at key points of the waveform (the amplitudes of harmonics are not drawn to scale). The square-wave has two points of phase congruence, at the edges, where all harmonics are in ±90° phase. For the triangle-wave, the harmonics are congruent at the apexes, where they have 0° or 180° phase. The trapezoid has no point of perfect phase congruence, but phases are maximally similar at the kneepoints, where the average phase is near 0° or 180°.

frequency of the trapezoid was too high, or the ramp width too small, or the contrast too low, Mach bands disappeared. An example of the results (reproduced in Fig. 18.4) will be discussed later, after a biologically plausible model for detection of phase congruency has been described.

The model

Several researchers have suggested that phase relationships of Fourier harmonics are important for vision (e.g. Oppenheim & Lim, 1981; Piotrowski & Campbell, 1982). The experiments with Mach bands provided further support for this assertion, and went on to suggest that it is not phase *per se*, but congruence of arrival-phase that determines visual features. In this section we describe a model of how visual mechanisms may act to detect phase congruence, and identify the feature associated with it. The model has two stages, one linear, the other non-linear.

We start with four sets of linear filters, of differing spatial frequency preference. For each spatial frequency, there are two matched filters of identical amplitude response but orthogonal in phase response: one has a constant phase spectrum of 0° that leaves the input phase untouched; the other has a constant phase spectrum of 90°, producing a 90° phase shift in all harmonics. Each filter has an associated receptive field, given by the inverse Fourier transform. The receptive fields of cosine filters will have even symmetry, those of the sine filters odd symmetry (see inset in Fig. 18.3). This assertion is reasonably consistent with most physiological observations of the structure of simple cell receptive fields (e.g. Hubel & Wiesel, 1962; Kulikowski & Bishop, 1981; but see also Field & Tolhurst, 1986). The receptive fields of the cosine filters are the Hilbert transforms of the sine filters.

The non-linear stage of the model is to square separately the output of the cosine and sine filters (or even- and odd-symmetric fields) and sum them at each scale (spatial frequency preference). This gives what we term the *local energy* profile, following Adelson & Bergen's (1985) terminology. Although the local energy operator is insensitive to the absolute phase of the input, it is highly sensitive to local phase organization. Morrone & Owens (1987) and Morrone & Burr (1988) have shown that maximum congruency of arrival-phases occurs at the peaks of the local maxima of the energy functions. Therefore, peaks in local energy will signal maximum congruence of phase.

Figure 18.3 illustrates the response of the model to a square, triangle and trapezoidal waveform. The lower profiles show the response of even-symmetric fields (solid lines) and odd-symmetric fields (dashed lines) at four scales. Because the filters are linear and span most of the frequency range of the image, most of the information about the image is preserved. However, at this first linear stage, the filters have not simplified the patterns. After the non-linear local energy operation, the output is simple to interpret. The local energy profiles (shown above the linear convolutions) do not exhibit the 'ringing' shown in the filtered response, but have clear unambiguous peaks. For all three patterns, the peaks in local energy occur at the points of interest: at the edges of the square, the apexes of the triangle and the kneepoints of the trapezoid.

Now return to the linear output (below), but consider the response only at the peaks in local energy. For the square-wave, the response of odd fields is strong at all scales, while the even response is zero. This is the signal for an edge, with the sign and contrast of the edge given by the sign and amplitude of the odd response. For the triangle and trapezoid the response at the peaks in local energy is primarily from the even-symmetric fields, particularly at higher scales. This is the signal for a line, even though there is no corresponding line in the luminance profile.

Figure 18.4 shows a sample of results of Mach band thresholds and the predictions of the energy model (taken from Ross, Morrone & Burr, 1989). The open circles are contrast thresholds for seeing Mach bands on a low-pass filtered trapezoid, as a function of the filter cut-off frequency. The closed circles show thresholds for detecting 'residual waveforms': high-pass waveforms derived from trapezoids by removing all the first block of harmonics that are congruent in phase at the mean-luminance cross (see Fig. 18.2). As the trapezoid is filtered more heavily, Mach bands become progressively more difficult to see. As the Mach bands become less visible, so do the residual waveforms, at a similar rate. That thresholds for Mach bands parallel those for detecting the higher harmonics (those that cause the phase congruence at the kneepoints) is a strong indication that phase congruence causes Mach bands.

But a stronger proof is provided by the quantitative predictions of the model. The solid curves of Fig. 18.4 reflect the predicted thresholds for seeing Mach bands and for detecting the residuals (see caption for details). The curves fit the data remarkably well, predicting not only the general shape of the curves, but also the slight differences in Mach band and residual thresholds. Thus local energy predicts where Mach bands should appear, and their contrast threshold: the strong response from even symmetric filters at those points predicts that the features should be bands rather than edges.

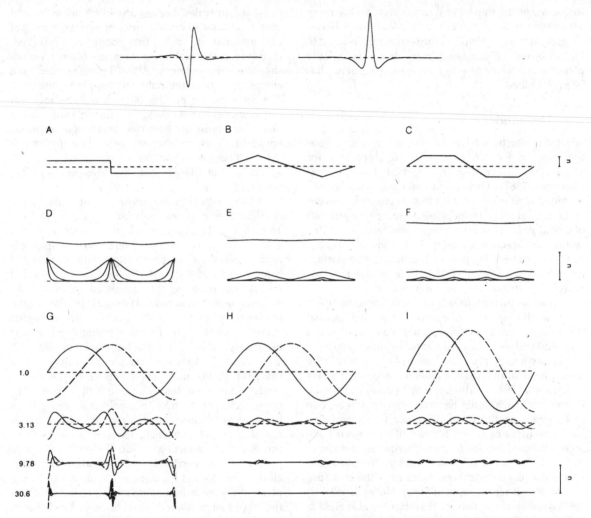

Fig. 18.3. The energy model applied to three input waveforms, a square (A), triangle (B) and trapezoidal (C) waveform. *Top*: Examples of the two types of receptive fields used for the linear stage of the model. The one on the right has even symmetry ($f(x) = f(-x)$), the one on the left odd symmetry ($f(x) = -f(-x)$). We assume four sizes of receptive field, each having a spatial frequency bandwidth of 1.2 octaves. The centre frequencies are 1.0, 3.1, 9.7 and 30.6 c/deg.

The lower curves (G, H & I) show the result of convolution with even-symmetric receptive fields (filled lines) and odd-symmetric receptive fields (dashed lines), of four sizes (spatial frequency preference). At each scale the square of the odd response is summed with the square of the even response to produce the local energy functions (D, E & F). These functions peak at the points of phase congruence, which occur at visually salient features. The response at the peaks is primarily from odd-symmetric detectors for the square-wave (leading to the perception of an edge), and primarily from even-symmetric detectors for the triangle and trapezoid, producing the perception of a line (or Mach band).

Craik–O'Brien illusion

According to our model, vision simplifies images by locating, identifying and encoding significant features such as lines and edges. These features provide key information about the whole image. A good example of how this can occur is the well known Craik–O'Brien illusion (Craik, 1966; O'Brien, 1958; Cornsweet, 1970), illustrated in Fig. 18.5. Except for a small region near the border, the luminance of this pattern does not vary: yet the centre region seems distinctly darker than the outer regions, particularly at low contrasts.

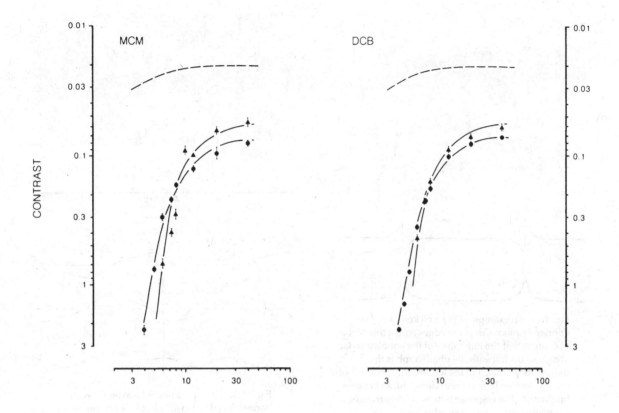

Fig. 18.4. Contrast thresholds for seeing Mach bands on a low-pass filtered trapezoidal waveform (of ratio ramp-width to period of 0.125) as a function of filter cut-off frequency (triangles). Also shown are detection thresholds for 'residual' waveforms, derived from trapezoids by removing the first two harmonics. Thresholds for both Mach bands and residuals increase with increasing blur at a commensurate rate. This suggests that Mach band thresholds are determined by thresholds for the higher harmonics, those that cause phase congruence to shift from the mean-luminance crossing point to the kneepoints. The curves are not best fits to the data, but predictions of the energy model (see Ross, Morrone & Burr, 1989 for details). The broken line above shows the predictions of lateral inhibition, assuming the same filter bandwidth, but only even-symmetric receptive fields.

Like Mach bands, researchers have sought to explain this illusion with lateral inhibition of adjacent detectors or high-pass filtering of the amplitude spectrum (e.g. Cornsweet, 1970; Campbell, Howell & Johnstone, 1978). However, like the Mach band explanation, this explanation fails quantitatively. The illusion is not restricted to low spatial frequencies where high-pass filters may be acting, but occurs at all spatial frequencies, at roughly equal strength (Burr, 1987).

Our explanation is different (see Burr, 1987 for details). We claim that significant features like edges encode information about the whole image. The visual system needs a system like this to signal brightness, as much information about luminance is lost at a peripheral stage of image processing (Shapley & Enroth-Cugell, 1984; Burr, Ross & Morrone, 1985). The local energy profile of the Craik–O'Brien pattern (shown below the profile) is similar to that of a real edge. There are only two peaks in the profile, and at those peaks only odd-symmetric detectors respond. This is the signal for an edge, and an edge is the signal for a brightness change. Therefore the visual system should perceive this image as three panels, the centre one darker than the outer two. Interestingly the illusion begins to fail at higher contrasts, almost vanishing at a contrast of 1 (Burr, 1987). This suggests that at higher contrasts, factors other than edge information influence brightness.

A

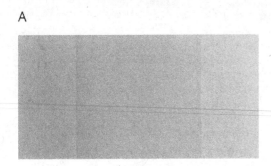

B

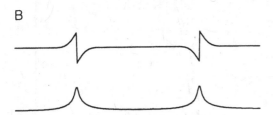

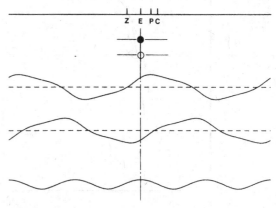

Fig. 18.5. An example of the well known Craik–O'Brien illusion. Cover the edges with a thin thread to confirm that the luminance of the panels is in fact identical. Underneath the photograph is the luminance profile, and the local energy profile. Local energy peaks where we see edges, and a change in brightness. The response here is entirely from odd-symmetric detectors, so an edge is seen, and interpreted as a signal for brightness change.

Monocular rivalry

An interesting pattern can be created by shifting the phases of all the harmonics of a square-wave by 45°, and blurring the image. This operation produces two points of phase congruence per period, where the phases are all 45°. Figure 18.6 shows an example of such a waveform. Observe it for some time and note that its appearance is unstable, alternating between a series of lines, and broad bars separated by edges. This alternation of appearances has been called *monocular rivalry* by Atkinson & Campbell (1974).

     While observing the pattern alternating in appearance, try to mark the apparent position of the central line (when it appears clearly as lines) and on the central edge (when it is clearly an edge). Under more controlled conditions than are possible here, observers reported that both lines and edges appear at very similar positions, indicated by the open and closed circles of Fig. 18.6. Both appear where the local energy (shown below) is maximal. Also shown on this graph are the peaks in luminance, usually associated with a line, and the point of maximal change in

Fig. 18.6. A low-pass filtered waveform with harmonics added in 45° phase. The luminance profile is given by:

$$L(x) = L_0 + a \sum_{(k=1)}^{\infty} \sin\left(2\pi k x/T + \pi/4\right) \exp\left(-k^2/18\right)$$

where L_0 is mean luminance, a amplitude, T the period and k odd integer. Observe the pattern for a while and notice it changing form from a series of broad bars with edges, to a series of thinner lines. The profiles show the luminance distribution (similar to the result of convolution with even-symmetric fields), its Hilbert Transform (the result of convolution with odd-receptive fields) and the local energy profile (below). The open circles show the average apparent position where observers report seeing lines (when the percept is one of lines), and the filled circles the average apparent position of edges (when broad bars were seen). Both these measures are close to the position predicted by the peak of the energy function (E), but quite different from the point of maximal slope (Z), the peak of the waveform (P) or centroid of positive going mass (C).

luminance (zero-crossing in the second derivative), usually associated with an edge (Marr, 1982). Yet the features, whether lines or edges do not correspond to those points, but to the peaks in local energy.

     Monocular rivalry is easily accommodated by

our model. The pattern produces responses from both even- and odd-symmetric detectors at the peaks in local energy, and these responses may vary randomly in strength over time. Although the nature of the feature is unstable, features are seen only where local energy peaks.

Perceptual structure from local energy

Figure 18.7 shows an example of how phase congruence, and hence local energy can dictate the perceptual organization of a pattern. The pattern was constructed from the harmonic components of a square-wave, shifting both relative and absolute phase systematically each row. The phase was organized so that it was equal at points which form an arrow pattern, pointing left. The value of the phases at these points varies systematically from +90° at the top and bottom through to −90° at the centre. Close up,

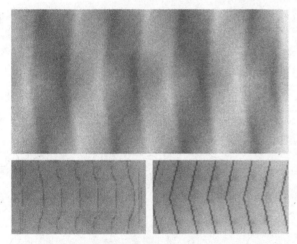

Fig. 18.7. A pattern in which harmonics were added to produce a phase congruency structure resembling an arrow pointing left. The luminance distribution $L(x, y)$ is given by:

$$L(x, y) = L_0 +$$

$$4a/\pi \sum_{k=1}^{\infty} \sin 2\pi[(y/2T - 1/4) + k(1/4 - y/4T) + kx/T]/k$$

for $y > 0$ and $L(x, y) = L(x, -y)$ for $y < 0$ (variables as for figure 6, y is vertical length: $-T \leqslant y \leqslant T$). Close to, the perceptual organization follows the peaks in phase congruence, and an arrow pointing left is seen. From a distance, however, the average luminance distribution is seen, and the arrow seems to point right. The lower figures show the peak of local energy for the blurred pattern (left) and for the unblurred pattern (right).

phase congruence dictates the perceptual organization, giving the appearance of an arrow pointing left. However, this is contrary to average luminance information in the figure, and the information at low spatial frequencies. View the pattern from a distance (or screw up your eyes), and the arrow points right. A similar illusion was described by Burr, Morrone & Ross (1986).

The lower sketches show the peaks in local energy for the original pattern, and for one which has been blurred. To obtain these the model was run in two dimensions, using receptive fields oriented in space. For each scale, there were four detectors of differing orientation preference. The lines marked by the model follow fairly accurately the perceptual structure of the blurred and unblurred images.

Another example of variable perceptual structure is coarse quantization, illustrated in Fig. 18.8. After an image has been quantized into a few blocks, it is not recognizable, even though there is sufficient low-frequency information in the image for recognition. The original explanation was that spurious high frequencies mask low frequencies which carry information about the face (Harmon & Julesz, 1973), this assertion has been disproved (Morrone, Burr & Ross, 1983). According to the model presented here, perceptual organization is dictated by peaks in the local energy function. The strong phase congruence at the edges of the blocks causes the peaks to occur there (see Fig. 18.7). Low frequency information about the face is present in the coarse quantized image, but this cannot be assessed. Like the wavering arrow of Fig. 18.7, it is phase congruence that dictates perceptual structure, not average luminance.

After low-pass filtering, the organization of the peaks in local energy is quite different. It follows roughly the features that are important for image recognition. This sketch is not itself recognizable, presumably because information about the nature and sign of features is not preserved in the energy profile.

Figure 18.8C shows the original portrait, with the local energy peak map. Here local energy peaks not only follow the important image features, but also provide a reasonable sketch of the face, much like an artist's line drawing. Unlike the output of the low-pass image, this sketch of local energy peaks provides a good, recognizable representation of the image, without having to code the nature and sign of the features. This is probably because most of the peaks occur at the higher scales, and at the higher scales the sign of contrast is less important than at lower scales (see Hayes, Morrone & Burr, 1986).

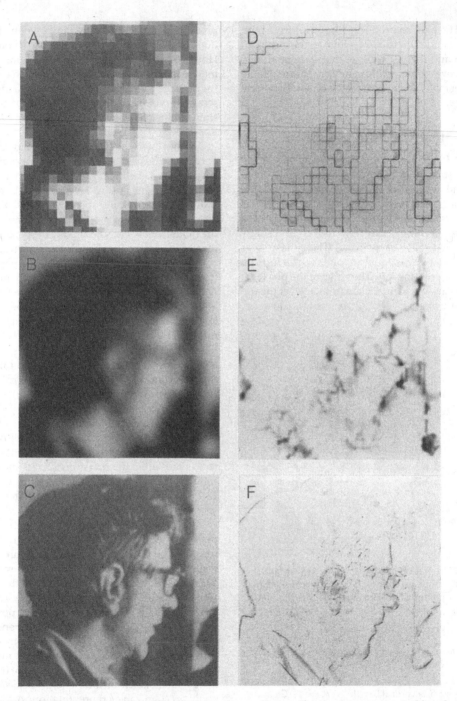

Fig. 18.8. A & D: Coarse quantized portrait of Professor Horace Barlow. The image is unrecognizable unless viewed from a distance, or blurred. The local energy profile (D) follows the block structure dictating the perceptual organization.

B & E: The coarse quantized imaged blurred with a Gaussian low-pass filter. The face is now recognizable from any viewing distance. Local energy peaks of this pattern follow far more closely the important image features.

C & F: Original photo from which figure A was derived. Local energy peaks (F) not only follow the important image features, but produce an acceptably recognizable sketch of the portrait.

Image encoding for artificial systems

Given the remarkable efficiency of human vision, it is likely that biological mechanisms for image simplification may also be applicable to artificial visual systems. Morrone & Owens (1987) have simplified the local energy model and applied it to computer vision. To accelerate computation, they used broad-band filters of only one spatial frequency and two orientations. The results when applied to natural scenes were very much like that of the lower figure of Fig. 18.7. The model marked the edges of objects, providing a convenient map for later processing (such as object recognition) or economical storage.

That the model worked adequately with broad-band filters suggests that spatial frequency filtering in the amplitude domain is not essential for visual processing. What is essential for our model is sets of orthogonal phase filters, matched in amplitude response. Spatial frequency filtering probably enhances efficiency and economy of processing, by matching the sampling grain of the filters to the spatial frequency response. We are currently considering whether algorithms such as Burt & Adelson's (1983) pyramid coding may enhance processing efficiency of the model.

Conclusions

To recapitulate: our model has two stages, linear and non-linear. The linear operators produce two functions of identical amplitude but differing phase spectra: one the Hilbert transform of the other. The non-linear operator squares the response of each and sums them, to produce a function that peaks where the local phase organization is maximal. Our experiments show that local phase organization signals features of interest to vision, either lines or edges. The linear operators determine whether the feature is a line or an edge, and also code its magnitude and sign.

Our present knowledge of the physiology of visual systems suggests that we have all the necessary neural hardware for both stages of the model. At all levels of visual processing there exist two classes of cells: quasi-linear and clearly non-linear cells. The separate role of the two classes of cells has been

debated for some time (see for example Lennie, 1980, for review). Our model allocates distinct roles to each cell class. The non-linear cells should detect and locate features, while linear cells may identify the type of feature at that point.

The known properties of simple cortical cells agree with the requirements of the linear stage of our model: they are quasi-linear filters (except for half-wave rectification) and their receptive fields tend to have either even or odd symmetry (Hubel & Wiesel, 1962; Kulikowski & Bishop, 1981; but see also Field & Tolhurst, 1986). Psychophysical studies support the existence of even- and odd-symmetric fields in central vision (Field & Nachmias, 1984; Burr, Morrone & Spinelli, 1989). Furthermore, adjacent pairs of simple cells tend to differ in phase response by 90° (Pollen & Ronner, 1981), making them matched filters in quadrature phase.

Non-linearities such as squaring (a second-order non-linearity) occur in many visual cells, including complex cortical cells (Spitzer & Hochstein, 1985). Complex cells could extract local energy. They could do so either by squaring and summing input from pairs of simple cells, or by computing the whole operation within the complex cell itself, if the quasi-linear sub-units (Movshon, Thompson & Tolhurst, 1978) could cause a 90° phase shift. These possibilities are testable by direct measurements of complex cell response to stimuli such as those described in this chapter.

The model is suggested as a means whereby the visual system may reduce significantly the redundancy of images. The local energy operator provides an efficient and biologically plausible means of detecting features rich in information, such as edges and bars. Vision can encode most image information by considering the linear response only at local maxima of the energy function. The model has successfully explained several mysteries of vision, including Mach bands, the importance of the Fourier phase spectrum, the Craik–O'Brien illusion, monocular rivalry, the perceived position of features and coarse quantizing. It may also prove to be a useful tool for artificial visual systems to simplify images for recognition and for economical storage.

References

Adelson, E. H. & Bergen, J. R. (1985) Spatio-temporal energy models for the perception of motion. *J. Opt. Soc. Am. A* **2**, 284–99.

Atkinson, J. & Campbell, F. W. (1974) The effect of phase on the perception of compound gratings. *Vision Res.*, **14**, 159–62.

Barlow, H. B. (1953) Summation and inhibition in the frog's retina. *J. Physiol. (Lond.)*, **119**, 69–88.

Barlow, H. B. (1957) Possible principles underlying the transformations of sensory messages. In *Sensory Communication*, ed. W. A. Rosenblith. Cambridge, Mass: MIT Press.

Burr, D. C. (1987) Implications of the Craik–O'Brien illusion for brightness perception. *Vision Res.*, **27**, 1903–13.

Burr, D. C., Ross, J. & Morrone, M. C. (1985) Local regulation of luminance gain. *Vision Res.*, **25**, 717–28.

Burr, D. C., Morrone, M. C. & Ross, J. (1986) Local and global visual analysis. *Vision Res.*, **26**, 749–57.

Burr, D. C., Morrone, M. C. & Spinelli, D. (1989) Evidence for edge and bar detectors in human vision. *Vision Res.*, **29**, 419–31.

Burt, P. J. & Adelson, E. H. (1983) The Laplacian pyramid as a compact image code. *IEEE Trans. Comm.*, **31**, 532–40.

Campbell, F. W., Howell, E. R. & Johnstone, J. R. (1978) A comparison of threshold and suprathreshold appearance of gratings with components in the low and high spatial frequency range. *J. Physiol.*, **284**, 193–201.

Campbell, F. W. & Robson, J. G. (1968) On the application of Fourier analysis to the visibility of gratings. *J. Physiol. (Lond.)*, **197**, 551–6.

Cornsweet, T. N. (1970) *Visual Perception*. New York: Academic Press.

Craik, K. J. W. (1966) *The Nature of Psychology*, ed. S. L. Sherwood. Cambridge: Cambridge University Press.

Field, D. J. & Nachmias, J. (1984) Phase reversal discrimination. *Vision Res.*, **24**, 333–40.

Field, D. J. & Tolhurst, D. J. (1986) The structure and symmetry of simple-cell receptive-field profiles in the cat's visual cortex. *Proc. Roy. Soc. Lond.*, B**226**, 379–99.

Fiorentini, A. (1972) Mach band phenomena. In *Handbook of Sensory Physiology*, Vol VII/4, ed. D. Jameson & L. M. Hurvich. Berlin: Springer-Verlag.

Harmon, L. D. & Julesz, B. (1973) Masking in visual recognition: effect of two-dimensional filtered noise. *Science*, **180**, 1194–7.

Hartline, H. K. (1949) Inhibition of activity of visual receptors by illuminating nearby retinal elements in the Limulus eye. *Fed. Proc.*, **8**, 69.

Hayes, T., Morrone, M. C. & Burr, D. C. (1986) Recognition of positive and negative bandpass-filtered images. *Perception*, **15**, 595–602.

Hubel, D. H. & Wiesel, T. N. (1962) Receptive fields, binocular interaction and functional architecture in the cat's visual cortex. *J. Physiol. (Lond.)*, **160**, 106–54.

Kuffler, S. W. (1953) Discharge patterns and functional organization of mammalian retina. *J. Neurophysiol.*, **16**, 37–68.

Kulikowski, J. J. & Bishop, P. O. (1981) Linear analysis of the responses of simple cells in the cat visual cortex. *Exp. Brain Res.*, **44**, 386–400.

Lennie, P. (1980) Parallel visual pathways: a review. *Vision Res.*, **20**, 561–94.

Mach, E. (1865) Uber die Wirkung der raumlichen Vertheilung des Lichtreizes auf di Neztzhaut. *I.S.-B. Akad. Wiss. Wien, math.-nat. K1.*, **54**, 303–22.

Mach, E. (1906) Uber den Einfluss Raumlich und zeitlich variierender Lichtreize auf die Gesichtswahrnehmung. *S.-B. Akad. Wiss. Wien, math.-nat. K1.*, **115**, 633–48.

Marr, D. (1982) *Vision*. San Francisco: Freeman.

Marr, D. & Hildreth, E. (1980) Theory of edge detection. *Proc. Roy. Soc. Lond.*, B**207**, 187–217.

Morrone, M. C. & Burr, D. C. (1988) Feature detection in human vision: a phase dependent energy model. *Proc. Roy. Soc. Lond.*, B**235**, 221–45.

Morrone, M. C., Burr, D. C. & Ross, J. (1983) Added noise restores recognition of coarse quantised images. *Nature*, **305**, 226–8.

Morrone, M. C. & Owens, R. (1987) Edge detection by local energy. *Pattern Recognition Letters*, **6**, 303–13.

Morrone, M. C., Ross, J., Burr, D. C. & Owens, R. (1986) Mach bands depend on spatial phase. *Nature*, **324**, 250–3.

Movshon, J. A., Thompson, I. D. & Tolhurst, D. J. (1978) Receptive field organization of complex cells in the cat's striate cortex. *J. Physiol.*, **283**, 79–99.

O'Brien, V. (1958) Contour perception, illusion and reality. *J. Opt. Soc. Am.*, **48**, 112–19.

Openheim, A. V. & Lim, J. S. (1981) The importance of phase in signals. *Proc. IEEE*, **69**, 529–41.

Piotrowski, L. N. & Campbell, F. W. (1982) A demonstration of the visual importance and flexibility of spatial-frequency amplitude and phase. *Perception*, **11**, 337–46.

Pollen, D. A. & Ronner, S. F. (1981) Phase relationships between adjacent simple cells in the visual cortex. *Science*, **212**, 1409–11.

Ratliff, F. (1965) *Mach Bands*. San Francisco: Holden–Day.

Robson, J. G. (1980) Neural images: the physiological basis of spatial vision. In *Visual Coding and Adaptability*, ed. L. S. Harris, L. Erlbaum & associates. New Jersey: Hillsborough.

Ross, J., Morrone, M. C. & Burr, D. C. (1989) The conditions under which Mach bands are visible. *Vision Res.* **29**, 699–715.

Ross, J., Holt, J. J. & Johnstone, J. R. (1981) High frequency limitations on Mach bands. *Vision Res.*, **21**, 1165–7.

Shapley, R. & Enroth-Cugell, C. (1984) Visual adaptation and retinal gain controls. In *Progress in Retinal Research 3*, ed. N. N. Osborne & G. J. Chader, pp. 263–346. Oxford: Pergamon Press.

Spitzer, H. & Hochstein, S. (1985) A complex-cell receptive field model. *J. Neurophysiol.*, **53**, 1266–86.

Watt, R. J. & Morgan, M. J. (1985) A theory of the primitive spatial code in human vision. *Vision Res.*, **25**, 1661–74.

Development of vision

19

On reformation of visual projection: cellular and molecular aspects

M. G. Yoon

Background

Development of the visual projection

The neural connections between the retinal ganglion cells and the higher order visual neurons in the midbrain (e.g. the optic tectum) or in the forebrain (e.g. lateral geniculate nucleus) develop in coherent topographic patterns. To establish the visual projections, individual ganglion cells send out their axons (the optic fibers) which grow towards the optic disc near the centre of the retina. The axons of ganglion cells exit the eyeball at its posterior pole and form a thick ensheathed bundle, the optic nerve. The growing tips of these axons select particular routes to reach their appropriate target zones along the visual pathways and eventually form synapses with higher order visual neurons.

Since the complexities of the visual pathways vary from one species to another we will discuss here a relatively simple example of visual projections in the goldfish. The optic fibers of goldfish make a complete cross at the optic chiasm and invade only the contralateral lobe of the optic tectum in the midbrain. Before they enter the rostral pole of the tectum the ingrowing axons from the ventral retina segregate from those originating from the dorsal area of the retina. The former select the medial branch of the optic tract and the latter the lateral branch. The optic fibers within the tectal tissue course through a superficial layer (the *stratum opticum*) towards the caudal pole along the spheroidal circumferences of the optic tectum. Most growing tips of retinal ganglion cell axons terminate in the subjacent layer (the *stratum fibrosum et griseum superficiale*) and form synapses with visual neurons of the tectum.

The pattern of neural connections between the retinal ganglion cells and tectal neurons has two essential topographic features. First, the retino-tectal projection is topographically coherent, in the sense that optic fibers originating from neighbouring ganglion cells in the retina connect with neighbouring visual neurons in the tectum. Second, the projection is topographically polarized, in the sense that a temporonasal sequence of retinal positions (or a nasotemporal sequence of their receptive fields in the external visual world) is represented by a rostrocaudal sequence on the tectum, and a ventrodorsal sequence of retinal positions (or superoinferior sequence in the visual field) by a mediolateral sequence on the tectum.

Recovery of vision after axotomy of the optic nerves in amphibia and teleosts

When the original visual projection is interrupted by injury of the optic fibers in birds and mammals, the animal suffers permanently a complete blindness or a partial scotoma for the injured part of the retina. In adult newts, however, Matthey (1925, 1926) discovered that their optic fibers can regenerate after axotomy and eventually restore normal vision following an initial period of transient blindness. The capability of retinal ganglion cells to regenerate their severed axons was confirmed in other species of amphibia (Stone & Zaur, 1940; Sperry, 1943a,b, 1944, 1945) and also in teleosts (Sperry, 1948). If the original neural connections between the retina and the tectum are interrupted by severing the axons of ganglion cells in these lower vertebrates, new neurites sprout out from the proximal stumps of the cut axons. The regenerating axons of retinal ganglion cells unsort themselves from the scramble and preferentially select particular routes to grow back to their appropriate destinations. They eventually reconnect with their previous target zones of the tectum in a correct topographic order and thus restore normal vision. Furthermore, if the eye is rotated by 180° and the optic fibers are cut to regenerate back to the brain, the restored visuomotor coordinations in these animals become systematically inverted and reversed. Their maladaptive visuomotor coordinations which correspond to the orientation of the 180° rotated retina persist without any sign of correction by some kind of learning process in the amphibia and teleosts (Sperry, 1943b, 1944, 1945, 1948).

Neuronal specificity

Sperry's pioneering experiments reveal that the reestablishment of neural connections between the retina and the visual centers of the brain in lower vertebrates is controlled by certain growth regulating factors rather than by functional readaptation processes such as learning. To explain the embryonic development and restoration of orderly visual projection, Sperry (1943b, 1945, 1948, 1951, 1963) proposed the chemoaffinity hypothesis of neuronal specificity as follows: the embryonic retinal ganglion cells undergo topographic differentiation (as well as cytologic and functional differentiations such as their receptive field properties) within the eye anlage. Each ganglion cell acquires an axially graded differential affinity marker of cytochemical nature for intercellular recognition, according to its relative position in the retinal field. The corresponding higher order visual neurons in the optic tectum (or in any other visual area) also undergo a congruent topographic differentiation and thus acquire matching or complementary differential chemoaffinity markers according to their relative positions in the tectal field. The ingrowing optic fiber is guided chemotactically to its appropriate target zone when it enters the tectum, and forms synapses with just those tectal neurons whose chemoaffinity matches its own.

Reorganization of retinotectal projection in goldfish

In addition to the ability of orderly regeneration of severed optic fibers, the visual system of an adult goldfish maintains a high degree of neural plasticity: it is capable of readjusting to various types of experimentally induced size-disparity between the retina and the tectum. For example, if the caudal half of the tectal lobe is ablated, the remaining rostral hemilobe accommodates ingrowing optic fibers not only from the proper temporal half of the retina but also from the previously inappropriate nasal half, in an orderly compressed retinotopic pattern (Gaze & Sharma, 1970; Yoon, 1971). Furthermore, the field

compression was found to be a reversible phenomenon (Yoon, 1972a): an orderly compression of the visual projection from the whole retina onto the rostral half of the tectum may be induced even in the presence of the caudal part of the tectum by surgical insertion of a mechanical barrier between the rostral half and the denervated caudal half of the tectum in adult goldfish. When the barrier is either later removed or absorbed, the field compression gradually reverts to a normal (decompressed) pattern of visual projections from the whole retina to the whole extent of the newly rejoined tectum. If the caudal part of the rejoined tectum is ablated in the same fish, the remaining rostral half-tectum eventually reacquires the visual projection from the whole retina in an orderly recompressed pattern (Yoon, 1972a).

Similar neural plasticity was also found after a partial ablation of the retina in adult goldfish (Horder, 1971; Yoon, 1972b; Schmidt, Cicerone & Easter, 1978). Following ablation of either nasal or temporal half of the retina, the visual projection from the surviving hemiretina expands over the entire extent of the whole tectal lobe in a correct retinotopic order. If ablation of the nasal hemiretina is combined with that of the caudal hemitectum, then the visual projection from the remaining temporal hemiretina becomes transposed to the entire extent of the previously inappropriate rostral hemitectum in a correct retinotopic order (Yoon, 1972b).

Further experiments which involve various types of tectal reimplantation show that the tectal tissue possesses a certain directional property, i.e. the topographic polarity, that does not change after excision and reimplantation in a different orientation. For instance, if a piece of tectal tissue is excised, and reimplanted into the same tectum after 90° or 180° rotation about the dorsoventral axis, the reestablished retinotectal projection shows a localized corresponding 90° or 180° rotation within the reimplanted area of the tectum (Sharma & Gaze, 1971; Yoon, 1973, 1975, 1976a, 1980). The topographic polarity of the reimplanted tectal tissue must have directed the ingrowing optic fibers to redistribute their terminals in accord with its original orientation regardless of the experimental rotation or inversion of the tectal tissue (Yoon, 1975). If two similar pieces of tectal tissue are reciprocally translocated either along the rostrocaudal or the mediolateral axis without rotation, the reestablished retinotectal projections onto these reimplants show corresponding reciprocal transpositions of receptive fields along the nasotemporal or the superoinferior axis (Hope, Hammond & Gaze, 1976;

Yoon, 1980). When the reciprocal translocation is combined with 180° rotation of both tectal reimplants, the reestablished retinotectal projection shows the corresponding reciprocal transposition and the localized 180° rotation within the tectal reimplants (Yoon, 1980). These results indicate that the translocated pieces of tectal tissue retain not only the topographic polarity, indicative of their normal orientation, but also the topographic addresses, indicative of their original positions in the tectum, with respect to their selective reinnervation by particular groups of incoming optic fiber terminals.

These dynamic reorganizations of visual projection following various experimental manipulations in adult goldfish indicate that the formation of neural connections between retinal ganglion cells and visual neurons of the tectum is regulated not by a rigid place-specific mechanism, but by adaptable, context-dependent mechanisms. The nature of the biological mechanisms is far from clear from these phenomenological experiments.

In the following sections, some details of the biological processes which are involved in the structural reconstruction of regenerating axons and their inter-cellular interactions with the target tissue are discussed at the cellular and molecular levels.

Trophic interactions between retinal neurites and the co-cultured tectal tissue *in vitro*

Under favorable culture conditions a piece of retinal tissue explanted from adult goldfish gives rise to vigorous outgrowths of neuronal processes *in vitro* (Landreth & Agranoff, 1976, 1979). The retinal neurites have bush-like growth cones with several microspikes protruding at their growing tips (Fig. 19.1). The trajectories of these outgrowing neurites can be monitored continuously with an inverted microscope. Thus the growth rate and pattern of these retinal neurites are studied under various experimental conditions. Landreth & Agranoff (1976, 1979) found that the growth index (based on the density and length of neurites growing from unit retinal area) is enhanced if the retinal ganglion cells are pre-conditioned by axotomy about two weeks prior to the explantation of the retinal tissue. When HRP is applied to the growing tips of these retinal neurites *in vitro*, only the ganglion cell bodies are found to be labeled by HRP (Johns, Heacock & Agranoff, 1978). These experiments show that the neurites growing

from the explanted retinal tissue are regenerating axons of retinal ganglion cells *in vitro*.

Possible trophic influences of tectal tissue upon the pattern of neuritic outgrowths from the goldfish retinal explant are tested during the course of their co-culture in a pre-designated topographic configuration. An elongated rectangular piece (about 0.75 mm× 3 mm) of the retinal tissue is dissected free from the nasal half of the right retina along the nasotemporal axis near the equator, 10–14 days after optic nerve crush in anaesthetized adult goldfish. The retinal piece is implanted such that the photoreceptor layer faced down on a culture dish. Most neurites begin to sprout from the centripetal edge of the retinal tissue in accordance with the radial orientation of optic fibers converging onto the optic disc *in situ* (Johns, Yoon & Agranoff, 1978). Figure 19.2(a) shows an example of such an asymmetric pattern of retinal neurites, most of which grew in the centripetal radial direction towards the phantom optic disc *in vitro*. In the absence of a proper target tissue, these retinal neurites tended to curl up to form clockwise spirals (Heacock & Agranoff, 1977) as they grew further on the poly-L-lysine coated culture dish. While the retinal culture was going, the same goldfish was revived for further experiment. Two and a half days after the retinal explantation a similar piece of tectal slab which contained the entire dorsoventral laminar structures was dissected from the caudal half of the left tectal lobe along the rostro-caudal axis near the lateral rim in the same goldfish (i.e. the co-cultured retinal and tectal tissues were approximately matched in their topographic relation). The tectal slab was implanted on the culture dish so that the *ependymal* layer was at the bottom and the *stratum marginale* faced upward. It was oriented in such a configuration that gave a maximal opportunity for the nearby growing tips of retinal neurites to contact the tectal tissue. Figure 19.2(b) shows the retinal and the rectal tissues co-cultured for three days. Note that the retinal neurites changed the pattern of their outgrowths after the delayed implantation of the tectal tissue: a majority of retinal neurites tended to grow preferentially more or less straight towards the tectal tissue as the co-culture progressed (see Fig. 19.2(c) & (d)). About five days after the co-culture, only those neurites which had succeeded in invading the tectal tissue remained and other retinal neurites eventually disappeared. Some of the retinal neurites which invaded the tectal explant detached from the substratum of the culture dish and appeared to form suspended cables that linked the retinal and tectal tissues. Histological examination of the tectal

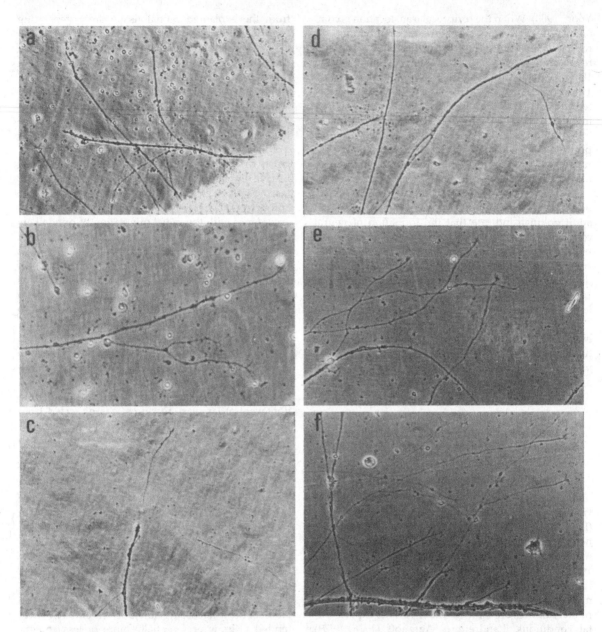

Fig. 19.1. Micrographs of neurites sprouting from retinal tissues *in vitro* after explantation from adult goldfish. (a) several neurites which grew *de novo* 12 hrs after retinal explantation. (b), (c) and (d) various patterns of branching in neuritic outgrowths at later stages. (e) mature growth cones with bush-like microspikes at the tips. (f) a fasciculation of several neurites a week after retinal explantation.

tissue revealed that some of the invaded retinal neurites coursed from the *stratum periventriculare* up to the *stratum opticum*. It was impossible, however, to determine the exact sites of termination of these invaded retinal neurites under the present experimental conditions.

Another example of the retino-tectal co-culture experiment is shown in Fig. 19.3 at a higher magnifica-

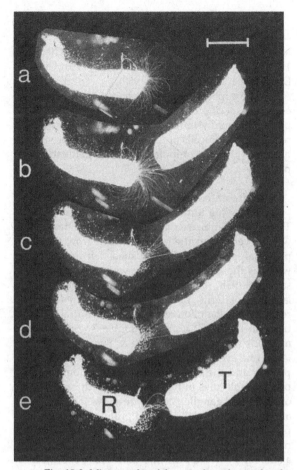

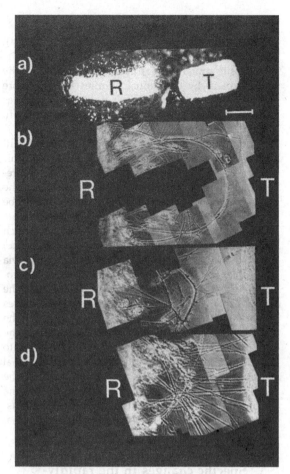

Fig. 19.2. Micrographs of the co-cultured retinal and tectal tissues, photographed under pseudo-dark field illumination of a Zeiss inverted microscope. (a) the pattern of neurite outgrowth from the centripetal edge of the retinal tissue (R) cultured for two days in the absence of any target tissue. (b) taken 3 days after co-culturing of a topographically matched tectal slab (T) with the retinal tissue. (c) the same pair at 5 days and (d) at 7 days after the co-culture. (e) the retinal and tectal tissues after fixation with Bodian fixative, 9 days after the co-culture. Both tissues detached afloat from the surface of the culture dish but their linkage by the invaded retinal neurites was not disrupted. Calibration bar: 1 mm.

Fig. 19.3. Photomicrographs of co-cultured retinal and tectal tissues. (a) taken under pseudo-dark field illumination at a low magnification. The calibration bar is 680 µm in (a). The tectal tissue (T) was just introduced to the retinal tissue (R), which had been cultured for 104.5 h. (b) a phase contrast micrograph of the same pair of retinal and tectal tissues at a higher magnification, 18 h after the co-culture. (c) the same pair at 26.5 h and (d) at 38.2 h after the co-culture. The calibration bar is 100 µm in (b), (c) and (d).

tion. In this case, the tectal tissue was introduced to the retinal culture 104.5 h after the initial explantation of the retinal tissue (Fig. 19.3(a)). At the beginning of the co-culture, the retinal neurites showed extensively curled clockwise spiral pattern. Some of them even formed loops, curling back towards the retinal tissue. The tectal tissue was implanted near one of these retinal loops. Figure 19.3(b) shows a close-up view of

this loop of retinal neurites and the nearby tectal tissue (on the right margin), examined under phase contrast 18 h after the co-culture. At this early stage only a few retinal neurites came off the loop and invaded the tectal tissue. As the co-culture progressed further, the same loop of retinal neurites underwent extensive changes. About 26.5 h after the co-culture, more and more retinal neurites were found to divert from the spiral course and tended to grow directly towards the tectal tissue (Fig. 19.3(c)). The loop of retinal neurites gradually diminished at around 38.2 h (Fig. 19.3(d)) and almost all surviving retinal neurites invaded the tectal tissue straightforwardly. As the invasion of the tectal explant by the retinal neurites became more extensive, the distance between the two tissues became shorter (from about 0.5 mm in Fig. 19.3(b) to about 0.37 mm in Fig. 19.3(d)).

The results of the present co-culture experiment suggest that the tectal tissue exerts a positive trophic influence which attracts retinal neurites to grow preferentially towards their main target tissue *in vitro*. The trophic influence from the tectal tissue seems to be mediated by initial contacts between the tectal tissue and the growth cones of a few retinal neurites (which happen to touch the nearby tectal explant by chance) rather than through interactions over a distance via diffusable factors. When a tectal tissue was co-cultured at a distance (greater than 5 mm) from the retinal explant such that none of the retinal neurites contacted it, the tectal explant had no influence on the retinal neurites. Furthermore, an addition of the supernatant fraction of homogenated tectal tissue into the culture medium did not affect the pattern of retinal neurite outgrowths. The attractive influence of the tectal tissue on the retinal neurites may be an outcome of complex sequences of mutual trophic interactions, mediated by molecular messages between the retinal ganglion cells and tectal cells.

Specific changes in the rapidly-transported proteins in the axons of retinal ganglion cells during their regrowth, interactions with their target tissue, and the compression of the visual projection

During the course of optic fiber regeneration in adult goldfish, the retinal ganglion cells undergo distinct changes in their metabolism and axoplasmic transport of proteins, ribonucleic acids (RNA), and lipids (for review see Grafstein & Forman, 1980; Ochs, 1983). The membrane constituents which will be incorporated into the growing tips of axons are synthesized in the cell bodies of the neurons and conveyed to the growth cones in the rapid phase of orthograde axoplasmic transport (McEwen & Grafstein, 1968; Droz, Rambourg & Koenig, 1975; Grafstein, Forman & McEwen, 1972; Forman, McEwen & Grafstein, 1971; Lorenz & Willard, 1978). During the course of axonal regeneration from the retinal ganglion cells in adult goldfish, the overall amount of various macromolecules increases as compared with the intact normal side (Grafstein & Murray, 1969; Forman, McEwen & Graf-

stein, 1971; Heacock & Agranoff, 1976, 1982; McQuarrie & Grafstein, 1982; Quitschke & Schechter, 1984; Quitschke, Francis & Schechter, 1980; Giulian, DesRuisseaux & Cowburn, 1980).

The following neurochemical experiments examine specific changes in the molecular spectral pattern of rapidly-transported proteins in the axons of retinal ganglion cells at different stages after various types of surgical manipulations of the goldfish visual pathways.

Differential changes in specific proteins following unilateral optic nerve crush

The axons of entire retinal ganglion cells in the left eye were severed and then allowed to regrow from the proximal stump of the crushed left optic nerve whereas those in the right eye were left intact in the same goldfish. At various post-operative periods, the labeling patterns of proteins transported in the regenerating ganglion cell axons were contrasted with those in the intact axons by double-isotope labeling methods (Benowitz, Shashoua & Yoon, 1981) as follows: one eye received an intraocular injection of ^{3}H-proline and the other eye the same amount of ^{14}C-proline molecules in the same fish. Both populations of the retinal ganglion cells were allowed to incorporate these differentially labeled proline molecules into proteins and to transport a minute fraction of the newly synthesized proteins from the soma into the axons for 4–5 h after the injection. This post-injection survival time was found to be optimal for collecting labeled retinal ganglion cell proteins that were transported in the rapid phase (Grafstein, Forman & McEwen, 1972). For each time-point studied, the two differentially labeled optic nerves, one containing the regenerating axons and the other the intact axons of retinal ganglion cells, were dissected free, combined and co-processed for gel electrophoretic separation of proteins according to their molecular weights (Benowitz *et al.*, 1981). Gel lanes containing experimental protein samples were calibrated for molecular weights and serially sectioned at 1 mm intervals. The rates of nuclear disintegration per minute (dpm) for ^{3}H and ^{14}C emitted from the differentially labeled retinal proteins in each gel slice were counted with a scintillation counter. The fraction of total radioactivity (in dpm) in every 1 mm gel slice of a given experimental time-point was computed for both isotopes ^{3}H and ^{14}C and their normalized labeling profiles along the molecular weight range were plotted for comparison (Fig. 19.4). The double-labeling method is used to detect a relative spectral difference in specific proteins at a particular molecular weight

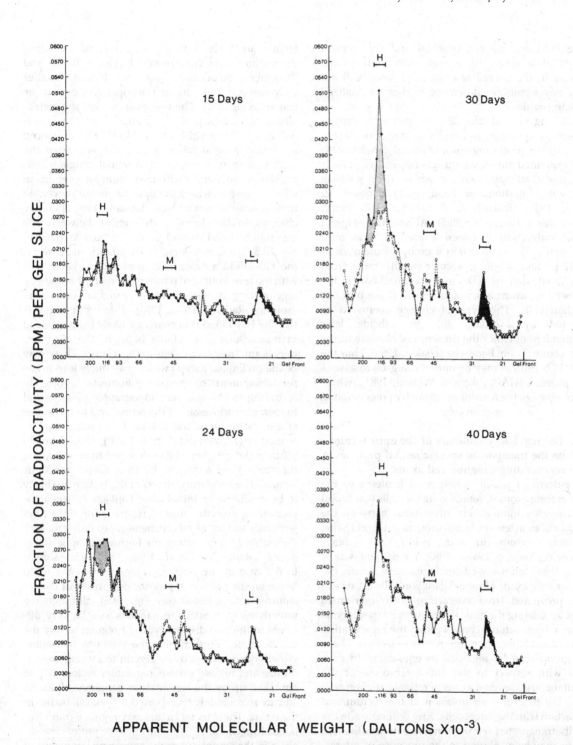

APPARENT MOLECULAR WEIGHT (DALTONS X10⁻³)

Fig. 19.4. Labeling profiles of ³H- and ¹⁴C-proline incorporated into rapidly-transported proteins in the optic fibers of the group R(T¹), denoted by filled circles (●), and of the group R(T⁰), denoted by open circles (○). The ordinate indicates the fraction of total radioactivity (dpm) for each gel slice (1 mm thick). The abscissa indicates the apparent molecular weight. H, the molecular weight range between 110 and 145 kDa; M, 43–49 kDa; and L, 24–27 kDa. The days indicate post-operative periods after bilateral optic nerve crush. (Reprinted from Yoon *et al.*, 1986).

range between the experimental and the control groups at a given time-point. Any non-specific changes in the overall amount of proteins will not show any significant difference in their normalized labeling profiles.

Using such double-labeling protocol, specific changes in rapidly-transported membrane bound proteins in the regenerating axons of retinal ganglion cells were examined during various post-operative periods after unilateral optic nerve crush in adult goldfish (Benowitz, Shashoua & Yoon, 1981; Benowitz & Lewis, 1983; Heacock & Agranoff, 1982; Perry, Burmeister & Grafstein, 1985). At an early stage of axonal outgrowth (between 8 and 15 days after unilateral optic nerve crush) a group of membrane-bound proteins whose molecular weights range from 43 to 49 kilo-daltons (kDa) increases markedly in the regenerating axons as compared with those of intact ganglion cells. This type of change seems to be activated by axotomy and to subside later independent of either the presence or absence of the optic tectum (Yoon, Benowitz & Baker, 1986). Thus the 43–49 kDa protein may be one of the growth associated proteins (GAP) (Skene & Willard, 1981), which are involved in the neuritic outgrowth of regenerating axons of retinal ganglion cells.

The regulatory influence of the optic tectum on the transport of specific retinal proteins in regenerating ganglion cell axons

The pattern of rapidly-transported proteins in the regenerating axons of retinal ganglion cells was found to change by intercellular interactions between the ingrowing axon terminals and their main target tissue, the optic tectum, in adult goldfish as follows (Benowitz, Yoon & Lewis, 1983; Yoon, Benowitz & Baker, 1986): following bilateral optic nerve crush, the regenerating axons of retinal ganglion cells in one eye were prevented from interacting with their main target by ablating the optic tectum in the experimental group, whereas in the control group the regenerating axons were allowed to reinnervate the tectum. These two groups can be regarded as equivalent to each other with respect to the initial regrowth of the simultaneously severed axons of retinal ganglion cells up to the time of their invasion of the tectum and interaction with the target cells. Any differences in the rapidly-transported retinal proteins between the two groups may be attributed to the presence of interactions between the ingrowing optic fibers and the tectum in one group and their absence in the other.

The rapidly-transported retinal proteins in the experimental group (axons regenerating without the tectum) and in the control group (axons reinnervating the tectum) were differentially labeled with ^{3}H- and ^{14}C-proline, respectively, and their labeling profiles were compared at various post-operative periods as shown in Fig. 19.4. The results show that the metabolism and/or transport of a group of retinal proteins with molecular weights of 110–145 kDa are enhanced maximally around 30 days after surgery when the regenerating axon terminals of retinal ganglion cells are allowed to interact with the tectum, in comparison with the case in which the optic fibers are prevented from interacting with the tectum. Post-operative changes in the labeling differences between the experimental and control groups are summarized in Fig. 19.5. The time-course of the specific increases in the 110–115 kDa proteins coincides remarkably well with the time-course of reinnervation of the tectum by regenerating axons of retinal ganglion cells after axotomy (Radel & Yoon, 1985). This result suggests that the 110–145 kDa proteins are likely to be involved in intercellular interactions between the axon terminals and their target cells in the tectum. These may be the preliminary steps which eventually lead to the reestablishment of proper retinotectal projection according to the coherent topographic polarity and topographic addresses of the retinal and tectal tissues (Yoon, 1980). Thus, the 110–145 kDa protein may be termed *target associated proteins* (TAP), whose metabolism in the ganglion cell bodies and transport along their axons are regulated by their target, the optic tectum. The regulatory effects of the tectum are likely to be mediated by initial close contacts between the pioneering growth cones of regenerating optic fiber terminals and the tectal cell membranes rather than by diffusable factors, acting on ingrowing optic fibers over a distance (Yoon *et al.*, 1986). This is quite similar to the case of the trophic influence from the tectal tissue on the pattern of neuritic outgrowth of the co-cultured retinal tissue (see Fig. 19.3), although the underlying molecular mechanisms may be very different in the two distinct types of regulations by the target tissue. Presumably, the contacts by retinal growth cones may activate certain tectal cells to synthesize and release various regulatory factors. These are taken up by the terminals of ganglion cell axons and are retrogradely transported to their cell bodies in the retina. These tectal factors may regulate transcriptions of specific *m*-RNA in the nuclei or protein metabolism in the cytoplasm or the axoplasmic transport of specific proteins, or any combinations of these events in the ganglion cell bodies.

Figures 19.4 and 19.5 also show an example of negative regulation of the tectum, which results in a

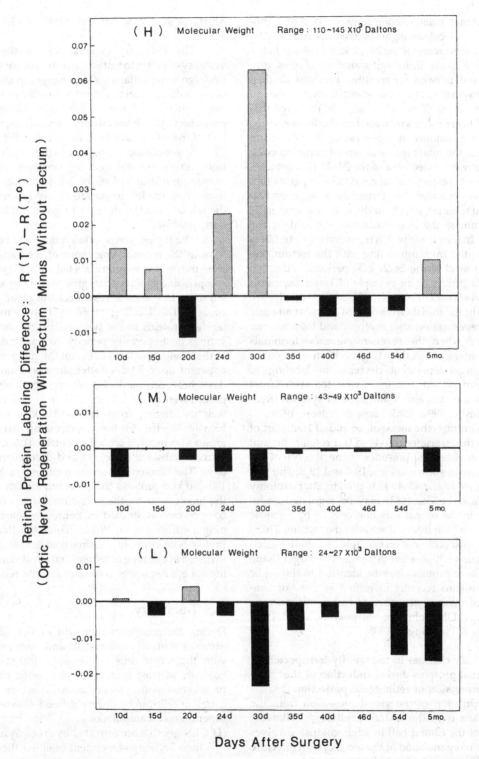

Fig. 19.5. Post-operative changes in labeling differences between the $R(T^1)$ group and $R(T^0)$ group. For the method of calculation of the labeling difference $[R(T^1) - R(T^0)]$ see the text. (Reprinted from Yoon *et al.*, 1986).

decreased metabolism and/or transport of retinal proteins with molecular weights between 24 and 27 kDa. The relative decrease of the 24–27 kDa proteins in the presence of the tectum begins around 30 days after surgery and persists for months. Previous double-labeling experiments on the goldfish after unilateral optic nerve crush (Benowitz et al., 1981) showed that the 24–27 kDa proteins increased markedly as early as 8 days after axotomy in regenerating axons as compared with the intact axons of retinal ganglion cells. Thus, the relative decrease of the 24–27 kDa proteins in the present experimental conditions suggests that interactions between the terminals of regenerating axons and their target cells in the tectum at around 30 days terminate the initial increase activated by the axotomy. In the case in which regenerating optic fibers are prevented from interacting with the tectum, the enhanced level of the 24–27 kDa persists. Thus, the 24–27 kDa protein is an example of *Target Dependent Growth Associated Proteins* (TD-GAP), which are involved in the initial outgrowth of axons at an early stage of regeneration after axotomy and they become terminated when the regenerating axon terminals begin to interact with their target cells in the tectum. Similar target-dependent decrease in labeling of rapidly-transported proteins, associated with target reinnervation, was also found in other systems (Redshaw & Bisby, 1984, 1985; Stone & Wilson, 1979).

In contrast, the metabolism and/or transport of the growth associated 43–49 kDa proteins do not depend on either the presence or the absence of the optic tectum as shown in Figs. 19.4 and 19.5. The 100-fold increase of the 43–49 kDa protein after axotomy (Benowitz & Lewis, 1983) may be regulated endogenously in the retinal ganglion cells or by extrinsic factors other than interactions with the tectum. Thus, the 43–49 kDa protein is an example of growth associated proteins which are independent of target tissue (GAP). These proteins may be identical to the acidic 46 kDa proteins recently identified as a major constituent of the growth cones of embryonic neurons (Pfenninger, Ellis, Johnson, Friedman & Somlo, 1983; Katz, Ellis & Pfenninger, 1985).

Specific changes in the rapidly-transported retinal proteins during induction of the compression of retinotectal projection

The compression of the visual projection from the entire retina onto the rostral hemitectum following excision of the caudal half in adult goldfish involves extensive reorganization of the tectal cytoarchitecture and the density and spatial distribution of retinotectal synapses within the hemitectum (Marotte, 1981, 1983;

Murray, Sharma & Edwards, 1982; Radel & Yoon, 1986).

The following experiments on the goldfish visual system aim to test whether retinal ganglion cells undergo certain characteristic changes in their metabolism and/or axonal transport of specific proteins during induction of the compression of retinotectal projection. After bilateral optic nerve crush, the caudal half of the left tectal lobe is excised in adult goldfish. Thus, regenerating axons of ganglion cells from the right retina are induced to compress within the remaining rostral half of the left tectal lobe whereas those from the left retina are allowed to reinnervate the whole extent of the intact right tectal lobe in the same goldfish.

The rapidly-transported membrane bound proteins in the regenerating axons of the ganglion cells from the right retina were labeled with ^{3}H-proline (the compressing experimental group) and those from the left retina (the uncompressed control group) with ^{14}C-proline. The labeling profiles of the differentially labeled proteins in the two groups are compared at various post-operative periods. No major differences in the labeling patterns between the two groups were apparent up to 30 days after surgery. From 40 to 55 days, however, marked differences between the two groups were observed: retinal proteins with molecular weights ranging from 180 to 210 kDa were more heavily labeled in the compressing experimental group as compared with the control. This differential increase subsided thereafter and disappeared by 120 days. The time-course of the relative changes in the 180–210 kDa proteins coincides remarkably well with the time-course for the induction of retinotectal field compression as studied by neurophysiological mapping methods (Yoon, 1976b). Thus, the 180–210 kDa protein is an example of retinal proteins which may be involved in one type of reorganization of visual projections, i.e. *Compression Associated Proteins* (CAP).

Summary

During the course of regrowth of the axotomized axons of retinal ganglion cells and their interactions with the target cells in the optic tectum in adult goldfish, at least four types of specific changes in protein metabolism and/or axonal transport of retinal ganglion cells can be distinguished following various experimental manipulations:

(1) Changes that are activated by axotomy and which then decline independent of either the presence or the absence of the target, the optic tectum (e.g. the GAP 43–49 kDa proteins)

(2) Changes that are activated by axotomy and then terminated by interactions between the regenerating terminals of retinal ganglion cells and their target cells in the tectum (e.g. the TD-GAP 24–27 kDa proteins)

(3) Changes that are initiated by intercellular interactions between the optic fiber terminals and their target cells in the tectum (e.g. the TAP 110–145 kDa proteins)

(4) Changes that are involved in the orderly compression of the visual projection from the whole retina onto the rostral hemitectum (e.g. the CAP 180–210 kDa)

The intricate mutual interactions between the presynaptic neurons and their target postsynaptic cells involve complex sequences of specific molecular changes which remain hidden beyond our present vision.

Acknowledgement

I thank Frank A. Baker for technical assistance and Dr Larry Benowitz for collaboration in neurochemical experiments. The research was supported by grants from MRC and NSERC of Canada.

References

Benowitz, L. I. & Lewis, E. R. (1983) Increased transport of 44–49,000 dalton acidic proteins during regeneration of the goldfish optic nerve: a 2-dimensional analysis. *J. Neurosci.*, **3**, 2153–63.

Benowitz, L. I., Shashoua, V. E. & Yoon, M. G. (1981) Specific changes in rapidly transported proteins during regeneration of the goldfish optic nerve. *J. Neurosci.*, **1**, 300–7.

Benowitz, L. I., Yoon, M. G. & Lewis, E. R. (1983) Transported proteins in the regenerating optic nerve: regulation by interactions with the optic tectum. *Science*, **222**, 185–8.

Droz, B., Rambourg, D. & Koenig, H. L. (1975) The smooth endoplasmic reticulum: structure and role in the renewal of axonal membrane and synaptic vesicles by fast axonal transport. *Brain Res.*, **93**, 1–13.

Forman, D. S., McEwen, B. S. & Grafstein, B. (1971) Rapid transport of radioactivity in goldfish optic nerve following injection of labeled glucosamine. *Brain Res.*, **28**, 119–30.

Gaze, R. M. & Sharma, S. C. (1970) Axial differences in the reinnervation of goldfish optic tectum by regenerating optic fibers. *Exp. Brain Res.*, **10**, 171–81.

Giulian, D., DesRuisseaux, H. & Cowburn, D. (1980) Biosynthesis and intraaxonal transport of proteins during neuronal regeneration. *J. Biol. Chem.*, **255**, 6494–501.

Grafstein, B. & Forman, D. S. (1980) Intracellular transport in neurons. *Physiol. Rev.*, **60**, 1167–283.

Grafstein, B. & Murray, M. (1969) Transport of protein in goldfish optic nerve during regeneration. *Exp. Neurol.*, **25**, 494–508.

Grafstein, B., Forman, D. S. & McEwen, B. S. (1972) Effects of temperature on axonal transport and turnover of protein in the goldfish visual system. *Exp. Neurol.*, **34**, 158–70.

Heacock, A. M. & Agranoff, B. W. (1976) Enhanced labeling of a retinal protein during regeneration of optic nerve in goldfish. *Proc. Natl. Acad. Sci. USA*, **73**, 828–32.

Heacock, A. M. & Agranoff, B. W. (1977) Clockwise growth of neurites from retinal explant. *Science*, **198**, 64–6.

Heacock, A. M. & Agranoff, B. W. (1982) Protein synthesis and transport in the regenerating goldfish visual system. *Neurochem. Res.*, **7**, 771–88.

Hope, R. A., Hammond, B. J. & Gaze, R. M. (1976) The arrow model: retinotectal specificity and map formation in the goldfish visual system. *Proc. Roy. Soc. Lond.*, **B194**, 447–66.

Horder, T. J. (1971) Retention by fish optic nerve fibers regenerating to new terminal sites in the tectum of 'chemospecific' affinity for their original sites. *J. Physiol.*, **216**, 53–5P.

Johns, P. R., Heacock, A. M. & Agranoff, B. W. (1978) Neurites in explant culturee of adult goldfish retina derived from ganglion cells. *Brain Res.*, **142**, 531–7.

Johns, P. R., Yoon, M. G. & Agranoff, B. W. (1978) Directed outgrowth of optic fibers regenerating in vitro. *Nature*, **271**, 360–2.

Katz, F., Ellis, L. & Pfenninger, K. H. (1985) Nerve growth cones isolated from fetal rat brain. III. Calcium-dependent protein phosphorylation. *J. Neurosci.*, **5**, 1402–11.

Landreth, G. E. & Agranoff, B. W. (1976) Explant culture of adult goldfish retina: effect of prior optic nerve crush. *Brain Res.*, **118**, 299–303.

Landreth, G. E. & Agranoff, B. W. (1979) Explant culture of goldfish retina: a model for the study of CNS regeneration. *Brain Res.*, **161**, 39–53.

Lorenz, T. & Willard, M. (1978) Subcellular fractionation of intra-axonally transported polypeptides in the rabbit visual system. *Proc. Natl. Acad. Sci. USA*, **75**, 505–9.

Marotte, L. R. (1981) Density of optic terminals in half tecta of goldfish with compressed retinotectal projections. *Neurosci.*, **6**, 697–702.

Marotte, L. R. (1983) Increase in synaptic sites in goldfish tectum after partial tectal ablation. *Neurosci. Lett.*, **36**, 261–6.

Matthey, R. (1925) Recuperation de la vue après résection des nerfs optiques chez le triton. *C. R. Soc. Biol.*, **93**, 904–6.

Matthey, R. (1926) La Greffe de l'oeil. I. Etude histologique sur la greffe de l'oeil chez la larve de salamandre (*Salamandre maculosa*). *Rev. Suisse. Zool.*, **33**, 327–34.

McEwen, B. S. & Grafstein, B. (1968) Fast and slow components in axonal transport of protein. *J. Cell Biol.*, **38**, 494–508.

McQuarrie, I. G. & Grafstein, B. (1982) Protein synthesis and fast axonal transport in regenerating goldfish retinal ganglion cells. *Brain Res.*, **235**, 213–23.

Murray, M., Sharma, S. C. & Edwards, M. A. (1982) Target regulation of synaptic number in the compressed retinotectal projection of goldfish. *J. Comp. Neurol.*, **207**, 45–60.

Ochs, S. (1983) *Axoplasmic Transport.* New York: Academic Press.

Perry, G. W., Burmeister, D. W. & Grafstein, B. (1985) Changes in protein content of goldfish optic nerve during degeneration and regeneration following nerve crush. *J. Neurochem.*, **44**, 1142–51.

Pfenninger, K. H., Ellis, L., Johnson, M. P., Friedman, L. B. & Somlo, S. (1983) Nerve growth cones isolated from fetal rat brain. I. Subcellular fractionation and characterization. *Cell*, **35**, 573–84.

Quitschke, W., Francis, A. & Schechter, N. (1980) Electrophoretic analysis of specific proteins in the regenerating goldfish retinotectal pathway. *Brain Res.*, **201**, 347–60.

Quitschke, W. & Schechter, N. (1984) 58,000 Dalton intermediate filament proteins of neuronal and non-neuronal origin in the goldfish visual pathway. *J. Neurochem.*, **42**, 569–76.

Radel, J. D. & Yoon, M. G. (1985) Time-course of ultrastructural changes in regenerated optic fiber terminals of goldfish. *Brain Res.*, **342**, 168–71.

Radel, J. D. & Yoon, M. G. (1986) Dorsoventral extension of the optic fiber termination zone in the rostral hemitectum after excision of the caudal portion in goldfish. *Neurosci. Abstr.*, **12**, 33.3.

Redshaw, J. D. & Bisby, M. A. (1984) Fast axonal transport in central nervous system and peripheral nervous system axons following axotomy. *J. Neurobiol.*, **15**, 109–17.

Redshaw, J. D. & Bisby, M. A. (1985) Comparison of the effects of sciatic nerve crush or resection on the proteins of fast axonal transport in rat dorsal root ganglion cell axons. *Exp. Neurol.*, **88**, 437–46.

Schmidt, J. T., Cicerone, C. M. & Easter, S. S. (1978) Expansion of the half-retinal projection to the tectum in goldfish: an electrophysiological and anatomical study. *J. Comp. Neurol.*, **177**, 257–77.

Sharma, S. C. & Gaze, R. M. (1971) The retinotopic organization of visual responses from tectal implants in adult goldfish. *Archs. ital. Biol.*, **190**, 357–66.

Skene, J. H. P. & Willard, M. (1981) Changes in axonally transported proteins during axon regeneration in toad retinal ganglion cells. *J. Cell Biol.*, **89**, 86–95.

Sperry, R. W. (1943a) Effects of 180 degree rotation of the retinal field on visuomotor coordination. *J. exp. Zool.*, **92**, 263–79.

Sperry, R. W. (1943b) Visuomotor coordination in the newt (*Triturus viridesens*) after regeneration of the optic nerves. *J. Comp. Neurol.*, **79**, 33–5.

Sperry, R. W. (1944) Optic nerve regeneration with return of vision in *Anurans. J. Neurophysiol.*, **7**, 57–70.

Sperry, R. W. (1945) Restoration of vision after crossing of optic nerves and after contralateral transplantation of eye. *J. Neurophysiol.*, **8**, 15–28.

Sperry, R. W. (1948) Patterning of central synapses in regeneration of optic nerve in teleosts. *Physiol. Zool.*, **28**, 351–61.

Sperry, R. W. (1951) Regulative factors in the orderly growth of neural circuits. *Growth*, **10**, 63–87.

Sperry, R. W. (1963) Chemoaffinity in the orderly growth of nerve fiber patterns and connections. *Proc. Natl. Acad. Sci. USA*, **50**, 703–10.

Stone, G. C. & Wilson, D. L. (1979) Qualitative analysis of proteins rapidly transported in ventral horn motoneurons and bidirectionally from dorsal root ganglia. *J. Neurobiol.*, **10**, 1–12.

Stone, L. & Zaur, I. (1940) Reimplantation and transplantation of adult eyes in the salamander (*Triturus viridescens*) with return of vision. *J. Exp. Zool.*, **85**, 243–69.

Yoon, M. G. (1971) Reorganization of retinotectal projection following surgical operations on the optic tectum in goldfish. *Exp. Neurol.*, **33**, 395–411.

Yoon, M. G. (1972a) Reversibility of the reorganization of retinotectal projection in goldfish. *Exp. Neurol.*, **35**, 565–77.

Yoon, M. G. (1972b) Transposition of the visual projection from the nasal hemiretina onto the foreign rostral zone of the optic tectum in goldfish. *Exp. Neurol.*, **37**, 451–62.

Yoon, M. G. (1973) Retention of the original topographic polarity by the 180° rotated tectal reimplant in young adult goldfish. *J. Physiol.*, **233**, 575–88.

Yoon, M. G. (1975) Re-adjustment of retinotectal projection following reimplantation of a rotated or inverted tectal tissue in adult goldfish. *J. Physiol.*, **252**, 137–58.

Yoon, M. G. (1976a) Topographic polarity of the optic tectum studied by reimplantation of the tectal tissue in adult goldfish. In *The Synapse. Cold Spring Harb. Symp. quant. Biol.*, **40**, 503–19.

Yoon, M. G. (1976b) Progress of topographic regulation of the visual projection in the halved optic tectum of adult goldfish. *J. Physiol.*, **257**, 621–43.

Yoon, M. G. (1977) Induction of compression in the re-established visual projections on to a rotated tectal reimplant that retains its original topographic polarity within the halved optic tectum of adult goldfish. *J. Physiol.*, **264**, 379–410.

Yoon, M. G. (1979) Reciprocal transplantations between the optic tectum and the cerebellum in adult goldfish. *J. Physiol.*, **288**, 211–25.

Yoon, M. G. (1980) Retention of topographic addresses by reciprocally translocated tectal re-implants in adult goldfish. *J. Physiol.*, **308**, 197–215.

Yoon, M. G., Benowitz, L. I. & Baker, F. A. (1986) The optic tectum regulates the transport of specific proteins in regenerating optic fibers of goldfish. *Brain Res.*, **382**, 339–51.

20

Retinal pathways and the developmental basis of binocular vision

I. D. Thompson

The study of binocular mechanisms in visual cortex is just one of the many areas of vision influenced by Horace Barlow. How do cortical neurons utilise positional disparities to signal depth (Barlow, Blakemore & Pettigrew, 1967) and what developmental processes regulate the binocularity of cortical neurons (e.g. Barlow, 1975)? Although cortex is the first site in the geniculo-striate pathway in which binocular neurons are found, the fundamental basis of binocular vision is established much earlier in the visual pathway. It is the existence of bilateral retinal projections that ensures one point in visual space projects to one locus in the brain and so achieves the binocular congruence that is exploited by cortical neurons.

The binocular representation of each visual hemifield on the opposite side of the brain depends on the partial decussation of the retinal projections. For visual congruence, not only must the retinal decussation line coincide with the representation of the vertical meridian of the visual field but also the mapping rules of the resulting crossed and uncrossed projections must differ (Thompson, 1979, 1984). As Sperry (1963) recognised, there has to be bilateral symmetry in the representation of the nasotemporal retinal axis and a developmental mechanism that ensures retinal ganglion cells from two different retinal regions, one nasal and one temporal, terminate in a common locus in the target nucleus. These rather stringent conditions for adult retinal projections are not fulfilled in the developing animal. In this chapter, I shall describe the features of retinal projections that permit binocular mappings, the development of some of these features and how they can be influenced by early experimental manipulations.

Introduction to the preparation

The establishment of orderly retinal projections occurs much earlier in development than the maturation of cortical binocularity. Indeed, for cats and monkeys, the process is essentially complete at the time of birth (see Shatz & Sretavan, 1986). The data presented here comes from hamsters and ferrets, which are both highly altricial species. They are also relatively laterally eyed, with small binocular fields of around 80°. Thus the uncrossed temporal crescent is relatively small and eccentric in the retina and the adult distribution of uncrossed terminals consequently restricted. These features can be defined in adult and neonatal animals by using the anatomical techniques illustrated in Fig. 20.1.

Tracer injected unilaterally into the subcortical visual pathways is taken up by retinal ganglion cell terminals and transported retrogradely to their cell bodies (Fig. 20.1A). If the retinae are prepared as flat-mounts, the relative contribution of ganglion cells to crossed and uncrossed pathways can be quantified. As indicated in the cartoon (see also Fig. 20.4A,B), the pattern of labelled cells divides the retina into two unequal parts: the uncrossed projection is almost entirely confined to the temporal crescent whereas the bulk of the crossed projection arises from nasal retina. The targets of the retinal axons can be revealed by injecting tracer into one eye, where it is taken up by the ganglion cells and transported anterogradely to their terminals (Fig. 20.1B). The label is distributed bilaterally and can be visualised either in brain sections or, as here, by making flat-mounts of the thalamus and mid-brain. Quantification of the terminal distribution is more complicated as axons as well as terminals can be labelled and the density of the label often varies from one reaction to another. But it is

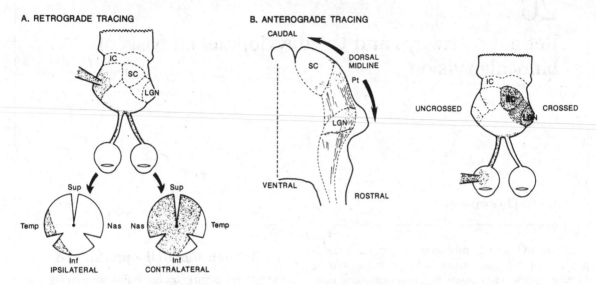

Fig. 20.1. The figure schematically illustrates the organisation of bilateral retinal pathways in carnivores and the anatomical procedures that can be used to characterise them. A. Retrograde transport of tracer unilaterally injected into the optic pathway reveals retinal decussation lines in the two retinae, which have been prepared as flatmounts. The majority of retinal ganglion cells labelled are found in the contralateral retina; only a small proportion are located in the ipsilateral retina, where they are packed into a discrete temporal crescent. Very few uncrossed cells are found outside this crescent and the crossed projection arising from temporal crescent is relatively weak. The abrupt changes in the density of labelled cells in the adult retinae are the crossed and uncrossed retinal decussation lines. They coincide with the retinal representation of the vertical meridian of the visual field, and thus are rather eccentric in laterally-eyed carnivores, such as the ferret. B. The anterograde transport of tracer injected into one eye reveals the projection zones of retinal axons: the lateral geniculate nucleus, pretectum and superior colliculus. Illustrated here are whole-brain and flat-mount preparations (in both cases, the cortical hemispheres have been removed). Reflecting the ganglion cell numbers, the crossed projection is much more extensive than the topographically restricted uncrossed projection. Abbreviations: LGN, lateral geniculate nucleus; SC, superior colliculus; IC, inferior colliculus; Pt, pretectum; Sup, superior; Inf, inferior; nas, nasal; temp, temporal.

possible to assess the proportion of the terminal nucleus occupied by the uncrossed terminals. When more precise topographical information is required, this can be obtained from electrophysiological mapping of the visual responses in the target nuclei.

Thus, the nature of the retinal decussation and of the uncrossed terminal distribution make good probes for examining mapping precision in the retinal pathways both in normal development and in animals manipulated early in postnatal life. The results presented in this chapter summarise changes in the numbers and distribution of retinal ganglion cells contributing to the partial retinal decussation and the associated changes in terminal distribution. Normal postnatal development is described first and then the consequences of three categories of manipulation are examined. The influence of the genome on map organisation is described; the albino mutation dramatically alters retinal decussation patterns (Guillery & Kaas, 1971; Guillery, 1986). Removal of one eye

has long been known to affect the organisation of the surviving retinal pathways (Lund et al., 1973; Rakic, 1981, 1986). Are the effects on cell death and on terminal distribution compatible and can they be explained as a disruption of binocular competition? Finally, neuronal activity plays a crucial role in normal cortical development (e.g. Barlow, 1975; Movshon & Van Sluyters, 1981): what is its involvement in the development of retinal pathways, when most adult aspects are attained prior to the onset of visual experience?

Normal development

When large unilateral injections of horseradish peroxidase (HRP) are made into the optic tract of adult pigmented ferrets a total of about 75 000 retinal ganglion cells are labelled of which only 6000 are found in the ipsilateral eye (Henderson, 1985; Morgan et al., 1987). These uncrossed cells are virtually all

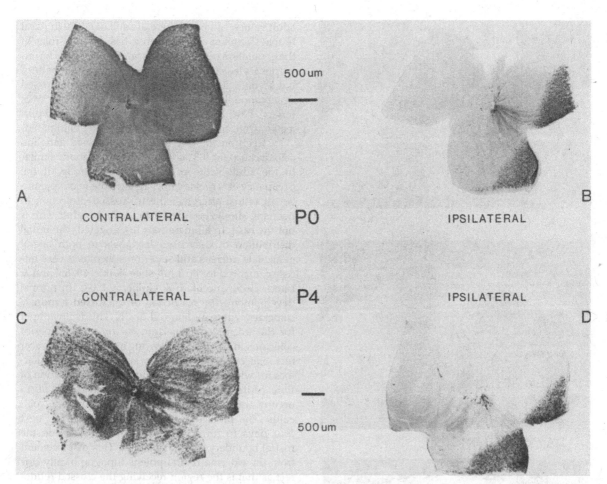

Fig. 20.2. Retinal decussation patterns in neonatal ferrets, following unilateral injections of wheatgerm agglutinin conjugated to horseradish peroxidase (WGA–HRP) into the optic pathway on P0 or P4. The retinae were prepared as flat-mounts, photographed in bright field and oriented so that superior is to the top of the figure and nasal is towards the centre. The condensed labelling of the temporal crescent ipsilateral to the injection is obvious (B, D). In both retinae, labelled axons can be observed exiting through the optic nerve head. A mirror-symmetric reduction of labelling in the crossed projection is marked only after injections on P4 (C); a strong crossed projection arises from temporal crescent on P0 (D).

packed into the temporal crescent where they constitute the majority of the ganglion cells – as in other carnivores, a small crossed projection does arise from the temporal crescent (Morgan *et al.*, 1987; see Fig. 20.4A,B). When similar injections are made into pigmented ferrets on the day of birth, there are marked differences in the retinal decussation pattern. Most dramatically, a total of around 160 000 ganglion cells are labelled with over 12 000 projecting ipsilaterally (Morgan & Thompson, 1985; Henderson *et al.*, 1988). As in the adult, the majority of these uncrossed cells are packed into the temporal crescent (see Fig. 20.2B). The decussation is not quite as precise in the newborn

as over 1700 uncrossed cells are found in nasal retina compared with an adult average of about 70. Quite unlike the adult, however, is the absence of an obvious decussation line in the crossed projection (Fig. 20.2A). This bilateral projection from the temporal crescent, which does not reflect bifurcating optic axons (fluorescent tracer studies), is quickly eliminated. By postnatal day 4 (P4), the excess of contralaterally projecting cells from temporal crescent has disappeared: a crossed decussation line is now discernible although many labelled cells persist at the retinal margin (Fig. 20.2C). Many uncrossed cells have also died; the number in temporal crescent (7000) is close to

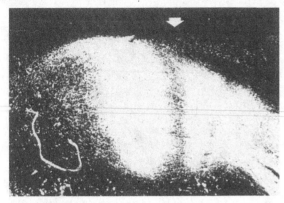

DAY 0

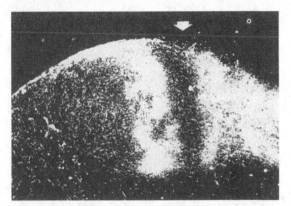

DAY 2

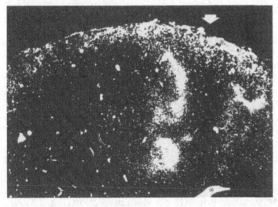

DAY 4

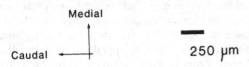

Medial

Caudal ←———

250 μm

Fig. 20.3. The uncrossed projection to the superior colliculus is shown in neonatal ferrets injected on day 0, day 2 and day 4. WGA–HRP was injected into one

adult values, although there are still over 600 in nasal retina. Ganglion cell death thus has different roles in the generation of retinal decussation lines in the ferret. It appears to establish the crossed decussation pattern but is only involved in fine tuning the uncrossed decussation line: as in the rodent (Martin *et al.*, 1983; Jeffery, 1984; Insausti *et al.*, 1984), the uncrossed projection from nasal retina is preferentially eliminated.

Even on the day of birth, uncrossed ganglion cells account for 9.3% of the total population, similar to the adult value of 8.1%. Consequently, if the occupancy of target territory reflects the relative number of retinal afferents, the uncrossed projection in neonates should be as restricted as in the adult. This is not the case. In all mammals investigated, the initial distribution of uncrossed terminals in both lateral geniculate nucleus and superior colliculus is very diffuse compared to the adult state (Rakic, 1976; Land & Lund, 1979; Cucchiaro & Guillery, 1984). In normal development, the restriction of uncrossed terminals coincides with ganglion cell death. This is illustrated for the uncrossed projection to the ferret superior colliculus in Fig. 20.3. Following an injection of tracer into one eye, the mid-brain is processed as a flat-mount, which reveals the topographic distribution of fibres. After injections on P0 (day 0), uncrossed fibres occupy the rostral two-thirds of the superior colliculus. The projection retracts rapidly over the next four days to form isolated clusters just inside the rostral boundary of the colliculus. This displacement from the extreme rostral pole is topographically correct as that is the region receiving the crossed retino-collicular projection from temporal crescent, corresponding to ipsilateral visual field. The pattern at P4 closely resembles that found in the adult, although the adult clusters are more circumscribed.

While ganglion cell death and terminal retraction obviously contribute to the normal development of binocular retinal projections, many puzzles about the process remain. Why is it that ganglion cell death appears to define the crossed decussation line but only refine the uncrossed one and what developmental mechanisms establish the retinal location of the latter? What is the exact relation between cell death and

eye, the brain reacted and prepared as a flat-mount; the superior colliculus was photographed through crossed polarizers under dark-field illumination. The terminal fibres, which appear white, progressively disappear from caudal colliculus to form small clusters just behind the rostral pole of the colliculus. The arrow indicates the rostral margin of the superior colliculus.

terminal retraction, events which are normally temporally coincident? Why are uncrossed terminals so initially exuberant when the proportion of ganglion cells giving rise to them is not?

Albinism and retinal pathways

In the adult pigmented carnivore, the uncrossed decussation line is more precisely specified than the crossed one (Fig. 20.4A,B). Very few ganglion cells project ipsilaterally from nasal retina whereas certain groups of ganglion cells in temporal crescent give rise to a crossed projection. The uncrossed decussation line is specified early in development, well before the phase of ganglion cell death. Whatever mechanisms are involved are dramatically disrupted by mutations that reduce the pigmentation of the retinal pigment epithelium. In adult albino ferrets, few ganglion cells in temporal crescent project ipsilaterally; instead they project contralaterally (Fig. 20.4C,D). It might be argued that the albino mutation merely alters the pattern of cell death such that the majority of cells dying in temporal retina come from the uncrossed projection rather than from the crossed projection, which is normally preferentially eliminated (Fig. 20.2). There are several lines of evidence against this hypothesis. First, the distribution of uncrossed terminals in albino mammals is reduced very early in development, before cell death (Cucchiaro & Guillery, 1984; Shatz & Kliot, 1982). Additionally, retrograde tracing studies reveal that this initially reduced distribution arises from a smaller population of ganglion cells, rather than diminished terminal arbors. The effect of albinism on the numbers of uncrossed cells in the ferret retina is shown in Table 20.1. Many fewer uncrossed ganglion cells are seen in newborn albino ferrets and about half of those will subsequently die. In neonatal albino ferrets, cell death in the crossed projection fails to create a crossed decussation line. The aberrant crossed projection in adult albino ferrets can also be revealed from electrophysiological mapping of the lateral geniculate where it gives rise to a representation of the ipsilateral visual hemifield that displays a retinotopic mapping appropriate for an *uncrossed* projection (Morgan, 1986), as in the Siamese cat (Guillery & Kaas, 1971).

It has been suggested that differential cell death was important in generating the albino anomaly in rodents (Land *et al.*, 1981), possibly because rodents do not show an obvious crossed decussation line (the majority of cells in temporal crescent project contralaterally). However, the reduction in albino hamsters does not seem to depend on cell death. Figure 20.5 shows the total number of uncrossed ganglion cells labelled after unilateral injections of tracer at various postnatal ages. At all ages, the mean number of uncrossed cells in albinos is lower than in pigmented animals and changes with a similar time-course. At the peak of the uncrossed projection (P2–P4), there is much more variability between animals: individual albino animals may show a larger uncrossed projection than individual pigmented neonates. The action of the albino mutation of uncrossed cell numbers is easier to quantify than its action on the extent of uncrossed terminal distributions.

While it is clear that the albino mutation shifts the retinal location of the initial uncrossed projection, it is not understood how this depends on the absence of melanin in the retinal pigment epithelium – nor are the mechanisms which relate the position of decussation lines to the laterality of the eyes, and thus degree of binocularity, in different species. However the topography of the re-routed temporal projection in albinos does suggest that mapping rules for most temporal retina cells are independent of the laterality of their projection.

The effects of unilateral eye removal

It has long been known that removal of one eye early in development leaves a much more extensive uncrossed terminal distribution than normal (Lund *et al.*, 1973; Rakic, 1981; Cucchiaro & Guillery, 1984), reflecting stabilisation of the early exuberant projection (Land & Lund, 1979). Enucleating also reduces the extent of retinal ganglion cell death (Jeffery, 1984; Insausti *et al.*, 1984; Williams *et al.*, 1983; Rakic & Riley, 1983). Does the extent and topography of the rescued retinal ganglion cells correlate with the stabilised terminal distribution?

The effects of enucleation on the uncrossed retino-geniculate projection in ferrets are illustrated in Fig. 20.6. In the normal pigmented animal, the terminals occupy discrete laminae in the lateral geniculate whereas, after removal of one eye on the day of birth, the terminals from the remaining eye now occupy the whole of the structure (Fig. 20.6A,B). The effect is even more dramatic in albinos (Fig. 20.6C,D). The intact adult has uncrossed label concentrated into discrete clusters scattered through the nucleus whereas in the enucleate the uncrossed terminals spread across the nucleus; the label is not completely continuous, obvious periodicities are apparent. Enucleation seems to stabilise the exuberant neonatal pattern of retinal projections (Cucchiaro & Guillery, 1984). Has it also stabilised the neonatal number of

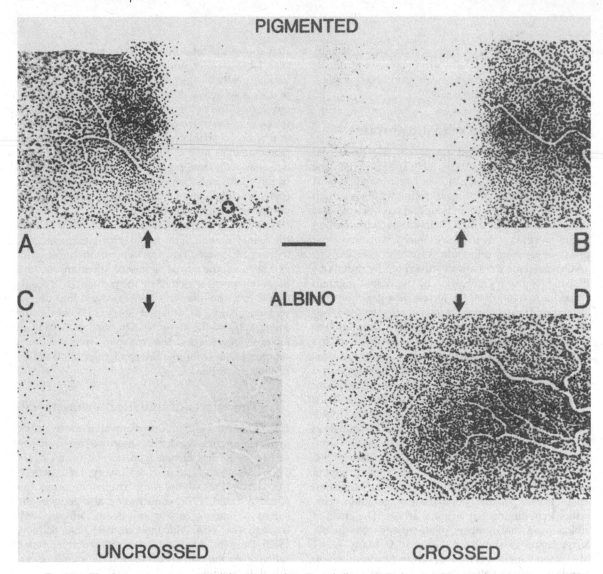

Fig. 20.4. The decussation pattern in adult pigmented (A, B) and albino (C, D) ferrets, after unilateral injections of HRP into the lateral geniculate nucleus and optic tract. Unlike Fig. 20.2, the retinae are not presented in mirror symmetry so that, in all four micrographs, temporal retina is to the left. The micrographs are of similar regions of retina, mid-way between optic disc and temporal retinal margin. (The arrows indicate the mid-point). Melanocytes in the underlying pigment epithelium are visible in A (asterisk). Scale = 500 μm. (Taken with permission from Morgan, Henderson & Thompson (1987) *Neuroscience* **20**:519–35).

uncrossed ganglion cells? The effects of enucleation on ganglion cell numbers are given in Table 20.1, from which it is clear that there are more uncrossed cells in the enucleate than in the normal adult. However, the effect is relatively small: the majority of uncrossed ganglion cells still die. Pigmented ferrets have about 1700 more cells and albino ferrets about 900. In both strains the increase in cells in nasal retina is the more marked. It would appear that removing one eye has a

greater effect on the distributions of terminals than on the survival of ganglion cells.

It might be argued that relatively few ganglion cells were rescued because the enucleation was performed relatively late in development: the bulk of cell death is complete within 4 days of birth. Perhaps prenatal enucleation would be more effective. This argument can be addressed by examining the effects of enucleation in the hamster, in which the number of

Table 20.1. *Ganglion cell numbers in the ferret uncrossed retinal projection*

	N	Temporal crescent	Nasal	Total
Pigmented ferrets:				
P0	3	12569 (1149)	1735 (464)	14304 (1451)
P4	5	7248 (449)	682 (280)	7930 (1273)
Adult	3	6029 (188)	71 (3)	6100 (191)
Enucleate	3	6765 (542)	1048 (360)	7813 (559)
Albino ferrets:				
P0	3	2567 (58)	3066 (1661)	5633 (1709)
P4	4	2452 (152)	1660 (449)	4112 (491)
Adult	5	1264 (212)	191 (62)	1455 (181)
Enucleate	3	1580 (161)	740 (91)	2319 (247)

The table gives the numbers (± standard errors) of ipsilaterally projecting retinal ganglion cells in pigmented and albino ferrets following large unilateral injections of horseradish peroxidase into the lateral geniculate nucleus and optic tract. The four groups of animals comprised neonates at two ages (injected on P0 and P4, perfused 1 day later), normal adults (1–2 days survival) and adult animals in which one eye had been removed on the day of birth (1–2 days survival after tracer application). The retinae were prepared as flat-mounts and labelled cell numbers counted within the temporal crescent and in nasal retina, outside the crescent.

uncrossed ganglion cells does not peak until 2–4 days after birth (Fig. 20.5). Removal of one eye in the hamster rescues a maximum of about 1000 ganglion cells, compared with normal loss of about 3000. The rescue is no greater, and may be less, if enucleation is performed on the day of birth rather than four days later. If the effects of enucleation are to be explained simply by the removal of binocular competition (e.g. Rakic, 1986), then early enucleation should be very effective – eliminating any possibility of competition. In fact very early eye removal actually *reduces* the uncrossed projection (Godement *et al.*, 1987; Guillery, 1989). Indeed, Fig. 20.7 suggests that the rescue may be related to the size of the projection at the time of eye removal: perhaps enucleation provides trophic action through the denervation of synaptic sites or the generation of axonal degeneration products?

The topographic expansion across the nucleus can be mapped electrophysiologically. In both pigmented and albino enucleated ferrets, the majority of receptive fields recorded in the lateral geniculate nucleus ipsilateral to the remaining eye correspond to input from temporal crescent, although fields in the ipsilateral hemifield (nasal retina) can be detected (Fig. 20.8A,B). After enucleation, the uncrossed projection in pigmented animals remains topographically ordered. A relatively orderly retinotopic map is also found in the expanded uncrossed projection of albino

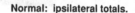

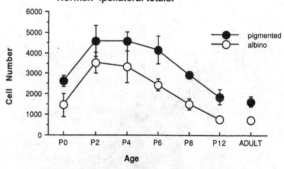

Fig. 20.5. The mean number (±standard error) of uncrossed ganglion cells are shown for both pigmented and albino hamsters at various ages. The injections were made into the lateral geniculate and optic tract on one side and the total number of labelled cells in the ipsilateral retina counted, both inside and outside the temporal crescent. Survival time was 1 day.

enucleates (Fig. 20.8C). In intact albinos, it is very difficult to record input from the ipsilateral eye even though the number of cells terminating is not much less than in the enucleate. In the intact albino, the terminals are densely clustered (Fig. 20.6B) and ganglion cells must be terminating in retino-topically inappropriate locations. Enucleation permits an

Normal

Enucleate

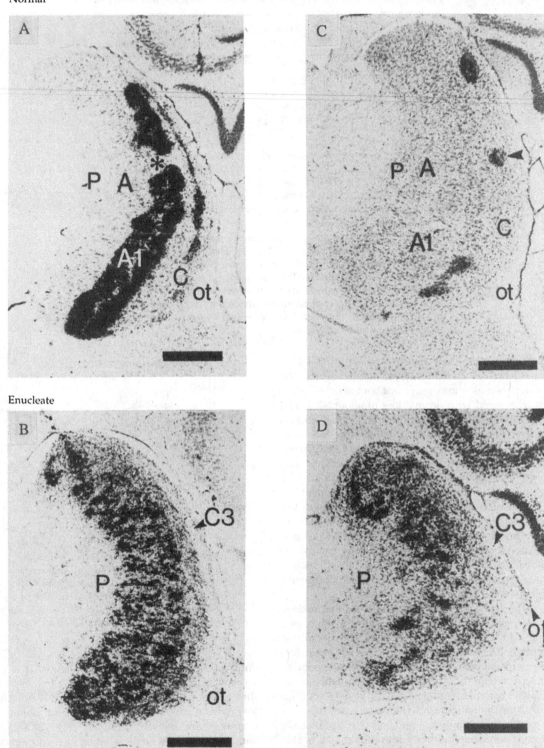

expansion of the projection which then forms a coherent map.

The consequences of unilateral eye removal seem to be more dramatic on the distribution of uncrossed terminals than on the numbers of the ganglion cells. Although the population of uncrossed cells in nasal retina is proportionately increased, from the evidence of physiological mapping, they do not explain the terminal expansion into topographically incorrect locations. Examination of the sensitive period for the effects of enucleation suggests that the observed phenomena may not depend simply on removal of binocular competition but also on the introduction, by eye removal, of novel trophic stimuli.

The role of neuronal activity

Changes in terminal distribution, in ganglion cell death and sensitivity to eye removal occur well before the onset of visual responsiveness in all mammals. Ferrets open their eyes at around 32 days of age and hamsters at 16 days, by which time the adult retinal projection pattern has been established. Although visual experience plays a significant role in establishing and refining cortical binocularity, it can therefore have no role in establishing the basic pattern of retinal projections that form the substrate for binocular vision. However, even in visual cortex, it is clear that patterns of spontaneous neuronal activity can affect its development (Swindale, 1981; Stryker & Harris, 1986; Chapman *et al.*, 1986). Could spontaneous activity in retinal ganglion cells play any role in controlling ganglion cell death and terminal retraction? If so, is this simply a trophic effect or could patterned spontaneous activity provide information useful to the ordering of projections?

Hamsters received daily injections, into one or both eyes, of the sodium channel blocker tetrodotoxin (TTX) between days 4 and 12. The dose was calculated to inhibit sodium-based action potentials and record-

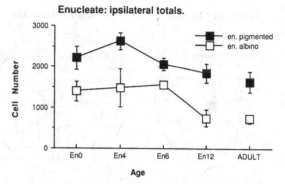

Fig. 20.7. The effects of uniocular enucleation at different neonatal ages on the number of ipsilaterally projecting ganglion cells is illustrated for both pigmented and albino hamsters. Neonatal hamsters had one eye removed under anaesthesia on P0, P4, P6 or P12. When adult, they received unilateral injections of tracer into the optic tract and the total number of uncrossed cells was counted. The graphs show means ±standard error.

ings from older animals demonstrated that the dose did indeed block visually elicited responses in the superior colliculus. The effects on ganglion cell numbers, on uncrossed terminal distribution and on individual terminal morphology were examined. The TTX treatment had little effect on the overall number of retinal ganglion cells in either the crossed or the uncrossed projection to the superior colliculus. Figure 20.9 illustrates the changes in uncrossed cell numbers after TTX treatment. The results indicate that blocking spontaneous activity alters the *pattern* rather than the *extent* of ganglion cell death.

There is a small increase in the total number of uncrossed ganglion cells (Fig. 20.9A) following TTX injections but this is not statistically significant compared to normals and is much less than that seen after enucleation on P4. However, the distribution of uncrossed retinal ganglion cells is altered in eyes that have received TTX injections: proportionately more are found in nasal retina (Fig. 20.9B). After binocular injections, the percentage of nasal cells approaches values seen in the enucleates. Interestingly, there is little change in untreated eyes when the other eye receives TTX. It would seem that uniocular TTX does not mimic uniocular enucleation.

As might be expected from the small changes in uncrossed cell number, the TTX treatment had relatively little effect on terminal distribution, certainly compared with the changes seen after enucleation. The uncrossed input to the hamster superior colliculus of normal and experimental

---

Fig. 20.6. Autoradiographs of the uncrossed retinogeniculate projection in ferrets. A, normal pigmented ferret; B, normal albino ferret; C, adult pigmented ferret that had one eye removed on the day of birth; D, adult albino ferret that had one eye removed on the day of birth. The animals received uniocular injections of ^{3}H-proline and survived for two days. The nucleus is sectioned parasagittally, dorsal is up and caudal to the right; bright field illumination, retinal terminals are dark. Scale = 500 μm.
Abbreviations: A, A1, C & C3, geniculate laminae; P, perigeniculate nucleus;) ot, optic tract.

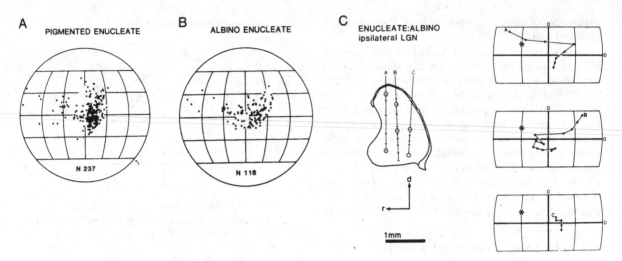

Fig. 20.8. Summary diagrams of the electrophysiological mapping of the uncrossed retino-geniculate input in enucleated ferrets, prepared as described by Price & Morgan (1987) and Morgan (1986). The positions of the optic discs were plotted and brought to a standard location, indicated by the asterisks (see Morgan et al., 1987). A. Pooled receptive field centre locations for 237 units activated through the ipsilateral eye in five pigmented enucleates. The majority of the fields are located in the binocular portion of contralateral visual hemifield, as in normal pigmented ferrets. However 21% of the receptive fields are scattered through the *ipsilateral* hemifield; these represent input from the uncrossed ganglion cells in *nasal* retina rescued by enucleation. B. Similar representation of 118 units activated through the ipsilateral eye in five albino enucleates. No such units were recorded in normal albino ferrets. In the enucleates, 26% of the fields were in the ipsilateral hemifield and the mean location of receptive fields in the contralateral hemifield was more peripheral than in pigmented enucleates. C. Examples of three electrode penetrations through the ipsilateral lateral geniculate of an albino enucleate. The penetrations are spaced rostrocaudally and indicate that visual responses could be recorded throughout the entire nucleus. The visuotopic order is not as precise as in a normal pigmented animal but overall trends can be seen. As the electrode moves ventrally the receptive fields move down in space. The representation of the nasotemporal retinal axis is more variable: there is a reversal on penetration A and some clustering of fields at the bottom of penetrations B and C.

animals is summarised in Fig. 20.10, which shows drawings of flat-mount preparations. Normally, the uncrossed label forms discrete clumps deep to the surface in rostro-lateral colliculus (Fig. 20.10A). After enucleation, the label remains spread across its whole extent (Fig. 20.10B) and extends into the superficial layers. TTX injections did not disrupt the normal process of terminal retraction from caudal and superficial superior colliculus but did affect the clustering of ipsilateral terminals. In projections from treated eyes (Fig. 20.10D), the label was both weaker and diffuse; very few animals had evidence of the discrete clumps seen in normals. These clumps were obvious in projections from the untreated eyes of uniocularly injected animals (Fig. 20.10C). The label in these animals was consistently stronger than in the treated projections and, sometimes, more clumps were seen than in normals.

This disparity in terminal label patterns with various TTX treatments is surprising, given the similarity in uncrossed cell numbers. A possible reason appeared on examination of the profiles of individual retinal axons after TTX treatment. After employing the same TTX injection schedules, small beads of HRP were placed in the brachium of the superior colliculus to label a few retinal axons. When axons from uninjected eyes are filled at P12, they show distinct, tightly clustered terminal arbors in the superficial collicular layers (Fig. 20.11A–C). Labelled axons from TTX-treated eyes were very different. They seemed to be less fasciculated in the *stratum opticum* and formed only weakly branching and diffuse terminal arbors (Fig. 20.11D–F). The axons labelled in this experiment come from the contralateral projection and showed a retarded pattern of arborisation, more like normal axons labelled at P4. The effect was similar whether the axons terminated in rostral (binocular) or caudal colliculus.

Abolishing spontaneous ganglion cell activity with TTX leaves the major phases of cell death and terminal retraction unaffected, although treated eyes no longer displayed preferential elimination of nasal

A

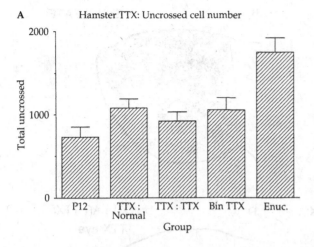

B

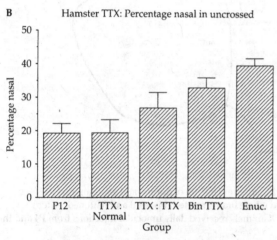

Fig. 20.9. The effects of intra-ocular TTX on ganglion cell numbers in the hamster uncrossed retino-collicular projects. Animals received injections of WGA–HRP into one superior colliculus on P12; after one day's survival the retinae were reacted, flat-mounted and the number of uncrossed cells counted. The experimental groups were: normal P12 animals (P12); animals enucleated at P4 (Enuc.); animals receiving daily uniocular injections of TTX (TTX:normal & TTX:TTX); animals receiving daily binocular injections of TTX (Bin TTX). The groups in which the uncrossed populations arose from TTX-treated eyes are TTX:TTX and Bin TTX. TTX injection schedules are as described in Thompson & Holt (1989). A. The total number of labelled cells in the retina ipsilateral to the injected colliculus. B. The percentage of the total number that were located outside temporal crescent, in nasal retina.

uncrossed cells. In addition to this effect on the pattern of cell death, it appears that TTX has a trophic effect in retarding the arborisation of individual retinal fibres.

Discussion

It is clear from a consideration of normal development that the adult pattern is not specified *ab initio*. Different aspects of binocular projections are shaped, to different extents, by regressive events, i.e. ganglion cell death and terminal retraction. Additionally, manipulations such as eye removal or intra-ocular TTX can disrupt the establishment of the normal pattern.

Ganglion cells

While the location of the uncrossed retinal decussation line is independent of cell death, how it is established and why it is so dramatically altered by the albino mutation is unclear. One hint may be in the relation between ganglion cell birthdates and decussation pattern in normally pigmented cats: there is a temporal shift of the decussation line and increased nasotemporal overlap for younger retinal ganglion cells (Walsh *et al.*, 1983). The albino abnormality can be described as an exaggerated version of this decussation pattern. Could lack of retinal melanin be delaying ganglion cell development (see Drager, 1985)? If the uncrossed decussation line is pre-specified, what is achieved by the phase of ganglion cell death in which over half all ganglion cells die. A crossed decussation line appears, the uncrossed cells in nasal retina are preferentially eliminated and topographical errors in the crossed projection die. The matching of the size of the retinal population to that of the target nuclei is another possibility (Cowan *et al.*, 1984). In this respect, the rescue of ganglion cells by early removal of one eye provides equivocal support: the number of cells rescued is relatively small considering that the uncrossed projection is given access to the entire target nucleus (Table 20.1; Fig. 20.7; Jeffery, 1984; Williams *et al.*, 1983; Rakic & Riley, 1983).

Although the overall extent of ganglion cell death is little affected by abolishing their spontaneous activity, the selective elimination of both crossed and uncrossed ganglion cells that make topographical errors is disrupted (O'Leary *et al.*, 1986a,b; Thompson & Holt, 1989). TTX treatment reduces the preferential loss of nasal uncrossed cells but not apparently by disrupting binocular competition (see also Van Sluyters *et al.*, this volume): the effect is specific to TTX-treated eyes. Coincidence of spontaneous activity indicates retinal neighbourliness (e.g. Mastronarde, 1983) and preservation of neighbourli-

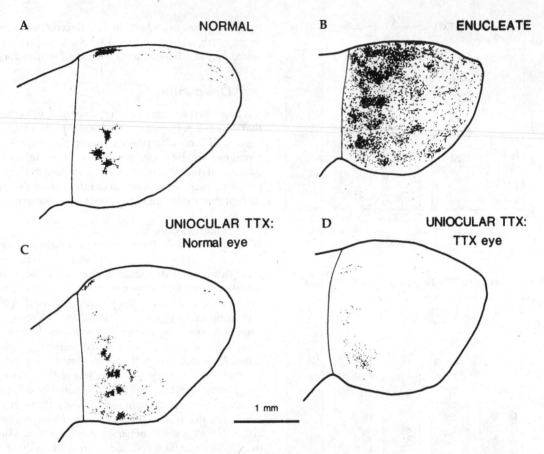

A   NORMAL   B   ENUCLEATE

UNIOCULAR TTX:
Normal eye

C

D   UNIOCULAR TTX:
TTX eye

1 mm

Fig. 20.10. Anterograde uncrossed label in flat-mounts of the superior colliculi of normal and experimental P12 hamsters. One eye was injected with HRP, the decorticated whole brains reacted, bisected and flattened. After clearing, the label was viewed in dark-field and drawn. TTX animals received daily uniocular injections from P4 and the enucleate had one eye removed under anaesthesia on P4.

ness is postulated as an important factor in map development (e.g. Willshaw & von der Malsburg, 1976, 1979; Schmidt & Edwards, 1983). Nasal uncrossed cells will be at a disadvantage in maintaining neighbour relations in the target nuclei, as they have a low retinal density at all stages of development. This relative disadvantage may disappear when all cells are silent, or when enucleation provides a new environment.

Retinal terminals

Consideration both of normal development and of the effects of manipulation indicate that ganglion cells display greater plasticity in the form and distribution of their terminals than in the number and distribution of their cell bodies. The distribution of terminals, of course, ultimately determines the retinotopic map in the target nuclei. Studies of the crossed projection indicate that, although some errors exist, the distribu-

tion of fibres is topographically appropriate even before the period of cell death (Jeffery, 1985; Thompson, unpublished observations). Establishment of early topographic order in retinal projections may well involve gradients of positional marker molecules (Bonhoeffer & Gierer, 1984; Constantine-Paton *et al.*, 1986). These marker systems cannot determine retinotopicity absolutely. For instance, although the earliest retinal projections in amphibia are ordered (Holt & Harris, 1983), the mismatch in the pattern of retinal and tectal growth means that retino-tectal connections cannot be fixed (Gaze *et al.*, 1979). Similarly, the topographic re-arrangements in the uncrossed retinal projection after enucleation (Thompson, 1979; Morgan, 1986; Fig. 20.8) indicate that markers cannot specify position invariantly in the mammalian visual pathway.

The mismatch between soma and terminal distributions is clearly seen early in the development of

NORMAL   TTX

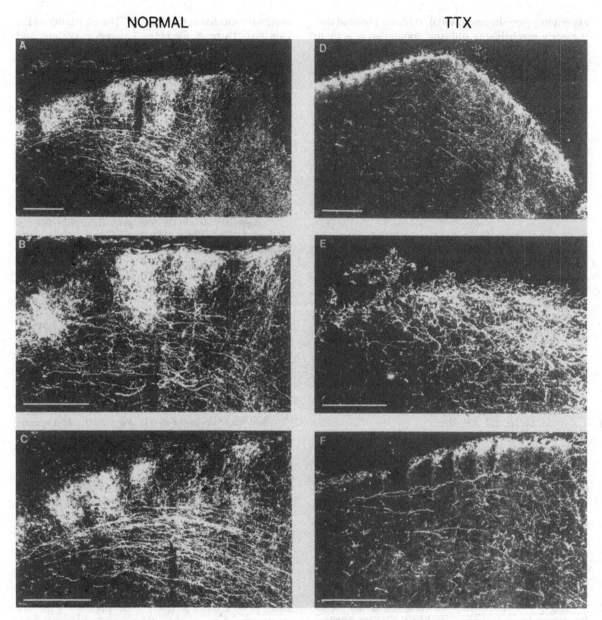

Fig. 20.11. The arbors of small numbers of retinal axons were labelled after daily uniocular injections of TTX by placing small beads of HRP bilaterally in the brachia of the superior colliculi (Cooper & Thompson, 1987). The colliculi were sectioned parasagittally and photographed under dark-field illumination. The photomicrographs in A–C come from the colliculus ipsilateral to the injected eye and show the dense, clustered arborisations of normal crossed axons. Micrographs D–F come from the colliculus contralateral to the injected eye; the TTX treated arbors are much sparser and do not form clusters. Scale = 200 μm.

uncrossed retinal projections. Prior to ganglion cell death, uncrossed terminals occupy more of the target nucleus than expected from the proportion of ganglion cells that project ipsilaterally. The expansion of terminals after enucleation is similarly greater than expected from the rescue of ganglion cells. TTX has a striking effect on terminal morphology, suggesting that normal activity is necessary for the maturation of axonal arbors (Fig. 20.11; Kalil *et al.*, 1986; Cooper & Thompson, 1987). Indeed, the fine details of the arbors of cat retinal ganglion cells are not established until after birth, when they depend on normal visual experience (see Sherman, 1985). It seems possible that the early mechanisms utilising spontaneous activity can be reiterated subsequently in both lateral geniculate and visual cortex to take advantage of the information present in patterned visual stimuli (see Barlow, 1975).

Acknowledgements

I am indebted to Anita Cooper, Zaineb Henderson, Christine Holt and James Morgan for much of the material included in this chapter. The assistance of Pat Cordery, Duncan Fleming, Lawrence Waters and Terry Richards is gratefully acknowledged. The work described was supported by grants from the MRC and E.P. Abrahams Fund to IDT. I am grateful for additional support from MRC Programme Grants to Prof. C. Blakemore.

References

Barlow, H. B. (1975) Visual experience and cortical development. *Nature*, **258**, 199–204.

Barlow, H. B., Blakemore, C. & Pettigrew, J. D. (1967) The neural mechanism of binocular depth discrimination. *J. Physiol.*, **193**, 327–42.

Bonhoeffer, F. & Gierer, A. (1984) How do retinal axons find their targets on the tectum? *Trends Neurosci.*, **7**, 378–81.

Chapman, B., Jacobson, M. D., Reiter, H. O. & Stryker, M. P. (1986) Ocular dominance shift in kitten visual cortex caused by imbalance in retinal electrical activity. *Nature*, **324**, 154–6.

Constantine-Paton, M., Blum, A. S., Mendez-Otero, R. & Barnstaple, C. J. (1986) A cell surface molecule distributed in a dorsoventral gradient in the perinatal rat retina. *Nature*, **324**, 459–62.

Cooper, A. M. & Thompson, I. D. (1987) Effects of intraocular injections of tetrodotoxin on the terminal arborization of retino-collicular axons in neonatal hamsters. *J. Physiol.*, **396**, 142P.

Cowan, W. M., Fawcett, J. W., O'Leary, D. D. M. & Stanfield, B. B. (1984) Regressive events in neurogenesis. *Science*, **225**, 1258–65.

Cucchiaro, J. & Guillery, R. W. (1984) The development of the retinogeniculate pathways in normal and albino ferrets. *Proc. Roy. Soc. Lond.*, B**223**, 141–64.

Drager, U. C. (1985) Calcium binding in pigmented and albino eyes. *Proc. Natl. Acad. Sci.* **82**, 6716–20.

Gaze, R. M., Keating, M. J., Ostberg, A. & Chung, S-H. (1979) The relationship between retinal and tectal growth in larval *Xenopus*: implications for the development of the retino-tectal projection. *Journal of Embryology and Experimental Morphology* **53**, 103–43.

Godement, P., Salaun, J. & Metin, C. (1987) Fate of uncrossed retinal projections following early or late prenatal monocular enucleation in the mouse. *J. Comp. Neurol.*, **255**, 97–109.

Guillery, R. W. (1986) Neural abnormalities of albinos. *Trends Neurosci.*, **9**, 364–7.

Guillery, R. W. (1989) Early monocular enucleations in foetal ferrets produce a decrease of uncrossed and an increase of crossed retinofugal components: a possible model for the albino abnormality. *J. Anat.*, **164**, 73–84.

Guillery, R. W. & Kaas, J. H. (1971) A study of normal and congenitally abnormal retinogeniculate projections in cats. *J. Comp. Neurol.*, **143**, 73–100.

Henderson, Z. (1985) Distribution of ganglion cells in the retina of adult pigmented ferret. *Brain Res.*, **358**, 221–8.

Henderson, Z., Finlay, B. L. & Winkler, K. C. (1988) Development of ganglion cell topography in ferret retina. *J. Neurosci.*, **8**, 1194–205.

Holt, C. E. & Harris, W. A. (1983) Order in the initial retinotectal map in *Xenopus*: a new technique for labelling growing nerve fibres. *Nature*, **301**, 150–2.

Insausti, R., Blakemore, C. & Cowan, W. M. (1984) Ganglion cell death during development of the ipsilateral retinocollicular projection in golden hamster. *Nature*, **308**, 362–5.

Jeffery, G. (1984) Retinal ganglion cell death and terminal field retraction in the developing rodent visual system. *Devel. Brain Res.*, **13**, 81–96.

Jeffery, G. (1985) Retinotopic order appears before ocular separation in developing visual pathways. *Nature*, **313**, 575–6.

Kalil, R. E., Dubin, M. W., Scott, G. & Stark, L. A. (1986) Elimination of action potentials blocks the structural development of retinogeniculate synapses. *Nature*, **323**, 156–8.

Land, P. W., Hargrove, K., Eldridge, J. & Lund, R. D. (1981) Differential reduction in the number of ipsilaterally projecting ganglion cells during the development of retinofugal projections in albino and pigmented rats. *Soc. Neurosci. Abstr.*, **7**, 141.

Land, P. W. & Lund, R. D. (1979) Development of the rat's uncrossed retinotectal pathway and its relation to plasticity studies. *Science*, **205**, 698–700.

Lund, R. D., Cunningham, T. J. & Lund, J. S. (1973) Modified optic projections after unilateral eye removal in young rats. *Brain, Behaviour and Evolution*, **8**, 51–72.

Martin, P. R., Sefton, A. J. & Dreher, B. (1983) The retinal location and fate of ganglion cells which project to the ipsilateral superior colliculus in neonatal hooded and albino rats. *Neurosci. Lett.*, **41**, 219–26.

Mastronarde, D. N. (1983) Correlated firing of cat retinal ganglion cells. I. Spontaneously active inputs to X- and Y-cells. *J. Neurophysiol.*, **49**, 303–24.

Morgan, J. E. (1986) *The Organization of the Retinogeniculate*

Pathway in Normal and Neonatally Enucleated Pigmented and Albino Ferrets. D. Phil. Thesis, University of Oxford (unpublished).

Morgan, J. E., Henderson, Z. & Thompson, I. D. (1987) Retinal decussation patterns in pigmented and albino ferrets. *Neurosci.*, **20**, 519–35.

Morgan, J. E. & Thompson, I. D. (1985) The distribution of ipsilaterally projecting retinal ganglion cells in neonatal pigmented and albino ferrets. *J. Physiol.*, **369**, 35P.

Movshon, J. A. & Van Sluyters, R. C. (1981) Visual neural development. *Ann. Rev. Psychol.*, **32**, 477–522.

O'Leary, D. D. M., Crespo, D., Fawcett, J. W. & Cowan, W. M. (1986a) The effect of intraocular tetrodotoxin on the postnatal reduction in the number of optic nerve axons in the rat. *Devel. Brain Res.*, **30**, 96–103.

O'Leary, D. D. M., Fawcett, J. W. & Cowan, W. M. (1986b) Topographic targeting errors in the retinocollicular projection and their elimination by selective ganglion cell death. *J. Neurosci.*, **6**, 3692–705.

Price, D. J. & Morgan, J. E. (1987) Spatial properties of neurones in the lateral geniculate nucleus of the pigmented ferret. *Exp. Brain Res.*, **68**, 28–36.

Rakic, P. (1976) Prenatal genesis of connections subserving ocular dominance in the rhesus monkey. *Nature*, **261**, 467–71.

Rakic, P. (1981) Development of visual centers in the primate brain depends on binocular competition before birth. *Science*, **214**, 928–31.

Rakic, P. (1986) Mechanism of ocular dominance segregation in the lateral geniculate nucleus: competitive elimination hypothesis. *Trends Neurosci.*, **9**, 11–15.

Rakic, P. & Riley, K. P. (1983) Regulation of axon number in primate optic nerve by prenatal binocular competition. *Nature*, **305**, 135–7.

Schmidt, J. T. & Edwards, D. L. (1983) Activity sharpens the map during the regeneration of the retinotectal projection in goldfish. *Brain Res.*, **269**, 29–39.

Shatz, C. J. & Kliot, M. (1982) Prenatal misrouting of the retinogeniculate pathway in Siamese cats. *Nature*, **300**, 525–9.

Shatz, C. J. & Sretavan, D. W. (1986) Interactions between retinal ganglion cells during the development of the mammalian visual system. *Ann. Rev. Neurosci.*, **9**, 171–207.

Sherman, S. M. (1985) Development of retinal projections to the cat's lateral geniculate nucleus. *Trends Neurosci.*, **8**, 350–5.

Sperry, R. W. (1963) Chemoaffinity in the orderly growth of nerve fibre patterns and connections. *Proc. Natl. Acad. Sci.*, **50**, 703–10.

Stryker, M. P. & Harris, W. A. (1986) Binocular impulse blockade prevents the formation of ocular dominance columns in cat visual cortex. *J. Neurosci.*, **6**, 2117–33.

Swindale, N. V. (1981) Absence of ocular dominance columns in dark-reared cats. *Nature*, **290**, 332–3.

Thompson, I. D. (1979) Changes in the uncrossed retinotectal projection after removal of the other eye at birth. *Nature*, **279**, 63–6.

Thompson, I. D. (1984) The generation of binocular maps in the hamster superior colliculus: normal and neonatally enucleated animals. In *Organizing Principles of Neural Development*, ed. S. C. Sharma, pp. 307–23. New York: The Plenum Press.

Thompson, I. D. & Holt, C. E. (1989) The effects of intraocular tetrodotoxin on the development of the retinocollicular pathway in the Syrian hamster. *J. Comp. Neurol.*, **282**, 371–88.

Walsh, C., Polley, E. H., Hickey, T. L. & Guillery, R. W. (1983) Generation of cat retinal ganglion cells in relation to central pathways. *Nature*, **302**, 611–14.

Williams, R. W., Bastiani, M. J. & Chalupa, L. M. (1983) Loss of axons in the cat optic nerve following fetal unilateral enucleation: an electron microscopic analysis. *J. Neurosci.*, **3**, 133–44.

Willshaw, D. J. & von der Malsburg, C. (1976) How patterned neural connections can be set up by self-organization. *Proc. Roy. Soc. Lond.*, **B194**, 431–45.

Willshaw, D. J. & von der Malsburg. C. (1979) A marker induction mechanism for the establishment of ordered neural mappings: its application to the retinotectal problem. *Phil. Trans. Roy. Soc. Lond.*, **B287**, 203–43.

21
Development of visual callosal connections

R. C. Van Sluyters, J. Olavarria and R. Malach

A prominent characteristic of the connections between cortical sensory areas is the close relationship that the overall pattern of these connections bears to the orderly representations of the sensory periphery that are a ubiquitous feature of these cortical areas. This relationship holds true not only for projections that arise and terminate within the same cerebral hemisphere, but also for the extensive system of interhemispheric cortico–cortical connections. For example, the topography of the interhemispheric pathway between cortical visual areas is such that the highest density of these connections is commonly found wherever the vertical meridian of the visual field is represented.

Although a great deal is known about the arrangement of visual cortico–cortical connections in the adult, our knowledge of the process by which this intricate pattern of connections is specified during development is much less complete. No doubt this is due at least in part to the abundant numbers and highly interwoven nature of the afferent and efferent cortical pathways, which makes it difficult to manipulate and study the development of any one set of projections in isolation. However, the interhemispheric visual cortico–cortical connections have a unique trajectory that carries them through the corpus callosum, a broad fiber tract that is visible in the interhemispheric fissure from an early stage of development onward. For this reason, much of what we know about the development of visual cortico–cortical connections comes from studies of the visual callosal pathway. Since it is reasonable to assume that similar mechanisms guide development of callosal and ipsilateral cortico–cortical connections, continued study of the more readily accessible interhemispheric pathway appears to offer the best chance for increasing our understanding of the factors responsible for

development of the other, less accessible, visual cortico–cortical projections.

The remainder of this chapter reviews the results of several of our recent experiments on development of the visual interhemispheric pathway in the rat. This work was undertaken in an effort to understand the mechanisms underlying the ontogeny of this highly organized cortico–cortical pathway. In performing these studies, we used enzymatic and autoradiographic tracing techniques to demonstrate the overall distribution of visual callosal connections in tangential and radial sections through the posterior neocortex of normally reared and neonatally enucleated pigmented (Long Evans) rats ranging in postnatal age from 3 days to adult. The details of this work, including complete descriptions of the methods used and the number of animals studied in each experimental condition, are presented in our recent publications (Olavarria & Van Sluyters, 1985; Olavarria *et al.*, 1987)

The pattern of visual callosal connections in the adult rat

At the beginning of our studies of the development of visual callosal connections, we examined the overall arrangement of connections in this pathway in normally reared adult rats, using the same anatomical techniques we would subsequently use to study newborn and neonatally enucleated rats. The results of this initial study were largely confirmatory in nature, and an example of our findings is shown in Fig. 21.1. Like a large number of previous workers (see Olavarria & Van Sluyters, 1985 for references), we found that callosal connections in the rat are densely and fairly homogeneously aggregated wherever there is a cortical representation of the visual vertical meridian. Thus, an elongated band of callosal connections strad-

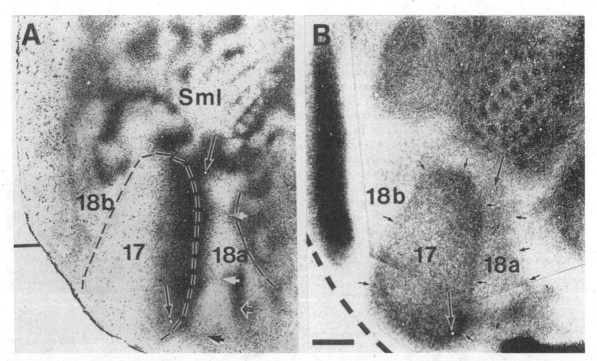

Fig. 21.1. Tangential distribution of callosal connections and its relationship to areas 17 and 18 in normally reared adult rat. Low-magnification brightfield views of adjacent 40-μm tangential sections through the flattened posterior neocortex of the right cerebral hemisphere following multiple injections of the tracer horseradish peroxidase (HRP) into the oppoiste hemisphere. Medial is to the left, and posterior is down. A. Unstained HRP-tested section through layer IV showing distribution of callosal cells and terminations in areas 17 and 18, and a portion of primary somatosensory cortex (SmI). Arrowheads and hollow arrow indicate callosal bands within the interior of area 18a. B. Montage of two myelin-stained sections separated by 40 μm, showing myeloarchitecture of areas 17, 18 and SmI. Honeycomb pattern related to SmI barrelfield in upper right portion of B is enhanced due to concomitant staining of cell bodies. Long arrows indicate locations of two penetrating blood vessels used to superimpose sections in A and B in a camera lucida. The borders of areas 17 and 18a in A (interrupted lines) were determined by tracing around the myelin patterns for these areas shown in B (small arrows). Scale bar = 1.0 mm. (Originally published in Olavarria & Van Sluyters, 1985.)

dles the border between area 17 and the lateral extrastriate visual areas that are contained within architectonic area 18a. This band is rather uniform in width (about 1.5 mm), and appears to be divided assymetrically by the 17/18a border, so that a greater portion of it lies in area 17 than in area 18a. Due to the ovate shape of area 17, the callosal band occupies a greater portion of the width of striate cortex anteriorly, where this area is fairly narrow, than it does posteriorly, where area 17 broadens noticeably.

In addition to the callosal connections along the 17/18a border, the normal callosal pattern features a ring-like configuration located just anterior to area 17 at the rostral end of the 17/18a band, a dense band of connections at the lateral border of area 18a, several narrow bands of connections that bridge area 18a at

various anteroposterior levels, and one or more callosal regions medial to area 17 in area 18b. In general, these other features of the visual callosal pattern correspond with the locations of the borders of the various extrastriate visual areas in the rat occipital cortex. Examination of similarly labeled sections cut in the coronal plane revealed that in each of the callosal regions described above labeled cells and terminations are densely accumulated in cortical layers II–III, Va and Vc–VIa, and less densely in layer IV and the remaining portions of layers V and VI. Finally, a significant number of callosally labeled cells can be seen in layers Vc–VIa spanning the full width of both area 17 and area 18a (see also Olavarria & Van Sluyters, 1983).

Normal development of visual callosal connections

It is well documented that the pattern of cortical interhemispheric connections in immature mammals differs markedly from that in the adult (see Olavarria & Van Sluyters, 1985 for references). When we examined the pattern of callosal connections in the posterior neocortex of neonatal rats, we found that until 5 days of age large numbers of retrogradely labeled callosal cells are distributed fairly uniformly across virtually the entire mediolateral extent of the posterior neocortex (see Fig. 21.2). Interestingly, experiments using an anterogradely transported tracer showed that the axons of these cells seem to be hovering in the white matter, just beneath the lower

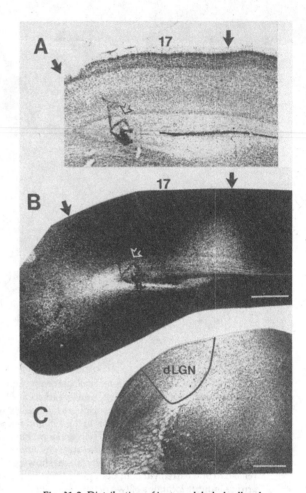

Fig. 21.3. Distribution of isotope-labeled callosal axons at 5 days of age. A, B. Bright- and darkfield views, respectively, of single coronal section through posterior neocortex of 5-day-old rat pup that received multiple injections of the anterogradely transported tracer ^{3}H-proline into the opposite cortex. This section was processed for autoradiography and counterstained with cresyl violet. Medial is to the left. Solid arrows indicate approximate location of the borders of area 17, estimated from pattern of Nissl staining shown in A. Hollow arrows indicate artifact that facilitates comparison of the two views of this section shown in A and B. Note in B that the presence of isotope-labeled axons in lower layers of cortical grey matter is restricted to region of the presumptive 17/18a border (indicated by more lateral of the solid arrows), at a time when distribution of callosal neurons is still widespread (see Fig. 21.2).
C. Autoradiograph showing pattern of isotope transported from injection sites to ipsilateral dorsal lateral geniculate nucleus (dLGN) in same rat pup. Scale bars = 0.5 mm. (Originally published in Olavarria & Van Sluyters, 1985.)

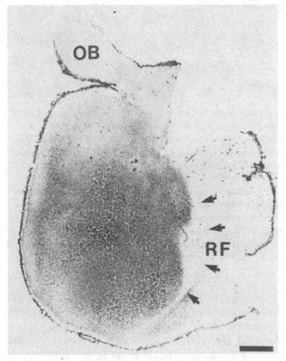

Fig. 21.2. Distribution of HRP-labeled callosal cells at 5 days of age. Brightfield view of HRP-tested tangential section through flattened cerebral cortex of 5-day-old rat pup following multiple injections of this tracer into the opposite hemisphere. Medial is to the left and posterior is down. Note dense accumulation of label that spreads over much of posterior neocortex, compared to restricted labeling pattern in adult rat shown in Fig. 21.1. OB = olfactory bulb, RF = rhinal fissure (arrows). Scale bar = 1.0 mm. (Originally published in Olavarria & Van Sluyters, 1985.)

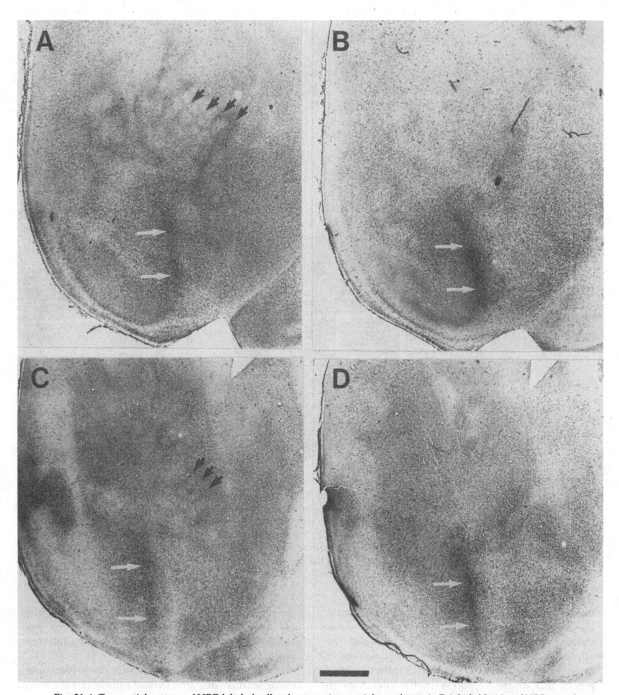

Fig. 21.4. Tangential pattern of HRP-labeled callosal connections at 6 days of age. A. Brightfield view of HRP-tested section taken through layer IV in 6-day-old rat pup following multiple injections of this tracer into the opposite cortex. B. Section from same pup taken 80 μm deeper into the cortex. C. Section taken through layer IV in second 6-day-old pup that was similarly injected. D. Section taken 80 μm beneath that in C. Medial is to the left, and posterior is down. Long white arrows indicate areas of enhanced labeling thought to represent an early stage in development of the callosal band at 17/18a border, and short black arrows indicate honeycomb callosal pattern in SmI. Another feature of the mature visual callosal pattern, reduced labeling in the interior of area 18a, is also apparent in these sections, just lateral to the emerging 17/18a callosal band. Scale bar = 1.0 mm. (Originally published in Olavarria & Van Sluyters, 1985.)

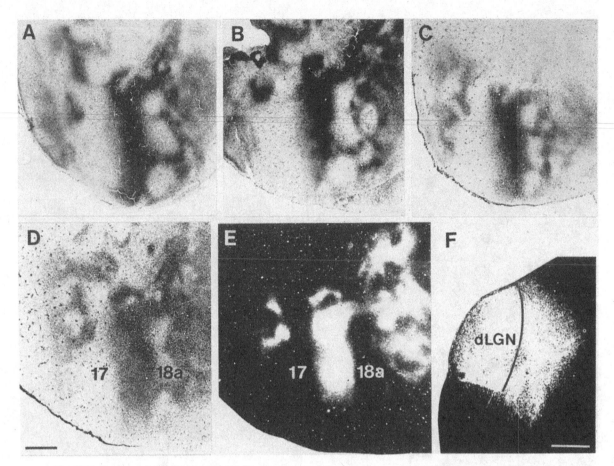

Fig. 21.5. Tangential distribution of callosal connections at 12 days of age. A–D. Brightfield views of HRP-tested tangential sections through posterior neocortex of four 12-day-old rat pups following multiple injections of this enzyme alone, or in combination with ³H-proline, into the opposite cerebral hemisphere. E. Autoradiograph of tangential section adjacent to that in D, showing distribution of anterogradely labeled callosal axons in this pup. Note that all features of adult visual callosal pattern shown in Fig. 21.1 are visible in these 12-day-old pups. Medial is to the left and posterior is down. F. Autoradiograph of pattern of isotope transported from cortical injection sites to ipsilateral dLGN in coronal section from pup shown in D and E. Scale bar for A–E (shown in D) = 1.0 mm, and scale bar for F = 0.5 mm. (Originally published in Olavarria & Van Sluyters, 1985.)

border of the developing cortical grey matter. However, at 5–6 days of age, the first of these callosal axons begin to invade the grey matter, and they appear to do so only in the *appropriate* regions of the developing visual cortex. Figure 21.3 shows an example of this invasion process in the region of the presumptive 17/18a border in a 5-day-old pup. As indicated by the data in Fig. 21.4, by 6 days of age the distribution of retrogradely labeled cell bodies also begins to change, as the first traces of the mature callosal pattern emerge from the immature widespread distribution of callosal cells. The visual callosal pattern rapidly matures over the next week or so, with

the result that by about 12 days of age the distribution of both anterogradely labeled terminations and retrogradely labeled cells has achieved the adult form (see Fig. 21.5).

The results of this study point out several interesting features of normal visual callosal development in the rat. First, there appear to be at least two distinct components to this process – an initial phase, during which axons from a widespread distribution of cells migrate through the corpus callosum, is followed by a second phase, during which there is highly selective invasion of the grey matter in the opposite hemisphere with the subsequent withdrawal of those axons that failed to make successful connections. Second, these two phases of development are separated by a brief waiting period – although visual callosal axons are present in the white matter of the opposite cortex at least as early as 3 days of age, invasion of the grey matter appears to be delayed until 5–6 days of age. Third, once invasion of the grey matter commences, the rest of callosal development proceeds quite rapidly, so that the overall pattern of connections appears mature within about a week. Finally, visual experience cannot be one of the factors responsible for guiding callosal axons to their proper cortical destinations in the rat, since callosal development is complete prior to the stage at which pups normally open their eyes (13–14 days of age).

Development of visual callosal connections in monocularly enucleated rats

Having studied the form and time course of normal visual callosal development in the rat, we next turned to the question of whether the precise relationship between visual callosal connections and cortical retinotopy described at the outset of this chapter is merely coincidental, or whether details of the cortical retinotopic pattern actually play a role in specifying the development of callosal connections. In an effort to examine this issue, we sought to induce formation of an abnormal pattern of connections in the developing retino-geniculo-cortical pathway in one hemisphere, and then to study the pattern of callosal connections that was specified for this hemisphere.

We knew from a variety of previous studies (see Olavarria *et al.*, 1987 for references) that, in rodents, removal of one eye at birth leads to marked anomalies in the pattern of projections from the surviving eye to the ipsilateral thalamus and tectum, and there was even preliminary evidence suggesting that these abnormalities might be passed on to the visual cortex by neurons in the dorsal lateral geniculate nucleus. Thus, in a number of rat pups we removed one eye at birth and then examined the distribution of callosal connections that subsequently formed in the visual cortex ipsilateral to the surviving eye.

Figure 21.6 displays the visual callosal pattern in the hemisphere ipsilateral to the surviving eye in several adult rats that were monocularly enucleated at birth. While all of the features of the normal callosal pattern are apparent in these animals (i.e., the 17/18a band, anterior ring, band at the lateral border of area 18a, bridges across area 18a, labeling in area 18b), an entirely new feature is also present – an extra band of

connections can be seen running anteroposteriorly through the middle of area 17. This extra callosal band, which is present in every rat enucleated at birth, usually appears to fluctuate regularly in width, so that it has a beaded appearance. In the opposite hemisphere of these animals, contralateral to the surviving eye, the callosal pattern appears entirely normal.

When we examined the callosal patterns in rat pups that had been allowed to survive for various periods of time following monocular enucleation, it was clear that the overall time course of postnatal callosal development was not affected by the loss of an eye at birth. Furthermore, the anomalous extra band of callosal connections was present continuously from the moment that features of the mature callosal pattern first became visible in the striate cortex (i.e., at 5–6 days of age) and, within this extra band, the laminar arrangement of callosal cells and terminations developed normally. This group of findings indicates that development of the extra callosal band in monocularly enucleated pups is caused neither by a general slowing down of callosal development, nor by an arrest of the normal developmental process at a premature stage (see Olavarria *et al.*, 1987).

At this point we performed a final experiment designed to determine the period of postnatal development during which formation of the callosal pattern was susceptible to the effects of monocular enucleation. Rat pups were monocularly enucleated on successive days between the ages of 1 and 6 days, and the arrangement of callosal connections in the hemisphere ipsilateral to their surviving eye was studied when they were adults. The data presented in Fig. 21.7 come from this final study and, as they indicate, susceptibility of the developing callosal pattern to unilateral eye removal ends abruptly at 6 days of age. Since development of the callosal pattern is not complete until pups reach about 12 days of age, and since individual features of the mature callosal pattern are just emerging from the widespread immature pattern at 6 days of age, the callosal pathway clearly becomes immune to the effects of monocular enucleation at a very early stage in its overall development.

Specification of the visual callosal pattern

What factors are normally responsible for specifying that certain parts of the developing visual cortex will become callosal regions? Our demonstration of the extra callosal band in monocularly enucleated rats clearly indicates that factors extrinsic to the visual cortex have the power to alter the pattern of callosal

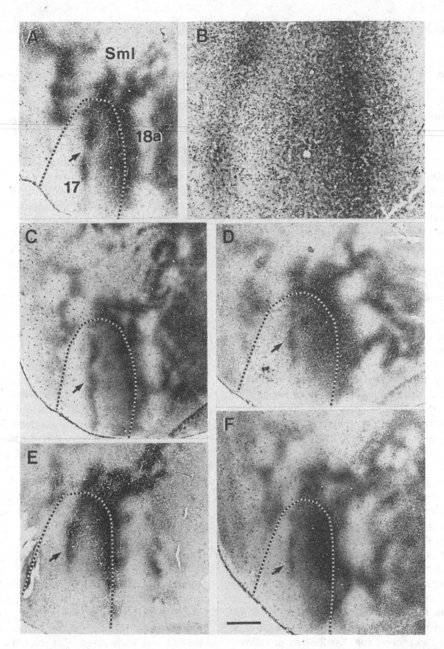

Fig. 21.6. Tangential distribution of callosal connection in monocularly enucleated rats. A, C–F. Brightfield views of HRP-tested tangential sections through layers III–IV in the hemisphere ipsilateral to the surviving eye in five adult rats that were monocularly enucleated at birth. Labeling patterns were produced by making multiple injections of the enzyme into the opposite cortical hemisphere. Medial is to the left, and posterior is down. Approximate location of the border of area 17 is indicated by interrupted line, and arrows indicate location of the anomalous beaded band of callosal connections within area 17. B. Higher magnification view of portion of the section in A, showing details of labeling pattern in region containing both the 17/18a band and the extra callosal band within area 17. Scale bar = 1.0 mm for A, C–F, and 0.5 mm for B. (Originally published in Olavarria *et al.*, 1987.)

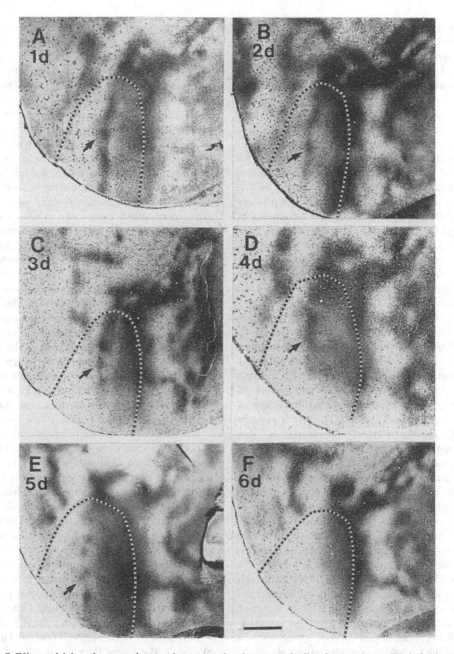

Fig. 21.7. Effects of delayed monocular enucleation on development of callosal connections. Brightfield views of HRP-tested tangential sections through layers III–IV in the hemisphere ipsilateral to the surviving eye in six monocularly enucleated rats. Labeling patterns were produced by making multiple injections of the enzyme into the opposite cortical hemisphere. A–F. Representative sections from adult rats monocularly enucleated at 1, 2, 3, 4, 5 or 6 days of age, respectively. Interrupted line indicates approximate location of border of area 17, and arrows indicate location of extra band of callosal labeling within area 17. Note normal appearance of callosal labeling pattern in rat enucleated at 6 days of age (e.g., cf with Fig. 21.1), and similarly abnormal labeling patterns in rats enucleated at 1 (A, and also see Fig. 21.6), 2, 3, 4 or 5 days of age (B–E, respectively). Scale bar = 1.0 mm. (Originally published in Olavarria *et al.*, 1987.)

connections that develops. We believe that the specification of this extra callosal band is related to the fact that the projection from the surviving retina to the ipsilateral dorsal lateral geniculate nucleus is markedly expanded in monocularly enucleated rats and that, as we have recently shown (Yee et al., 1987), this abnormality is also present in the ipsilateral geniculo-cortical pathway. Thus, development of a markedly abnormal feature in the visual callosal pattern of monocularly enucleated rats is correlated with an anomalous pattern of connections in their retino-geniculo-cortical pathway. Another example of this same relationship between anomalies in the primary visual and callosal pathways comes from studies of Siamese cats (e.g., Shatz, 1977; Shatz & Kliot, 1982), in which early misrouting of retino-geniculate axons, and the consequent changes in the retinotopy of the developing visual cortex, have been shown to be associated with the formation of a distinctly abnormal visual callosal pattern.

Is visual callosal development regulated entirely by the pattern of connections that forms in the developing retino-geniculo-cortical pathway, or do intrinsic cortical factors also play a role in guiding callosal axons to their destinations? Two lines of evidence indicate that intrinsic factors also may be important for callosal development. We have found that a crude version of the normal visual callosal pattern is present even in congenitally eyeless rodents (Olavarria & Van Sluyters, 1984), indicating that at least the basic instructions for callosal development reside in central nervous structures. However, this finding does not clarify whether these instructions are contained in the cortex itself. That the developing neocortex appears to have at least some innate ability to induce interhemispheric axons to invade its grey matter is suggested by studies of callosal development in rodents with lesions of the thalamo-cortical pathway (Wise & Jones, 1978; Cusick & Lund, 1982; Rhoades et al., 1987). Although there are discrepancies in the specific results reported in these studies, it seems clear that while removal of thalamic input early in postnatal life does not completely block the formation of callosal connections, it does prevent the formation of a normal visual callosal pattern.

In reviewing these various findings on the development of interhemispheric connections, it seems likely to us that specification of the visual callosal pattern normally is what might be termed a 'hand and glove' phenomenon. That is, a crude set of instructions for specifying the callosal pattern resides somewhere in the extraretinal portion of the central visual pathway, although probably not entirely within the cortex itself. These intrinsic instructions are designed in such a way as to 'anticipate' the establishment of a normal pattern of connections in the retino-geniculo-cortical pathway, and the retinotopy of the geniculo-cortical projection is used to refine the features of the developing callosal pattern. For their part, callosal axons apparently are innately programmed to grow across the midline in markedly exuberant numbers, and then to lie in wait in the white matter of the opposite hemisphere. One way this could be accomplished would be for the axons of presumptive callosal cells simply to take the shortest route to the midline, where they would encounter axons originating from cells in the corresponding region of cortex in the opposite hemisphere (see Olavarria & Van Sluyters, 1986). At this point the growing callosal axons would only have to retrace the paths taken by their fellows from the opposite hemisphere to arrive in white matter beneath approximately the appropriate region of the cortex (see Olavarria et al., 1988). In rodents, the signal for these waiting axons to begin their invasion of cortical grey matter comes at about 5 days of age. The fact that this is the stage of development at which the mature pattern of thalamo-cortical connections first becomes established (Lund & Mustari, 1977; Wise & Jones, 1978), is consonant with the idea that thalamic axons help to specify callosal regions of the cortex.

Admittedly, these speculations about the course of normal callosal development fail to address several important issues. One of these is our understanding of the process by which neonatal monocular enucleation disrupts development of the pathway from the surviving eye in such a way as to cause formation of an extra callosal band. For example, is it actually necessary to remove an eye at birth to cause the extra band to form, or would it be sufficient simply to eliminate retinal activity monocularly during the period of postnatal callosal development? To answer this question, we recently examined the visual callosal pattern in 12-day-old rat pups in which repeated intraocular injections of tetrodotoxin had been used to block neural activity in one eye throughout postnatal life (Chang et al., 1987). We found that visual callosal connections developed normally in these animals, indicating that a unilateral loss of retinal activity alone is not sufficient to promote development of the extra callosal band.

We also need to learn more about the retinotopic organization of area 17 in monocularly enucleated animals. Although our anatomical data show that the distribution of projections in the pathway from the surviving eye to the ipsilateral striate cortex is markedly expanded (Yee et al., 1987), they reveal nothing about the detailed organization of this abnormal projection. In normal animals visual callosal connections are concentrated in regions representing the visual vertical meridian, but it remains to be seen whether the presence of an extra band of connections in monocularly enucleated rats is somehow related to a remapping of the vertical meridian in area 17.

Yet another unresolved issue is the nature of the process by which thalamo-cortical axons 'instruct' callosal axons to grow into the appropriate regions of the cortex (e.g., see Olavarria & Van Sluyters, 1984, 1985). One way in which thalamic input could guide interhemispheric axons involves a possible role for the layer of 'subplate cells' found in the white matter of the developing neocortex (e.g., Luskin & Shatz, 1985). These cells receive transient synapses during development, and they may serve to provide an initial postsynaptic substrate for 'waiting axons' in white matter (e.g., Shatz & Luskin, 1986; Shatz et al., 1988). If this is the case, then the thalamic axons could use these subplate cells as a conveniently located postsynaptic

surface upon which to leave markers for the later arriving callosal axons to follow in innervating the grey matter above. The answer to this and many other interesting questions about the ontogeny of cortico–cortical connections remains forthcoming. Hopefully, study of the visual callosal pathway will continue to yield significant new information about the development of this important class of connections in the mammalian brain.

Acknowledgements

The research described in this chapter was supported by research grants to RCVS from the Developmental Neuroscience Program of the National Science Foundation (BNS 8418738) and the Eye Institute of National Institutes of Health (EY02193), and by a Core Facilities Grant from the National Eye Institute (EY03176). We are grateful to J. Fiorillo, A. Halperin, P. Lee, P. Leondis, and K. Yee for their skilled technical assistance.

References

Chang, C.-Y., Van Sluyters, R. C. & Olavarria, J. (1987) Effects of intraocular injections of tetrodotoxin in newborn rats on the development of the visual callosal pattern. *Invest. Ophthal. and Vis. Sci., ARVO Abstracts Supplement*, **28**, 236.

Cusick, C. G. & Lund, R. D. (1982) Modification of visual callosal projections in rats. *J. Comp. Neurol.*, **212**, 385–98.

Lund, R. D. & Mustari, M. J. (1977) Development of the geniculocortical pathway in rats. *J. Comp. Neurol.*, **173**, 289–306.

Luskin, M. B. & Shatz, C. J. (1985) Studies of the earliest generated cells of the cat's visual cortex: cogeneration of the subplate and marginal zones. *J. Neurosci.*, **5**, 1062–75.

Olavarria, J., Malach, R. & Van Sluyters, R. C. (1987) Development of visual callosal connections in neonatally enucleated rats. *J. Comp. Neurol.*, **260**, 321–48.

Olavarria, J., Serra-Oller, M. M., Yee, K. T. & Van Sluyters, R. C. (1988) Topography of interhemispheric connections in the neocortex of mice with congenital deficiencies of the callosal commisure. *J. Comp. Neurol.*, **270**, 575–90.

Olavarria, J. & Van Sluyters, R. C. (1983) Widespread callosal connections in infragranular visual cortex of the rat. *Brain Res.*, **279**, 233–7.

Olavarria, J. & Van Sluyters, R. C. (1984) Callosal connections of the posterior neocortex in normal-eyed, congenitally anophthalmic, and neonatally enucleated mice. *J. Comp. Neurol.*, **230**, 249–68.

Olavarria, J. & Van Sluyters, R. C. (1985) Organization and postnatal development of callosal connections in the visual cortex of the rat. *J. Comp. Neurol.*, **239**, 1–26.

Olavarria, J. & Van Sluyters, R. C. (1986) Axons from restricted regions of the cortex pass through restricted regions of the corpus callosum in adult and neonatal rats. *Devel. Brain Res.*, **25**, 309–13.

Rhoades, R. W., Fish, S. E., Mooney, R. D. & Chiaia, N. L. (1987) Distribution of visual callosal projection neurons in hamsters subjected to transection of the optic radiations on the day of birth. *Devel. Brain Res.*, **32**, 217–32.

Shatz, C. J. (1977) Anatomy of visual interhemispheric connections in the visual system of Boston Siamese and ordinary cats. *J. Comp. Neurol.*, **173**, 497–518.

Shatz, C. J., Chun, J. J. M. & Luskin, M. B. (1988) The role of the subplate in the development of the mammalian telencephalon. In *The Cerebral Cortex*, ed. E. G. Jones & A. Peters, pp. 35–58. New York: Plenum Press.

Shatz, C. J. & Kliot, M. (1982) Prenatal misrouting of the retinogeniculate pathway in Siamese cats. *Nature*, **300**, 525–9.

Shatz, C. J. & Luskin, M. B. (1986) The relationship between the geniculocortical afferents and their cortical target cells during development of the cat's primary visual cortex. *J. Neurosci.*, **6**, 3655–68.

Wise, S. P. & Jones, E. G. (1978) Developmental studies of thalamocortical and commissural connections in the rat somatic sensory cortex. *J. Comp. Neurol.*, **178**, 187–208.

Yee, K. T., Murphy, K. M. & Van Sluyters, R. C. (1987) Expansion of the ipsilateral primary visual pathway in rats monocularly enucleated at birth. *Invest. Ophthal. and Vis. Sci., ARVO Abstracts Supplement*, **27**, 335.

22

Sensitive periods in visual development: insights gained from studies of recovery of visual function in cats following early monocular deprivation or cortical lesions

D. E. Mitchell

On the basis of clinical experience with treatment of amblyopia, it had been long been suspected that the central visual pathways possessed a degree of plasticity in early life that did not exist in adulthood (Duke-Elder & Wybar, 1973). The first insight into the site and nature of this plasticity was obtained by Wiesel & Hubel (1963) in their pioneering study of the effects of early monocular deprivation on the kitten visual cortex. Whereas periods of deprivation imposed in the first months of life caused very substantial shifts of ocular dominance of cortical cells towards the nondeprived eye, similar periods of deprivation imposed on adult cats caused no measurable changes of ocular dominance. The time course of the sensitive period for the effects of monocular deprivation was documented more precisely in subsequent investigations that examined in a more systematic fashion the effects of short periods of deprivation imposed on both cats (Hubel & Wiesel, 1970; Olson & Freeman, 1980; Cynader, Timney & Mitchell, 1980; Jones, Spear & Tong, 1984) and monkeys (e.g. Hubel, Wiesel & LeVay, 1977; Blakemore, Garey & Vital-Durand, 1978; Von Noorden & Crawford, 1979; LeVay, Wiesel & Hubel, 1980) of different ages. While there is general consensus that the visual cortex of the cat is most sensitive to monocular deprivation during the fourth week of postnatal life, there is substantial disagreement concerning the rate of decline of susceptibility beyond this point. Early studies (Hubel & Wiesel, 1970) suggest that the cat cortex becomes immutable to monocular deprivation during the fourth month, but later investigations that employed longer periods of deprivation indicated that the cortex retained some susceptibility to this form of deprivation until 8 or even 10 months of age (Cynader et al., 1980; Jones et al., 1984).

The discovery by Blakemore & Van Sluyters (1974) that it was possible to reverse the effects of monocular deprivation by early reversal of occlusion lead to a broadened concept of a sensitive period as an interval in the animal's life during which it is possible, by suitable manipulation of the early visual input, to both disrupt and to re-establish functional cortical connections lost during a prior period of deprivation. The experiments of Blakemore & Van Sluyters (1974) also introduced a new way to document the declining plasticity of the visual cortex. The extent to which ocular dominance can be shifted back towards the originally deprived eye by reverse occlusion gradually declines with age such that beyond about 4 months the physiological effects of an early period of monocular deprivation are permanent. At the peak of the sensitive period for the cat, at about 4 or 5 weeks of age, cortical ocular dominance can be switched from complete dominance by the nondeprived eye to total dominance by the formerly deprived eye by only 9 days of reverse occlusion (Movshon, 1976). A similar fast reversal of the physiological effects of monocular deprivation is also observed in monocularly deprived monkeys (Blakemore, Vital-Durand & Garey, 1981). While the restoration of functional connections with the deprived eye by reversal of occlusion represented the first demonstration of recovery of function in the central nervous system (Movshon, 1976), it is important to recognize that this recovery occurs at the expense of functional connections with the formerly nondeprived eye, which in extreme situations (where reverse occlusion is imposed early and for a sufficiently long time) could be completely lost. From a clinical perspective such an extreme outcome is clearly far from satisfactory since one functional defect has been replaced by another of equal severity. It might be thought that a more desirable final outcome could be achieved by simply restoring normal visual input to

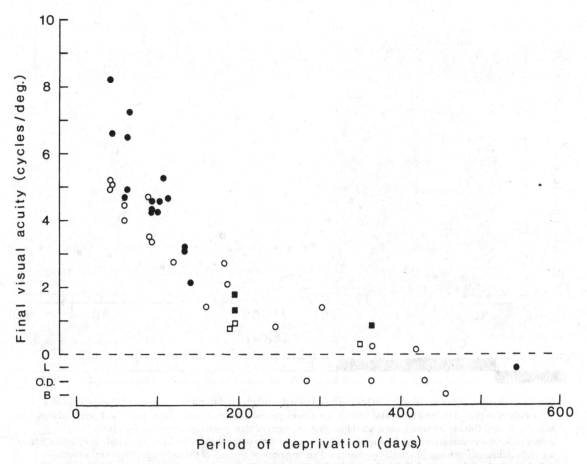

Fig. 22.1. The grating acuity that was eventually achieved by the deprived eye of a large number of monocularly deprived kittens as a function of the duration of the prior period of occlusion. Filled symbols indicate the results from animals that were reverse occluded following the initial period of monocular deprivation, while open symbols depict results from animals that had both eyes open during recovery. Animals that never recovered any useful vision as tested on a jumping stand are signified by the letter 'B', while those denoted as 'O.D.' were able to discriminate by visual cues alone an open from a closed door on the jumping stand. Animals that could in addition pass a formal luminance discrimination are signified by the letter 'L'. The square symbols show data of Smith & Holdefer (1985). Reproduced with permission from Mitchell (1988).

the deprived eye without occluding the other eye at the same time (binocular recovery). However, although some physiological recovery can occur in this situation in kittens (Mitchell, Cynader & Movshon, 1977; Olson & Freeman, 1978), little or no recovery occurs in monkeys under analogous conditions (Blakemore *et al.*, 1981), and even in kittens the extent of this recovery is considerably less than that which occurs during reverse occlusion. On the other hand, a much smaller difference in outcome is observed on some behavioural measures where, for example, the extent of recovery of visual acuity of the deprived eye is only slightly worse with binocular recovery than

with reverse occlusion. This point is illustrated by Fig. 22.1 which displays the visual acuity that was eventually recovered by the deprived eye in these two recovery conditions by animals that were monocularly deprived from birth for various periods. It is also apparent from Fig. 22.1 that some animals that were deprived to 1 year of age showed limited visual recovery which suggests that some residual plasticity may remain at some location(s) in the visual pathway for a longer time than indicated by experiments that examine the physiological effects of monocular deprivation on various visual cortical structures.

Impressed by the speed with which functional

236   D. E. Mitchell

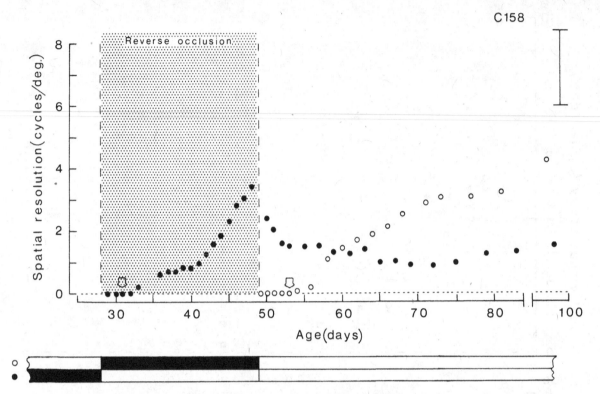

Fig. 22.2. Changes in the visual acuity of the deprived (filled symbols) and nondeprived (open symbols) eyes of a monocularly deprived kitten during and following a 3 week period of reverse occlusion imposed at 4 weeks of age. The arrow indicated the day on which the animal first showed signs of vision with the deprived eye (during reverse occlusion) or the nondeprived eye (in the period following reverse occlusion) on the jumping stand. The vertical bar on the right indicates the range of acuities encountered among normal animals of the same age. Reproduced with permission from Mitchell, Murphy & Kaye (1984b).

connections are re-established with the deprived eye following reverse occlusion, my colleagues and I reasoned that by combining the two recovery conditions in suitable ways it might be possible to achieve a greater degree of recovery of vision by the deprived eye than can occur with binocular recovery alone, and at the same time prevent the detrimental changes to the vision of the nondeprived eye that occurs with prolonged reverse occlusion. In order to set the stage for a test of this idea, we decided that it was necessary to investigate, in a systematic manner, the events that occurred immediately after termination of periods of reverse occlusion of various durations upon introduction of simultaneous visual input to the two eyes. Monocular measurements were made of the visual acuity for gratings at frequent intervals throughout the period of reverse occlusion and afterwards by use of a simple behavioural technique that employs a jumping stand (Mitchell, Griffin & Timney, 1977). To our sur-

prise we found that in general the substantial improvement of the vision of the formerly deprived eye that occurred during reverse occlusion was not retained afterwards (Mitchell, Murphy & Kaye, 1984a). A representative example of this phenomenon is illustrated in Fig. 22.2 for an animal that was monocularly deprived to 4 weeks of age and then reverse occluded for 3 weeks. During the latter period, the vision of the initially deprived eye improved from blindness to 3.4 c/deg. However, upon termination of reverse occlusion, and introduction of simultaneous visual input to both eyes, an interesting reciprocal change occurred in the vision of the two eyes. Concurrent with an improvement of the vision of the initially nondeprived eye, which had been rendered blind by the 3 weeks of reverse occlusion, the vision of the initially deprived eye dropped rapidly to about 1.0 c/deg in only 3 weeks, after which it showed only very slight improvement. Although the vision of the

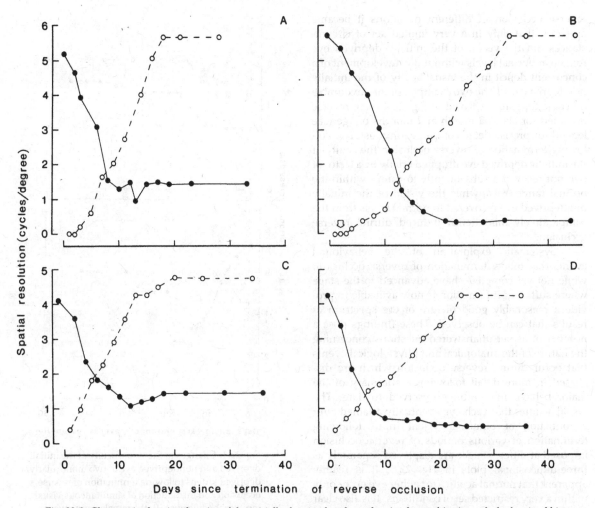

Fig. 22.3. Changes in the visual acuity of the initially deprived and nondeprived eye of 4 monocularly deprived kittens following termination of reverse occlusion and introduction of simultaneous visual input to the two eyes. The individual deprivation conditions were as follows: A. reverse occlusion for 38 days begun at 35 days of age. B. reverse occlusion for 44 days begun at 42 days of age. C. reverse occlusion for 91 days begun at 103 days of age. D. reverse occlusion for 102 days begun at 101 days of age. Symbols as in Fig. 22.2. Reproduced with permission from Mitchell, Murphy & Kaye (1984a).

initially nondeprived eye improved considerably in this time, it never acquired an acuity within the normal range. Subsequently, my colleagues and I have demonstrated that similar reciprocal changes in the vision of the two eyes can be observed at any time in the first 4 months of life following termination of periods of reverse occlusion of widely different durations. A further four examples of this phenomenon are provided in Fig. 22.3. Although the initially nondeprived eye of the two animals (A and B) that were reverse occluded at 5 or 6 weeks of age eventually acquired an acuity that was just below the normal

range, the two animals (C and D) that were reverse occluded when about 14 weeks old exhibited a much more substantial deficit in the vision of this eye.

Comparison with Fig. 22.1 indicates that the common outcome that followed termination of reverse occlusion was a state of affairs in which the acuity of the initially deprived eye was worse than it would have been if the animal had not been subjected to reverse occlusion at all! Moreover, the vision of the initially nondeprived eye was frequently compromised as well. Early in our systematic exploration of the events that follow termination of periods of reverse occlusion of different durations it became apparent that only in a very limited set of circumstances did the vision of the initially deprived eye remain at normal levels without the development of a concurrent deficit in the visual acuity of the initially nondeprived eye. The two examples of this favourable outcome that are displayed in Fig. 22.4 were reverse occluded for about a month at 2 months of age (see legend for precise details of the rearing history). Following termination of reverse occlusion the acuity of the initially deprived eye dropped briefly by a factor of two but recovered subsequently to values within the normal range. Meanwhile the vision of the initially nondeprived eye recovered to normal levels from the comparatively mild deficit induced during reverse occlusion.

Systematic exploration of the behavioural events that follow termination of reverse occlusion, while not yet complete, have advanced to the stage where sufficient information is now available to provide a reasonably good picture of the spectrum of results that can be observed. These findings pose a number of as yet unanswered questions concerning the nature of the anatomical and physiological events that occur during reverse occlusion which are discussed in more detail following a summary of the major behavioural findings observed to date. The visual acuities that each eye eventually attained after introduction of binocular visual input following termination of various periods of reverse occlusion imposed at different ages are displayed separately as three-dimensional plots in Fig. 22.5. It is readily apparent that normal acuities for either eye occur only within a very restricted set of conditions. It is also clear from Fig. 22.5 that apart from this very narrow set of conditions, the acuity of the initially deprived eye is very poor in every other condition that has been surveyed. Although the acuity of the initially nondeprived eye was in general better than that of the other eye, in nearly all conditions it never quite attained normal levels. Two other aspects of these results deserve to be highlighted.

The first notable findings relate to the results obtained from animals that were reverse occluded at 4,5, or 6 weeks of age for periods that were short (9 to 21 days), but yet known from previous work (Movshon, 1976) to be sufficiently long to permit a complete shift of ocular dominance in the visual cortex towards the formerly deprived eye at these particular ages. This particular set of conditions was examined in some detail (Murphy & Mitchell, 1987) since it was thought that they might afford an excellent opportunity for recovery of good vision in both eyes because of the

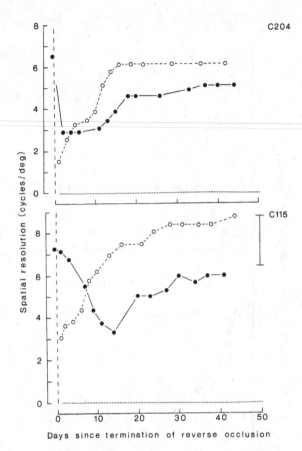

Fig. 22.4. Changes in the visual acuity of the initially deprived and nondeprived eye of two monocularly deprived kittens following termination of reverse occlusion and introduction of simultaneous visual input to the two eyes. Both animals were reverse occluded for 35 days beginning at either 64 (C204) or 66 (C115) days of age. The vertical bar to the right of the data for C115 represents the range of acuities observed among a large sample of normal animals of the same age. Symbols as in Fig. 22.2.

early age at which binocular visual input was introduced. Surprisingly the eventual outcome of this rearing procedure was exactly the opposite, namely a severe bilateral amblyopia, in which the acuity of both eyes was very poor. Examples of this finding are displayed in Fig. 22.6 which shows the changes in visual acuity of the two eyes during the periods of binocular vision for two kittens that were previously monocularly deprived to 5 weeks of age and then reverse occluded for just 18 days. Measurements of contrast sensitivity functions for the two eyes of a limited number of animals reared in this manner

a) Deprived Eye

b) Non-deprived Eye

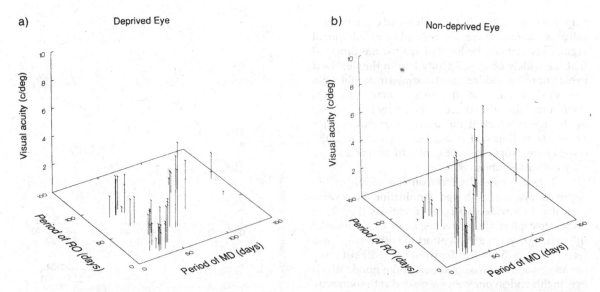

Fig. 22.5. The height of each bar represents the visual acuity that was eventually attained by the deprived eye (a) and non-deprived eye (b) of a large sample of kittens that were monocularly deprived from near birth to the ages indicated and which then received various periods of reverse occlusion followed by several months of binocular visual exposure. Short horizontal bars indicate the data from individual animals in the situation where several animals were reared with the same deprivation regimen.

revealed that the contrast sensitivities were reduced from normal values by a factor of about 10 at all spatial frequencies (Murphy & Mitchell, 1987). The severity of the bilateral amblyopia was even more evident in measures of vernier acuity, which were 16 to 70 times worse than normal values (Murphy & Mitchell, in preparation).

The second interesting finding was obtained from animals reared in the situation where the period of reverse occlusion was initiated early for an extended period of time. It was anticipated that under these rearing conditions the substantial recovery of vision by the initially deprived eye that occurred during the long period of reverse occlusion would be maintained afterwards because binocular visual input would be introduced when the animals were 4 months of age or older. Surprisingly, the visual acuity of the initially deprived eye, which recovered to near normal levels during the long period of reverse occlusion, dropped rapidly afterwards while at the same time the acuity of the initially nondeprived eye recovered only to very poor levels. Once again, the final result was a severe bilateral amblyopia. A particularly noteworthy example of this finding obtained from a monocularly deprived kitten that was reverse occluded for 12 weeks at 5 weeks of age is shown in Fig. 22.7.

The rapid decline in the visual acuity of the initially deprived eye was a common and surprising finding following termination of reverse occlusion (Fig. 22.5). One simple explanation for this finding that immediately springs to mind is that this acuity loss represents the sudden onset of strabismic amblyopia. On the basis of common experience following termination of a period of monocular deprivation, where a wide scatter of eye positions are observed, it is quite likely that a substantial proportion of the reverse occluded animals may also have had a strabismus, at least for a few weeks following introduction of simultaneous visual input to the two eyes. However, as with the former situation, the distribution of binocular alignment among a sample of reverse occluded animals would in all probability be centered on zero misalignment but with a large standard deviation around this mean. Quantitative measures of eye alignment (measured under paralysis) were made on only a few animals, but to casual inspection many appeared to have normal eye alignment. Although this issue has not yet been examined quantitatively, no obvious relationship was apparent between the nature of eye alignment and the final visual acuity of the deprived eye. This point can be highlighted by citing the fact that one animal (C115) that manifested a very obvious convergent strabismus from the time that simultaneous binocular visual input was first introduced, was one of the few animals in which the initially deprived eye eventually achieved very good vision. In addition to this and other empirical observations, there are a number of additional arguments that can be levelled against the proposal that the widely observed acuity loss in the deprived eye is due to the sudden onset of strabismic amblyopia (see Mitchell *et al.*, 1984a). Foremost among these is the fact that the time course of the acuity loss, as well as the age at which it can occur, does not fit with known facts (Mitchell *et al.*, 1984c) concerning the onset of amblyopia following introduction of a surgically induced strabismus.

The detrimental effects on the vision of the deprived eye that followed termination of reverse occlusion in a wide variety of conditions (Fig. 22.5) lead us to explore alternative regimens of occlusion of the nondeprived eye in an effort to both recover and retain good vision in the deprived eye, without causing any concurrent loss of vision in the nondeprived eye. In this endeavour we were guided at the outset by the common clinical procedure of part-time occlusion for treatment of amblyopia where the nonamblyopic eye is occluded for only part of each day in order to allow a few hours of daily binocular visual experience. Our initial thought was that functional connections established with the deprived eye during occlusion of the nondeprived eye might be reinforced in a Hebbian sense (Hebb, 1949) by simultaneous activity through the nondeprived eye during the daily periods of binocular visual exposure. In order to achieve part-time occlusion of the nondeprived eye, a form-fitting helmet of closed-cell neoprene foam was devised (Dzioba *et al.*, 1986). The first experiments were conducted on kittens that had been monocularly deprived to 6 weeks of age. From this point onwards the daily visual experience of each kitten was restricted to 7 hours in order that they could be monitored closely during the daily period of occlusion of the nondeprived eye by the helmet. Following the 7 hours of visual experience they were placed with their mother in a darkroom. Daily monocular tests of the grating acuity of the two eyes were made during and after a 6 week period of part-time occlusion. The total daily period of visual exposure was maintained at 7 hours after the 6 week period of part-time occlusion until the vision of the two eyes had stablized (typically within 4 weeks).

It became apparent very early in these studies that daily periods of occlusion of the nondeprived eye of 2 hours or less caused little or no improvement in the vision of the deprived eye over that which occurred with no occlusion at all. However, when the length of daily occlusion was extended to 3½ (50% of the daily period of visual exposure) or 5 hours (70%)

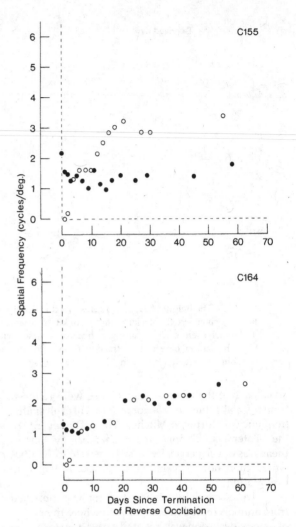

Fig. 22.6. Changes in the visual acuity of the deprived (filled symbols) and nondeprived (open symbols) eye of two monocularly deprived kittens during the period of binocular vision that followed termination of a short period of reverse occlusion. The kittens had previously been monocularly deprived from near birth until 5 weeks of age following which they were reverse occluded for 18 days. Reproduced with permission from Murphy & Mitchell (1987).

each day, the vision of the deprived eye improved substantially more during the 6 weeks of occlusion and moreover, continued to improve afterward toward normal levels in only a month. At the same time, the vision of the nondeprived eye, which was depressed during the 6 week period this eye was occluded for part of each day, also improved rapidly afterwards so that one month later the acuities of the two eyes were both equal and normal. Representative

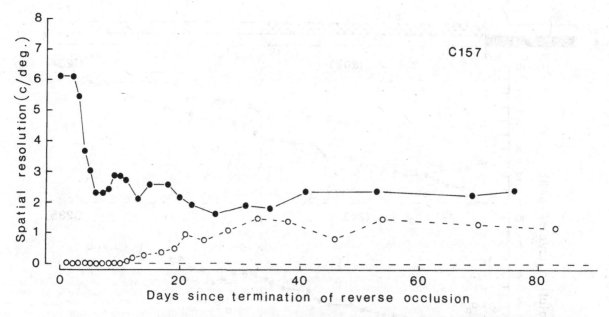

Fig. 22.7. Changes in the visual acuity of the initially deprived and nondeprived eye of a monocularly deprived kitten following termination of 12 weeks of reverse occlusion that had been imposed when the animal was 5 weeks of age. Symbols as in Fig. 22.7. Reproduced with permission from Murphy & Mitchell (1987).

results from three animals that received either 3½, 5, or 7 (effectively full-time) hours of occlusion during the 7 hours of daily visual exposure are displayed in Fig. 22.8. As observed earlier in kittens that were reverse occluded by eyelid suture (Figs. 22.2 and 22.3), following full-time reverse occlusion with a helmet there were reciprocal changes in the vision of the two eyes so that much of the substantial gain in the vision of the deprived eye that occurred during the period of occlusion was not retained afterwards.

Following collection of the data of Fig. 22.8, measurements were made of the contrast sensitivity functions of the two eyes followed by assessment of vernier acuity. Results of the former measurements for three kittens of Fig. 22.8 are displayed in Fig. 22.9. Whereas the contrast sensitivity functions of the two eyes of the animals that received daily periods of part-time occlusion for 3½ or 5 hours were equal and normal, the animal that received effective full-time occlusion exhibited poor contrast sensitivities in both eyes. Indeed the contrast sensitivity function for the deprived eye of this kitten was worse than that of the equivalent eye of the control animal that received no occlusion. A similar picture emerged from the measurements of vernier acuity; the kittens that received 3½ or 5 hours occlusion exhibited normal vernier acuities in both eyes (1.2 minutes), while the

acuities of both eyes of the animal that was occluded for all 7 hours each day were substantially lower.

The depth perception of some of the animals that recovered normal visual acuity in both eyes has been assessed in order to ascertain whether they may have acquired stereoscopic vision. While some animals assessed according to the procedure of Mitchell *et al.* (1979) appeared to have acquired a unique binocular cue to depth consistent with the presence of stereopsis, preliminary data obtained in collaboration with M. Ptito and F. Leporé indicate that these same animals may be unable to pass more rigorous tests for stereopsis that employ anaglyphic presentation of random-dot stimuli that effectively eliminate all monocular cues and provide only retinal disparity cues to depth. These preliminary data can be tentatively interpreted to mean that these animals may have acquired local but not global stereopsis.

Subsequently, the effectiveness of part-time reverse occlusion has been examined on animals that were monocularly deprived to 8, 10, or 12 weeks of age. The only regimen of occlusion that appeared effective in animals deprived to 8 weeks was the situation where the nondeprived eye was occluded for 5 hours each day. No regimen of part-time occlusion produced beneficial results in kittens monocularly deprived for longer periods, indicating that this pro-

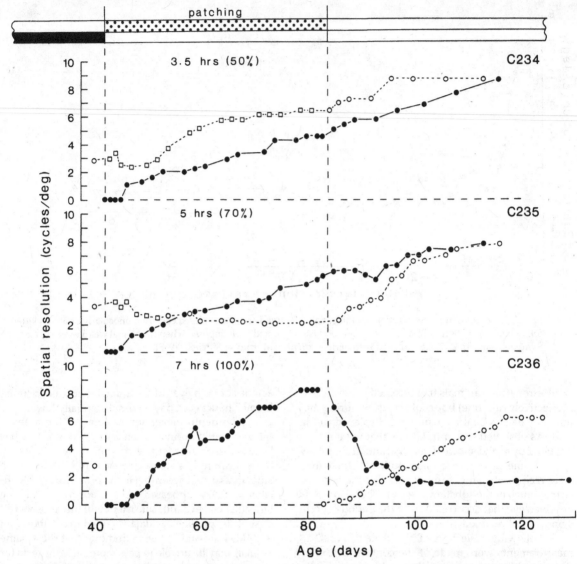

Fig. 22.8. Changes in the visual acuity of the two eyes of three monocularly deprived kittens during and following various regimens of part-time occlusion of the formerly nondeprived eye that were imposed for 6 weeks at 6 weeks of age. As in earlier figures, solid and open circles indicate the monocular acuities of, respectively, the formerly deprived and nondeprived eyes, while open squares depict the binocular visual acuity which earlier work had shown is equal to the monocular acuity of the better of the two eyes. A mask occluded the formerly nondeprived eye for either 3.5 (C234), 5 (C235) or 7 (C236) hours each day which represented respectively, 50, 70, and 100% of the period of daily visual exposure. Reproduced with permission from Mitchell *et al.* (1986).

cedure is only effective in a very limited range of conditions. As mentioned earlier, our initial explanation for the success of certain regimens of part-time occlusion was in terms proposed first by Hebb (1949), namely that functional connections established with the deprived eye during reverse occlusion were reinforced and stabilized by synchronous activity through the nondeprived eye that occurred during the daily periods of binocular vision. This simple explanation was examined in experiments in which kittens wore prisms during the daily period of binocular visual exposure which displaced the images vertically in opposite directions in the two eyes by 10 or 20 prism dioptres (approx. 5 or 10 deg). Despite the highly

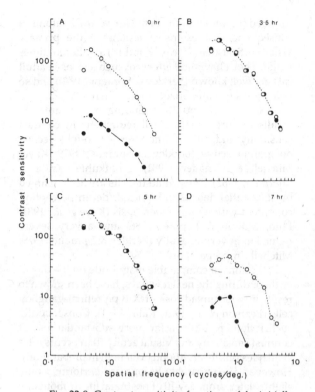

Fig. 22.9. Contrast sensitivity functions of the initially deprived (filled symbols) and nondeprived (open symbols) eyes of 4 cats that had been monocularly deprived from near birth to 6 weeks of age and which had then received various regimens of part-time occlusion of the initially nondeprived eye for 6 weeks followed by 3 months of binocular visual exposure. The individual regimens of occlusion were as follows. A. No occlusion (binocular recovery). B. 3.5 hours of daily occlusion. C. 5 hours of daily occlusion. D. 7 hours of daily occlusion (equivalent to full-time occlusion). Reproduced with permission from Mitchell *et al.* (1986).

discordant vision, animals that had been monocularly deprived to 6 weeks of age and which subsequently received either 3½ or 5 hours of occlusion of the nondeprived eye still recovered normal vision in both eyes! This surprising result casts doubt on explanations in such simple Hebbian terms.

Preliminary examinations have been made of the effectiveness of a number of different regimens of part-time occlusion that are currently employed in the clinical treatment of amblyopia. One successful variant of the 50% occlusion regimen is to alternate on a daily basis, full-time occlusion with no occlusion. On the other hand, another common procedure (Enoch & Campos, 1985) that combines, for equal periods each

day, occlusion of the nondeprived eye with occlusion of the deprived eye followed by a period of binocular exposure was found to be quite ineffective. It appears that, at least for kittens monocularly deprived from birth to 6 weeks of age, the regimens of occlusion that promote recovery of good vision in both eyes are very limited.

Neural substrates of the behavioural events

Current knowledge of the anatomical and physiological events that occur in the visual cortex during reverse occlusion is insufficient at present to account for either the variety of effects observed on termination of full-time reverse occlusion (Fig. 22.5), or for the behavioural effectiveness of certain regimens of part-time reverse occlusion. However, certain of the behavioural findings as well as the results of electrophysiological recordings made in the visual cortex of a very limited number of animals, permit a number of preliminary conclusions to be drawn which are enumerated below.

1. The major finding of a sudden loss of vision in the deprived eye following termination of reverse occlusion in a wide variety of conditions suggests that functional neural connections established in the initial period of monocular occlusion must be fundamentally different and in some way more robust than functional connections formed later with the initially deprived eye during the period of reverse occlusion. In other words, the shifts of ocular dominance observed in electrophysiological investigations of the visual cortex during reverse occlusion which appear identical to those observed earlier at the end of the initial period of monocular deprivation, must reflect quite different underlying anatomical events. One anatomical difference that is already known and which may contribute to the behavioural findings is the fact that the ocular dominance of cells in layer IV of area 17 can be influenced by monocular occlusion over a much shorter period than cells in other cortical layers (Shatz & Stryker, 1978). As a consequence the shifts of ocular dominance observed in the latter layers during reverse occlusion must be accompanied by much smaller effects in layer IV than would have occurred earlier during the prior period of monocular deprivation.

2. The second point emerges from physiological studies of 4 kittens that had been subjected to part-time reverse occlusion and which had recovered normal visual acuity in both eyes. The preliminary data from four animals such as these indicated that in animals that received 5 hours daily occlusion of the

nondeprived eye an equal proportion of cells were dominated by each eye, a result that to a first approximation fits well with the behavioural findings (Mitchell & Cynader, 1987). However in animals that received only $3\frac{1}{2}$ hours of daily occlusion (who also recovered normal acuity in the two eyes), the distribution of cortical ocular dominance was still highly biased towards the initially nondeprived eye. From this it must be concluded that good vision can be mediated by a relatively small number of cortical cells.

It is apparent that explanations for the behavioural findings require a much more detailed knowledge than is presently available of the anatomical and physiological events that occur in the visual cortex during reverse occlusion. As a first step it is important to document the sequence of anatomical events that occur during reverse occlusion as functional connections are established with the initially deprived eye. Anatomical investigations are required at different levels of resolution, that range, for example, from gross studies of the changes in the dimensions of ocular dominance columns in cortical areas 17 and 18 to detailed examination of the changes in the pattern of dendritic arborization of geniculate X- and Y-type axons from the two eyes in the visual cortex.

Despite the lack of detailed knowledge of the nature of the anatomical events that occur in the visual cortex during reverse occlusion, it is already apparent from the behavioural results described here that these changes must be fundamentally different from those that occur during the initial period of monocular deprivation. Thus, in contrast to the conclusion that could be easily and mistakenly drawn from knowledge of just the magnitude of the shifts of cortical ocular dominance prior to and following reverse occlusion, the neural plasticity during this period reflects different events and mechanisms than those responsible for the biased ocular dominance distributions during the initial period of monocular deprivation. Consequently, it is apparent that the complex effects of monocular occlusion on the visual cortex at different ages may eventually be understood in terms of a series of interactions between the timing of the period(s) of occlusion with the time course of a number of different developmental events of an anatomical, neurochemical or physiological nature.

Insights on neural plasticity gained from studies of the effects of cortical lesions at different ages

An additional dimension to the plasticity that exists in the central visual pathways in early life has been revealed by studies of the behavioural and anatomical consequences of extensive lesions of the primary visual cortical areas (areas 17 and 18) at different times in life. The behavioural effects of such lesions in adult cats are well known (Berkley & Sprague, 1979) and so will only be summarized briefly here. Ablation of cortical areas 17 and 18 (including part of area 19) results in surprisingly small reductions in contrast sensitivity and only a little over a two-fold decline on grating acuity (Berkley & Sprague, 1979; Kaye, Mitchell & Cynader, 1981; Lehmkuhle, Kratz & Sherman, 1982). These mild deficits are accompanied by substantial deficits in binocular depth perception consistent with a loss of stereopsis (Kaye et al., 1981; Ptito, Moisan & Leporé, 1986) and a very severe reduction in vernier acuity (Berkley & Sprague, 1979; Mitchell, in preparation).

Lesions of comparable magnitude on the day of birth, or during the next few days, have been shown to result in widespread loss of X-type retinal ganglion cells (Pearson et al., 1981; Kalil, 1984). Consequently such lesions result in a far more substantial loss of contrast sensitivity and visual acuity than occurs after similar lesions in adulthood (Mitchell, in preparation). However, if comparable lesions are performed only slightly later, from day 10 of postnatal life to about day 26, the behavioural consequences are surprisingly small. As indicated by the histograms of Fig. 22.10, which show the grating acuities of cats with cortical lesions performed within this narrow interval of time, as well as data from cats with comparable lesions made when they were over one year old, the acuities of the former are substantially better than the latter with some animals achieving grating acuities within the normal range (Kaye, Mitchell & Cynader, 1982). Preliminary data from a single animal with a cortical lesion performed at 12 days of age revealed both normal contrast sensitivity functions and visual acuity. However, the vernier acuity of this animal was significantly reduced from normal values. Despite the negligible deficits in grating acuity and contrast sensitivity, animals with lesions induced after day 10 of postnatal life possess poor depth perception which is no better binocularly than with monocular viewing (Kaye et al., 1982). Like animals with similar lesions performed in adulthood, it would appear that cats with neonatal lesions also lack stereoscopic vision.

The surprisingly small deficits in grating acuity and contrast sensitivity in animals with ablation of area 17 and 18 performed at between days 10 and 26 of postnatal life suggests that such lesions could not have caused the sort of widespread loss of X-type retinal ganglion cells that are observed in animals that

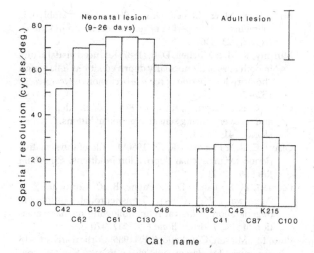

Fig. 22.10. Histograms that depict the visual acuity of two groups of adult cats in which cortical areas 17 and 18 (including part of area 19) had been ablated either in adulthood or very early in life, at between 9 and 26 days of age. The scale bar (top right) indicates the range of acuities of normal animals.

received comparable lesions near the day of birth. It must be concluded that the very different outcome observed in the former group of animals must result from a substantial reorganization of the visual pathway that can occur only within a narrow window of time. Explanations for the very different findings obtained from the animals with cortical lesions imposed at different ages may best be sought in terms of the relationship between the timing of the lesion and the development of normal and transitory exuberant projection patterns in the visual system.

Acknowledgements

The experiments described in this chapter were supported by a grant (A7660) from the Natural Sciences and Engineering Research Council of Canada, and by a Program grant (PG-29) from the Medical Research Council of Canada. Many of the experiments were performed in collaboration with Dr K. Murphy. Much of the behavioural testing was conducted by Heather Dzioba, Jane-Anne Horne and Dawn Pickering.

References

Berkley, M. A. & Sprague, J. (1979) Striate cortex and visual aucity functions in the cat. *J. Comp. Neurol.*, **187**, 679–702.

Blakemore, C., Garey, L. J. & Vital-Durand, F. (1978) The physiological effects of monocular deprivation and their reversal in the monkey's visual cortex. *J. Physiol.*, **283**, 223–62.

Blakemore, C. & Van Sluyters, R. C. (1974) Reversal of the physiological effects of monocular deprivation in kittens: further evidence for a critical period. *J. Physiol.*, **237**, 195–216.

Blakemore, C., Vital-Durand, F. & Garey, L. J. (1981) Recovery from monocular deprivation in the monkey. I. Recovery of physiological effects in the visual cortex. *Proc. Roy. Soc. Lond.*, **B213**, 399–423.

Cynader, M., Timney, B. N. & Mitchell, D. E. (1980) Period of susceptibility of kitten visual cortex to the effects of monocular deprivation extends beyond six months of age. *Brain Res.*, **191**, 545–50.

Duke-Elder, S. & Wybar, K. (1973) Ocular motility and strabismus. In *System of Ophthalmology*, Vol. 6, ed. S. Duke-Elder. London: Henry Kimpton.

Dzioba, H. A., Murphy, K. M., Horne, J. A. & Mitchell, D. E. (1986) A precautionary note concerning the use of contact lens occluders in developmental studies on kittens, together with a description of an alternative occlusion procedure, *Clinical Vision Sciences*, **1**, 191–6.

Enoch, J. M. & Campos, E. C. (1985) Helping the aphakic neonate to see. *International Ophthalmology*, **8**, 237–48.

Hebb, D. D. (1949) *The Organization of Behaviour*, New York: John Wiley.

Hubel, D. H. & Wiesel, T. N. (1970) The period of susceptibility to the physiological effects of unilateral eye closure in kittens. *J. Physiol.*, **206**, 419–36.

Hubel, D. H., Wiesel, T. N. & LeVay, S. (1977) Plasticity of ocular dominance columns in monkey striate cortex. *Phil. Trans. Roy. Soc. Lond.*, **B278**, 377–409.

Jones, K. R., Spear, P. D. & Tong, L. (1984) Critical periods for effects of monocular deprivation: differences between striate and extrastriate cortex. *J. Neurosci.*, **4**, 2543–52.

Kalil, R. E. (1984) Removal of the visual cortex in the cat: effects on the morphological development of the retino-geniculo-cortical pathway. In *Development of Visual Pathways in Mammals*, ed. J. Stone, B. Dreher & D. H. Rapaport, pp. 257–74. New York: Alan R. Liss.

Kaye, M., Mitchell, D. E. & Cynader, M. (1981) Selective loss of binocular depth perception following ablation of cat visual cortex. *Nature*, **293**, 60–2.

Kaye, M., Mitchell, D. E. & Cynader, M. (1982) Consequences for binocular depth perception of neonatal and adult lesions of cat visual cortex. *Invest. Ophthal. and Vis. Sci.*, *ARVO Supplement*, **22**(3), 125.

LeVay, S., Wiesel, T. N. & Hubel, D. H. (1980) The development of ocular dominance columns in normal and visually deprived monkeys. *J. Comp. Neurol.*, **191**, 1–51.

Lehmkule, S., Kratz, K. E. & Sherman, S. M. (1982) Spatial and temporal sensitivity of normal and amblyopic cats. *J. Neurophysiol.*, **48**, 372–87.

Mitchell, D. E. (1988) The extent of visual recovery from early monocular or binocular deprivation in kittens. *J. Physiol.*, **395**, 639–60.

Mitchell, D. E. & Cynader, M. (1987) Enhanced physiological

recovery in the visual cortex of monocularly deprived kittens promoted by certain regimens of part-time reverse occlusion. *Soc. Neurosci. Abstr.*, **13**, 1242.

Mitchell, D. E., Cynader, M. & Movshon, J. A. (1977) Recovery from the effects of monocular deprivation in kittens. *J. Comp. Neurol.*, **176**, 53–64.

Mitchell, D. E., Griffin, F. & Timney, B. (1977) A behavioural technique for the rapid assessment of the visual capabilities of kittens. *Perception*, **6**, 181–93.

Mitchell, D. E., Kaye, M. & Timney, B. (1979) Assessment of depth perception in cats. *Perception*, **8**, 389–96.

Mitchell, D. E., Murphy, K. M., Dzioba, H. A. & Horne, J. A. (1986) Optimization of visual recovery from early monocular deprivation in kittens: implications for occlusion therapy in the treatment of amblyopia. *Clinical Vision Sciences*, **1**, 173–7.

Mitchell, D. E., Murphy, K. M. & Kaye, M. G. (1984a) Labile nature of the visual recovery promoted by reverse occlusion in monocularly deprived kittens. *Proc. Nat. Acad. Sci., Washington*, **81**, 286–8.

Mitchell, D. E., Murphy, K. M. & Kaye, M. G. (1984b) The permanence of the visual recovery that follows reverse occlusion of monocularly deprived kittens. *Invest. Ophthal. and Vis. Sci.* **25**, 908–17.

Mitchell, D. E., Ruck, M., Kaye, M. G. & Kirby, S. (1984c) Immediate and long-term effects on visual acuity of surgically induced strabismus in kittens. *Exp. Brain Res.*, **55**, 420–30.

Movshon, J. A. (1976) Reversal of the physiological effects of monocular deprivation on the kitten's visual cortex. *J. Physiol.*, **261**, 125–74.

Murphy, K. M. & Mitchell, D. E. (1986) Bilateral amblyopia following a short period of reverse occlusion in kittens. *Nature*, **323**, 536–8.

Murphy, K. M. & Mitchell, D. E. (1987) Reduced visual acuity in both eyes of monocularly deprived kittens following a short or a long period of reverse occlusion. *J. Neurosci.*, **7**, 1526–36.

Olson, C. R. & Freeman, R. D. (1978) Monocular deprivation and recovery during sensitive period in kittens. *J. Neurophysiol.*, **41**, 65–74.

Olson, C. R. & Freeman, R. D. (1980) Profile of the sensitive period for monocular deprivation in kittens. *Exp. Brain Res.*, **39**, 17–21.

Pearson, H. E., Labar, D. R., Payne, B. R., Cornwall, P. & Aggarwal, N. (1981) Transneuronal retrograde degeneration in the cat retina following neonatal ablation of visual cortex. *Brain Res.*, **212**, 470–5.

Ptito, M., Moisan, C. & Leporé, F. (1986) Cortical areas 17–18 are crucial for stereoscopic vision in cats. *Soc. Neurosci. Abstr.*, **12**, 432.

Shatz, C. T. & Stryker, M. P. (1978) Ocular dominance in layer IV of the cat's visual cortex and the effects of monocular deprivation. *J. Physiol.*, **281**, 267–83.

Smith, D. C. & Holdefer, R. N. (1985) Binocular competitive interaction and recovery of visual acuity in long-term monocularly deprived cats. *Vision Res.*, **25**, 1783–94.

Von Noorden, G. K. & Crawford, M. L. J. (1979) The sensitive period. *Trans. Ophthal. Soc. UK.*, **99**, 442–6.

Wiesel, T. N. & Hubel, D. H. (1963) Single-cell responses in striate cortex of kittens deprived of vision in one eye. *J. Neurophysiol.*, **26**, 1003–17.

23
The developmental course of cortical processing streams in the human infant

J. Atkinson and O. J. Braddick

Introduction

The work of Horace Barlow, his colleagues and his students has not only made us consider the efficiency of the visual system in encoding significant properties of the visual world it has also focused attention on the question: how did the visual system get that way? Initially, the most promising approach appeared to be through experimental manipulations in the visual development of animals, and the continuing fruits of that approach can be sampled elsewhere in this volume. However, in the last decade and a half it has also been realized that human infants can tell us a great deal about the development of their visual systems, if we use the right techniques. It turns out that this development is particularly rapid over the first few months of life. One aspect of this is a quantitative improvement in many aspects of visual performance. However, there are also radical qualitative changes, which we will argue show the progressive emergence of functions of the visual cortex.

The basis of developments in spatial visual performance

Visual scientists' first questions about infant development were concerned with acuity and contrast sensitivity, and used measures of grating detection from behaviour in forced-choice preferential looking (FPL) and from visual evoked potentials (see reviews by Dobson & Teller, 1978; Atkinson & Braddick 1981; Atkinson, 1984; Banks & Salapatek, 1983). There are some differences still to be resolved, particularly between earlier estimates of newborn performance and those recently reported from the 'sweep VEP' method (Norcia & Tyler, 1985). It is uncertain how far these apparent discrepancies can be attributed to different spatio-temporal interactions in different studies, or to differences in adaptation and other dynamic effects between the sweep method and steady-state methods (Regan, 1980). Nonetheless, it should be emphasized that the general finding from FPL and VEP studies of acuity around 1 c/deg in the first month, and Norcia & Tyler's finding of 4.5 c/deg, both imply that the newborn acuity is at least an order of magnitude below the adult. There is general agreement that the greater part of the infant's 'deficit' relative to the adult has been made up by 6–9 months. The picture for contrast sensitivity is similar. The most obvious developmental question, then, concerns the changes that underly this rapid improvement.

Possible limiting factors on acuity and contrast sensitivity may arise from the optics of the eye, the receptor mosaic, or subsequent neural processing. So far as optics are concerned, there is no evidence that the infant eye has any markedly greater aberrations than the adult. Studies using photorefractive techniques (Howland et al., 1983) allow the refractive state of infants to be readily assessed (see Fig. 23.1). These and other methods indicate that very young infants show errors of accommodation, but the conclusion from depth of field calculations (Braddick et al., 1979; Banks, 1980) has been that any resulting defocus is not the limiting factor on acuity in the first few months. However, acuity values obtained using a single orientation of grating, from either VEP or FPL methods on infants in at least the first postnatal year, may be limited by optical blur due to the common problem of infant astigmatism (Howland et al., 1978; Mohindra, et al., 1978).

Although there is recent anatomical evidence on the immaturity of the foveal cones at birth (Yuodelis & Hendricksen, 1986) there is essentially no quantitative information on morphological development over the

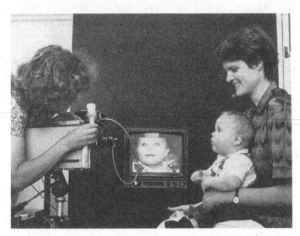

Fig. 23.1. A Barlow of a new generation (Oscar Barlow, seated on the knee of Miranda Barlow) making a contribution of his own to visual research. Videorefraction uses light reflected from the fundus to measure the refractive state of the eye, and thus to investigate accommodative control, the distribution of refraction in the infant population, and the process by which the infant eye develops towards emmetropia.

period between 0 and 6 months. Nonetheless, there have been several attempts to analyse newborn/adult differences in terms of photoreceptor packing and morphology. Wilson (1988) assumed that the quantum catch of the receptors should be proportional to outer-segment length, and in combination with the newborn's greater foveal cone spacing and smaller eye size calculated that the newborn's acuity should be reduced from an adult value taken as 35 c/deg to about 7 c/deg. Banks (1989) calculates on a different and rather fuller basis (using a model of the outer-segment's efficiency which includes its waveguide properties, and an ideal-observer model of detection). However, for acuity, the adult/newborn ratio he derives is quite similar to Wilson's. (A large part of the apparent difference in their results is due to differences in the estimates they take for adult sensitivity with Banks taking 60 c/deg as the adult acuity value.) These calculations indicate that receptor changes determine a considerable developmental improvement in acuity, but neither yields a limit as low as 4–5 c/deg which is the highest value obtained for newborn acuity (Norcia & Tyler, 1985). Similarly, Jacobs & Blakemore's (1988) calculations for the developing monkey retina (see chapter 24), which consider only the effects of receptor spacing on the Nyquist sampling limit, account for about two-thirds of the improvement of acuity measured in lateral geniculate

nucleus (LGN) cells (and a smaller fraction of the behaviourally measured improvement). The conclusion seems to be that receptoral changes can account for a substantial improvement in performance between birth and adult-hood, but that post-receptoral changes, in the neural organization of the retina or higher in the visual pathway, are also an essential component. How much these different levels contribute to the especially rapid changes in early infancy, will remain unknown until we have more data on the course of human photoreceptor development during the first six months postnatally.

Postnatal cortical development

While retinal development may play a major role in determining the limits on spatial information transmitted by the infant's visual system, the ability to encode that information in the ways needed to perform any visual task must depend on central processing. We know that in the human visual cortex there is a great increase in neural connectivity in the first six months of life (Garey & De Courten, 1983) and presumably these new synapses are defining and refining the stimuli to which cortical cells respond. We have discussed elsewhere the wide range of evidence which implies that the cortex may play a minor role in neonatal visual function, but come to achieve dominance over subcortical vision between about 2 and 4 months (Atkinson, 1984; Braddick & Atkinson, 1988). Here we outline a particular approach, using stimuli that are specially designed to elicit a response only from cortical neurons that have developed particular selective properties. These responses may be detected either by means of visual evoked potentials or by behavioural discriminations.

Binocularity

Signals from the two eyes first interact in the cortex, and probably the strongest body of evidence for the postnatal development of a visual cortical function comes from studies of responses that depend on binocular interaction. An example of such a response is the VEP elicited by a random dot correlogram (Julesz, Kropfl & Petrig, 1980); any signal locked to alternations of a dynamic pattern between binocular correlation and anticorrelation must arise from neurons with binocular input. Such responses are first seen on average around 3–4 months of age (Braddick et al., 1980; Petrig et al., 1981; Braddick et al., 1983; Wattam-Bell et al., 1987b). The ability to detect binocular correlation does not necessarily imply stereopsis,

DYNAMIC ORIENTATION-REVERSAL STIMULUS

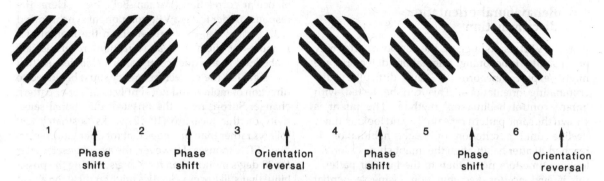

1		2		3		4		5		6	

Phase shift   Phase shift   Orientation reversal   Phase shift   Phase shift   Orientation reversal

Fig. 23.2. A sample from the stimulus used in the dynamic double orientation stimulus pattern. With each new frame the pattern undergoes a random position displacement (phase shift), and between frames 3 and 4 its orientation is changed. The single orientation stimulus was similar but with the same orientation in frames 4, 5, 6 as in 1, 2, 3.

but work from a number of laboratories agrees that by around four months postnatally most infants can be shown to discriminate disparities (Atkinson & Braddick, 1974; Fox, Aslin, Shea, & Dumais, 1980; Held, Birch & Gwiazda, 1980; Birch, Gwiazda & Held, 1983; Birch, Shimojo & Held, 1985; see review by Braddick and Atkinson, 1983). However, there is quite a wide range of individual differences found in onset times for both functions (ranging from 2 to 6 months). Current work by Jocelyn Smith in our laboratory is comparing correlation and disparity detection by the same infants under the same conditions; so far she has found no systematic difference in age of onset, or between VEP and behavioural measures of detection using similar stimuli (Smith *et al.*, 1988).

Orientation selectivity

Besides binocularity, a property that is not found in primate visual neurons prior to the cortex is orientation selectivity. A recently developed VEP technique can identify this selectivity in infants (Braddick, Wattam-Bell & Atkinson, 1986). The infant views a grating which changes in position on each frame and in orientation every third frame (see Fig. 23.2). A significant VEP, time locked to the orientation changes, indicates that the infant's cortex has produced a response specific to orientation change and not just to local contrast changes. This orientation-specific VEP is usually first seen at around 6 weeks postnatal age, even though significant pattern-appearance VEP responses can be recorded from infants in the first few days of life. Figure 23.3 shows an example of an

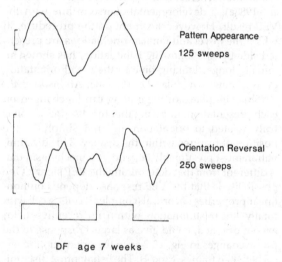

Pattern Appearance
125 sweeps

Orientation Reversal
250 sweeps

DF age 7 weeks

Fig. 23.3. Orientation VEP response and pattern-appearance VEP, from a normal 7-week old infant. The bottom trace indicates the timing of the stimulus alternations (total duration = 0.5 s). Each record is the averaged response of the number of sweeps indicated. Vertical scale = 5 microvolts.

orientation VEP response in a normal 7-week old. These results were obtained with orthogonal oblique orientations; however, we do not find any different age of onset for the response to horizontal/vertical orientations (Wattam-Bell *et al.*, 1987a). Anisotropies between horizontal/vertical and oblique responses do occur with this response, but they emerge later (3–5 months) and may be associated with the differential significance of vertical and horizontal contours for stereopsis.

Behavioural orientation discrimination

If, as the VEP results suggest, the newborn cortex may not contain functioning orientation detectors, we might expect newborns to have difficulties discriminating orientations. This can be tested with 'infant control habituation' method. The infant is shown the same pattern repeatedly, and looking times decline until a criterion of visual habituation is reached. If after habituation the infant shows a longer looking time to a novel than to the familiar pattern, this is evidence for discrimination. Using sequential presentation of familiar and novel patterns, with the distinctive feature of the new pattern being a change in orientation, we found that newborns showed no discrimination whereas 5- to 6-week olds did (Atkinson et al., 1988a), a developmental course in line with the VEP result. However, a variant on the procedure, in which the novel and familiar orientations are presented side by side following habituation, has shown an initially longer looking time to the novel orientation even in newborns (Slater et al., 1988; Atkinson et al., 1988b). The phase of the grating can be changed on each presentation, implying that the discrimination is truly related to orientation and not simply to the position of features within the display. This discrimination must presumably depend on a mechanism that is different from that determining the VEP signal. One possibility is that the VEP response depends on non-linear properties of cortical (complex?) cells (a cell with totally linear summation within its receptive field, even if oriented, could give as large a response to the phase changes in Fig. 23.2 as to the orientation reversal between frames 3 and 4). The behavioural discrimination by neonates might then depend on simple cells which behaved in a near-linear way and so were relatively silent in the VEP. This possible dissociation is discussed further below.

Directionality

A third property of many visual cortical neurons, absent at lower levels of the primate geniculostriate pathway, is selective responsiveness to motion in a particular direction. Sensitivity to motion is often thought of as a very primitive visual function, which might therefore be expected to be present earlier in development than discriminations of purely spatial pattern properties. The developmental course of direction selectivity can be studied by VEP method quite analogous to those used for orientation and binocular correlation (Wattam-Bell, 1987). Here, the response under test is a VEP component synchronized with periodic up-down reversals in the motion of a random-dot field. These direction reversals are embedded in a sequence of pattern changes, so that any signal at the correct frequency must be linked to direction of motion and not simply to flicker or pattern change. Surprisingly, the onset of directional selectivity on this measure (10–12 weeks postnatal age) follows rather than precedes that for orientation selective VEP responses. However, the age of onset is later for 20 deg/s motion than for 5 deg/s, raising the possibility that still lower velocities might reduce the age at which directional responses can be measured. This direction of development, with slower velocities (i.e. smaller displacements) detected earlier, is an interesting contrast to the general picture that spatial vision develops from coarse to fine, or low to high acuity.

Directionality, then, provides another visual cortical function which appears to emerge in the course of the immediately postnatal months of human development. In the mature cortex, orientation- and direction-selectivity are closely associated. Some findings in cat (Pettigrew, 1974) suggested that neurons in the newborn cortex were more direction- than orientation-selective, raising the possibility that a directional preference might be the foundation on which a cell built its orientation-selectivity. Our results make it doubtful whether this can be the sequence in human development. The developmental co-ordination of orientation- and direction-selectivity has to allow for the fact that, orthogonal to any one contour orientation, there are two opposed directions of motion. Topographic studies of cat cortex (Swindale et al., 1987) show discontinuities between such opposed directions in the direction map, within regions of continuity in the orientation map; this is consistent with the idea that the spatial organization of orientation-selectivity is prior to that of direction in the development of the columnar layout of the visual cortex. Hopefully, more detailed study of the developmental sequence may help us understand better how these properties of visual cortex become established and organized.

Other aspects of cortical function

This chapter has concentrated on the development of selectivity for various stimulus properties, which are known to be characteristic of the visual cortex. Over the same developmental period, infants start to show behavioural evidence of discriminations of spatial patterns which can be described in terms of spatial phase (Braddick, Atkinson, & Wattam-Bell, 1986) or in terms of the presence of pattern primitives or 'textons' (Atkinson, Wattam-Bell, & Braddick, 1986). These abilities may reflect the emergence of new classes of specific cortical detector, or they may reflect the capacity to combine information across detectors. In any case, it is clear that to use cortical encoding mechanisms effectively, they cannot simply be used as passive receptors. Control processes are necessary and must develop (Braddick & Atkinson, 1988). The cross-channel integration of visual information presumably involves controlling the flow of information within the cortex. Equally important is the developing control of the visual cortex over its own input. One way in which this is reflected is the development, over the early months, of the ability to select for fixation one of several competing targets (Atkinson & Braddick, 1985; Atkinson *et al.*, 1988a). Another, longer-term process, is the visual control over ocular development by which an emmetropic eye is achieved. Although this mechanism is not yet understood, it is likely that central control is at least partly involved (Troilo & Wallman, 1988). In the follow-up of our infant refractive screening programme (Atkinson & Braddick, 1988; Atkinson *et al.*, 1987) we have identified groups of infants in whom emmetropization is slow or imperfect, and we must consider how far this may be due to deficits in specific or general central control processes, as well as in the initial optical parameters.

Overview

The results we have outlined show that some essential aspects of visual cortical function, namely binocularity, orientation-, and direction-selectivity, are at least extremely immature at birth and develop greatly over the first few months of human life. There may be significant differences from other primates in this respect, given that the first month or so of cranial and brain development in humans may be analogous to the final prenatal period in other primates (Prechtl, 1984). However, there are a number of possibilities for the nature and degree of this immaturity. The simplest and most radical suggestion is that the visual behaviour seen before about six weeks is subcortically mediated – a suggestion first made by Bronson (1974) and developed by Atkinson (1984). This view has to be reconciled with the finding of orientation-based

behavioural discriminations at birth. A key element of Atkinson's (1984) proposal was the development of pathways by which visual cortical activity could control subcortical oculomotor and orienting function. Immaturity in this aspect of visual function might explain why the demonstration of orientation-selectivity is so sensitive to the behavioural test procedures, but it is difficult to see how neonates could perform our discriminations without some kind of orientation-selective, presumably cortical, structures.

Developmental dissociations: parvocellular and magnocellular pathways?

It is possible that discriminative behaviour can occur with a very small number, or very weak activity, of orientation-selective neurons, while a measurable VEP depends more strongly on mass activity. Alternatively, the two methods may depend on different specific populations of neurons. We have already raised the possibility that our VEP technique may measure primarily the activity of complex cells. Some years ago, Maurer & Lewis (1979) speculated, largely on the basis of evidence from cat, that neonatal vision might reflect an absence of Y-cell input to the cortex. We now know that the primate system is not quite analogous, but does include an apparently far-reaching separation of different kinds of visual information between parvo- and magnocellular pathways (see e.g. Livingstone & Hubel, 1988). The relatively late development of directional responses, especially for higher velocities, raises the possibility that the magnocellular pathway, which is believed to be the primary route for motion information, may be slower in development. If so, the non-linear response reflected in the orientation VEP might also arise in this pathway, albeit at a somewhat earlier age. The thick CO-staining stripes in area V2, which receive input largely from the magnocellular system, are also reported to be the predominant location of disparity-selective cells. This raises the possibility that the development of sensitivity to binocular correlation and disparity around 3–4 months may also be a function of the development of the magno pathway. It is also worth noting that high contrast sensitivity appears to require the magno pathway (Shapley, Kaplan, & Soodak, 1981).

To evaluate any of these hypotheses, we shall need a fuller understanding of the contribution of different classes of cortical cell to adult human vision, and of the development of their functions in other primates. We believe that the developmental dissociation of functions in human infancy can also help us to understand the organization of the adult system.

Acknowledgements

The research of the Visual Development Unit described here is supported by the Medical Research Council and the East Anglia Regional Health Authority.

References

Atkinson, J. (1984) Human visual development over the first 6 months of life: a review and a hypothesis. *Human Neurobiol.*, **3**, 61–74.

Atkinson, J. & Braddick, O. J. (1974) Stereoscopic discrimination in infants. *Perception*, **5**, 29–38.

Atkinson, J. & Braddick, O. J. (1981) Acuity, contrast sensitivity and accommodation in infancy. In *The Development of Perception: Psychobiological Perspectives. Vol. 2: The Visual System*, ed. R. N. Aslin, J. R. Alberts & M. R. Petersen, pp. 245–77. New York: Academic Press.

Atkinson, J. & Braddick, O. J. (1985) Early development of the control of visual attention. *Perception*, **14**, A25.

Atkinson, J. & Braddick, O. J. (1988) Infant precursors of later visual disorders: correlation or causality. In *20th Minnesota Symposium on Child Psychology*, ed. A. Yonas. Hillsdale, NJ: Lawrence Erlbaum.

Atkinson, J., Braddick, O.J., Wattam-Bell, J., Durden, K., Bobier, W. & Pointer, J. (1987) Photorefractive screening of infants and effects of refractive correction. *Invest. Ophthal. and Vis. Sci. (Suppl.)*, **28**, 399.

Atkinson, J., Hood, B., Braddick, O. J. & Wattam-Bell, J. (1988a) Infants' control of fixation shifts with single and competing targets: mechanisms of shifting attention. *Perception*, **17**, 367.

Atkinson, J., Hood, B., Wattam-Bell, J., Anker, S. & Tricklebank, J. (1988b) Development of orientation discrimination in infancy. *Perception*, **17**, 587–96.

Atkinson, J., Wattam-Bell, J. & Braddick, O. J. (1986) Infants' development of sensitivity to pattern 'textons'. *Invest. Ophthal. and Vis. Sci. (Suppl.)*, **27**, 265.

Banks, M. S. (1980) Infant refraction and accommodation. *International Ophthalmology Clinics*, **20**, 205–32.

Banks, M. S. (1989) The role of optical and retinal factors in the development of human visual performance. In *The Neurophysiological Foundations of Visual Perception*, ed. L. Spillmann & J. S. Werner. San Diego: Academic Press.

Banks, M. & Salapatek, P. (1983) Infant visual perception. In *Handbook of Child Psychology, vol 2: Biology and Infancy*, ed. M. M. Haith & J. Campos, pp. 435–571. New York: John Wiley.

Birch, E. E., Gwiazda, J. & Held, R. (1983) The development of vergence does not account for the development of stereopsis. *Perception*, **12**, 331–6.

Birch, E. E., Shimojo, S. & Held, R. (1985) Preferential-looking assessment of fusion and stereopsis in infants aged 1–6 months. *Invest. Ophthal. and Vis. Sci.*, **26**, 366–70.

Braddick, O. J. & Atkinson, J. (1983) Some recent findings on the development of human binocularity: a review. *Behavioural Brain Research*, **10**, 71–80.

Braddick, O. J. & Atkinson, J. (1988) Sensory selectivity, attentional control, and cross-channel integration in early visual development. In *20th Minnesota Symposium on Child Psychology*, ed. A. Yonas. Hillsdale, NJ: Lawrence Erlbaum.

Braddick, O. J., Atkinson, J., French, J. & Howland, H. C. (1979) A photorefractive study of infant accommodation. *Vision Res.*, **19**, 319–30.

Braddick, O. J., Atkinson, J., Julesz, B., Kropfl, W., Bodis-Wollner, I. & Raab, E. (1980) Cortical binocularity in infants. *Nature*, **288**, 363–5.

Braddick, O. J., Atkinson, J. & Wattam-Bell, J. R. (1986) Development of the discrimination of spatial phase in infancy. *Vision Res.*, **26**, 1223–39.

Braddick, O. J., Wattam-Bell, J. & Atkinson, J. (1986) Orientation-specific cortical responses develop in early infancy. *Nature*, **320**, 617–19.

Braddick, O., Wattam-Bell, J., Day, J. & Atkinson, J. (1983) The onset of binocular function in human infants. *Human Neurobiol.*, **2**, 65–9.

Bronson, G. W. (1974) The postnatal growth of visual capacity. *Child Development*, **45**, 873–90.

Dobson, V. & Teller, D. Y. (1978) Visual acuity in human infants: a review and comparison of behavioral and electrophysiological studies. *Vision Res.*, **18**, 1469–83.

Fox, R., Aslin, R. N., Shea, S. L. & Dumais, S. T. (1980) Stereopsis in human infants. *Science*, **207**, 323–4.

Garey, L. & De Courten, C. (1983) Structural development of the lateral geniculate nucleus and visual cortex in monkey and man. *Behavioural Brain Research*, **10**, 3–15.

Held, R., Birch, E. E., & Gwiazda, J. (1980) Stereoacuity of human infants. *Proc. Natl. Acad. Sci. USA*, **77**, 5572–4.

Howland, H. C., Atkinson, J., Braddick, O. & French, J. (1978) Infant astigmatism measured by photorefraction. *Science*, **202**, 331–3.

Howland, H. C., Braddick, O. J., Atkinson, J. & Howland, B. (1983) Optics of photorefraction: orthogonal and isotropic methods. *J. Opt. Soc. Am.*, **73**, 1701–8.

Jacobs, D. & Blakemore, C. B. (1988) Factors limiting the postnatal development of visual acuity in the monkey. *Vision Res.*, **28**, 947–58.

Julesz, B., Kropfl, W. & Petrig, B. (1980) Large evoked potentials of dynamic random-dot correlograms and stereograms permit quick determination of stereopsis. *Proc. Natl. Acad. Sci. USA*, **77**, 2348–51.

Livingstone, M. & Hubel, D. H. (1988) Segregation of form,

color, movement, and depth: anatomy, physiology and perception. *Science*, **240**, 740–9.

Maurer, D. & Lewis, T. L. (1979) A physiological explanation of infants' early visual development. *Canad. J. of Psychol.*, **33**, 232–52.

Mohindra, I., Held, R., Gwiazda, J. & Brill, S. (1978) Astigmatism in infants. *Science*, **202**, 329–31.

Norcia, A. M. & Tyler, C. W. (1985) Spatial frequency sweep VEP: visual acuity in the first year of life. *Vision Res.*, **25**, 1399–408.

Petrig, B., Julesz, B., Kropfl, W., Baumgartner, G. & Anliker, M. (1981) Development of stereopsis and cortical binocularity in human infants: electrophysiological evidence. *Science*, **213**, 1402–5.

Pettigrew, J. D. (1974) The effect of visual experience on the development of stimulus specificity by kitten cortical neurones. *J. Physiol.*, **237**, 49–74.

Prechtl, H. (ed.) (1984) *Continuity of Neural Functions from Prenatal to Postnatal Life* London: Spastics International Medical Publications.

Regan, D. M. (1980) Speedy evoked potential methods for assessing vision in normal and amblyopic eyes: pros and cons. *Vision Res.*, **20**, 265–9.

Shapley, R., Kaplan, E. & Soodak, R. (1981) Spatial summation and contrast sensitivity of X and Y cells in the lateral geniculate nucleus of the macaque. *Nature*, **292**, 543–5.

Slater, A., Morison, V. & Somers, M. (1988) Orientation discrimination and cortical function in the human newborn. *Perception*, **17**, 597–602.

Smith, J., Atkinson, J., Braddick, O. J. & Wattam-Bell, J. (1988) Development of sensitivity to binocular correlation and disparity in infancy. *Perception*, **17**, 395–6.

Swindale, N. V., Matsubara, J. A. & Cynader, M. S. (1987) Surface organization of orientation and direction selectivity in cat area 18. *J. Neurosci.*, **7**, 1414–27.

Troilo, D. & Wallman, J. (1988) Experimental emmetropization in chicks. *Invest. Ophthal. and Vis. Sci (Suppl.)*, **29**, 76.

Wattam-Bell, J. (1987) Motion-specific VEPs in adults and infants. *Perception*, **16**, 231.

Wattam-Bell, J., Braddick, O. J., Marshall, G. and Atkinson, J. (1987a) Development and anisotropy of the orientation-specific VEP. *Invest. Ophthal. and Vis. Sci. (Suppl.)*, **28**, 5.

Wattam-Bell, J., Braddick, O., Atkinson, J. & Day, J. (1987b) Measures of infant binocularity in a group at risk for strabismus. *Clinical Vision Sciences*, **1**, 327–36.

Wilson, H. (1988) Development of spatiotemporal mechanisms in infant vision. *Vision Res.*, **28**, 611–28.

Yuodelis, C. & Hendrickson, A. (1986) A qualitative and quantitative analysis of the human fovea during development. *Vision Res.*, **26**, 847–55.

24

Maturation of mechanisms for efficient spatial vision

C. Blakemore

Introduction

One of the most remarkable achievements of the human visual system is the capacity to resolve fine detail in the retinal image and efficiently to detect contrast between neighbouring regions of the image. In the central visual field these perceptual abilities appear to be limited by the physical properties of the photoreceptors themselves. The development of spatial vision provides a fine example of the way in which the efficiency of coding in the visual system emerges through an interplay between innate (presumably genetically determined) organization and plasticity of synaptic organization at the level of the visual cortex. As Barlow (1972) pointed out, developmental plasticity might allow the visual cortex to discover, in the pattern of stimulation it receives, important associations and coincidences in the retinal image that relate to the nature of the visual world.

Efficiency of spatial vision in the adult

Factors that might limit spatial vision

The resolution of spatial detail and the detection of contrast in the retinal image might, in principle, be limited by one of a number of factors. Obviously, the optical quality cf the image could determine spatial performance and certainly does so in states of refractive error. Even when the eye is accurately focused, chromatic and spherical aberration degrade the image, as does the effect of diffraction, which is dependent on the size of the pupil. Interestingly, under photopic conditions, the pupil of the human eye tends to adopt a diameter that optimizes visual acuity: a larger pupil size would augment the effects of aberrations and a smaller one would increase diffraction, as well as decreasing retinal illumination (Campbell & Gregory, 1960).

The retinal image, whose magnification depends on the size of the eyeball, is then sampled by the distribution of the outer segments of the photoreceptors. Recent work has shown that, under conditions of optimum focus, the quality of the image in a wide variety of species is superior to the limit of sampling imposed by the mosaic of photoreceptors (Wehner, 1981; Land & Snyder, 1985; Snyder et al., 1986). Therefore, in well focused eyes optical factors do not normally limit visual resolution. This seems to be the case even for the very centre of the human fovea, where the outer segments of the cones are exceptionally slim and tightly packed, with a centre-to-centre spacing of as little as 2.8–3.0 μm (Østerberg, 1935; Miller, 1979). This is equivalent to an angular spacing ($\triangle\phi$) of about 0.5–0.6 min arc.

According to the sampling theorem, an array of detectors can just reliably encode a repetitive distribution of light and dark when the spacing of neighbouring receptors is equal to one half-period of the pattern. Thus, the highest spatial frequency that can be correctly encoded (the Nyquist limit) is $\frac{1}{2}\triangle\phi$, which gives a predicted resolution of 50–52 cycles deg^{-1} (cycles of a grating pattern per degree of visual angle) for the central human fovea. However, in the adult primate eye, foveal cones are arranged in local domains, each of which has a regular, hexagonal array (or, more exactly, a triangular lattice; see Williams, 1986). In such an array, neighbouring *rows* are separated by $\sqrt{3}/2\cdot\triangle\phi$, which produces a Nyquist limit:

$$\nu_s = 1/\sqrt{3}\cdot\triangle\phi \quad \text{(Snyder \& Miller, 1977).}$$

For the human eye this row-to-row Nyquist limit

predicts a bandwidth for the identification of extended high-contrast gratings of 58–60 cycles deg^{-1}. The maximum human acuity, measured as the cut-off spatial frequency for gratings of high mean luminance, is in fact about 55–60 cycles deg^{-1} (see Campbell & Green, 1965; Miller, 1979). By comparison, the bandwidth of the optics of the eye is just a little better (65–70 cycles deg^{-1}) at the fovea (Campbell & Gubisch, 1966; Westheimer, 1977).

The fact that we can resolve gratings whose individual bars are the same size as single photoreceptors implies that we have access, at the level of perception, to independent signals from neighbouring foveal cones. This requires the preservation of spatial information, from at least some fraction of those cones, through the whole of the visual pathway. In the primate retina, there are in fact more bipolar cells and ganglion cells representing the central fovea than there are foveal photoreceptors, and some cones undoubtedly have 'private lines' to their own midget ganglion cells (Dowling & Boycott, 1966), each one probably contributing the entire centre mechanism of the receptive field of such a ganglion cell.

There is further anatomical and physiological evidence for the effective preservation of 1:1 connectivity for the centre mechanisms of the receptive fields of neurons in the foveal representation area of both the lateral geniculate nucleus (LGN) and the pimary visual cortex. Some individual neurons in the LGN and the cortex of monkeys can detect the presence of drifting gratings up to a spatial frequency close to the receptor and optical limits for the monkey eye, which are similar to those of the human (Derrington & Lennie, 1984; Parker & Hawken, 1985; Blakemore & Vital-Durand, 1986a; M. J. Hawken & A. J. Parker, this volume). In the visual cortex, many neurons in the lower part of layer 4, where the bulk of LGN axons arrive, have circular, concentrically organized receptive fields, with centre dimensions similar to those of LGN cells representing the same part of the visual field.

Outside layer 4c, most cells are orientation selective (Hubel & Wiesel, 1977) and have elongated receptive fields with a length equivalent to many photoreceptors. However, for at least some cells of the 'simple' class, the receptive field centre can be the same width (orthogonal to the preferred orientation) as for geniculate cells representing the same retinal eccentricity, i.e. equivalent to approximately a single cone for the very centre of the fovea.

The preservation of spatial information beyond the level of 'simple' cells in the primary visual cortex is not well understood. However, we can make an unequivocal inference, from the perceptual abilities of human beings and monkeys, that the spatial sampling imposed by the foveal photoreceptors is somehow maintained through the system. Of course, this cannot be true for the whole of the visual field since the *total* number of photoreceptors in the retina far outnumbers that of ganglion cells. Only 10 deg from the human fovea, where the optical bandpass may still be as high as 60 cycles deg^{-1}, the cones are much more coarsely spaced and the Nyquist limit of their mosaic is only 13 cycles deg^{-1} (see Snyder *et al.*, 1986). However, the psychophysical visual acuity is even worse than the value predicted by the cone mosaic. Thus, we can be sure that visual resolution in the peripheral field is limited by spatial pooling or under-sampling within the retina and visual pathway.

Under ideal conditions, at high mean illumination, in the central visual field, less than 0.5% intensity difference is needed between the bars of a grating of about 5 cycles deg^{-1} for the detection of the pattern. This remarkable ability to detect contrast in patterns of intermediate spatial frequency may well be ultimately limited by the physical properties of the photoreceptors making up the receptive fields of neurons in the visual pathway; it may depend on the efficiency with which quanta are caught and signalled by the photoreceptors, and on the stochastic nature of quantal absorption (Barlow & Levick, 1969; see also Wilson, 1988).

Development of spatial vision

Postnatal improvement in resolution and contrast sensitivity

There is now a wealth of behavioural evidence that the spatial resolution and contrast sensitivity of human babies and young primates are grossly inferior to those of the adult (e.g. Atkinson, Braddick & Moar, 1977; Dobson & Teller, 1978; Teller *et al.*, 1978; Boothe, Dobson & Teller, 1985). The natural tendency of babies and young monkeys to look at visual stimuli containing contour and contrast rather than at areas of unmodulated luminance has been exploited, through the so-called *preferential looking* technique, to assess both visual acuity and contrast sensitivity. In neonatal primates (human and non-human), visual acuity determined by this technique is less than 1 cycle deg^{-1} and contrast sensitivity is at least ten times worse than in the adult, even in the optimal range of spatial frequencies. Thus, the young animal views the visual world through a severe spatial filter, which restricts its vision to the high-contrast, low spatial-frequency components of any image. The visual capability of a newborn baby, judged in terms of its spatial performance, is substantially worse than that of an adult cat and is even inferior to the vision of a rat!

In both monkeys and human beings, there is a surprisingly slow improvement in spatial performance, involving at least a 30-fold increase in visual acuity and an enormous overall improvement in contrast sensitivity. In humans this process may take as long as ten years, and even in monkeys, where maturation is considerably faster, behavioural acuity and contrast sensitivity probably do not reach their adult values until the end of the second year.

Neurophysiological correlates

These perceptual improvements in spatial vision are qualitatively paralleled by the physiological maturation of neurons in the primate visual pathway. A rather direct comparison between psychophysical ability and neurophysiological performance can be obtained by testing the ability of single cells, recorded in the anaesthetized monkey, to detect the presence of briefly presented grating patterns, drifting across the receptive field. Even on the day of birth, most if not all neurons in the LGN are already responsive to visual stimuli (Blakemore & Vital-Durand, 1986a), and so too are the majority of cells in the primary visual cortex. However, the spatial structure of their receptive fields is extremely immature: the receptive field centres of LGN cells and the spatially summating sub-units of the receptive fields of cortical cells are unusually large and the neurons respond sluggishly even to a spot or bar of optimum position and size. In both LGN and cortex, the best-performing neurons can detect the presence of high-contrast gratings up to a spatial frequency of only about 5 cycles deg^{-1}. Figure 24.1 shows the way in which the spatial resolution of LGN cells, measured in this fashion, improves with age in monkeys (Blakemore & Vital-Durand, 1986a). There is an approximately seven-fold increase in the average spatial resolution of LGN cells in the foveal representation area, over the first year or so of life. The best-performing cells improve from about 5 cycles deg^{-1} to more than 35 cycles deg^{-1} (under the conditions of this experiment, which are described in the legend to Fig. 24.1).

Comparison with behavioural results (unfilled squares in Fig. 24.1) shows a general similarity in the improvement of neuronal and perceptual performance; however, the best LGN neurons in a neonatal monkey are substantially superior in their ability to resolve high-contrast gratings compared with the

whole animal (as judged by the preferential looking method). By about ten weeks of age behavioural acuity is close to the resolution of the best cells in the population, as it is in adult monkeys (Parker & Hawken, 1985; M. J. Hawken & A. J. Parker, this volume).

The spatial resolution of neurons, for any particular eccentricity in the visual field, varies over a much greater range in the primary visual cortex than in the LGN. However, at every age in normal monkeys, the best-performing cortical cells in the foveal representation are similar in their spatial resolution to the best LGN cells (Blakemore & Vital-Durand, 1983; see Fig. 24.4 below). Thus, it seems likely that in normal monkeys some fraction of cortical cells is effectively excited by a small ensemble of incoming geniculate fibres, providing the cortical cell with a receptive field whose spatial summating area (measured orthogonal to the preferred orientation) is similar in size to the centre region of geniculate receptive fields.

The contrast sensitivity of individual neurons in LGN and cortex also matures in a way that mimics the improvement in behavioural performance (Blakemore & Hawken, 1985; Blakemore & Vital-Durand, 1983). Cells in neonatal monkeys typically require gratings of high contrast. Figure 24.2 shows representative contrast sensitivity functions for two individual cortical neurons, one recorded in a newborn monkey (filled circles), the other in a normal adult (unfilled circles). In each case, the receptive field was presented with drifting gratings (of optimum orientation and direction of movement) at different spatial frequencies. For each stimulus, the contrast was adjusted between successive brief exposures, in order to determine the threshold contrast at which the cell just responded to the presence of the grating. The cell from the adult has a high 'acuity', responding to gratings of high contrast up to more than 30 cycles deg^{-1}. It has a pronounced peak of high contrast sensitivity around 8 cycles deg^{-1}, with attenuation of sensitivity at lower spatial frequencies (presumably due to the presence of strong inhibitory side-bands flanking the spatially summating sub-unit). By comparison, the resolution and peak contrast-sensitivity of the cell from the newborn animal are much inferior, and low-frequency attenuation is less exaggerated.

Development of spatial vision depends on visual experience

The common clinical condition of *amblyopia* (see R. F. Hess, D. J. Field & R. J. Watt, chapter 25) provides strong evidence that the maturation of spatial vision is itself dependent on visual experience. Young babies

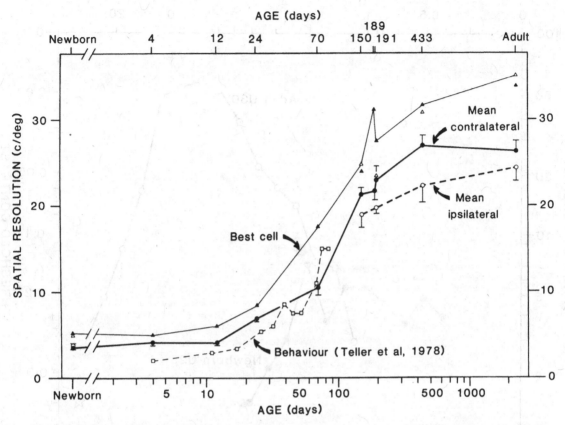

Fig. 24.1. Spatial resolution is plotted against age (on a logarithmic scale) for these results from Old-World monkeys. The unfilled squares, joined by interrupted thin lines, plot the behavioural visual acuity of a pigtail monkey, determined with the preferential looking technique by Teller *et al.* (1978). The rest of the points come from Blakemore & Vital-Durand's (1986a) study of single neurons in the LGN. The animals were anaesthetized and, with each eye optimally refracted and viewing through a 4 mm artificial pupil, the receptive fields of cells were stimulated with drifting gratings of high contrast (0.75) and a mean luminance of 45 cd m^{-2}, generated on a television display. The highest spatial frequency for which each cell gave a just detectable response was taken as its spatial resolution. Recordings were always taken from the right LGN. The filled circles, joined by thick lines, show the mean resolution (+ or − 1 standard error) for all LGN cells with linear spatial summation (X cells) that were responsive through the contralateral (left) eye, with receptive fields centred within 2 deg of the middle of the fovea. Some of these results come from completely normal animals, others from the non-deprived layers of monocularly deprived monkeys. For the animals that were not deprived, there are corresponding unfilled circles joined by dashed thick lines, which plot the mean resolution for similar samples of receptive fields connected to the ipsilateral (right) eye. The number of cells, in each sample ranges between 5 and 22. The triangles (filled for the left eye, open for the right) show the neuronal 'acuity' for the best-performing cell in each sample. The thin line is, then, the upper envelope of performance for this series of animals.

who suffer deprivation of pattern vision (because of cataract, corneal opacity, drooping of the eyelid, etc.), anisometropia (a difference in the refractive error of the two eyes) or squint (deviation, especially inward turning, of one eye) early in life often subsequently suffer from abnormally low visual acuity in one eye, which is not explained by any obvious pathology in the eye itself and which persists even when the eye is optimally refracted. This condition of amblyopia is commonly characterized by poor contrast sensitivity, especially for relatively high spatial frequencies, and also by more subtle disturbances of visual perception, in addition to the classical reduction in visual acuity (see R. F. Hess *et al.*, chapter 25).

It is tempting to think, then, that amblyopia is due to a *failure* of normal maturation, precipitated by

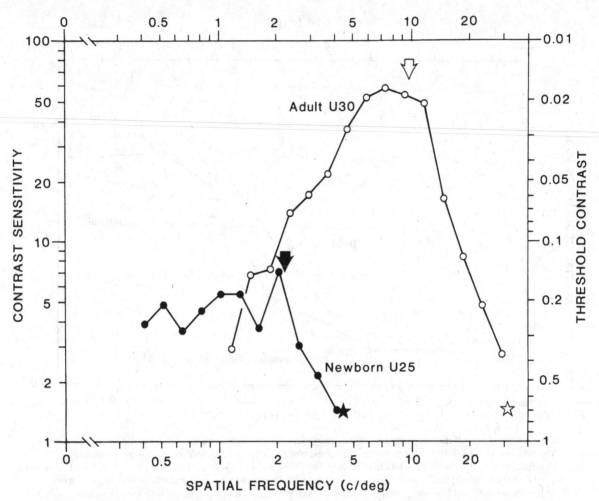

Fig. 24.2. These unpublished results of C. Blakemore & F. Vital-Durand show the ability of two individual neurons recorded in the primary visual cortex of monkeys to detect contrast. One cell (unfilled circles) was recorded in a normal adult animal, the other (filled circles) in a newborn monkey. A drifting grating of optimal orientation, generated on a television display (mean luminance about $280\,\text{cd}\,\text{m}^{-2}$), was centred on the receptive field of the cell, with the non-dominant eye covered. For each spatial frequency of grating, the contrast was varied, while the experimenter listened to the cell's response, in order to determine a threshold contrast (plotted on the right ordinate) below which the cell did not reliably respond to the grating. Each circle is the mean of four determinations. The left ordinate is the reciprocal of threshold contrast, i.e. contrast sensitivity. (Contrast $= (L_{\text{max}} - L_{\text{min}})/(L_{\text{max}} + L_{\text{min}})$.) The arrows indicate the optimal spatial frequency, judged by ear, for drifting gratings of high contrast, while the stars show the visual resolution (mean of four estimates) for a grating of high contrast, determined as for the LGN cells in Fig. 24.1.

the difference in stimulation of the two eyes resulting from the predisposing conditions. A parsimonious account of both the normal development of spatial vision and amblyopia would suggest that some sort of reorganization of spatial sampling in the retina (perhaps a change in the anatomical convergence between photoreceptors and ganglion cells) underlies the natural improvement in spatial resolution and

contrast sensitivity, and that conditions leading to amblyopia retard this process of neuronal reorganization. It turns out that this explanation, attractive though it is, does not account for the facts: normal maturation is indeed restricted by peripheral factors, but the origin of amblyopia (at least deprivation amblyopia in the monkey) seems to lie at the level of the visual cortex.

Limiting factors during normal maturation

The very poor behavioural acuity of neonatal monkeys and human beings is unlikely to be limited by inferior optical quality or inaccurate accommodation of the eyes. Williams & Boothe (1981) have shown that there is only a slight postnatal improvement in the optical quality of the monkey's eye, which reaches the adult state by about 13 weeks of age, whereas behavioural acuity is not fully mature for well over a year. Accommodation is somewhat inaccurate in young monkeys (Howland *et al.*, 1982), but, again, the degradation of the image caused by incorrect accommodation is unlikely to be serious enough to account for the poor performance in preferential looking tasks. In neurophysiological experiments (see Blakemore & Vital-Durand, 1986a), accommodation is paralysed and the optical state of the eye is optimized with spherical refractive correction and an artificial pupil, so errors of accommodation cannot possibly explain the relatively poor spatial performance of LGN and cortical neurons in young monkeys. It seems, then, that the substantial improvement in the properties of individual neurons in the visual pathway can be accounted for only by changes in spatial sampling within the retina itself or at the input to geniculate cells.

The most likely candidate factor for the production of such a large change in the receptive field structure of neurons would seem to be an alteration in the degree of synaptic convergence in the peripheral part of the visual pathway, perhaps a reduction in the number of cones contributing to the centre mechanisms of the receptive fields of foveal ganglion cells. However, Jacobs & Blakemore (1988) have suggested that the bulk of the neurophysiological changes can be accounted for by simple alterations (presumably passive) in the array of photoreceptors themselves.

During the first two years or so of life, the primate eyeball grows, thus increasing the axial length and hence the magnification of the retinal image (Blakemore & Vital-Durand, 1986a). If the retina were simply to be uniformly stretched as the eye grows, there would, of course, be no change in the spatial sampling of the image by the photoreceptors, expressed in angular terms. However, in both monkeys and human beings, the central fovea actually *decreases* in linear dimensions (almost a three-fold reduction in diameter) over the first two years or so of life (Hendrickson & Kupfer, 1976; Yuodelis & Hendrickson, 1986). The total number of cones within the rod-free area remains roughly constant during this shrinkage of the macular area, so cone spacing changes *pari passu*

with the reduction in the diameter of the rod-free area. Thus, there appears to be a roughly three-fold *reduction* in the linear spacing of central cones, while the magnification of the retinal image is *increasing* by about 50%. These two factors combine to predict a substantial (roughly five-fold) increase in the theoretical Nyquist limit of the photoreceptor array.

The analysis in Fig. 24.3 suggests that the Nyquist limit for reliable sampling of the retinal image may be as low as 8–9 cycles deg^{-1} at birth in monkeys and that it rises slowly during the first year or two of life. Figure 24.4 provides a direct comparison between the developmental change in the photoreceptor sampling limit and the improvement in spatial resolution (on a logarithmic scale) of the best-performing LGN and cortical cells. Neurophysiological performance is definitely worse than the limit of the photoreceptor array during the first few months of life, but at most by only a factor of two or so. And, beyond about ten weeks of age, the functions describing the improvement in geniculate and cortical performance run virtually parallel to the change in the receptor mosaic. Thus, any change in spatial convergence beyond the photoreceptors, if it occurs at all, seems to be minor in magnitude and restricted to the first two or three months of life. Fig. 24.4 again reproduces Teller *et al.*'s (1978) behavioural determinations of acuity, using the preferential looking method. Behavioural resolution is substantially inferior to the theoretical photoreceptor limit in young monkeys, but reaches the level of performance of the best cortical neurons by about ten weeks of age. The discrepancy between neuronal resolution and behavioural performance at younger ages suggests either that there is initially excessive spatial pooling or under-sampling in the visual pathway beyond the primary cortex, which is gradually eliminated during development, or that the preferential looking method fails to press young animals to the true limit of their spatial resolution.

The meaning of spatial resolution

So far, this analysis has glossed over an important distinction between the prediction of the Nyquist limit and the index of resolution provided by neurophysiological experiments (and by most behavioural studies). The sampling theorem predicts the limit to accurate *identification* of the periodicity of a stimulus by a detector array. But the cut-off spatial frequency of an individual neuron, responding to high-contrast, drifting gratings, is a measure of *detection* rather than identification. It should depend only on the spatial transfer characteristics of the centre mechanism of the receptive field.

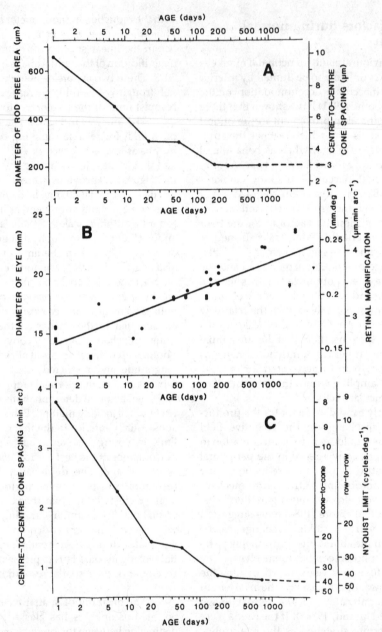

Fig. 24.3. These graphs from Jacobs & Blakemore (1988) derive a prediction of the Nyquist limit for the foveal photoreceptor array in Old-World monkeys, as a function of age. A. The diameter of the rod-free area of the pigtail macaque (Hendrickson & Kupfer, 1976) is plotted against postnatal age (on a logarithmic abscissa). The right-hand ordinate shows the predicted centre-to-centre spacing of foveal cones, based on a value of 3 μm (corrected for shrinkage) for adult monkeys (see Miller, 1979). B. The equatorial diameter of the eye is plotted against log age, with different symbols representing different species of Old-World monkey (Blakemore & Vital-Durand, 1986a). A regression line is fitted to the points. The right-hand ordinates convert these results to retinal magnification, expressed as mm deg^{-1} and μm min arc^{-1}. C. The results of A and B are combined to derive the *angular* centre-to-centre spacing of foveal cones against log age. The right-hand ordinates convert these results to the predicted spatial bandwidth. The inner scale shows the cone-to-cone Nyquist limit, while the right-most scale shows the improved predicted limit of resolution based on row-to-row sampling, assuming a hexagonal lattice of cones.

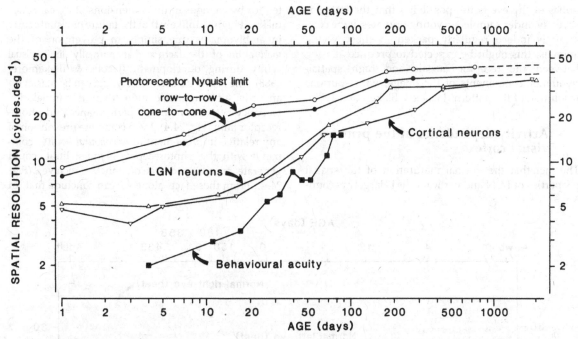

Fig. 24.4. The cone-to-cone Nyquist limit (filled circles) and the slightly higher row-to-row limit (unfilled circles) for foveal photoreceptors (see Fig. 24.3C) are compared with the performance of individual neurons in the LGN (unfilled upright triangles) and the primary visual cortex (unfilled, inverted triangles), as well as with the behavioural determinations of visual acuity already presented in Fig. 24.1 (filled squares). For the neurophysiological results, each point shows the highest spatial frequency that could be detected by the best performing cell in the foveal representation area of the LGN or the cortex (mean of four determinations).

Imagine an eye with only a single photoreceptor, corresponding in size to the dimensions of a foveal cone. Cells in the visual pathway connected to this single receptor should, under ideal conditions, be able to detect the presence of gratings up to the spatial bandwidth of that photoreceptor. Equally, the whole animal, using that photoreceptor for its vision, could theoretically *detect* gratings up to that same cut-off frequency, but would obviously be incapable of correctly identifying and discriminating the periodicities and orientations of different gratings.

Although an *absolute* comparison between the photoreceptor Nyquist limit and neuronal and behavioural resolution is, then, invalid, their *relative* changes with age can certainly be compared, on the assumption that the transfer function of each individual cone changes in proportion to the alteration in the centre-to-centre spacing between cones. In fact, the diameter of the inner segment of cones is a somewhat smaller fraction of the centre-to-centre spacing in very young monkeys, compared with adults (Hendrickson & Kupfer, 1976), which might be expected to produce a cone cut-off frequency that is

relatively higher in young animals, when compared with the Nyquist limit (Snyder & Miller, 1977). However, this expected relative superiority might well be more than counteracted by the shorter length of the outer segments of cones in young animals (Hendrickson & Kupfer, 1976), which would be expected to reduce their quantal catch, and by the general sluggishness of LGN and cortical neurons in young monkeys (Blakemore & Vital-Durand, 1986a). The change in receptor length, and hence quantum efficiency, and the possible increase in synaptic gain at synapses in the pathway might well account for the general improvement in contrast sensitivity during development, without any change in spatial pooling (Wilson, 1988).

Jacobs & Blakemore's (1988) overall conclusion from this analysis is that the changes in the spatial properties of neurons in the visual pathway, at least up to the level of the primary visual cortex, are largely, if not completely, accounted for by anatomical changes in the dimensions of the photoreceptors. One consequence of the relative coarseness of the foveal mosaic compared with the relative maturity of the optics of the eye is the possibility that the image is severely under-sampled in young primates; if the cone array is indeed regularly packed in these young animals, this might be expected to produce aliasing between the receptor mosaic and high spatial-frequency components of the image, with spurious resolution of the pattern (Jacobs & Blakemore, 1988).

Activity-dependence at the primary visual cortex

The fact that the normal maturation of the spatial properties of LGN and cortical cells is largely accoun-

ted for by changes in the dimensions of foveal cones makes it highly unlikely that the failure of visual acuity in amblyopia is due simply to prevention of the maturation of the factors that normally limit visual acuity during development (Jacobs & Blakemore, 1988). The acuity defect in amblyopia can be massive – an order of magnitude more than the initial discrepancy between neuronal performance and photoreceptor limit (Fig. 24.4). Even complete prevention of any relative improvement in *behavioural* acuity, compared with the photoreceptor Nyquist limit, could generate an acuity defect of only 2–3 octaves (Fig. 24.4). From these facts alone we can conclude that, in

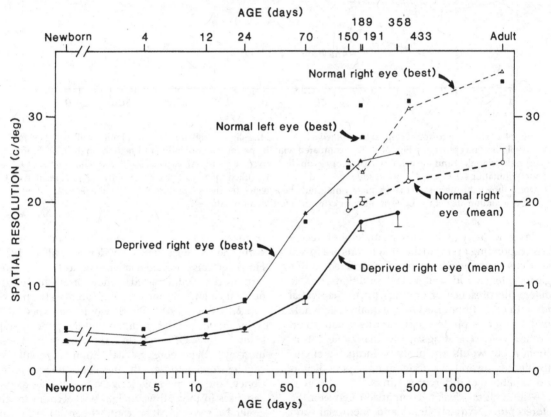

Fig. 24.5. These results of Blakemore & Vital-Durand (1986b) showing the effects of visual deprivation on the development of the LGN are plotted as in Fig. 24.1. Again, all data came from linear (X-type) cells with receptive fields in the central 2 deg of the visual field. The open circles joined by dashed thick lines show the mean resolution (+1 standard error) for cells with receptive fields in the ipsilateral (right) eye in normal monkeys. For comparison, the filled circles joined by thick lines plot the mean resolution for neurons connected to the *deprived* ipsilateral eye in a series of monocularly deprived monkeys, as well as results from right-eye cells in a newborn animal and in a monkey that was continuously *binocularly* deprived for the first year of life (plotted at 358 days on the abscissa). For each normal animal, an open triangle (joined by thin interrupted lines) plots the spatial resolution of the best performing right-eye cell. Filled triangles, connected with thin lines, show the best deprived right-eye cell. Filled squares plot the resolution of the best cell found in layers connected to the non-deprived left eye.

primates at least, amblyopia involves a *positive* degradation of spatial coding (excessive spatial pooling, under-sampling or 'scrambling' of spatial signals) and it could be primarily a central as opposed to a retinal phenomenon. Blakemore & Vital-Durand (1981; 1984; 1986b) have employed deprivation of form vision, by closure of the eyelids, to determine the locus of the functional defect underlying deprivation amblyopia in monkeys. As little as a few days of monocular deprivation, during the first few weeks of life, precipitates a profound amblyopia in primates (Boothe *et al.*, 1985). But, in line with the arguments above, even continuous deprivation, from the day of birth for as long as 27 weeks hardly affects the maturation of the spatial properties of LGN neurons.

Comparison of the effects of deprivation on LGN and primary visual cortex

Fig. 24.5 shows Blakemore & Vital-Durand's (1986b) determinations of neuronal 'acuity' for cells in the foveal representation of the LGN in deprived monkeys, plotted in the same form as Fig. 24.1. Despite the lack of patterned visual stimulation, the average spatial resolution for foveal LGN neurons increases by at least a factor of five, and even after 27 weeks of continuous deprivation, the best-performing cells in the deprived layers can resolve gratings up to more than 25 cycles deg^{-1}, very similar to the resolution of the best cells in the non-deprived layers.

On the other hand, deprivation by lid suture has several dramatic effects on the visual cortex. Monocular deprivation results in a failure of establishment of the normal pattern of anatomical input from the two eyes to layer 4c of the cortex; the terminal distribution from the cells of the deprived layers of the LGN comes to occupy only about a quarter of the area of the cortical input layer (LeVay *et al.*, 1980; Swindale *et al.*, 1981). This anatomical change in terminal distribution, which is considered to be the result of some kind of competitive interaction between the two eyes' sets of fibres, is accompanied by (and presumably partially causes) the well-known change in physiological properties of the visual cortex in monocularly deprived animals: cortical cells, the majority of which can normally be excited through either eye, mostly become completely dominated by input from the non-deprived eye (see Blakemore, 1988). In the monkey cortex, *binocular* deprivation also causes changes in binocularity: cells again tend to become monocularly driven with only about 20% being binocularly driven, but there are roughly equal proportions of cells domin-

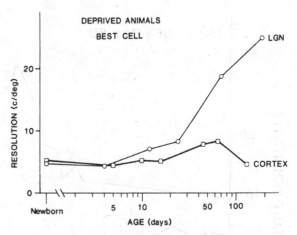

Fig. 24.6. For each of a series of visually deprived monkeys of different age, the symbols plot the resolution, for a drifting high-contrast grating, of the best performing cell found in the foveal representation. Circles plot results for the LGN, squares for the primary visual cortex. All of these cells had receptive fields in eyes that had been deprived of visual experience by closure of the lids from the day of birth until the recording experiment. The LGN cells came from monocularly deprived monkeys while the cortical data came from binocularly deprived animals.

ated by the right eye and the left eye (Wiesel & Hubel, 1974; Blakemore & Vital-Durand, 1984).

Blakemore & Vital-Durand (1981, 1984) have studied the effects of deprivation on the maturation of the spatial properties of the receptive fields of cortical cells. They used binocular deprivation because of the difficulty of finding any cells responding through the deprived eye in monocularly deprived animals. Although the majority of cortical neurons remain visually responsive, even after prolonged periods of binocular deprivation from the day of birth, there are clear effects on receptive field structure. Whereas on the day of birth fully 40% of cells in the primary visual cortex are already clearly selective for orientation, virtually no orientational cells can be found after a few weeks of binocular deprivation. With prolonged deprivation, the receptive fields of cortical cells become relatively large and diffuse, and the responses of the cells more sluggish.

These qualitative observations are matched by defects in spatial resolution and contrast sensitivity. Figure 24.6 shows a direct comparison between the spatial resolution of LGN cells recorded in the deprived layers of monocularly deprived monkeys

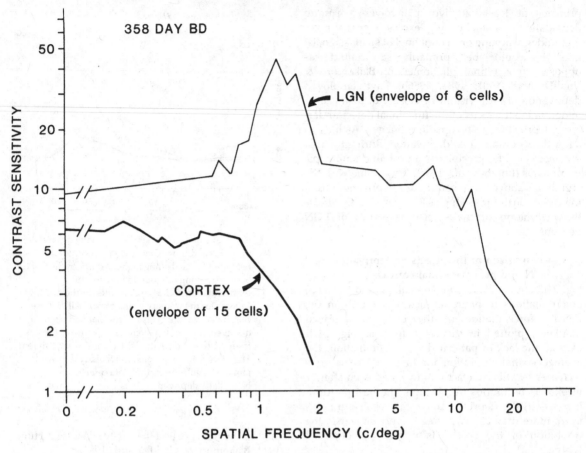

Fig. 24.7. Contrast sensitivity is plotted against spatial frequency for samples of neurons from the primary visual cortex (thick line) and the LGN (thin line) of a single monkey which had been binocularly deprived from the day of birth until recording at almost a year of age. Contrast sensitivity was determined (as in Fig. 24.2) for 15 representative cells in the cortex and the thick line describes the envelope of all these data combined. It thus represents the highest contrast sensitivity found at each spatial frequency among the entire sample of cortical cells. After this long period of deprivation, both neuronal 'acuity' and contrast sensitivity are very low. By comparison, the envelope of sensitivity for the six neurons recorded in the LGN shows much higher resolution and contrast sensitivity.

and cortical neurons recorded in binocularly deprived animals. In each case, only the very best cell from the foveal representation area is shown for each animal at each particular age. However, these 'best' cells reflect the properties of the population as a whole (see Figs 24.1 and 24.5 for the LGN), and they give a reasonable indication of the behavioural performance that might be expected from the animal if it were able, perceptually, to consult the neurons with highest spatial resolution in order to determine its visual acuity. Figure 24.6 shows quite clearly that, whereas the improvement of resolution in the LGN is little affected by deprivation, there is a failure of normal maturation

at the cortex. Indeed, more recent experiments have shown that if deprivation is continued for as long as a year (see Fig. 24.7), the highest spatial resolution seen in the cortex is only about 2 cycles deg^{-1}, substantially lower than at birth, despite the fact that the photo-receptor mosaic itself should have increased its sampling limit by a factor of four over the same period of time (Fig. 24.4).

The defect in spatial properties of cortical neurons caused by deprivation seems to apply even at the first-order cells in layer 4c and therefore it seems that the transmission of spatial information across the geniculo-cortical synapse is established and maintained by an activity-dependent process early in life. In deprived animals, cortical cells have poor spatial performance despite the fact that they receive their input from geniculate axons that can have fine spatial resolution and/or high contrast sensitivity. It is not only the resolution of cortical cells that is affected by deprivation; their contrast sensitivity is also markedly depressed.

Figure 24.7 provides convincing evidence of this failure of spatial transmission between LGN and cortex. It shows results for a single animal, binocularly deprived for the first year of life. In this animal spatial resolution was determined in a substantial number of cortical neurons and the highest value found was about 2 cycles deg^{-1}. In a regular sub-sample of those cells, contrast sensitivity was also determined over a range of spatial frequencies (as in Fig. 24.2). In Fig. 24.7, the thick line is the *envelope* of all the individual contrast sensitivity functions of cortical neurons. This function thus describes the highest contrast sensitivity found amongst this sample of cortical cells, over the whole range of spatial frequencies. These cells were grossly insensitive and the best sensitivities found were similar to, or even lower than the typical values of neurons in the cortex of newborn monkeys (see Fig. 24.2). At the end of the cortical recording in this animal, a microelectrode was introduced into the foveal representation area of the LGN and just six LGN cells were studied. The thin line in Fig. 24.7 shows the envelope of the contrast sensitivity functions for this very small sample of geniculate neurons. Some of them responded to high-contrast gratings up to a spatial frequency of almost 30 cycles deg^{-1} and the contrast sensitivities of the population extended to much higher values than for the larger sample of cortical cells.

Conclusions

These results strongly suggest that the synaptic connexions between geniculate axons and cortical cells have properties quite different from the earlier synapses in the pathway. The connectivity between foveal cones and retinal cells and between retinal ganglion cells and LGN cells seems to be specified with extraordinary precision on the basis of innate instructions in the developing monkey. Moreover, the peripheral part of the visual pathway is capable of preserving its exquisite spatial organization even in the absence of visual stimulation. However, at the level of the cortex, the selection of afferent input by neurons appears to depend on the pattern of activity in those afferent axons. Deprivation by lid suture presumably results in a retinal image which, at best, contains patterns of only very low spatial frequency with very poor contrast. Such images presumably result in cortical cells receiving correlated, though weak input from large ensembles of geniculate axons, rather than from well localized, spatially coherent, small clusters of axons, as in the normal animal. Under conditions of deprivation, cortical neurons fail to maintain and complete the maturation of their orientation selectivity (presumably because of the absence of sharply defined, oriented contours in the image) and they seem to take input from a diffuse array of geniculate axons, giving them only poor resolution and low contrast sensitivity. The synaptic plasticity that underlies the activity-dependent maturation of spatial properties provides an excellent example of the way in which coincidence or correlation detection may be used by cortical neurons to optimize their efficient encoding of the visual scene (Barlow, 1972).

Acknowledgements

Much of the experimental work described here was done in collaboration with François Vital-Durand and was supported by grants from the Medical Research Council and INSERM, as well as by Twinning Grants from NATO, the French Government and the International Brain Research Organization.

References

Atkinson, J., Braddick, O. & Moar, K. (1977) Development of contrast sensitivity over the first three months of life in the human infant. *Vision Res.*, **17**, 1037–44.

Barlow, H. B. (1972) Single units and sensation: a neuron doctrine for perceptual psychology? *Perception*, **1**, 371–94.

Barlow, H. B. & Levick, W. R. (1969) Three factors limiting the reliable detection of light by retinal ganglion cells of the cat. *J. Physiol.*, **200**, 1–24.

Blakemore, C. (1988) The sensitive periods of the monkey's visual cortex. In *Strabismus and Amblyopia* (Wenner-Gren International Symposium Series Vol. 49), ed. G. Lennerstrand, G. K. von Noorden & E. C. Campos, pp. 219–34. London: Macmillan Press.

Blakemore, C. & Hawken, M. (1985) Contrast sensitivity of neurones in the lateral geniculate nucleus of the neonatal monkey. *J. Physiol.*, **369**, 37P.

Blakemore, C. & Vital-Durand, F. (1981) Postnatal development of the monkey's visual system. In *The Fetus and*

Independent Life (Ciba Foundation Symposium 86). pp. 152–71. London: Pitman.

Blakemore, C. & Vital-Durand, F. (1983) Development of contrast sensitivity by neurones in monkey striate cortex. *J. Physiol.*, **334**, 18–19P.

Blakemore, C. & Vital-Durand, F. (1984) Development of the monkey's geniculo-cortical system. In *Development of Visual Pathways in Mammals (Neurology and Neurobiology, vol. 9)*, ed J. Stone, B. Dreher & D. H. Rapaport, pp. 463–7. New York: Alan R. Liss.

Blakemore, C. & Vital-Durand, F. (1986a) Organization and post-natal development of the monkey's lateral geniculate nucleus. *J. Physiol.*, **380**, 453–91.

Blakemore, C. & Vital-Durand, F. (1986b) Effects of visual deprivation on the development of the monkey's lateral geniculate nucleus. *J. Physiol.*, **380**, 493–511.

Boothe, R. G., Dobson, V. & Teller, D. Y. (1985) Postnatal development of vision in human and non-human primates. *Ann. Rev. Neurosci.*, **8**, 495–545.

Campbell, F. W. & Green, D. G. (1965) Optical and retinal factors affecting visual resolution. *J. Physiol.*, **181**, 576–93.

Campbell, F. W. & Gregory, A. H. (1960) Effect of size of pupil on visual acuity. *Nature*, **187**, 1121–3.

Campbell, F. W. & Gubisch, R. W. (1966) Optical quality of the human eye. *J. Physiol.*, **186**, 558–78.

Derrington, A. M. & Lennie, P. (1984) Spatial and temporal contrast sensitivities of neurones in lateral geniculate nucleus of macaque. *J. Physiol.*, **357**, 219–40.

Dobson, M. V. & Teller, D. Y. (1978) Visual acuity in human infants: a review and comparison of behavioral and electrophysiological studies. *Vision Res.*, **18**, 1469–83.

Dowling, J. E. & Boycott, B. B. (1966) Organization of the primate retina: electron microscopy. *Proc. Roy. Soc. Lond.*, B**166**, 80–111.

Hendrickson, A. E. & Kupfer, C. (1976) The histogenesis of the fovea in the macaque monkey. *Invest. Ophthal.*, **15**, 746–56.

Howland, H., Boothe, R. G. & Kiorpes, L. (1982) Accommodative defocus does not limit development of acuity in infant *Macaca nemestrina* monkeys. *Science*, **215**, 1409–11.

Hubel, D. H. & Wiesel, T. N. (1977) Functional architecture of macaque monkey visual cortex,. *Proc. Roy. Soc. Lond.*, B**198**, 1–59.

Jacobs, D. S. & Blakemore, C. (1988) Factors limiting the postnatal development of visual acuity in the monkey. *Vision Res.*, **28**, 947–58.

Land, M. F. & Snyder, A. W. (1985) Cone mosaic observed directly through natural pupil of live vertebrate. *Vision Res.*, **25**, 1519–23.

LeVay, S., Wiesel, T. N. & Hubel, D. H. (1980) The development of ocular dominance columns in normal and visually deprived monkeys. *J. comp. Neurol.*, **191**, 1–51.

Miller, W. H. (1979) Ocular optical filtering. In *Handbook of Sensory Physiology*, Vol. 7, Part 6A, ed. H. Autrum, pp. 69–143. Berlin: Springer Verlag.

Østerberg, G. (1935) Topography of the layer of rods and cones in the human retina. *Acta Ophthal. (Suppl.)*, **65**, 1–102.

Parker, A. J. & Hawken, M. J. (1985) The capabilities of monkey cortical cells in spatial resolution tasks. *J. opt. Soc. Amer. A*, **2**, 1101–14.

Snyder, A. W., Bossomaier, T. R. J. & Hughes, A. (1986) Optical image quality and the cone mosaic. *Science*, **231**, 499–501.

Snyder, A. W. & Miller, W. H. (1977) Photoreceptor diameter and spacing for highest resolving power. *J. opt. Soc. Amer.*, **67**, 696–8.

Swindale, N. V., Vital-Durand, F. & Blakemore, C. (1981) Recovery from monocular deprivation in the monkey. III. Reversal of anatomical effects in the visual cortex. *Proc. Roy. Soc. Lond.*, B**213**, 435–50.

Teller, D. Y., Regal, D. M., Videen, T. O. & Pulos, E. (1978) Development of visual acuity in infant monkeys (*Macaca nemestrina*) during the early postnatal weeks. *Vision Res.*, **18**, 561–6.

Wehner, R. (1981) Spatial vision in arthropods. In *Handbook of Sensory Physiology*, Vol. 7, Part 6C, ed. H. Autrum, pp. 287–616. New York: Springer Verlag.

Westheimer, G. (1977) Visual acuity and spatial modulation thresholds. In *Handbook of Sensory Physiology*, Vol. 7, Part 4, ed. D. Jameson and L. M. Hurvich, pp. 170–87. New York: Springer Verlag.

Wiesel, T. N. & Hubel, D. H. (1974) Ordered arrangement of orientation columns in monkeys lacking visual experience. *J. comp. Neurol.*, **158**, 307–18.

Williams, D. R. (1986) Seeing through the photoreceptor mosaic. *Trends Neurosci.*, **9(5)**, 193–8.

Williams, D. R. & Boothe, R. G. (1981) Development of optical quality in the infant monkey (*Macaca nemestrina*) eye. *Invest. Ophthal. and Vis. Sci.*, **21**, 728–36.

Wilson, H. R. (1988) Development of spatiotemporal mechanisms in infant vision. *Vision Res.*, **28**, 611–28.

Yuodelis, C. & Hendrickson, A. (1986) A qualitative and quantitative analysis of the human fovea during development. *Vision Res.*, **26**, 847–55.

25
The puzzle of amblyopia

R. F. Hess, D. J. Field and R. J. Watt

Introduction

Science is analogous to doing a jig-saw puzzle where the overall picture is unknown. One of two strategies can be adopted. The obvious one is first to see which individual pieces best fit together and hope to obtain a better idea of the overall picture as more of the puzzle is completed. However if there are many pieces and the picture very complicated then this may not be successful. Another method is to hazard a guess at what the overall picture might be and then to segregate pieces on the basis of this, only then beginning to put individual pieces together. While the initial guess might not turn out to be totally correct, as time goes on and more pieces are segregated, it can be further refined.

Research into amblyopia has so far followed the first of these two strategies. Over the past decade or so a number of workers have been busy seeing how individual pieces to the amblyopia puzzle fit without much regard for what the overall completed picture might look like. Initially this might be a sensible approach but we have now reached the point where it might be useful to hazard a guess at what the overall picture might look like so that more key pieces can be sought. In this paper we will consider three different types of pictures of amblyopia and assess into which the already collected pieces best fit. We stress that these are 'pictures' in the broadest sense, for not enough pieces have been collected to be able to assess them in the detail that we would like. In each case we attempt to portray what information might be available to the amblyopic visual system according to each 'picture' by a simple computational model. In some cases these cannot be regarded as accurate descriptions because the assumptions that we have chosen for our computations may not coincide with those that

our creator has chosen for our visual systems. While bearing this in mind they at least give some idea, albeit crude, of what restricted information is available to the amblyopic visual system, according to each model. They really act as starting points and they give us a glimpse of the number of different possible shades that occur even within the same picture. The correct shade depends a lot on the computations used by the normal visual system which in turn suggests that while we might now be on the right track to understanding amblyopia we are somewhere nearer to the beginning than the end.

One puzzle or many?

There are probably at least four different types of amblyopia in terms of its clinical identity and so there may be four or more different 'pictures' for amblyopia. About one third of amblyopes have a strabismus (strabismic amblyopia), one third have unequal refractive error (anisometropic amblyopia) and the remaining third have a mixture of the two. The fourth category is very rare (<1% of amblyopes) and results from severe pattern deprivation in early life (deprivation amblyopia). The bulk of the available psychophysical data suggest that the first three categories can be collapsed into two depending upon whether the amblyope has a strabismus or not (Hess *et al.*, 1981, Sireteanu & Fronius, 1981, Hess & Pointer, 1985). The visual loss in monocular deprivation amblyopia is very severe (Hess *et al.*, 1981; Maurer, Lewis & Brent, 1990) and it is as yet impossible to tell whether it is a separate category or merely an end point of one of the other two categories. The main difference between strabismic and, let us call it, non-strabismic amblyopia is how the neural deficit is distributed across the visual field. In non-strabismic

amblyopia it is more evenly distributed than it is in strabismic amblyopia where it mainly affects central vision. Whether the neural deficit *per se* is different is still an open question (Lampert & Howland, 1987).

Throughout this paper we will endeavour where possible to keep the strabismic pieces of the puzzle separate from the non-strabismic pieces but let us keep an open mind on the possibility that the two pictures they eventually complete may only be subtly different.

Which picture?

It may be easy enough to come up with a set of possible pictures to describe amblyopia but how should one evaluate them? One possibility is the following. Let us consider that the amblyopic visual system contains some unknown variability E_I which we wish to identify. If we introduce the right variability into our stimulus, let us call this E_S then it should be possible to titrate the internal amblyopic error or variability with the external stimulus error or variability. If this is successful we have taken the first steps towards identifying the nature of the internal variability and hence which 'picture' is the correct one.

This is illustrated graphically in Fig. 25.1. Here a measure of visual sensitivity is plotted against a stimulus error or variability E_S. Initially the normal eye's sensitivity is not affected by the small magnitudes of the stimulus error but eventually it

varies directly with the stimulus error. Consider two extreme scenarios, one where the external error is a good model of the internal error and one where it is not.

The first case is illustrated by the amblyopic curve in Fig. 25.1A. Here amblyopic sensitivity remains constant until it coincides with that of the normal eye. At this $E_S=E_I$ and all of the original amblyopic deficit can be accounted for by a raised level of E_I. In the second case (Fig. 25.1B) the sensitivity of the amblyopic's eye shows the same dependence on E as does the normal eye. In this case none of the original deficit (i.e. the deficit of $E_S=0$) is accounted for by the type of stimulus error used. The underlying assumption is that if we have chosen the right error to put in the stimulus it will add to the internal amblyopic error and allow us to titrate one against the other. We will use this titration test to assess which picture best describes amblyopia. Possible limitations of this method are discussed in a later section.

The weak signal picture

Initially this was the implicit assumption that those who applied the contrast sensitivity approach to amblyopia must have had. Up until the sixties, amblyopia had been thought of only in terms of acuity. This new approach offered the possibility of quantifying the weak signal hypothesis in terms of contrast and spatial frequency. Numerous reports emerged of

A

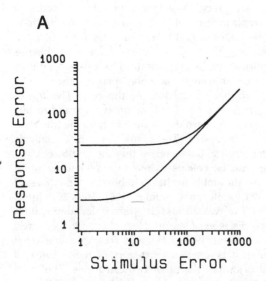

B

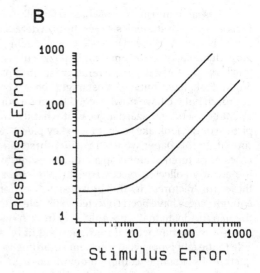

Fig. 25.1. Two different models of amblyopia. In each case, the sensitivity to some visual task is plotted against the magnitude of stimulus error or variability. In A the stimulus error is a good model of the resident neural error whereas in B it is not (see text).

the type of the contrast sensitivity defect that characterized amblyopia (Gstalder & Green, 1971; Mitchell *et al.*, 1973; Hess & Howell, 1977; Levi & Harwerth, 1977; Rentschler *et al.*, 1977; Sjostrand, 1978; Bradley & Freeman, 1981). While the magnitude of the contrast deficit depended on the severity of the amblyopia both strabismic and non-strabismic amblyopes exhibited similar *types* of deficit. In general, the higher the frequency the greater the contrast sensitivity deficit. This is depicted in Fig. 25.2. The results were accepted by all of us on face value to mean that the contrast gain of the amblyopic visual system was reduced accordingly.

What perceptual effect should this have? Let us consider the case where we reduce the contrast gain evenly at all spatial scales. The effect of this can be seen in Fig. 25.3 which depicts two well-known vision scientists vying for the attention of the camera. In the upper frame is the original photograph and below it

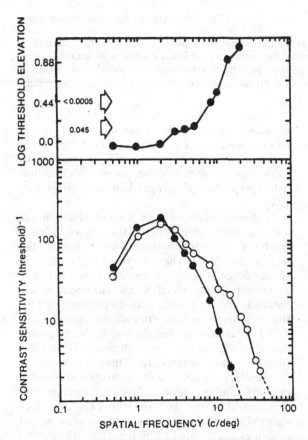

Fig. 25.2. The typical type of contrast sensitivity loss in amblyopia. Contrast sensitivity is plotted against spatial frequency for the normal (filled symbols) and fellow amblyopic eye. The higher the spatial frequency the larger the sensitivity loss (From Hess & Howell, 1977).

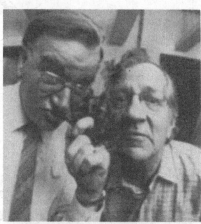
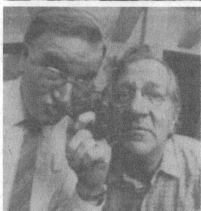
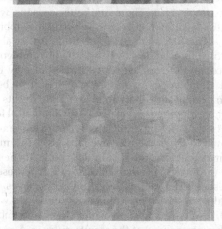

Fig. 25.3. The perceptual effect of reduced contrast gain with a flat frequency response. The original is seen at the top and below it two reduced contrast versions (50% and 90% reductions).

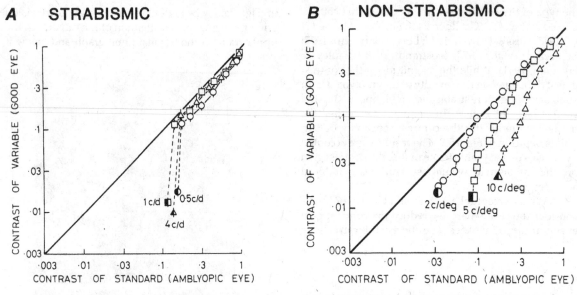

Fig. 25.4. Interocular contrast matching results for a strabismic (A) and non-strabismic (B) amblyope. The contrast of a fixed standard shown to the amblyopic eye is plotted against the contrast of a variable test stimulus shown to the fellow normal eye. The solid sloping line represents veridical matches. The initial thresholds are represented by half filled symbols. For both types of amblyopia thresholds are raised but suprathreshold contrast perceptions are approximately normal (From Hess et al., 1983).

two reduced contrast versions. In the middle picture the luminance deviation from the mean level has been reduced by 50% and on the bottom by 90%. The perceptual effect is quite minor and one would expect the amblyopic disability to be correspondingly slight if it were, in fact, due to this. However, amblyopes express great difficulties when they are forced to rely on their amblyopic vision which seem out of step with this simple idea. There are better reasons why the contrast gain notion is inappropriate for amblyopia.

The first of these is the finding that although contrast thresholds may be elevated in amblyopia the perception of contrast above threshold may be normal. If amblyopes are asked to match contrast between their normal and fellow amblyopic eye, results similar to those depicted in Fig. 25.4 are obtained. Here the contrast of a standard, fixed contrast stimulus is shown to the amblyopic eye (abscissa) and matched with a variable, contrast stimulus shown to the normal eye (ordinate). The half filled symbols represent the thresholds for normal and amblyopic eyes. In A, results are shown for a strabismic amblyope whereas in B, results are shown for a non-strabismic amblyope. Although the *form* of the results differ in A and B the overall result is the same – the higher the contrast level, the less is the contrast deficit. In other words contrast deficits in amblyopia are mainly restricted to

threshold and do not mean that the overall contrast *gain* has been reduced. The second point against the notion that the contrast gain is reduced is that there are amblyopes who do not exhibit a measurable threshold deficit yet do have a perceptual disability (Hess et al., 1978).

Recently there has been a report which showed a strong relationship between the vernier deficit in amblyopia and the contrast sensitivity deficit (Bradley & Freeman, 1985). These workers found that the vernier deficit in amblyopia could be accounted for by a contrast scaling equal to the threshold deficit. Results leading to a conclusion of a different kind but still involving a hyperacuity task are shown in Fig. 25.5. Here we are plotting the amplitude of a second derivative of a Gaussian perturbation (d^2G) in a line stimulus against its intensity relative to threshold. If the vernier acuity deficit is due to an attenuated signal resulting from an elevated threshold then the performance of normal and amblyopic eye should be identical as a function of signal strength when plotted as multiples of threshold. This is not the case for either strabismic (Fig. 25.5A) or non-strabismic amblyopes (Fig. 25.5B).

Thus the idea that first led us to investigate amblyopia with new and more refined methods seems not to be a good candidate for the overall picture of

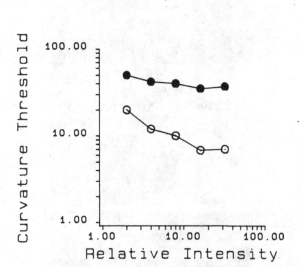
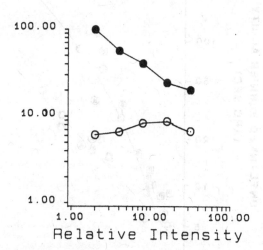

Fig. 25.5. Curvature threshold (see text) is plotted against the intensity of the line stimulus relative to its threshold for the normal (open circles) and fellow amblyopic (filled circles) eye. Results are shown for a strabismic (A) and a non-strabismic (B) amblyopia. These results do not support the weak signal model of amblyopia as outlined in the text.

amblyopia in terms of the pieces of the puzzle that we have at present.

The blur picture

Another proposal that has been put forward is that it is the selective *loss* of the high frequency filters in amblyopia that account for their perceptual disability. This suggestion has been particularly applied to non-strabismic amblyopia (Levi & Klein, 1982, 1983, 1985; Flom & Bedell, 1985). Support for this comes from the strong correlation found between hyperacuity bisection sensitivity and grating resolution in amblyopia (Levi & Klein, 1982, 1983, 1985). This result is displayed in Fig. 25.6 for strabismic (S) and non-strabismic (A) amblyopes. Figure 25.7 shows what information may be available to the amblyopic visual system according to this notion. The upper photograph is the original and below it are two blurred replicas. The blur functions are Gaussian having space constants of 1/25 and 1/8 of the picture width.

This notion is open to direct test along the lines of that outlined earlier (p. 268) (see Watt & Hess, 1987). If the amblyopic visual system has an internal blur which reduces performance on, let us say hyperacuity tasks, then it should be possible to titrate it by introducing a similar blur error into the stimulus.

The results of such an experiment are displayed in Fig. 25.8 for a strabismic (A) and non-strabismic (B)

amblyope. The task is one involving curvature detection of a bright line with a d^2G perturbation. The intensity of the line is at a constant fraction above the threshold of the normal and fellow amblyopic eye and the space constant was chosen to produce optimal sensitivity for both eyes. The normal eye's sensitivity is relatively independent of the one-dimensional Gaussian blur until it reaches 3 arc minutes standard deviation. After this point sensitivity is reduced. For non-strabismic amblyopia (Fig. 25.8B) similar results are seen. The solid curve is a least squares fit to a model in which the internal and external errors are independent and additive such that

$$B_E = B_I + B_S$$

where B_E is the effective blur, B_I the internal blur and B_S the stimulus blur. It is clear from Fig. 25.8B that the initial hyperacuity curvature deficit in this amblyopic eye (i.e. at low blurs) is not able to be accounted for by any level of stimulus blur – the two functions remain essentially parallel for all stimulus blurs. A slightly different picture is seen in strabismic amblyopia (Fig. 25.8A). Here a significant part of the 'in focus' deficit can be accounted for by titrating it with stimulus blur. Hence the internal blur in strabismic visual systems is contributing to reduced performance in tasks such as these. It is however not the sole problem as we will see in the next section.

Thus the blur model is not adequate for non-

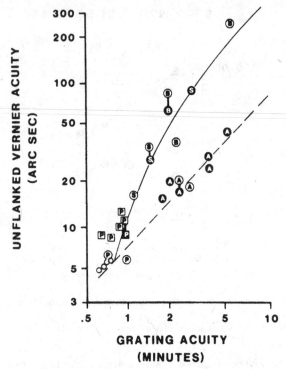

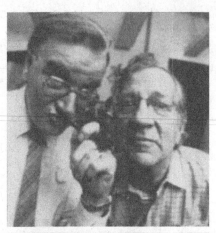

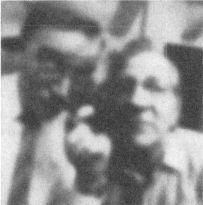

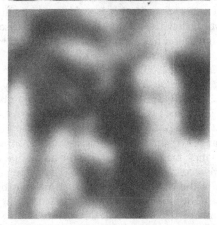

Fig. 25.6. The correlation between acuity on reduced performance for a so-called hyperacuity task is depicted for a group of strabismic and non-strabismic amblyopes (From Levi & Klein, 1982). This supports the blur model of amblyopia (see text). ○ – normal observers; Ⓟ – preferred eyes of anisometropic amblyopes; ☐P – preferred eyes of strabismic amblyopes; S – amblyopic eyes of strabismics; A – amblyopic eyes of anisometropes; B – amblyopic eyes of strabismic-anisometropes. Solid line is for the normal periphery. (From Levi *et al.*, 1985 Fig. 9.).

strabismic amblyopia and at best only partially adequate for strabismic amblyopia.

The spatial scrambling picture

The importance of this fact in amblyopia was brought home forceably to one of us (RFH) by the results of just one amblyopic subject at a time when the weak signal hypothesis was the only one considered. Trisha Greenhalgh, Cambridge undergraduate and strabismic amblyope, had essentially normal contrast sensitivity but reported that grating stimuli appeared distorted at and above threshold when viewing with her amblyopic eye. These distortions, which were neural, increased with spatial frequency, as is illustrated in Fig. 25.9 along with her contrast sen-

Fig. 25.7. The information available to the amblyopic visual system according to the blur model. Here an original photograph (top) has been subjected to Gaussian blurring of two different degrees (space contents of 1/25 and 1/8 of the picture width).

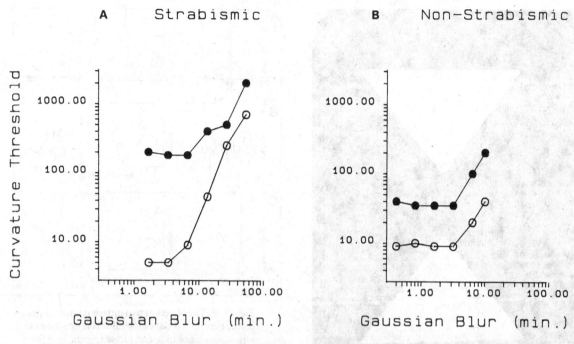

Fig. 25.8. Curvature threshold is plotted against Gaussian blur of the stimulus for the amblyopic (filled circles) and fellow normal eye (open circles) of a strabismic (A) and non-strabismic amblyope (B). Blur is not a good model for non-strabismic amblyopia and is only partially successful for strabismic amblyopia (see text).

sitivity results, which are normal (filled symbols for amblyopic eye). Subsequent assessment of other amlyopes (Hess *et al.*, 1978) who exhibited contrast sensitivity losses, particularly strabismic amblyopes, showed that these distortions were an important aspect of amblyopia which, although known for some time (Pugh, 1958), had not received their due attention. This suggests that at least for these amblyopes the weak signal and blur models are inappropriate because there is no evidence from contrast sensitivity that they have either a weak signal or a loss of high spatial frequency filters. Bedell and Flom documented similar distortions using a variety of spatial bisection tasks. They found that strabismics exhibited relatively large constant errors in spatial alignment and partitioning (Bedell & Flom, 1981, 1983; Flom & Bedell, 1985). An example of their spatial alignment stimulus is shown in Fig. 25.10. This led to the suggestion that *amblyopia* which means blunt sight might be more accurately thought of as *tarachopia* which means distorted sight (Hess, 1982). The next question was simply whether it should best be measured in the frequency domain as in Fig. 25.9 or the space domain as in Fig. 25.10. In the frequency domain it could be translated into a phase coding problem somewhat

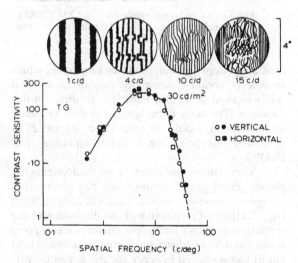

Fig. 25.9. Spatial contrast sensitivity is seen to be normal even at high spatial frequencies in this amblyope even though letter acuity is subnormal. The reason is because there are severe spatial distortions which are illustrated in the top of the figure. These are drawings made by the amblyope of how the one-dimensional gratings appear above detection threshold (From Hess *et al.*, 1978).

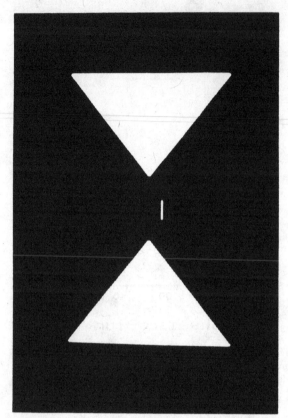

Fig. 25.10. One type of spatial bisection and aligning task found to produce abnormal results in strabismic amblyopes (From Flom & Bedell, 1985).

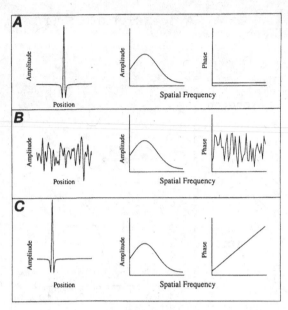

Fig. 25.11. The effects of two different kinds of phase disruption. In A a Gabor stimulus is represented in terms of its amplitude and phase spectra. In B the effect of a local randomizing of the phase values is seen to produce a global spatial dispersion. In C a local spatial displacement of the stimulus is seen to produce a rotation of the phase spectrum. In both cases the amplitude spectrum is undisturbed.

separately from the amplitude coding upon which previously contrast sensitivity measurements had solely focused. It seemed natural to continue in this direction. The next issue was what sort of phase randomization should be considered. Figure 25.11 illustrates this point for a Gabor stimulus (Fig. 25.11A).

There are two possible ways of randomizing the phase. First phase values can be randomized independently at each spatial frequency as depicted in Fig. 25.11B. This results in a global dispersion of the spatial energy. Since amblyopes do not perceive point sources as diffusely distributed across their visual field but in fact displaced in space (Bedell & Flom, 1981, 1983; Flom & Bedell, 1985) this did not seem to be the correct choice. In the second case the phase spectrum can be altered as a systematic function of spatial frequency and this produces a local spatial displacement. This seemed the appropriate direction in which to proceed because, as Fig. 25.9 illustrates, the distortions reported by amblyopes are spatially localized.

Phase distortions?

A number of studies showed that amblyopes exhibited selective deficits for tasks in which either the global phase of globally transformed images (Weiss *et al.*, 1985) or global phase values of local images (Lawden, *et al.*, 1982; Pass & Levi, 1982) were manipulated. One of these was intentionally designed to investigate the model outlined in Fig. 25.11C. It involved the discrimination of whether a spatially localized, low contrast $\langle 3f \rangle$ sinewave component was added in peaks-add or peaks-subtract phase to a higher contrast $\langle f \rangle$ sinewave component (Lawden *et al.*, 1982). This seemed to be an ideal task for one could measure both the detectability of the $\langle 3f \rangle$ alone as well as in the presence of the higher contrast $\langle f \rangle$ component. The results showed that amblyopes needed much more contrast to discriminate how the $\langle 3f \rangle$ component was mixed, than to detect its presence in either of the above conditions. For the normal visual system the opposite was true, less contrast was needed to do the phase discrimination than for either of the control detection tasks. Thus amblyopes seemed to exhibit a selective defect for which the variable was local spatial phase. Does this mean that the amblyopic deficit was due to a phase encoding abnormality? The answer must be No! As a later analysis revealed (Hess & Pointer, 1987) the normal visual system uses other local spatial cues such as edge-blur and contrast to make these judgements and so the inability of amblyopic eyes to do these tasks is most likely due to their inability to utilize the same spatial cues and not to a phase deficit *per se*. Similar conclusions have been reached by Badcock (1984a,b) and Field (1984) for other types of experiments that initially had been designed to evaluate the phase coding properties of normal vision. Thus the main obstacle to understanding the amblyopic deficit in terms of a global phase distortion is that there is as yet no satisfactory method by which we can measure phase sensitivity for normal vision.

Spatial distortions?

An alternative approach is to consider the distortions reported by amblyopes purely in space domain terms (i.e. as displacements, see Fig. 25.11C). Let us also assume that the visual system has only spatial information with which to interpret its image. In these terms let us consider that the retinal image is sampled with a fixed spatial error, e, which is small for the normal visual system but large in amblyopia. The standard deviation of the distribution of values of e

corresponds to the variable error or what we will refer to as the *spatial uncertainty* of the system. Let us now introduce *positional uncertainty* or static spatial jitter into the elements making up our stimulus and assume that the internal uncertainty and the stimulus positional jitter are independent and additive sources of error. It then should be possible, via the method outlined earlier (p. 268), to assess whether the internal spatial uncertainty is elevated in amblyopia using the titration method. Thus

$$J = (J_I^2 + J_S^2)^{1/2}$$

where J is the overall standard deviation of internal spatial uncertainty resulting from an internal spatial uncertainty of J_I and an added stimulus positional uncertainty or jitter of J_S. In Fig. 25.12 results are displayed in which the amplitude of d^2G perturbation in a thin bright line is plotted against the magnitude of positional jitter added to the stimulus. By positional jitter we mean that each dot making up the stimulus was subjected to a positional change according to a Gaussian probability rule. Using this method it is possible in non-strabismic amblyopia to tritrate the internal error with stimulus positional jitter (Fig. 25.12B). In strabismic amblyopia it is however only partially successful (Fig. 25.12A). Therefore in both forms of amblyopia, spatial scrambling is an important aspect of the visual disorder. In non-strabismic

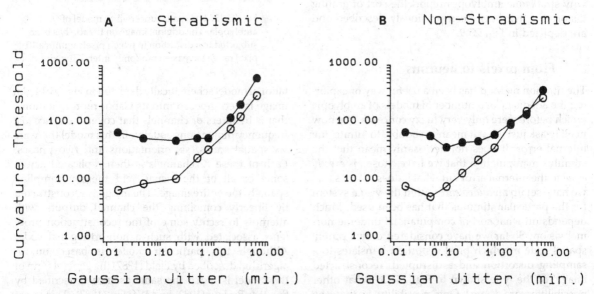

Fig. 25.12. Curvature threshold is plotted against Gaussian positional jitter (see text) of the stimulus for the normal (open circles) and fellow amblyopic (filled symbols) eye of a strabismic (A) and non-strabismic (B) amblyope. For the non-strabismic amblyope, positional uncertainty is a good model of amblyopia, as in strabismic amblyopia it is only partially successful.

amblyopia is can account for all of the performance deficit. In strabismic amblyopia the internal error involves both spatial scrambling and internal blur. In an attempt to represent the implications of this for non-strabismic amblyopia we have perturbed the photograph on the top in Fig. 25.13 in the following way. Pixels were randomly interchanged in the range of 1 to 10 with a flat probability distribution. This produces a broad band scrambling of the image.

Similar results using a different spatial task have been reported by Bedell & Flom (1981, 1983; Flom & Bedell, 1985). Their task involved either vernier alignment or space bisection. For each task both strabismic and non-strabismic amblyopes are defective. However their interpretation of this in the case of non-strabismic amblyopia is quite different from that presented here. They attribute the reduced spatial localization accuracy to a raised level of internal blur. However the argument is not a very secure one since they only show that a blurred normal eye can exhibit similar loss of spatial localization. This does not resolve the issue, for what we really need to know is how the performance of the amblyopic eye varies with stimulus blur (see Figs. 25.1 and 25.8). One interesting difference that Bedell & Flom found between strabismic and non-strabismic amblyopia is that, in the former, there are large *absolute* spatial errors. This means that these amblyopes exhibit constant distortions in their spatial map. This is probably the reason why strabismic amblyopes report the sort of grating distortions that have been previously described and are depicted in Fig. 25.9.

From pixels to neurons

The titration method has been a useful way of exploring the adequacy of a number of models of amblyopia which before were only very fuzzy concepts. We now need to ask just what it means to be able to 'titrate' the internal error. It does not necessarily mean that the stimulus manipulation that we have chosen is *exactly equal* to the internal error but what it does mean is that we have set up an *equivalence* within the visual system for the particular stimulus that has been used. Much depends on what sort of computations underlie normal vision. So far we have considered only a purely spatial code in which pixel distortion translates to a sampling distortion and a disrupted 'reconstructed image' of the type shown in Fig. 25.13. What other possibilities are there? One possibility is that the retinal image is transformed into a channel code along the lines of a Gabor transform. Consider the compu-

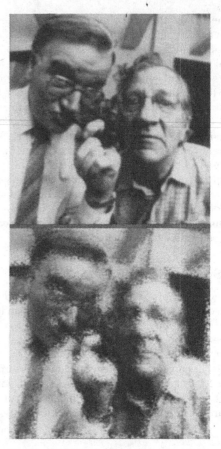

Fig. 25.13. The spatial uncertainty model of amblyopia. The original image on the top has been subjected to a distortion in which pixels within a 10 pixel range have been randomly interchanged.

tational model schematically depicted in Fig. 25.14. An image is decomposed into its Gabor representations, that is by filters or channels that cover the space *and* frequency dimensions equally. In this model there are six spatial scales, six orientations and two phases. Each of these 72 channels is then replicated across some or all of the visual field thereby sampling spatially the entire image. The image is reconstructed by linearly combining the channel outputs with attempts to rectify some of the reconstruction problems associated with such a non-orthogonal code. Although this particular model is based on an algorithm described by Field (1987) the general form of the model is much the same as those described by Sakitt & Barlow (1982) and Watson (1983). This is not intended to be a full description of all visual processing but it can be used as a means to illustrate a concept.

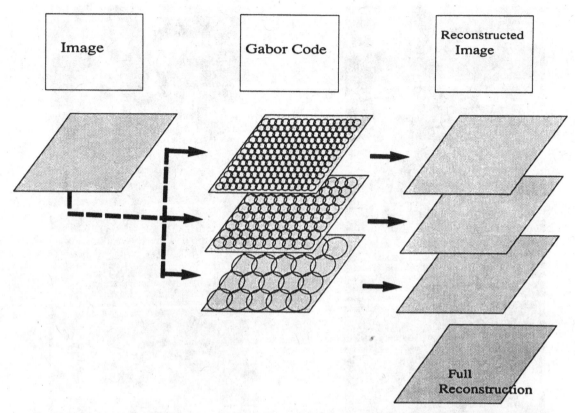

Fig. 25.14. A channel model of picture processing. The image is decomposed into its channel representation which are here represented by different planes each containing an array of channel elements. The image is reconstructed by a linear combination of the channel outputs with correction for the non-orthogonal nature of this type of transform.

The image is reconstructed not because the visual system reconstructs but to demonstrate what information is available to an amblyopic visual system as a result of certain effects. What is important is that a distortion or scrambling within such a code would not be best represented by a pixel distortion but by a scrambling of the filter (or receptive field) outputs within the transform. Exchanging two pixels which is by definition a local event cannot be mimicked by exchanging two filter outputs which are concerned with neighbourhood operations in the scene. Within such a framework the distortion could take on many different forms. For example, channel scrambling could involve either a constant distance in the transform or a constant fraction of the channel size. In the former case the disruption is greater for the high frequency information compared with the low frequency information. In the latter case, the same relative disruption is seen at each scale in the transform. An example of the first case is shown in Fig.

25.15 and of the second case in Fig. 25.16 (see Fig. captions for details). The disruption is very different to that of pixel distortion (Fig. 25.13). These are only two examples out of many possibilities whose visual effect depends as much on the manipulation chosen as on the nature of the transform employed to reconstruct the image. Hence their usefulness at this stage is only as an illustration of the possibilities that are yet to be investigated for the spatial distortion model of amblyopia.

Another possibility is that of undersampling. Within the purely spatial transform this is equivalent to blurring but in the channel transform its effects could be different from blurring since an undersampling by even the highest frequency filters need not mean a complete loss of high frequency information in the 'reconstructed image'. For this to be the case the visual system would need to have identified where samples were missing and taken appropriate action. The effects of undersampling on a channel model are

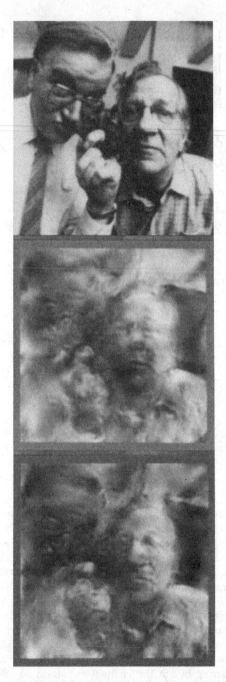
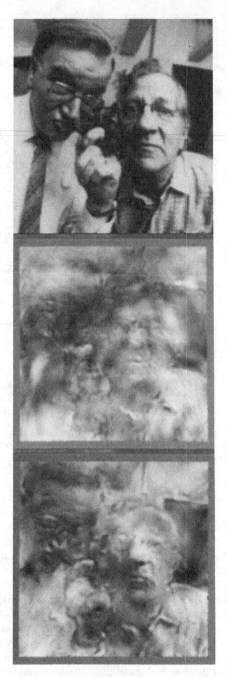

Fig. 25.15. Filter-jitter within the channel model of Fig. 25.14. The original image (top) is reconstructed with two different magnitudes of filter-jitter (±1/25 and ±2/25 of the picture width) which corresponds to a fixed distance in the transform.

Fig. 25.16. As in Fig. 25.15 but with a filter-jitter which corresponds to a constant fraction of the filter size (±1/5 and ±2/5 of the filter size).

difficult to predict in the absence of such a specific assumption about how filter outputs are used to combine and what rules determine regions of the image for which no filter responds. For example consider the case of the optic disc where there is known to be severe undersampling. One does not perceive a black spot in this region of the field, instead the visual system performs a filling in operation. Without a precise model of this filling in procedure one cannot derive what an undersampled image would look like. Nonetheless it remains another interesting possibility for the distortions in amblyopia.

Concluding remarks

In this review we have intentionally kept away from much of the fine detail that surrounds amblyopia. Instead we have tried to assess which of a number of plausible schemes might best describe the overall amblyopia picture. We have looked into the weak signal picture, the elevated internal blur picture and the neural scrambling picture. The available evidence suggests that a different picture might best describe strabismic and non-strabismic amblyopia. In the former, there are relatively large absolute distortions combined with spatial inaccuracy which results from a combination of an elevated internal blur and neural scrambling. In the non-strabismic form of amblyopia the spatial inaccuracy seems to be simply due to neural scrambling.

The exact nature of this neural scrambling is not known. The pixel manipulations described in this paper with their accompanying spatial model is a strong candidate but there are also other, yet unexplored, possibilities based on channel models of visual processing. We give a number of examples, not as serious contenders but merely to show that any particular picture of amblyopia comes in many shades. Some, like undersampling, are so model dependent that they are difficult to evaluate at the moment.

It is clear that we are just at the beginning of understanding what this neural scrambling entails and how it might best be measured. We now know what type of general picture describes amblyopia without having a clear idea of its exact details. Hopefully, this will make us more discriminating when selecting new pieces to complete the puzzle.

Acknowledgements

We gratefully acknowledge the financial assistance of the Medical Research Council of Great Britain and The Wellcome Trust. RFH is a Wellcome Senior Lecturer.

References

Badcock, D. R. (1984a) Spatial phase of luminance profile discrimination? *Vision Res.*, **24**, 613–23.

Badcock, D. R. (1984b) How do we discriminate relative spatial phase? *Vision Res.*, **24**, 1847–57.

Bedell, H. E. & Flom, M. C. (1981) Monocular spatial distortion in strabismic amblyopia. *Invest. Ophthal. and Vis. Sci.*, **20**, 263–8.

Bedell, H. E. & Flom, M. C. (1983) Normal and abnormal space perception. *Am. J. Optom. Physiol. Opt.*, **60**, 426–35.

Bradley, A. & Freeman, R. D. (1981) Contrast sensitivity in anisometropic amblyopia. *Invest. Ophthal. and Vis. Sci.*, **21**, 466–76.

Bradley, A. & Freeman, R. D. (1985) Is reduced vernier acuity in amblyopia due to position, contrast or fixation defects. *Vision Res.*, **25**, 55–66.

Field, D. (1984) A space domain approach to pattern vision. An investigation of phase discrimination and masking. Ph.D. Thesis, University of Pennsylvania (unpublished).

Field, D. J. (1987) Relations between the statistics of natural images and the response properties of cortical cells. *J. Opt. Soc. Am. A*, **4**, 2379–94.

Flom, M. C. & Bedell, H. E. (1985) Identifying amblyopia using associated conditions, acuity and non-acuity features. *Am. J. Optom. Physiol. Opt.*, **62**, 153–60.

Gstalder, R. J. & Green, D. G. (1971) Laser interferometric acuity in amblyopia. *J. Ped. Ophthal.*, **8**, 251–5.

Hess, R. F. (1982) Developmental sensory impairment: amblyopia or tarachopia? *Human Neurobiol.*, **1**, 17–29.

Hess R. F., Bradley, A. & Piotrowski, L. (1983) Contrast coding in amblyopia. I. Differences in the neural basis of amblyopia. *Proc. Roy. Soc. Lond.*, **B217**, 309–30.

Hess, R. F., Campbell, F. W. & Greenhalgh, T. (1978) On the nature of the neural abnormality in human amblyopia: neural aberrations and neural sensitivity loss. *Pflugers Arch. Ges. Physiol.*, **377**, 201–7.

Hess, R. F., France, T. D. & Keesey, U. T. (1981) Residual vision in humans who have been monocularly deprived of pattern vision in early life. *Exp. Brain Res.*, **44**, 295–311.

Hess, R. F. & Howell, E. R. (1977) The thresholds contrast sensitivity function in strabismic amblyopia: evidence for a two-type classification. *Vision Res.*, **17**, 1049–55.

Hess, R. F. & Pointer, J. S. (1985) Differences in the neural basis of human amblyopia. The distribution of the anomaly across the visual field. *Vision Res.*, **25**, 1577–94.

Hess, R. F. & Pointer, J. S. (1987) Evidence for spatially local computations underlying discrimination of periodic patterns in fovea and periphery. *Vision Res.*, **27**, 1343–60.

Lawden, M. C., Hess, R. F. & Campbell, F. W. (1982) The discriminability of spatial phase relationships in Amblyopia. *Vision Res.*, **22**, 1005–16.

Lampert, P. & Howland, H. C. (1987) A comparison of contrast acuity measurements in individuals with amblyopia due to anisometropia or strabismus. *Invest. Ophthal. and Vis. Sci. (Suppl.)*, **28**, (3) 37.

Levi, D. M. & Harwerth, R. S. (1977) Spatio-temporal interactions in anisometropic and strabismic amblyopia. *Invest. Ophthal. and Vis. Sci.*, **16**, 90–5.

Levi, D. M. & Klein, S. (1982) Differences in vernier discrimination for gratings between strabismic and anisometropic amblyopia. *Invest. Ophthal. and Vis. Sci.*, **23**, 398–407.

Levi, D. M. & Klein, S. (1983) Spatial localization in normal and amblyopic vision. *Vision Res.*, **23**, 1005–17.

Levi, D. M. & Klein, S. (1985) Vernier acuity, crowding and amblyopia. *Vision Res.*, **25**, 979–91.

Levi, D. M., Klein, S. A. & Aitsebaonao, P. (1985) Vernier acuity, crowding and cortical magnification. *Vision Res.*, **25**, 963–77.

Maurer, D., Lewis, T. L. & Brent, H. P. (1990) The effects of deprivation on human visual development. In *Applied Developmental Psychology*, Vol. 3, ed. F. J. Morrison, C. E. Lord & D. P. Keating. London: Academic Press.

Mitchell, D. E., Freeman, R. D., Millidot, M. & Haegerstrom, G. (1973) Meridional amblyopia: evidence for modification of the human visual system by early visual experience. *Vision Res.*, **13**, 535–58.

Pass, A. F. & Levi, D. M. (1982) Spatial processing of complex visual stimuli in A.V.S. *Invest. Ophthal. and Vis. Sci.*, **23**, 780–6.

Pugh, M. (1958) Visual distortion in amblyopia. *Brit. J. Ophthal.*, **42**, 449–60.

Rentschler, I., Hilz, R. & Brettel, A. (1977) Myopic and strabismic amblyopia: substantial differences in human visual development. *Exp. Brain Res.*, **30**, 445–6.

Sakitt, B. & Barlow, H. B. (1982) A model for the economical encoding of the visual image in cerebral cortex. *Biol. Cybern.*, **43**, 97–108.

Sireteanu, R. & Fronius, M. (1981) Naso-temporal asymmetries in human amblyopia: consequence of long term interocular suppression. *Vision Res.*, **21**, 1055–63.

Sjostrand, J. (1978) Contrast sensitivity in amblyopia: a preliminary report. *J. Metab. Ophthal.*, **2**, 135–7.

Watson, A. B. (1983) Detection and recognition of sample spatial forms. In *Physical and Biological Processing of Images*, ed. O. J. Braddick & A. C. Slade. Berlin: Springer-Verlag.

Watt, R. J. & Hess, R. F. (1987) Spatial information and uncertainty in anisometropic amblyopia. *Vision. Res.*, **27**, 661–74.

Weiss, C., Rentschler, I. & Caelli, T. (1985) Amblyopic processing of positional information. Part II. Sensitivity to phase distortion. *Exp. Brain Res.*, **60**, 279–88.

Depth and texture

26
Is there a single, most-efficient algorithm for stereopsis?

J. D. Pettigrew

Introduction

It can be argued that stereopsis has evolved on at least three separate occasions; in mammals, in birds and in machines (see Bishop & Pettigrew, 1986; Pettigrew, 1986). While the evolution of machine algorithms for stereopsis is still occurring, such algorithms have reached a level of sophistication where comparison with animals can be made (see Poggio & Poggio, 1984). When the mammalian, avian and machine systems for stereopsis are compared, some fundamental similarities in organisation emerge despite the many structural differences. In particular, all three systems appear to delay image processing until after information from both eyes is brought together. The surprising fact that stereopsis can occur without prior monocular pattern recognition was already recognised from psychophysical studies on humans and was reinforced by detailed studies of the neural machinery underlying stereopsis in both mammals and birds, not to mention the more recent machine algorithms which also avoid complex form analysis prior to extraction of the stereoscopic information.

This chapter deals with the possible reasons behind this common feature of successful stereoscopic systems. Two general lines of argument will be advanced;

i. If the primary role of stereopsis is not the judgement of depth but rather the detection of edges which are invisible to monocular inspection, it is necessary that this edge-detection step precede any attempts at form analysis. This is a teleological argument which can be supported by an examination of the evolutionary context within which some avian groups have acquired stereopsis while other close relatives have not.

ii. Alternatively, there may be a single, most-effi-

cient algorithm for achieving stereopsis and this is the one which has been discovered independently by the mammalian visual system, the avian visual system and by designers of artificial intelligence systems. There are a number of reasons why it might be more efficient to start the process of binocular interaction before advancing too far with pattern analysis of the monocular image.

A summary of our present understanding of avian and mammalian stereoscopic analysis is followed by a brief account of some of the recent developments in machine stereopsis, with special emphasis on the similarities which can be found in all three systems. The surprisingly-scattered phylogenetic distribution of avian stereopsis is considered in the light of the likely ecological pressures responsible for the emergence of stereopsis in birds. Finally, there is discussion of the possible reasons for the similarities in organisation of all three systems, including the possibility that there may be a single, most-efficient solution to the problem of stereopsis.

Similarities between mammalian and avian stereopsis

Triple, parallel processing

The W-, X- and Y- subsystems which have been so well characterised in the cat with respect to the processing of form and motion also have functionally-distinct roles in stereopsis. The W-subsystem is involved with the detection of circumscribed targets (end-stopped receptive fields), moving at low angular speed (nondirectional, low cut-off velocity fields) in the far plane (divergent receptive field disparities); the X-subsystem is involved in high-resolution tasks (receptive fields with high spatial frequency and linear summation) in the fixation plane (receptive fields slightly more convergent than those of the W-subsystem); the Y-subsystem is involved in the detection of indistinct targets (large receptive fields with high tolerance for blur and 'glitch-enchancing' non-linearities) moving at high speed in near space (convergent receptive field disparities) (Pettigrew & Dreher, 1987).

There is not much information on this point in primates, where the W-subsystem in particular (koniocellular laminae) is variable from species to species, never prominent and certainly not readily amenable to analysis (see for example, Kaas, 1986). Psychophysical evidence in humans argues that similar mechanisms are likely to apply in primates to those found in cats. Such evidence includes one's own introspective appreciation of the power of motion parallax to generate a stereoscopic impression in which angular velocity and depth are closely tied. The following qualification is necessary concerning the possible role of a W-like system for stereopsis in primates. In the very-high-resolution system of primates one would not expect to find the difference between the far plane and the fixation plane to be as large as in the cat where it is small enough to be contentious in any case (around 1 deg). Based on other cat–human comparisons, my expectation would be a difference around 6 min arc between the zero reference for binocular fixation and the centre of the fovea, a margin presently close to the limits of measurability.

In the owl there is striking evidence for the separation of stereo-processing into three streams (this was where I obtained the first convincing evidence, in fact), because the separation on the tangent screen of receptive fields recorded from binocular neurons in the Wulst (whose major inputs seem to correspond to the X- and Y- systems of mammals) is always more convergent than the separation of the precisely-defined foveal projections. Only after an extensive search was I able to find any binocular neurons with receptive field separations equal to that of the foveae. These all had properties (difficult to activate, end-stopped, slow movement in the far plane) and a location (tecto-fugal pathway rather than geniculo-striate) consistent with a connection to a heterogeneous, small cell system akin to the W-system of mammals. This impression of a phylogenetically-old, koniocellular system which is associated with the detection of distant, slowly-moving targets also receives support from studies of binocular receptive fields in the optic tectum of the toad (Finch & Collett, 1983).

Concentric fields as 'raw material' for binocular receptive fields

Perhaps the most striking feature shared in common by both avian and mammalian systems is the avoidance of abstract feature analysis until after pathways from both eyes have converged. Birds and mammals both have retinal ganglion cells which take feature extraction to quite high levels, such as the abstraction of direction of movement or edge orientation (although it should be noted in this context that it was once popular to think that a high degree of retinal pre-processing was a feature only of 'lower vertebrates' and 'lower mammals' such as the rabbit). Yet despite the fact that feature extraction is an important early aspect of a binocular neuron's function, whether it be avian or mammalian, no use is apparently made of the feature-extracting retinal ganglion cells by the pathways underlying binocular vision. This was first noted by Levick (1967; 1977) for the rabbit and is true for all of the many species in which stereoscopic visual processing has now been shown to occur (see summary in Pettigrew, 1986). It is possible to make the generalisation that binocular receptive fields, despite their complexity, are 'constructed' from monocular inputs of the concentrically-organised variety and not from the more-specialised retinal outputs which appear to project to targets not primarily concerned with binocular vision. One possible exception to this rule may occur in development of the kitten visual cortex when horizontally- and vertically-oriented monocular units may play a role in 'seeding' the developing orientation array. The origin of these units is not clear so a retinal one is a possibility, however unlikely (seé Pettigrew, 1978 for a discussion).

End-stopped fields

Once thought to represent a higher level of processing than edge detection (hence the term, 'hypercomplex'), end-stopped fields are a common class of units in the earliest stages of visual cortical processing in all species so far examined with their possible existence in mind. The proportions reported vary considerably between studies, probably because these cells readily escape detection on account of their strong inhibitory input for most visual stimuli except a precisely-positioned terminator. They play an important role in the detection of the horizontal disparities of horizontally-oriented edges (Maske et al., 1986) as well as the detection of an 'obscuring edge' which is visible only as an alignment of the interruptions of other contours (cf. illusory contours, Peterhans et al., 1986). In view of the failure of simple cells in monkey striate cortex to respond to random-dot stereograms when complex cells do so (Poggio, 1984), one could speculate that disparity-selective, end-stopped cells provide the raw material for such 'global' complex cells. An array of binocular end-stopped neurons with the same preferred orientation and disparity (perhaps difficult to discover in the behaving monkey preparation because of their tiny receptive field size and specific requirements) would then provide the input to a particular complex cell coding for one global depth plane in the stereogram. Such a system may also be present in the owl (Pettigrew, 1979).

Binocular inhibition of monocular concentric fields

A little-studied but important feature of stereoscopic visual systems is the presence at the earliest stages of processing in an inhibitory field in the otherwise unresponsive eye opposite to the eye which provides the monocular excitation. Thus, at the level of the lateral geniculate nucleus (LGN) or lamina IV of striate cortex a concentrically-organised excitatory field in the 'dominant' eye has a corresponding, horizontally-elongated inhibitory field in the other eye. There are species differences here, since the binocular inhibition is a feature of almost all neurons in the cat LGN (Sanderson *et al.*, 1969) but only of the Y-like cells in the magnocellular layers of the monkey LGN (Dreher *et al.*, 1976). These differences are not likely to be of great significance when it is recalled that the monkey has a much higher proportion of monocular concentric fields at the level of lamina IV of striate cortex (it can be looked upon as having 'encephalised' to a hierarchical level one synapse higher than the cat) and that the cortical monocular fields may have an inhibitory counterpart in the non-exciting eye when this is examined with appropriate techniques. This is the case in the owl, whose visual cortex has two layers of monocular concentric units, each excited by one eye but with an inhibitory field in the other (Pettigrew, 1979 and unpublished observations).

The importance of these observations on binocular inhibition is the very early stage at which this kind of binocular interaction takes place . . . well before the stage at which feature extraction or excitatory binocular interaction take place.

Similarities between avian and mammalian stereopsis: logical consequences

There are two general lines of thought which follow once one accepts that there is a remarkable degree of similarity between the avian and mammalian solutions to stereopsis despite the rather different 'wiring diagrams' of their respective visual pathways.

The first line of thought is that the similar hierarchical arrangement, with binocular interaction occurring early before any attempt at feature extraction, is a trivial consequence of the fact that both systems have evolved stereopsis to aid in the process of edge detection preceding form analysis. In other words, if the prime purpose of stereopsis is the detection of a stereoscopic edge which is invisible to monocular inspection and NOT the determination of the depth of an edge which may be visible monocularly, it is logically necessary for such a system to set about the process of binocular comparison first. This is not a viewpoint which I find easy to adopt because of the prevailing wisdom that stereopsis is the most accurate basis for distance judgements which is available to the visual system. Yet I am compelled toward that viewpoint on the basis of mounting evidence derived from the very scattered phylogenetic distribution of stereopsis among birds. This evidence is summarised below, where one can see that evolution of stereopsis in the interests of edge detection *per se*, rather than accurate distance judgements, is the most parsimonious explanation.

The second line of thought is more in keeping with the spirit of this volume and Horace Barlow's interest in the efficiency of visual coding. It also receives some support from the 'convergent evolution' of some of the machine algorithms for stereopsis if we make the questionable assumption that they have evolved in environments rather different from the ones in which 'camouflage breaking' was important for predatory birds. (In fact, the almost-universal use of Julesz random-dot stereograms in benchmark tests of such algorithms makes it more likely that this assumption is wrong and that there is 'ecological pressure' operating on machine algorithms to break camouflage too!) According to this line of reasoning, there may be a single, most-efficient solution to the problem of stereopsis and it is this solution to which the avian, mammalian and machine systems have all converged.

Formulating this hypothesis in a sufficiently mathematical way to be able to test it from first principles is probably beyond reach at the moment (at least as far as my limited abilities go!), but there are a number of arguments which can be made in its favour.

Flexibility of the search for a match using different 'primitives'

Prior monocular processing implies that a decision has been made about which kinds of features to 'extract' in the interest of comparing both images in the search for matching parts. Such feature extraction can lead to 'blind spots', like the legendary difficulties suffered by anurans in the detection of non-moving prey as a result of the specific properties of their retinal neurons. Accordingly, it would seem wise to avoid 'jumping to conclusions' about the features to be used for matching, instead delaying this process as long as possible. Feedback from higher centres to the binocular inhibitory process at the monocular concentric level would enable even a very-high-order match (e.g. that based on randomly-oriented line segments in the experiment of Frisby & Julesz, 1975) to be used to aid the disparity-detection task at lower levels.

Statistics of the 'window' of acceptable disparity

A problem which dogs many machine algorithms for stereopsis is the interaction between the size of receptive field used to filter the image and the range of disparities within which false matches no longer occur (see Poggio & Poggio, 1984 for a discussion of this problem). A cautious, progressive approach to the choice of the matching primitives to be used, with this decision delayed until after the first preliminary comparison of the monocular images has been made, could be the best approach to this problem. After all, the choice of the matching primitive is based fundamentally on some measure of similarity between the images, a goal which is diametrically opposed to the difference-measuring task which depends so critically upon the establishment of the match. Walking this tight-rope would seem to require the avoidance of too early a commitment to a particular matching strategy and perhaps therefore to require a hierarchy where increasingly-sophisticated analysis goes hand-in-hand with increasing binocular interaction.

Scattered phylogenetic distribution of avian stereopsis

If one is prepared to accept neurobiological criteria for the presence of stereopsis in a particular species without waiting for full behavioural demonstrations, one can draw some interesting conclusions about the phylogenetic distribution of avian stereopsis. The criteria I have adopted admittedly reflect my chauvinistic bias for the economical answers one can obtain with a microelectrode, but in defence of this approach one must point out the long latency which can intervene between a neurobiological demonstration of stereopsis in single binocular neurons and an

unequivocal behavioural demonstration with Julesz patterns in the whole cantankerous animal. In the case of the cat, for example, the latency was 15 years! (see Pettigrew, 1986).

The criteria I have adopted for the diagnosis of stereopsis in a given species are the following:
(1) A mechanism for the decussation of the pathways from each eye so that a precise retinotopic registration can be established between hemifield maps for each eye
(2) Binocularly-activated neurons with precisely-defined receptive fields which are exactly matched with respect to preferred orientation and orientation tuning, direction selectivity, structure of sub-regions etc
(3) Disparity-selectivity with neuron-to-neuron variation in the peak of the disparity tuning curve.
Having found all of these features in the visual Wulst of the owl (Pettigrew & Konishi, 1976; Pettigrew, 1979; Cooper & Pettigrew, 1979), I predict that this bird will have stereopsis equal to that enjoyed by a primate. There are as yet no behavioural studies of owls using random-dot stereograms, but there is a report that another avian predator, the kestrel, shows behavioural evidence of stereopsis (Fox et al., 1977). I initially expected that other birds would show comparable neurobiological substrates for stereopsis, even if not to the same elaborate degree that is evident in owls. That expectation has not been fulfilled. Amongst the avian groups which I have been able to study so far, only a minority have a neural substrate for stereopsis.

Avian orders surveyed
In an electrophysiological survey of 21 species in eight avian orders, the above-listed criteria for stereopsis were found in only nine species, five of which were owls in the families Strigidae and Tytonidae (Pettigrew, Frost & Konishi, in prep.) In addition to the Strigiformes, the orders Caprimulgiformes, Falconiformes and Passeriformes had some representatives, but the orders Columbiformes, Anseriformes, Psittaciformes and Apodiformes all appeared to lack the necessary neural substrate within the visual Wulst. Based on the presence of a greatly enlarged visual Wulst like that found in owls, I think it possible that ratites and coucals will subsequently prove to have stereopsis, but not shorebirds or galliforms.

There has been some suggestion that pigeons have stereopsis, but I reject this possibility on the basis that there is no appropriate neural substrate, despite the presence of a crossed visual thalamo-cortical pathway which might enable the degree of binocular inter-action sufficient to account for inter-ocular transfer of some learned discrimination. Neither anatomical nor physiological studies (Frost *et al.*, 1983) have been able to demonstrate any of the three criteria for stereopsis laid out above and behavioural studies of pigeons are consistent with depth judgements being based on vergence, motion parallax and accommodative cues rather than those based on stereopsis (e.g. Martinoya *et al.*, 1988; Martinoya & Bloch, 1980; McFadden & Wild, 1986). Like many bird families, the Columbi-formes appear to have the rudiments of binocular vision, with some degree of vergence eye movements, but without the necessary machinery to achieve local stereopsis (Frost *et al.*, 1983). The presence of this machinery in a few avian families, such as the owl, raises the question why fully-fledged stereopsis should be so restricted amongst birds.

There are a number of reasons why the Caprimulgiformes are of special interest in this regard. First, these birds, all of which are nocturnal, are believed to be the closest relatives of the owls (Sibley & Ahlquist, 1972). Second, they show a whole spectrum of visual behaviour and foraging abilities, from aerial insect-catching, like swifts, to the capture of live vertebrates from the ground in a way which is not far removed from the owls except for the absence of talons. Third, only two of the five families which I surveyed showed evidence of stereopsis, the family Podargidae (Frogmouths) and the family Aegothe-lidae (Owlet-nightjars). These two families are the only two within the Caprimulgiformes which have the ability to capture prey from the substrate. The other families all forage in mid-air.

There is, therefore, a strong link between the presence of stereopsis and the advanced ability to capture prey from a substrate as opposed to the air. In both cases precise depth judgements are required, but these are presumably mediated in the case of the stereoblind, aerial prey-catchers by monocular cues such as movement parallax (which would be powerful in a swiftly-moving bird) and accommodation (which would also be a powerful cue, given the extra-ordinarily rapid ciliary muscle response in birds – Murphy & Howland, 1983). In the case of the owlet-nightjars and frogmouths feeding from the substrate, binocular cues have assumed greater prominence and both of these families have an elaborate stereoscopic system which is quite comparable to that of the owl. In fact, the only discernible difference between the visual system of owls and that of frogmouths and owlet-nightjars is the presence of large eye-movements in

the latter two groups compared with their virtual absence in the owl (Wallman & Pettigrew, 1985). A formal cladistic analysis of the distribution of a wide range of attributes, including stereopsis, across the owls, Caprimulgiformes and swifts (which are the nearest relatives to the Caprimulgiformes apart from owls), indicates that prey capture from the substrate and stereopsis are both derived features which have evolved together at a later stage and are not likely to have been present in the ancestors of these birds (Pettigrew, in prep.).

In the light of these data on the restricted dis-tribution of avian stereopsis, it is possible to consider in more detail some of the reasons for the evolution of stereopsis.

Evolutionary pressures for the emergence of stereopsis

Camouflage breaking

Stereopsis may have evolved to aid the primary task of image analysis by defining those edges invisible to monocular inspection but derivable from retinal dis-parity cues. This scenario has been proposed by Julesz (1971) amongst others, and although not as popular as the view that stereopsis evolved primarily for precise depth judgements (see below), it is now supported by considerable weight of evidence from the phylogeny of stereopsis in birds, as already outlined above. Acceptance of the camouflage-breaking viewpoint becomes easier when one is made to realise the diffi-culties inherent in the delineation of object boundaries in real images (Pettigrew, 1986). The use of retinal disparity cues to find an object boundary in an image can then be viewed as a fourth mechanism equal in importance to the use of (i) movement parallax cues (cf. the detection of edges in kinematograms, Frost *et al.*, 1988), (ii) phase congruence in the detection of edges in a spatial Fourier spectrum (Morrone *et al.*, 1987) and (iii) chromaticity as a cue to iso-luminant colour boundaries (Livingstone & Hubel, 1984).

For a nocturnal predator attempting to detect prey against a substrate, disparity cues would be all important in edge detection because of problems with each of the other three mechanisms: (i) movement parallax cues may be absent if the prey is relatively immobile and in any case will be particularly subject to noise limitations at low levels of illumination (of which more below), (ii) 'conventional' edges in the phase congruence–orientation domain may be absent because of the prey's attempts to mask these with cryptic patterning and (iii) light levels will be outside the operating range of cones, thereby eliminating the use of spectral cues to define edges.

Precise distance judgements

The extraordinary precision of stereopsis certainly provides a mechanism superior to the depth judgements available from monocular movement parallax, accommodation, size constancy and the other monocular cues (Collett & Harkness, 1982). Improved precision *per se* is unlikely to provide a good account of the evolutionary origins of stereopsis, however, since it seems unlikely that stereopsis originated in the fully-fledged, 'hyperacute' form currently seen in the higher primates. In any case, many primates and owls supplement binocular depth judgements with monocular parallax by the use of 'head bobbing', so it is hard to argue for the superiority of the binocular system on the grounds of precision alone.

The emergence of stereopsis in the early nocturnal predators seems more likely to be related to three other aspects in which binocular parallax does better than monocular parallax:

(i) Absence of the need for the predator to move   Those who have watched the wild gyrations and bobbings of an owl's head while locating its prey will not be impressed with the need of a nocturnal predator to avoid detection by remaining immobile. Nevertheless, furtiveness can be of considerable help in the capture of prey, particularly at close quarters (cf. prey-catching by the slow loris, *Nycticebus*, Jolly, 1987). It is also a clear advantage to be able to keep a camouflaged target continuously in view without the need to 'refresh' it at regular intervals by head movement.

(ii) Absence of the need for the prey to move   This is the other side of the coin to the first advantage of stereopsis over movement parallax. It is easy to imagine the value of a system which circumvented the disappearance of a camouflaged prey at the moment when it stopped moving. The gradual emergence of such a system from a pre-existing system for detecting camouflaged moving targets (as in kinematograms) is therefore a likely scenario. This is reinforced by the fact that the detection of camouflaged moving targets is an ability characteristic of the tecto-fugal pathway (Frost *et al.*, 1988). The tecto-fugal system is phylogenetically universal in vertebrates and almost certainly preceded the specialised geniculo-cortical pathways subserving binocular vision because of the latters' scattered occurrence and heterogeneity of mechanism. We can be reasonably confident on these bases that the use of motion parallax to 'disambiguate'

a prey object from its surroundings was a prior skill from which the use of binocular parallax emerged so as to extend the process to stationary targets.

(iii) Lower susceptibility to photonic noise   Quantal fluctuations at low light levels reduce the detectability of a target in a way which is more severe the faster the target is moving. There would thus be pressure on a nocturnal predator to achieve detection of camouflaged prey at lower and lower prey velocities. At the limit where the prey is stationary and disparity cues are the only ones available, this alternative is no different from the previous one, but it does provide a further argument to show how ecological pressure might favour the emergence of stereopsis from a pre-existing, movement-parallax system.

Probability summation

The two channels of information about the same visual scene provided by binocular vision have the potential to increase the signal/noise ratio by the square root of two, the number of channels over which probability summation takes place. This advantage would accrue to any kind of binocular vision, whether it was capable of achieving stereopsis or not, but could have been a factor in the emergence of stereopsis in a nocturnal predator. For the reason already pointed out, the noise-free operation of movement parallax becomes increasingly limited to low target velocities as light levels fall. In other words, in dim light, the use of monocular parallax becomes problematical except at the low target velocities best suited for binocular parallax which has the added advantage that photonic noise can be averaged between the two eyes. The use of binocular vision can thus be seen as the means by which visibility of a camouflaged target can be improved at low light levels, even when monocular parallax cues are also available.

Conclusion

The present comparison between different stereoscopic systems has been qualitative and would have been facilitated if there were accepted measures of the efficiency with which each system could solve problems such as random-dot stereograms with specified amounts of noise, size anisotropy, contrast reversal etc. Nevertheless, it seems undeniable that there has been a remarkable degree of convergence toward a solution which makes the binocular comparison well in advance of complex form analysis. The two explanations offered for this notable feature are not incompatible if looked at in the following way.

A solution which enables the discrimination of a monocularly-invisible boundary is clearly preferable to one which does not have this power, so long as the price paid for this 'camouflage breaking' ability of stereopsis is not high. On the other hand, this very early comparison of the information from each eye does not preclude the use of later comparisons between the high level descriptions of each image, provided that there is an opportunity for feedback to the early comparison when necessary (see: cortico-geniculate feedback). There does not seem to be any incompatibility, therefore, between a 'camouflage breaking' algorithm and other solutions involving higher-level comparisons between the eyes. Acceptance of this fact leads to the conclusion that a stereoscopic system which incorporates both the low-level ('camouflage breaking') and higher-level comparisons will be superior to one lacking in the first stage, even if 'camouflage breaking' is regarded as a facultative, rather than obligatory, function of stereopsis.

On this basis I believe that it is possible to conclude that the solution to the problem of stereopsis which has been adopted by some mammals, some birds and some machines IS the most efficient one. Bringing together information from both eyes at the earliest possible opportunity enables camouflage breaking, if necessary, without at the same time precluding a range of comparisons between the descriptions of each eye's image at subsequent stages of processing.

References

Bishop, P. O. & Pettigrew, J. D. (1986) Neural mechanisms of binocular vision. *Vision Res.*, **26**, 1587–1600.

Cooper, M. C. & Pettigrew, J. D. (1979) A neurophysiological determination of the vertical horopter in the cat and owl. *J. Comp. Neurol.*, **184**, 1–26.

Collett, T. S. & Harkness, L. I. K. (1982) Depth vision in animals. In *Analysis of Visual Behavior*, ed. D. Ingle, M. A. Goodale & R. Mansfield, pp. 111–77. Cambridge, Mass: MIT Press.

Dreher, B., Fukada, Y. & Rodieck, R. W. (1976) Identification, classification and anatomical segregation of cells with X-like and Y-like properties in the lateral geniculate nucleus of old world monkeys. *J. Physiol.*, **258**, 433–52.

Finch, D. J. & Collett T. S. (1983) Small-field, binocular neurons in the superficial layers of the frog optic tectum. *Proc. Roy. Soc. Lond.*, B**217**, 491–7.

Fox, R., Lemkuhle, S. W. & Bush, R. C. (1977) Stereopsis in the falcon. *Science*, **197**, 79–81.

Frisby, J. P. & Julesz, B. (1975) The effect of orientation difference on stereopsis as a function of line length. *Perception*, **41**, 179–86.

Frost, B. J., Goodale, M. A. & Pettigrew, J. D. (1983) A search for functional binocularity in the pigeon. *Proc. Soc. Neurosci.*, **9**, 823.

Frost, B. J., Cavanagh, P. & Morgan, B. (1988) Deep tectal cells in pigeons respond to kinematograms. *J. Comp. Physiol.*, A**162**, 639–47.

Kaas, J. H. (1986) The structural basis of information processing in the primate visual system. In *Visual Neuroscience*, ed. J. D. Pettigrew, K. J. Sanderson & W. R. Levick, pp. 315–40. Cambridge: Cambridge University Press.

Jolly, A. S. (1987) *The Evolution of Primate Behaviour*. London: Livingstone.

Julesz, B. (1971) *The Foundations of Cyclopean Perception*. Chicago: University of Chicago Press.

Levick, W. R. (1967) Receptive fields and trigger features of ganglion cells in the visual streak of the rabbit's retina. *J. Physiol.*, **188**, 285–307.

Levick, W. R. (1977) Participation of brisk-transient retinal ganglion cells in binocular vision – an hypothesis. *Proc. Aust. Physiol. Pharmacol. Soc.*, **8**, 9–16.

Livingstone, M. S. & Hubel, D. H. (1984) Anatomy and physiology of a color system in the primate visual cortex. *J. Neurosci.*, **4**, 309–56.

Martinoya, C. & Bloch, S. (1980) Depth perception in the pigeon: looking for the participation of binocular cues. In *Sensory Functions, Advances in Physiological Sciences* 16, ed. E. Grastyan & P. Molnar, pp. 477–82. Oxford: Pergamon Press.

Martinoya, C., Le Houezec, J. & Bloch, S. (1988) Depth resolution in the pigeon. *J. Comp. Physiol.*, A**163**, 33–42.

Maske, R., Yamane, S. & Bishop, P. O. (1986) End-stopped cells and binocular depth discrimination in cat striate cortex. *Proc. Roy. Soc. Lond.*, B**229**, 257–76.

McFadden, S. A. & Wild, J. M. (1986) Binocular depth discrimination in the pigeon (*Columba livia*). *J. Exp. Analysis Behav.*, **45**, 148–60.

Morrone, M. C., Ross, J. & Burr, D. C. (1987) Mach bands are phase dependent. *Nature*, **324**, 250–3.

Murphy, C. J. & Howland, H. C. (1983) Owl eyes: accommodation, corneal curvature and refractive state. *J. Comp. Physiol.*, A**151**: 277–84.

Peterhans, E., Von der Heydt, R. & Baumgartner, G. (1986) Neuronal responses to illusory contour stimuli reveal stages of visual cortical processing. In *Visual Neuroscience*, ed. J. D. Pettigrew, K. J. Sanderson & W. R. Levick, pp. 343–51. Cambridge: Cambridge University Press.

Pettigrew, J. D. (1978) The paradox of the critical period for striate cortex. In *Neuronal Plasticity*, ed. C. W. Cotman, pp. 321–30. New York: Raven Press.

Pettigrew, J. D. (1979) Binocular visual processing in the owl's telencephalon. *Proc. Roy. Soc. Lond.*, B**204**, 435–54.

Pettigrew, J. D. (1986) The evolution of binocular vision. In

Visual Neuroscience, ed, J. D. Pettigrew, K. J. Sanderson & W. R. Levick, pp. 208–22. Cambridge: Cambridge University Press.

Pettigrew, J. D. & Dreher, B. (1987) Parallel processing of binocular disparity in the cat's retino-geniculo-cortical pathways. *Proc. Roy. Soc. Lond.*, B**232**, 297–321.

Pettigrew, J. D. & Konishi, M. (1976) Neurons selective for orientation and binocular disparity in the visual Wulst of the barn owl (*Tyto alba*). *Science*, **193**, 675–8.

Poggio, G. F. (1984) Processing of stereoscopic information in primate visual cortex. In *Dynamical Aspects of Cortical Function*, ed. G. M. Edelman, W. E. Gall & W. M. Cowan, pp. 613–35. New York: Wiley.

Poggio, G. F. & Poggio, T. (1984) The analysis of stereopsis. *Ann. Rev. Neurosci.*, **7**, 379–412.

Sanderson, K. J., Darian-Smith, I. & Bishop, P. O. (1969) Binocular corresponding receptive fields of single units in the cat dorsal lateral geniculate nucleus. *Vision Res.*, **9**, 1297–303.

Sibley, C. G., & Ahlquist, J. E. (1972) A comparative study of the egg white proteins of non-passerine birds. *Bull. Peabody Mus. Nat. Hist.*, **39**, 1–276.

Wallman J. & Pettigrew, J. D. (1985) Conjugate and disjunctive saccades in two avian species with contrasting oculomotor strategies. *J. Neurosci.*, **6**, 1418–28.

27

Binocular mechanisms in the normal and abnormal visual cortex of the cat

R. D. Freeman and I. Ohzawa

Introduction

We have considered the following three questions regarding the physiological organization of binocular pathways in the visual cortex of the cat. First, what are the rules by which signals from left and right eyes are combined in the visual cortex? Second, how are these rules affected when normal visual experience is prevented during an early stage of development? Third, how early in the development process is the physiological apparatus for binocular vision established?

These questions have been examined by use of a technique that differs from other physiological procedures that have been employed to study binocular vision. The major feature of our method is use of large, bright, sinusoidal gratings which are varied in relative phase between the two eyes so that retinal disparity is systematically changed. Aside from the analytical advantage of this stimulus, the large spatial extent of the gratings increases the likelihood that receptive fields are stimulated. We have found, for example, that 56% of cortical cells in normal cats exhibit disparity-dependent binocular interaction. In another study in which a thorough examination was made of binocular properties of cortical cells by use of single bars of light, only 37% displayed disparity selectivity (Ferster, 1981).

With respect to the questions we have addressed, our results are as follows. First, most simple cells and around half the sample of complex cells show phase-specific binocular interaction. This leads to the conclusion that most binocular interaction in striate cortex can be accounted for by linear summation of signals from each eye. Second, monocularly deprived kittens retain input from the occluded eye to visual cortex for a much longer time than previously

thought. In the case of binocular deprivation, a surprising degree of phase-specific binocular interaction occurs, suggesting that receptive field organization is irregular but the balance of excitatory and inhibitory components does not differ from that of normal cats. Third, a normal physiological pattern of binocular interaction is present for cortical cells of very young kittens. By 3 weeks postnatal, cortical cells of kittens exhibit all aspects of binocular interaction properties that are observed in adults.

Methods

Cats were obtained mainly from a closed colony. Normal adults were used according to standard procedures as described in detail in other papers (e.g., Ohzawa & Freeman, 1986a; Freeman & Ohzawa, 1988). In the cases of monocular or binocular deprivation, one or both eyes, respectively, were sutured closed at 2 to 3 weeks postnatal. These kittens were monitored until they were studied physiologically at 6 months of age or later. For the question of the developmental status of binocular vision, kittens were studied physiologically at 2, 3, or 4 weeks postnatal.

Our procedures for physiological study are as follows. Initially, after preanaesthetic delivery of a tranquilizer and atropine, the cat is anaesthetized with halothane. Venous and tracheal cannulae are positioned, anaesthesia is continued with sodium thiamylal, and a cranial hole is made for placement of a tungsten-in-glass electrode in striate cortex. After all surgical procedures are completed, the animal is positioned in front of a screen, paralyzed with gallamine triethiodide, and artificially ventilated with a mixture of N_2O, O_2, and CO_2 (approximately 70%, 29%, and 1%, respectively). Contact lenses are positioned on the corneas. Vital signs are monitored throughout the experiment (EKG, EEG, heart rate, temperature, and intratracheal pressure).

Once a cell is isolated, its receptive fields are explored manually with slits and bars of light. Then quantitative runs are made with sinusoidal gratings presented to each eye to determine optimal parameters of orientation and spatial frequency. Temporal frequency and contrast are nearly always set at 2 Hz and 50%, respectively. Once optimal parameters for each eye are determined, a binocular test is run in which relative phase of the gratings presented to the eyes is varied in 30° steps. All tests are run in randomly interleaved fashion. A schematic diagram of the apparatus used for these experiments is shown in Fig. 27.1.

Results

Normal cats

The visual cortex is the primary site at which signals from left and right eyes are mixed. The mixture is not complete, as evidenced by varying degrees of ocular dominance among the cells. The notion has been put forward that visual cortex is the main site at which information about retinal disparity is processed, as required for stereoscopic depth discrimination (Barlow *et al.*, 1967). An alternative view is that retinal disparity selectivity is an inevitable feature of the receptive field organization of most cortical cells. Although this is not in conflict with the other idea, the disparity selectivity observed could be independent of the main mechanism of stereopsis. In either case, one should be able to define rules by which left and right eye inputs are combined. Specifically, we wish to consider alternative models of binocular convergence to simple or complex type cortical cells. Summation of left and right eye signals could occur with pre or postsynaptic inhibition or with both. In this case, a non-linear convergence would be likely. Alternatively, the combination of inputs could be multiplicative. This type of convergence is likely in cases where neither eye, when stimulated alone, results in a response, but the cell is activated when stimuli are presented to both eyes together. Another possibility is that of linear summation by which inputs from left and right eyes converge by simple addition. This latter possibility is supported by most of our data.

An example of results from a representative simple cell is shown in Fig. 27.2. In A and B, tuning curves are given for orientation, and spatial frequency of gratings presented at a temporal frequency of 2 Hz and a contrast of 50%. The two curves in each case, represent results for left and right eyes. Response

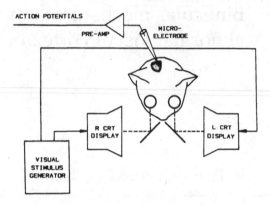

Fig. 27.1. Dichoptic stimulation set-up used in the experiments is shown schematically at the top. At the bottom are disparity varying stimuli produced by changing the interocular phase of the two gratings presented to the eyes. Here, the four conditions depict 90°-step phase shifts, but in the actual experiments, 12 phase angles separated by 30° were used.

patterns are typical and show well-tuned functions for each parameter, with one eye somewhat more dominant than the other. Optimal orientation and spatial frequency are 80% and 0.3 cycles/deg, respectively. These values are used for the binocular run in which phase between the eyes is varied in 30° steps. Results of this test are shown as PSTH (peri-stimulus-time histograms) data in C. In addition to results for a variety of relative interocular phases, responses are shown for tests of each eye alone and for a blank run to determine spontaneous discharge levels. The histograms in C are modulated so that regular bursts of discharge occur with a period corresponding to the temporal cycle of the stimulus. Results of harmonic

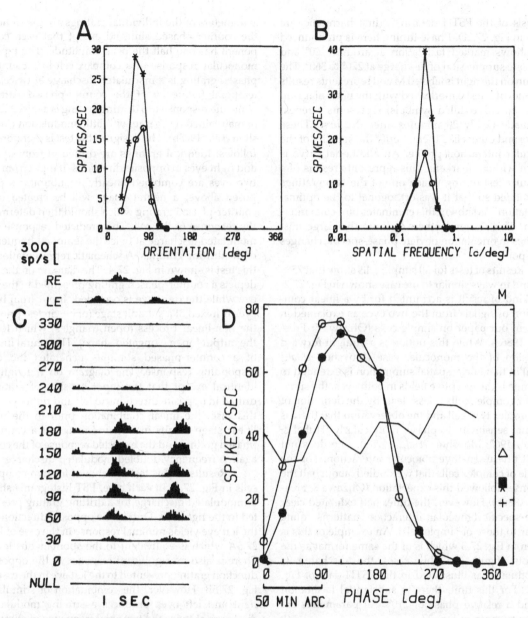

Fig. 27.2. Responses of a simple cell are shown. A and B, respectively, show orientation and spatial frequency tuning curves. Open circles and asterisks indicate responses to stimulation of the left and right eyes, respectively. Values of the orientation angle also indicate the direction of grating drift. For example, 90° and 270° denote opposite directions of motion of the vertical grating. Using the optimal orientation and spatial frequency determined by these tests, dichoptic phase-shift runs are performed. Results of these tests are shown as PSTH data in C. Interocular phase values are shown at the left of each histogram, and at the top, responses to a monocular stimulus are shown as RE and LE for right and left eyes, respectively. At the bottom is the response to a null condition in which a patternless mean luminance screen was shown to each eye. In D, response amplitudes (first harmonic) are plotted as functions of interocular phase. Two curves (open and filled circles) show results from repeated runs. The curve with no data points shows the result when one orientation of the dichoptically presented gratings was orthogonal to the optimal.

analysis of the PSTH data in C (first harmonic) are given in Fig. 27.2D. Phase-tuning here is pronounced and shows marked facilitation at around 120° and complete suppression of discharge at 270° to 360°. The column on the right is labeled M and represents results of monocular tests interleaved with the binocular run. A second curve (filled symbols) represents a repeat run made nearly 20 minutes after the first. These results and others like them, verify the stability of the binocular interaction profile. An additional curve is shown without markers. This represents results of a binocular test during which one of the two gratings was rotated so that it was orthogonal to the optimal orientation. As shown, this eliminates binocular interaction. This test and others indicate that large mismatches in orientation obviate phase-specific changes in response.

Results of tests for all simple cells show that 75% respond in ways similar to the case shown in Fig. 27.2. This kind of result is accounted for by a linear combination of signals from the two eyes as explained in detail in our paper on simple cells (Ohzawa & Freeman, 1986a). While this notion is a straight-forward extension of the monocular case (Movshon *et al.*, 1978a) in that linear spatial summation is extended to encompass the receptive fields in both eyes, the situation for complex cells is less clear. By the definition of the complex type cell and the observation that there is minimal sensitivity to phase, monocularly (Hubel & Wiesel, 1962; Movshon *et al.*, 1978b), one does not expect phase-sensitive binocular interaction. For the sample of complex cells that we studied, about half the responses followed this expectation (Ohzawa & Freeman, 1986b). However, the other half exhibited clear phase-specific binocular interaction patterns, quite similar to those of simple cells. An example of this is shown in Fig. 27.3 which is of the same format as the previous figure. In this case, the discharge is unmodulated as illustrated in the PSTH data of Fig. 27.3C. For this unit, there is substantial facilitation around a relative phase of 210°. All parameters are similar to those of Fig. 27.2.

To account for phase-specific binocular interaction in complex cells, there must be some sort of an internal structure which is not apparent by standard receptive field mapping. One possibility is that, within a complex receptive field structure, there are binocular subunits that combine input from the two eyes linearly as if they are simple cells. We devised a test of this supposition by noting a mathematical relationship used in wave theory which allows a decomposition of a counter-phased sinusoid into two drifting grating components moving in opposite directions. All parameters of the individual gratings are the same as the counter-phased sinusoid except that each component has one half the peak amplitude. The typical monocular response of a complex cell to a counter-phased grating is a modulated discharge at twice the temporal frequency of the counter-phased pattern while the response to a drifting grating is a raised level of maintained discharge with little modulation (Movshon *et al.*, 1978b). The design of the test is therefore as follows. Identical gratings are drifted in front of left and right eyes in opposite directions. If input from the two eyes are combined linearly at subunits as proposed above, a neural image will be created of a counter-phased grating which should then determine the response of the cell. The predicted response is a modulated discharge at twice the temporal frequency of the drifting gratings. A schematic representation of this test is shown in Fig. 27.4. The diagram on the left depicts a counter-phased grating presented to the left eye while the right eye is occluded. Input from both eyes is mixed at a subunit stage (open circles) prior to the non-linear process (open triangles) which feeds the output (open elongated shape). The neural image of a counter-phased stimulus generates the corresponding response. The diagram on the right is identical except that the input consists of gratings drifted in opposite directions to left and right eyes. In this case, the linear combination prior to the non-linear stage results in a neural image of a counter-phased grating and the expected response of the cell is again a frequency-doubled modulated discharge.

Results of this test are shown for two complex cells in Fig. 27.5. In each case, PST histograms show unmodulated discharge for a drifting grating presented to the right eye. Drift in the opposite direction for the left eye yields minimal response in the case of Fig. 27.5A which is equivalent to the spontaneous level. There is also no significant response to the opposite direction grating presented to the left eye in the case of Fig. 27.5B. However, the combination of stimuli to right and left eyes produces a striking modulated discharge at twice the temporal frequency of stimulation. The response is exactly what is predicted by the model of Fig. 27.4. These kinds of tests suggest that around half of the complex cells in the cat's striate cortex have a receptive field organization with underlying binocular subunits which are responsible for a linear combination of signals from left and right eyes. Since this rule applies to virtually all simple cells, we conclude that the binocular combination of afferent inputs from the two eyes, for the majority of cells in the visual cortex, is by linear summation.

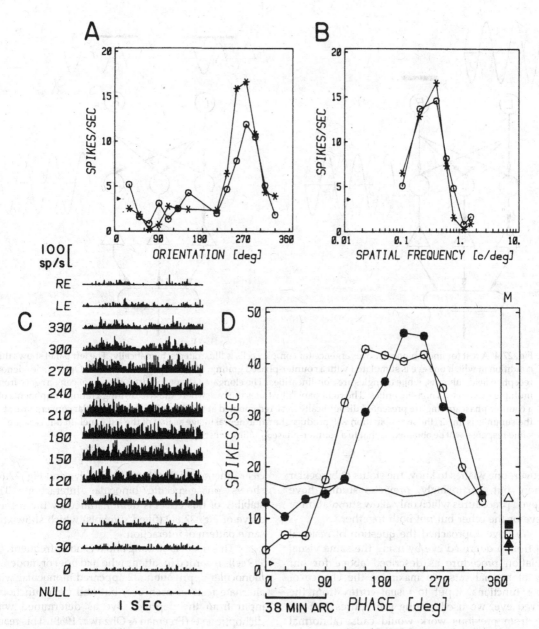

Fig. 27.3. Responses of a complex cell are shown in the same format as that of Fig. 27.2, except that the mean discharge rate (d.c. component) is plotted in A, B, and D. For this cell, optimal orientation and spatial frequency were 270° and 0.4 c/deg, respectively.

Monocularly deprived cats

The physiological, anatomical, and behavioral consequences of monocular deprivation have been studied extensively. However, little is known about the process of disconnection of the deprived eye from the visual cortex. One fundamental question is whether input remains even when a cell cannot be activated by visual stimulation. Although this question has been addressed previously (see Mitchell & Timney, 1984; Frégnac & Imbert, 1984 for reviews), some of the results appear inconsistent with each other, the methods involve population studies before and after a procedure, and there is a lack of quantitative data.

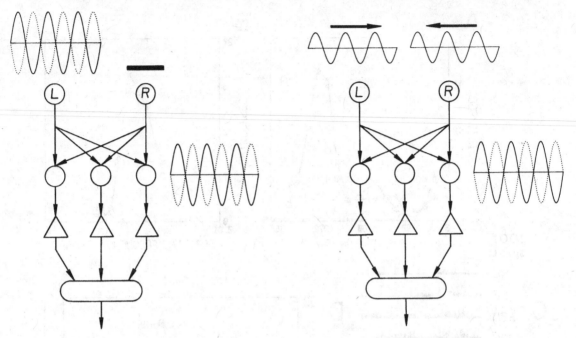

Fig. 27.4. A test for linear binocular convergence for complex cells is illustrated schematically. The left panel shows the condition in which one eye is stimulated with a counter-phased grating. The other eye is occluded. Open circles denote receptive field subunits, while triangles are non-linearities. The elongated shape indicates the site of convergence from multiple subunits via non-linearities. The right panel illustrates the case where the two drifting grating components of a counter-phase grating are presented dichoptically to be recombined at the subunits. If the binocular convergence at the subunits is linear, the recombination will produce the same neural image as that of the left panel. In this case the same response will be obtained as that to a counter-phased grating presented monocularly.

Moreover, one wishes to know the status of binocular function, but, surprisingly, previous studies have employed procedures which only allow stimulation of one eye or the other but not both together.

We have approached the question of residual input from a deprived eye by using the same visual stimulation procedure as described above for our study of normal cats. To maximize the chance of finding functional input to visual cortex from the deprived eye, we used rearing procedures that we knew from previous work would cause abnormal ocular dominance histograms, but would leave some cells with intact afferent connections from each eye. An example of a result from one of these experiments is shown in Fig. 27.6. The format is the same as that of previous figures. In this case, the cell is from a kitten whose left eye was monocularly deprived for 3 days at 5 weeks postnatal. The upper panels show tuning curves for orientation and spatial frequency and there is clearly no response through the deprived (left) eye. This is illustrated again in the PSTH data which show a silent left eye. However, the binocular tests reveal

clear functional input from the left eye and Fig. 27.6D shows phase-specific binocular interaction. The stability of this effect is demonstrated by the second curve of Fig. 27.6D (filled symbols) which shows the same pattern of interaction.

This result is striking and it is not infrequent. Of 119 cells recorded in kittens who had brief or moderate monocular deprivation, 32 appeared monocular with alternate tests of each eye, but had clear functional input from the deprived eye as determined with dichoptic tests (Freeman & Ohzawa, 1988). This result shows that the process of disconnection of the deprived eye from visual cortex takes considerably longer than previously thought. However, these residual connections are rare in animals deprived for long periods of time.

Binocularly deprived cats
Binocular deprivation has also been studied extensively, but this process is inherently more difficult to assess because many cells are either unresponsive or erratic. Of the cells from which responses are

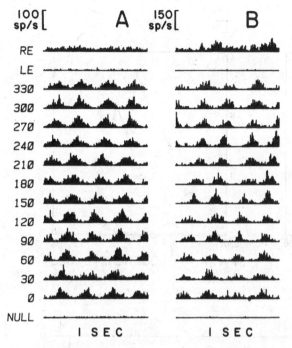

Fig. 27.5. Responses are shown of two complex cells to the stimuli described in the right panel of Fig. 27.4. Responses shown in A are for the cell in Fig. 27.3. All conditions for which gratings are drifted in opposite directions to the two eyes (as noted by phase angles 0° to 330°) show characteristic responses of complex cells to a counter-phased grating.

obtained, patterns of discharge are often irregular and standard tuning curves (e.g., for orientation and spatial frequency) are difficult to obtain. One possible explanation for the physiological characteristics of cortical cells in binocularly deprived cats is as follows. With normal visual exposure, ON and OFF areas in receptive field structure form regular patterns. When the visual system is deprived of form vision, these patterns become irregular so that ON and OFF areas are scrambled. However, if the overall balance of inhibitory and excitatory connections remains nearly constant so that linear combination is still maintained, then binocular interaction profiles would appear essentially normal with our tests using sinusoidal gratings, and one would observe phase-specific changes in response patterns. This is a property of a linearly summing receptive field stimulated with a sinusoid.

The data we have obtained from binocularly deprived cats support this notion (Ohzawa & Freeman 1988). Cells which could be held and from which recordings could be made reliably, were tested with

the same general protocol as that used for the other experiments described above. Examples of binocular interaction tests are shown in Fig. 27.7. The four sets of curves all display phase-specific binocular interaction with both suppression and facilitation of discharge. It is difficult to determine if there are exceptions to this pattern since the rearing procedure produces many cells that are not amenable to quantitative measurements, and we are selecting units that can be held and that give reliable responses. However, of the sample which fits in this category (66 cells), 55% gave normal phase-specific responses to dichoptically presented gratings. This finding is striking because it is somewhat counter-intuitive that highly regular response patterns are exhibited by cortical cells whose monocular tuning properties are abnormal. However, the finding is consistent with the suggestion that the primary result of binocular deprivation is an irregular pattern of ON–OFF regions of receptive fields. Synaptic functions which support linear summation are retained by a maintained balance of excitation and inhibition.

Development of binocular interaction in kittens

The developmental time course of binocular vision in the kitten has been studied previously, but results are not in accord (Pettigrew, 1974; Hubel & Wiesel, 1963). The time course of development of binocular vision is of fundamental importance to questions of plasticity, and our dichoptic grating stimulation procedure is well suited for the study. We examined responses of cells in visual cortex of normally reared kittens at ages 2, 3 or 4 weeks postnatal. Procedures are identical to those described above with the exception that special techniques are required to record from 2-week-old kittens. The main additional requirement in this case is that structural support must be used to position the kitten in the stereotaxic apparatus.

Our main results from these experiments are as follows. Kittens recorded at ages 3 or 4 weeks postnatal, display response characteristics that are largely indistinguishable from those of adults. Tuning curves for orientation and spatial frequency are similar to those for adults, but mean optimal spatial frequency increases from around 0.3 cycles/deg at 3 weeks to about 0.65 cycles/deg in adults. An example of a set of responses from a cell recorded in a 3-week-old kitten is shown in Fig. 27.8. In this case, the right eye is dominant but there are clear tuning curves for each eye with respect to orientation and spatial frequency. The PSTH data shown in Fig. 27.8C exhibit modulated discharge patterns along with substantial facilitation

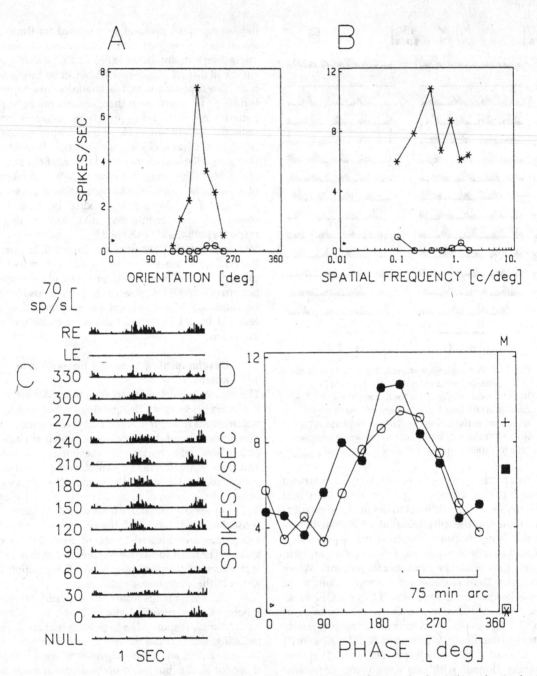

Fig. 27.6. Responses are shown of a simple cell from a kitten reared with brief monocular deprivation (deprived at 5 weeks postnatal for 3 days and physiologically studied immediately after the deprivation period). Results are shown in the same format as that of Fig. 27.2. Optimal spatial frequency and orientation were 0.2 c/deg and 170°, respectively.

at around 0° and 300° and complete suppression at 120° to 180° relative phase. The second curve in Fig. 27.8D represents data from a second complete run. Here, as in other cases, the pattern is closely similar to that of the first run.

At 2 weeks, the situation is more difficult to determine because of the fragility of the preparation and the non-neural factors (i.e., optics) that become problematic. In general, responses of cells in this group are weak but when units could be studied, they

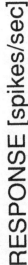
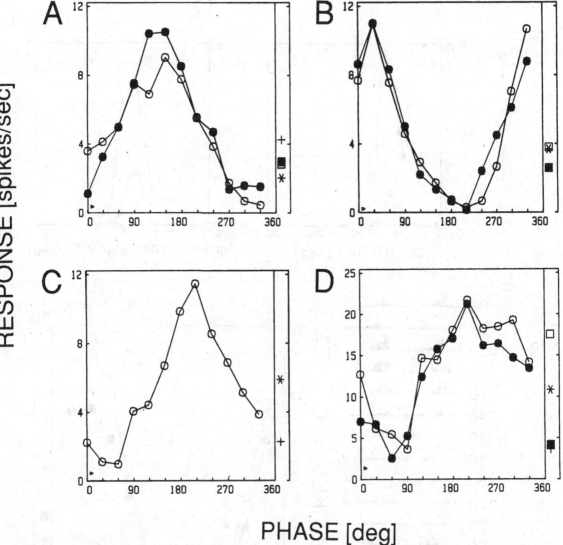

Fig. 27.7. Results of dichoptic phase shift experiments are shown for four cells from binocularly deprived cats, in the same format as that of Fig. 27.2D. The two curves in A, B, and D are results of repeated measurements. The orientation and spatial frequency for each cell were: A 25°, 0.8 c/deg; B 209°, 1.2 c/deg; C 0°, 0.8 c/deg; D 167°, 0.6 c/deg.

were invariably tuned for orientation and spatial frequency. Furthermore, about a half of these units were clearly binocular and displayed phase-tuned responses. We conclude that the physiological apparatus for binocular vision is present and functional at an age between 2 to 3 weeks postnatal.

Discussion

The three questions we have considered here have to do with the physiological organization of binocular

vision in normal and visually deprived cats and kittens. With respect to normal adults, we find that virtually all simple cells and half of the complex cells studied, receive inputs from each eye by linear summation. This holds even for cells which are dominated by one eye. This represents an extension of the notion of receptive field organization from the monocular to the binocular case and allows a unified view of the convergence of input to striate cortex.

In the case of monocular deprivation, we find that cells which appear monocular when tests consist

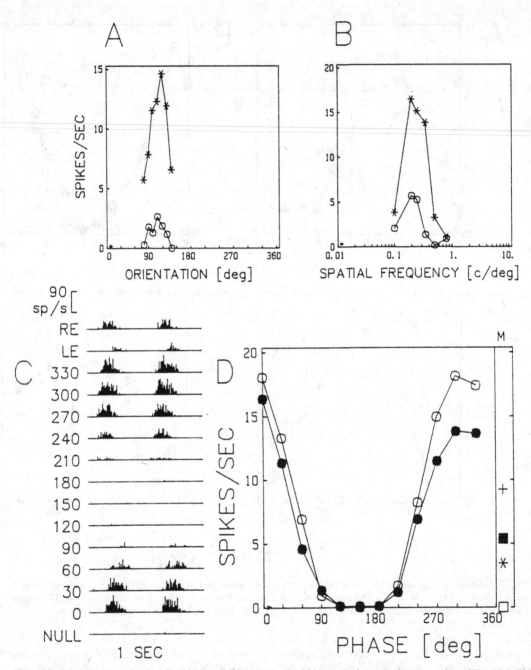

Fig. 27.8. Responses are shown of a simple cell from a 3-week-old kitten in the same format as that of Fig. 27.2. The spatial frequency and orientation used in tests shown in C and D were 0.25 c/deg and 109°, respectively.

of alternate presentation of gratings to each eye, are often binocular. Input from the silent eye is expressed in the form of suppression or phase-specific interaction when gratings varying in interocular phase are presented dichoptically. The process of functional disconnection from the deprived eye during monocular deprivation is, therefore, more gradual than previously thought. The first stage may simply be that of threshold elevation so that any excitatory influence to offset this, could result in measurable discharge from the cell when the apparently silent eye is activated simultaneously with the dominant eye.

The study of binocular deprivation with dichoptic stimulation also reveals a pattern of response that suggests how cortical cells in this preparation are organized. With monocular tests, we obtain the expected result of erratic or unresponsive cells, and those with abnormal monocular tuning characteristics. However, dichoptic stimulation with phase-varying gratings often reveals a remarkable pattern of regular phase-specific binocular interaction. This result strongly suggests that binocular deprivation causes a scrambling of receptive field organization which in the normal animal is highly regular. If the balance of inhibitory and excitatory connections remains approximately constant, phase-specific binocular interaction

is predicted based on responses of a linear system to sinusoidal input.

Finally, we have attempted to define the youngest age at which kittens are physiologically developed for binocular vision. Our experiments demonstrate that this apparatus is functional at 2 to 3 weeks postnatal. Practically, this is the earliest that one can effectively measure this function. It is likely that the physiological substrate for binocular interaction is an innate facility which develops and is refined during postnatal visual experience.

Acknowledgement

This work was supported by grant EY01175 from the US National Eye Institute.

References

Barlow, H. B., Blakemore, C. & Pettigrew, J. D. (1967) The neural mechanism of binocular depth discrimination. *J. Physiol. (Lond.)*, **193**, 327–42.

Ferster, D. (1981) A comparison of binocular depth mechanisms in areas 17 and 18 of the cat visual cortex. *J. Physiol. (Lond.)*, **311**, 623–55.

Freeman, R. D. & Ohzawa, I. (1988) Monocularly deprived cats; binocular tests of cortical cells reveal functional connections from the deprived eye. *J. Neurosci.*, **8**, 2491–506.

Frégnac, Y. & Imbert, M. (1984) Development of neuronal selectivity in primary visual cortex of cat. *Physiol. Rev.*, **64**, 325–434.

Hubel, D. H. & Wiesel, T. N. (1962) Receptive fields, binocular interaction and functional architecture in the cat's visual cortex. *J. Physiol. (Lond.)*, **160**, 106–54.

Hubel, D. H. & Wiesel, T. N. (1963) Receptive fields of cells in striate cortex of very young, visually inexperienced kittens. *J. Neurophysiol.*, **26**, 994–1002.

Mitchell, D. E. & Timney, B. (1984) Postnatal development of function in the mammalian visual system. In *Nervous system III, Handbook of physiology, Vol. III, Sect. I*, pp. 507–55. Washington DC: American Physiological Society.

Movshon, J. A., Thompson, I. D. & Tolhurst, D. J. (1978a) Spatial summation in the receptive fields of simple cells in the cat's striate cortex. *J. Physiol. (Lond.)*, **283**, 53–77.

Movshon, J. A., Thompson, I. D. & Tolhurst, D. J. (1978b) Receptive field organization of complex cells in the cat's striate cortex. *J. Physiol. (Lond.)*, **283**, 79–99.

Ohzawa, I. & Freeman, R. D. (1986a) The binocular organization of simple cells in the cat's visual cortex. *J. Neurophysiol.* **56**, 221–42.

Ohzawa, I. & Freeman, R. D. (1986b) The binocular organization of complex cells in the cat's visual cortex. *J. Neurophysiol.*, **56**, 243–59.

Ohzawa, I. & Freeman, R. D. (1988) Binocularly deprived cats: binocular tests of cortical cells show regular patterns of interaction. *J. Neurosci.*, **8**, 2507–16.

Pettigrew, J. D. (1974) The effect of visual experience on the development of stimulus specificity by kitten cortical neurones. *J. Physiol. (Lond.)* **237**, 49–74.

28

Viewing geometry and gradients of horizontal disparity

G. J. Mitchison and G. Westheimer

Introduction

Though stereoscopic vision is often regarded as a means of gauging distance, human stereo depth judgements depart strikingly from the predictions of geometry. Not only are judgements of absolute distance highly inaccurate, as shown by Helmholtz's experiments using a single vertical thread against a featureless background (Helmholtz, 1909), but also the perceived distance of an object is strongly affected by other objects nearby (Gogel, 1963; Gogel & Mershon, 1977), with the result that relative distance is often incorrectly estimated.

In the case of horizontal rows of features, what stereo vision seems to deliver is a measure of local protrusion or curvature (Mitchison & Westheimer, 1984). For instance, a linear horizontal gradient of disparity generates no curvature and is therefore poorly perceived. However, the same is not true of a vertical gradient of (horizontal) disparity, and indeed there is known to be a marked horizontal/vertical anisotropy in stereo perception (Rogers & Graham, 1983). We suggest here a rationale for some of these phenomena. It turns out that oblique viewing introduces gradients of horizontal disparity which are largely eliminated by the curvature measure, thereby allowing a stable percept under changing viewing conditions. These disparity gradients are present only in the horizontal direction, and this may be the basis of the horizontal/vertical anisotropy.

Depth judgements in horizontal rows of features

We first review the experiments which show how stereo depth judgements are made in figures consisting of horizontal rows of lines or dotted lines (Mitch-ison & Westheimer, 1984). These figures were presented as stereograms with no other depth cues, viewed by subjects at a distance of 3 metres for $\frac{1}{2}$ second. The subjects were required to make relative depth judgements (e.g. 'the left line lies in front of the right') which were signalled by pressing a button. From these judgements, a threshold was derived (for details of this procedure, see legend to Fig. 28.1).

When subjects were asked to judge the relative depths of two dotted columns (Fig. 28.1a), they all obtained the low thresholds characteristic of those with good stereo vision. When presented with a grid of dots with a horizontally oriented, linear gradient of disparity (Fig. 28.1b), the thresholds, expressed as the disparity between an adjacent pair of columns in the grid, were very much higher. This was true whether the subjects attended to an adjacent pair of columns or whether they used every cue available, such as the (larger) disparities between non-adjacent columns, or the perceived tilt of the whole grid. It is remarkable that embedding a pair of columns in a larger figure should make depth judgement so very much harder; the naive expectation might have been that the task would have been easier. The fact that horizontal disparity gradients are very poorly perceived has also been reported by Gillam et al. (1984), who noted that a perception of tilt does eventually emerge, but only slowly, taking tens of seconds.

In a further experiment, we placed two lines in front of a grid identical to that used in the preceding experiment, and the subject was asked to judge the relative depth of these two lines. The background grid was given a horizontal disparity gradient which took, randomly, one of two equal and opposite values. The responses for these two conditions were collected separately, and the disparities at which the two lines appeared at equal depth calculated for each condition.

This enabled us to ask whether the background tilt affected the relative depths of the lines, and this turned out to be the case. In fact, the lines appeared at equal depth when they were approximately lined up with the background plane (Fig. 28.1d).

These results have a slight air of paradox: the tilt of a grid cannot be perceived, and yet it is evidently used in aligning the test pair. However, a possible explanation is that what is perceived is relative depth, an idea which goes back to Gogel (1963) and Gogel & Mershon (1977). We can cast this in a numerically testable form by postulating that perceived depth of a line is measured by the sum of the disparities between that line and its neighbours. If d is the disparity, relative to the fixation plane, of the line, and d_L, d_R those of the adjacent lines on either side, then we define a formal measure of perceived depth D by

$$D = -[(d-d_L)+(d-d_R)] . \qquad (1)$$

None of our experiments attempt to quantify perceived depth; all are concerned only with judging which of two features lie nearer. We therefore include no constant of proportionality in (1); the minus sign is introduced because, close to the fixation plane, disparity varies negatively with distance.

In the case of the grid with a linear horizontal disparity gradient, (1) predicts that the perceived depths of all columns will be equal (except for the two end columns, a point we return to later). The perceived depths will in fact be zero, since the two terms in (1) have equal and opposite values for a linear disparity gradient. This explains the high thresholds in this situation. Similarly, one can easily see that, when two test lines lie in front of a tilted plane, they will have the same value of D only when the disparities between the test lines and the nearest lines in the plane have the same values, which implies that the test lines are tilted parallel to the background plane. Note finally that, for an isolated pair of lines, the difference in perceived depth should be proportional to their disparity, so that correct depth judgements can be made in this case (assuming that, if no neighbour is present, the corresponding difference in (1) is omitted).

This formula therefore accounts for the results described so far. By using horizontal rows of lines with various spacings, we were able to see how far the formula held true. As an example, consider the experiment shown in Fig. 28.1d. A subject was asked to judge which of the two inner lines lay nearest. These two lines were given disparities of d and $-d$ relative to the fixation plane while the two outer lines were given disparities of nd and $-nd$, where n is an integer.

Then, according to (1), for the left inner line $D = -(d+d)-(d-nd)=(n-3)d$; for the other line $D=(3-n)d$. These are equal when $(n-3)d=0$ or $n=3$, in which case the four lines follow a linear disparity gradient.

For two subjects, the prediction from (1) seemed correct (Fig. 28.1d), but for three other subjects n was larger than the expected value. This could be accounted for by modifying the sum in (1) to include not just nearest neighbours but also next nearest neighbours with weaker weightings. From this and other experiments a rule emerged, which was that the nearest neighbour sum of (1) should be replaced by an extended sum of disparities, so the perceived depth of a feature F is given by

$$D = -\Sigma w_i(d-d_i), \qquad (2)$$

where $(d-d_i)$ is the disparity between F and a feature F_i. The weight w_i varies inversely with (retinotopic) distance and by a factor μ with each feature interposed between F and F_i. Formally, $w_i=\mu^k/\text{dist}(F,F_i)$, where k features intervene between F and F_i, and $\text{dist}(F,F_i)$ is the distance between F and F_i. We called μ a 'masking factor', since it indicates how much the effect of a feature is attenuated or masked by intervening features.

In the experiment of Fig. 28.1d, the condition for equal perceived depth becomes $D=-(d+d)-(d-nd)-\mu(d+nd)=0$, or $n=(3+\mu/2)/(1-\mu/2)$. For the two subjects with $n=3$ the best fit was obtained with $\mu=0$, and for the other three, $\mu=0.4$, $\mu=0.57$ and $\mu=1$ were the best choices. The existence of masking could be demonstrated by extending this experiment to the situation shown in Fig. 28.1e. The top configuration is the same as that in Fig. 28.1d. In the second down, the outer lines were twice as far from the inner pair as in Fig. 28.1d, and here the condition for equal perceived depth of the central pair, $n=(5+2\mu/3)/(1-2\mu/3)$, was quite accurately fulfilled. In the third configuration, the disparities of the inner four lines were as in Fig. 28.1d. Even when the outermost lines were given very large disparities (ten times those of the test pair), they had no effect on the perceived depth of the test pair for the two subjects with a masking factor of 1, even though these same lines were strongly effective in the second experiment. Their influence had been entirely masked by the two nearest neighbours of the test pair (for more details, see Mitchison & Westheimer, 1984, Table 1). For the other subjects, the outermost lines did have an influence which could be accurately predicted from (2) using the appropriate masking factor.

A good fit to the results of a variety of experi-

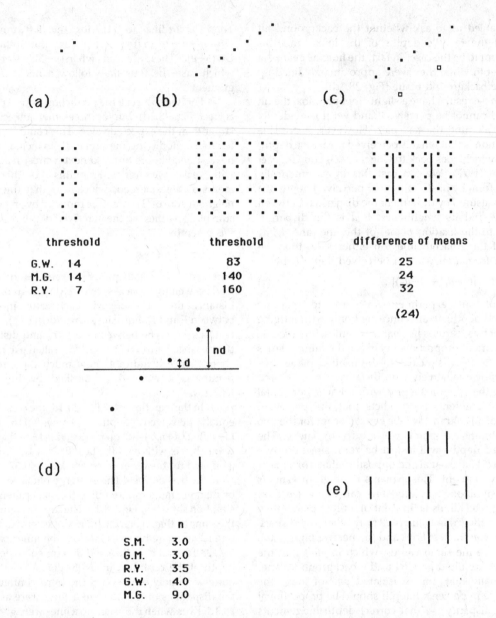

(a)   (b)   (c)

threshold	threshold	difference of means
G.W. 14	83	25
M.G. 14	140	24
R.Y. 7	160	32
		(24)

(d)   (e)

	n
S.M.	3.0
G.M.	3.0
R.Y.	3.5
G.W.	4.0
M.G.	9.0

Fig. 28.1. In all the experiments described here, the stereograms were generated by two Tektronix 602 cathode-ray display units with short-acting white phosphor (P4). An arrangement of beam-splitting pellicle and polaroid filters ensured that each eye saw only one of the display units. Patterns were composed of dots about 30 second of arc in diameter. Luminance was equivalent to about 40 mL, seen against a uniform background of about 1 mL. A fixation pattern, consisting of a small (5 min arc) cross and four brackets of similar size outlining a square 45 min of arc side length, was shown at all times except for the 1/2 second when the test stimulus was presented. (a) A pair of columns made of 7 dots spaced 8 min of arc apart, the columns separated by 8 min of arc horizontally and given equal and opposite disparities relative to the fixation plane. The appearance of the columns when viewed by the subject is shown, with a schematic view from above assuming that disparities are interpreted according to the usual geometry. The disparities randomly took one of seven values of disparity (equally spaced and zeroed on the fixation plane), and the subject's resposes were fitted to a cumulative Gaussian psychometric function using the probit method (Finney, 1952). From this, the threshold (the point where judgements are 75% correct) could be obtained, and also the mean (the 50%

ments like those shown in Fig. 28.1 was obtained by using (2) with a suitable choice of masking factor for each subject (Mitchison & Westheimer, 1984, Tables 1 & 2). We called D defined by (2) the *salience* of the feature F, indicating that it measures the prominence or curvature at F. Despite the greater complexity of (2) compared to (1), the expression only requires one free parameter (the masking factor μ). Moreover, it has a natural interpretation as a kind of second derivative of disparity d. For suppose d is regarded as a continuous function of position, and F_i and F_j are features on either side of a feature F with an equal number, k, of features intervening between F and each of F_i, F_j. Then the contribution of these two features to the sum (2) is $w_i(d-d_i)+w_j(d-d_j)=w_i[d(0)-d(x_i)]+w_j[d(0)-d(-x_j)]$. Expanding in a Taylor series gives $w_i(d-d_i)+w_j(d-d_j)$ $=\mu^k[d'(0)x_i+\tfrac{1}{2}d''(0)x_i^2+\ldots]/x_i+\mu^k[-d'(0)x_j+\tfrac{1}{2}d''(0)x_j^2+\ldots]/x_j\approx\mu^k(x+x_i)d''(0)$. The complete sum will therefore be a product of the second derivative of disparity, $d''(0)$, at the feature F, with a term depending on the distances x_i.

There is a formal analogy between this and balanced centre-surround operators such as the second derivative of a Gaussian $\nabla^2 G$ (Marr & Hildreth, 1980). However, unlike the centre-surround operator which has a fixed spatial extent, the salience operator varies its range according to the distribution of neighbouring features. In our experiments, the features were high contrast lines; presumably weaker features would mask less strongly, and the sum of the salience operator would therefore extend over more features. In this way, masking would allow a flexible use of neighbouring features, weighting them according to their reliability and proximity. In principle, the definition of salience could be generalized to grey level images by assigning an appropriate weighting to primitives derived from the image, but whether this would give a correct measure of perceived depth remains to be seen.

Horizontal/vertical anisotropy and stereo viewing geometry

When the same type of experiment was carried out with vertical rows of features, quite different results were often obtained. The most striking contrast between horizontal and vertical was found with the tilted grid (Fig. 28.1b, 28.2a). If this grid was given a linear vertical gradient of (horizontal) disparity, the threshold for perception of tilt was, for most subjects, considerably lower than that for a horizontal gradient (Fig. 28.2b). One trivial explanation for this phenomenon might be that subjects could perceive the shear distortion in each monocular image produced by the vertical disparity gradient. This was guarded against by introducing a random shear into all the grids before adding disparity (Fig. 28.2b).

Differences between percepts of horizontal and

---

point), which measures the point of equal perceived depth of the two columns. The thresholds for three subjects (in seconds of arc) are shown below. (b) A grid constructed from seven columns like those shown in (a), with the disparities varying linearly in a horizontal direction. The grid therefore defines a tilted plane, as indicated in the schematic view from above. The thresholds for judgements of relative depth of any pair of columns in the figures or for any perceived tilt are shown below (in seconds of arc). (c) A grid of dots identical to that in (b) was shown as a background to a pair of lines whose relative depth the subject was required to judge (solid lines and hollow squares in the schematic diagram above). The two test lines were 24 min of arc long and 24 min of arc apart, and were placed at a disparity of 1 min of arc in front of the grid. The tilt of the grid was given two equal and opposite values, randomly interspersed in the experiments, and the two sets of judgements were collected separately and analysed afterwards. If the two test lines were aligned parallel to the grid, the difference of the means between the two sets should have been 24 arc seconds. Values obtained by the subjects are shown below. (d) Four lines, 20 min of arc high, separated by 10 min of arc, were given disparities as shown in the top part of the diagram. The horizontal line here represents the plane of the fixation pattern, relative to which disparities are measured for convenience of calculation. The subject judged which of the two inner lines lay closer. Several conditions, corresponding to choices of integral values of n, were randomly intermingled so that the subject was unaware of the configuration in each trial. Afterwards, thresholds for each n were calculated. It was found that some critical value of n gave an infinite threshold (this value might lie, by interpolation, between integers). At this value the two test lines should appear at equal depth. Critical values of n for five subjects (from Mitchison & Westheimer, 1984) are shown below. (e) Three experiments demonstrating the effects of masking. The top figure is the experiment shown in (d). In the second figure, the spacing between the outer lines and the nearest test line is doubled. In the third, two lines have been added outside the flanking lines in (d) to give six equally spaced lines. The outermost lines are given disparities which are large multiples (e.g. 10) of the disparity of the test lines. For SM and GM these outer lines had little effect upon the perceived relative depth of the test pair, even though they had a large influence in the second configuration, where there were no intervening lines.

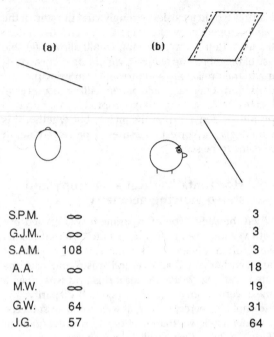

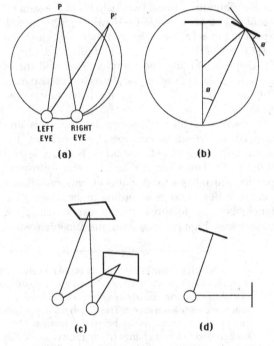

through the two eyes is shown in Fig. 28.3, the loci of equal disparities being the Vieth–Müller circles. Suppose that an observer looks straight ahead, fixating a point P, then rotates his head about a vertical axis while keeping his gaze fixed on P. We can represent this in the coordinate system of the observer's head by drawing OP straight ahead and a line of equal length OP' making an angle ϕ with OP (Fig. 28.3a). As observed by Ogle (1950), the normal plane at P' makes an angle ϕ with the tangent to the Vieth–Müller circle through P (Fig. 28.3b). This means that the effect of

S.P.M.	∞	3
G.J.M..	∞	3
S.A.M.	108	3
A.A.	∞	18
M.W.	∞	19
G.W.	64	31
J.G.	57	64

Fig. 28.2. Thresholds (in seconds of arc) for the perception of disparity gradients where the gradients are (a) horizontal (view from above) or (b) vertical (view from the side). In the second experiment, it was necessary to rule out the possibility that shear distortions due to the disparity gradient were detected by subjects. Accordingly, the rectangular grid was given a random shear, as indicated in the upper part of (b) (where solid lines indicate the figure shown to the right eye, dotted lines that shown to the left). This ensured that monocularly perceived shear could not provide a reliable cue, though of course binocular shear (change of horizontal disparity in a vertical direction) was present.

Fig. 28.3. (a) Loci of constant disparity (Vieth–Müller circles) in a plane through the eyes. The distances from P and P' to the mid-point of the arc between the eyes are equal. This represents (approximately) the transformation which occurs when the head is rotated in the plane of the Vieth–Müller circle keeping the eyes fixed at a point. The circle through P' has a larger radius than that through P, signifying that the disparity at P' is less than that at P. (b) The circle shown here is that through P'. A normal plane (heavy line) is shown at P and P'. If the head is rotated through an angle ϕ, the normal plane at P' makes an angle ϕ with the tangent to the Vieth–Müller circle. This implies that there is disparity gradient, to a first approximation linear, introduced by the rotation. (c) A vertical rotation causes no change in the geometry of a plane viewed straight ahead. (d) shows a side view of (c).

vertical disparity profiles have previously been reported by Rogers & Graham (1983). In particular, they observed that thresholds for depth perception in slow changing sinusoidal disparity profiles were higher when the orientation of the profile was horizontal than when it is vertical, a result which has similarities with the tilt experiments described above.

Why does this anisotropy exist? We give an explanation below, the essence of which is that the stereo system must try to obtain a measure of depth which is stable under eye and head movements. We shall see that linear disparity gradients are introduced by oblique viewing, but these gradients are predominantly horizontal, so only in the horizontal direction is a second derivative operation like salience required.

The geometry of stereo viewing in a plane

rotation is to add a linear disparity gradient. Suppose now that the head is rotated up or down. In that case there is no induced disparity gradient because any plane through the two eyes has identical geometry (Figs. 28.3c, 28.3d). A plane which is tangent at P will remain tangent at P'.

To back up this intuitive argument, consider a plane through the eyes. Take as origin O the point midway between eyes, and let r, β be polar coordinates, with β measured from the straight forward viewing direction. Then it is easily checked that this disparity ϕ (measured in the plane through the eyes) is given by $\tan\phi=2wr\cos\beta/(r^2-w^2)$, where $2w$ is the distance between the eyes. If $w^2<<r^2$ and β is small we get $\phi\approx2w\cos\beta/r$. Suppose that r is given as a function $r(\beta)$ of β in a neighbourhood of $\beta=0$. This defines $\phi(\beta)=2w\cos(\beta)/r(\beta)\approx2w/r(\beta)$. If we now rotate by an angle β_o we get a new function $\phi_o(\beta)=2w\cos(\beta_o+\beta)/r(\beta)$. Expanding around $\beta=0$, $(\phi_o-\phi)=2w/r\cdot[(\cos\beta_o-1)-\sin\beta_o\beta-(\cos\beta_o-1)\beta^2/2+\ldots)-r'(\cos\beta_o-1)\beta/r+$other terms in derivatiees of r]. If β_o is small and r not too small, only the constant and linear terms are significant, and all the terms in derivatives of r can be ignored because of the factor $1/r$. For instance, taking $2w=6$ cm, $r=100$ cm, $\beta_o=15°$ and expressing $(\phi_o-\phi)$ and β in minutes of arc we get $(\phi_o-\phi)=7.2-1.5\times10^{-2}\beta-2.5\times10^{-7}\beta^2$, showing that the effect of rotation is to add an absolute disparity of about 7 minutes, a linear disparity gradient of about 1 minute of arc disparity per degree of viewing angle, and only small quadratic and higher terms.

As salience is only a discrete approximation to a second derivative, its effect on $(\phi_o-\phi)$ cannot be accurately predicted by differentiating the equation given above. Calculations for various distance profiles can give a feel for its behaviour, an example of this being shown in Fig. 28.4. A set of features (shown as dots) is viewed at 100 cm (Fig. 28.4a) and the two functions ϕ and ϕ_o for $\beta=15°$ are shown in Fig. 28.4b. As can be seen, the functions differ by a significant linear disparity gradient. The effect of the salience operator is shown in Fig. 28.4c; here the masking factor $\mu=0.4$, and only the nearest and next-nearest neighbours were used. It is striking that the saliences derived from ϕ and ϕ_o are almost indistinguishable. For this to be true, the ratio r'/r must not be too large; in this example it never exceeds 1/10.

We have considered only pure horizontal or vertical head rotations so far. The geometry of full three dimensional head movements is more complex. Breaking down a rotation into a vertical followed by a horizontal rotation suggests that only horizontal disparity gradients will be created. But eye movements

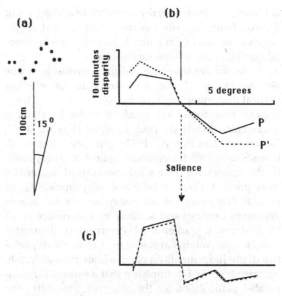

Fig. 28.4. A calculation showing the effectiveness of salience at removing disparities introduced by a horizontal rotation. (a) A set of 11 features (marked as dots) is viewed at a distance of 100 cm. (b) The disparities of these features when viewed directly ahead are shown (joined by solid line, labelled P), and also their disparities after the head has been rotated through 15° (dotted line, labelled P'). Only 7 of the 11 features are plotted, to avoid edge effects. There are two principal consequences of the rotation from P to P'. First, there is a constant decrease in the disparity by about 7 min of arc; the size of this is indicated by the vertical bar above the graph. Second, a linear gradient is introduced which manifests itself as a gradually increasing separation of the two graphs. (c) The salience operator, (2), with a masking factor $\mu=0.4$, summed over the two nearest neighbours on each side of each point, is applied to the two graphs in (b) to yield the almost superimposing graphs shown here. In order to include only points with two neighbours on both sides, only 7 of the 11 points in (a) have been plotted here and in (b).

are governed by Listing's Law, so the orientation of the eyes in the oblique position is obtained by rotation about an axis orthogonal to the plane through the two lines of sight and not by the successive vertical and horizontal rotations. However, the effect of this is quite small, at least in the region of ±15° where most eye movements are confined.

Cyclotorsional eye movements can introduce vertical gradients of disparity. In fact, the disparity at vertical angle β has an added component βv, where v is the cyclotorsion angle. If v is 5 minutes of arc (a large amount of cyclotorsion) this amounts to adding about 5 seconds of disparity per degree of vertical angle, which is an order of magnitude less than the horizontal gradients due to oblique viewing.

As we are invoking oblique viewing as a key element in our scheme, it is natural to ask whether vertical disparities might play a rôle, since it has been argued that these are used to estimate viewing parameters (Mayhew, 1982; Longuet-Higgins, 1982; Gillam & Lawergren, 1983; but see Rogers & Koenderink, 1986 for evidence against this proposal). In the figures we have used, no vertical disparities were present. Could it be that an appropriate set of vertical disparities are necessary to give the stereo system its bearings and so allow an assignment of tilt to horizontal gradients of (horizontal) disparity? Several observations argue against this. Firstly, relative depth judgements on pairs of lines are reasonably accurate (Fig. 28.1a), implying that a notional fronto-parallel plane exists for the observer. Secondly, the vertical disparities expected at a viewing distance of 3 metres from the stereograms in our displays would be tiny, less than half a second of arc (and considerably below the resolution of our display apparatus). Thirdly, it is difficult to show any effect of vertical disparities in the highly simplified figures used in these experiments (Westheimer, 1978, 1984).

Discussion

There is a parallel between the theory of lightness computation (Horn, 1974, Blake, 1985) and the argument we are putting forward here, in that both invoke a second derivative-like operator to remove unwanted added components, these being illumination gradients in the case of lightness and disparity gradients in the situation considered here. However, there are some important differences.

Firstly, unlike illumination gradients, the viewing parameters are not unknowns, as is indicated by the fact that good judgements can be made on isolated pairs of lines. If we say that the absence of a reasonably close feature leads to the appropriate difference term in equation (2) being omitted, then this result is formally accounted for by the salience operator. In effect, this says that the stereo system relies upon neighbouring objects to obtain a more stable relative depth measure, but must abandon this strategy when isolated test lines float in a featureless void, as happens in the somewhat contrived conditions of Fig. 28.1a.

Secondly, the final percept is not integrated to restore an approximation to the true distance profile (Horn, 1974; Blake, 1985), but comes as a raw second derivative. This points towards a different strategy, which is to use other cues, such as perspective, shading, or texture gradients, to supply the tilt information removed by salience. There is some evidence in support of this (Stevens & Brookes, 1987), which is of considerable interest because it suggests that different depth cues may sometimes be assigned complementary rôles rather than being required to seek a compromise by averaging.

Our argument suggests that a second derivative-like operator should be required in the horizontal direction, but has little to say about stereo processing in the vertical direction. There is evidence for depth contrast effects in figures with vertically changing disparities (Graham & Rogers, 1982; Westheimer, 1986), but we know that these cannot be explained by salience because of the detectability of linear vertical gradients of disparity. One possibility is that there exists an underlying second derivative operation in the vertical direction which is supplemented by a measure of tilt about a horizontal axis. However, this is far from being well understood at present. Though the state of our knowledge is somewhat better for horizontal rows of features, salience falls short of being a perfect description. As mentioned above, salience implies that there should be a depth difference between the outermost columns in the grid of Fig. 28.1b, yet this is not perceived. Other instances of this kind of failure are given in Mitchison & Westheimer (1984); they can all be loosely accounted for by saying that some estimate of local tilt is formed, and it is departures from the expectations of this tilt which signal depth changes. Salience may therefore be only a convenient numerical measure which often gives a good approximation to the interactions in a system of local oriented surface elements, a point of view which receives some indirect support from recent work of Rogers, Cagenello & Rogers (1987).

There is clearly much that remains to be done in exploring stereoscopic depth perception. Our hope is that, by finding a suitable set of constraints and goals for depth perception, we can guide ourselves through this complex and fascinating area.

Postscript:

Several relevant articles have been published since this chapter was written. Stevens & Brookes (*Vision Res.*, **28**, 371–86, 1988), Gillam, Chambers & Russo (*J. Exp. Psych.: Human Perception & Perf.*, **14**, 163–75,

1988), and Rogers & Cagenello (*Nature* **339**, 135–7, 1989) discuss the rôle of second derivative operations in stereo vision, and Brookes & Stevens (*Perception* **18**, 601–14, 1989) discuss the analogy between stereo depth and brightness.

References

Blake, A. (1985) Boundary conditions for lightness computation in Mondrian world. *Comput. Vision, Graphics and Image Processing*, **32**, 314–27.

Finney, D. J. (1952) *Probit Analysis*. Cambridge: Cambridge University Press.

Gillam, B. & Lawergren, B. (1983) The induced effect, vertical disparity, and stereoscopic theory. *Perception & Psychophysics*, **34**, 121–30.

Gillam, B., Flagg, T. & Finlay, D. (1984) Evidence for disparity change as the primary stimulus for stereoscopic processing. *Perception & Psychophysics*, **36**, 559–64.

Gogel, W. C. (1963) The visual perception of size and distance. *Vision Res.*, **3**, 101–20.

Gogel, W. C. & Mershon, D. H. (1977) Local autonomy in visual space. *Scand. J. Psychol.*, **18**, 237–50.

Graham, M. & Rogers, B. (1982) Simultaneous and successive contrast effects in the perception of depth from motion parallax and stereoscopic information. *Perception*, **11**, 247–62.

Helmholtz, H. (1909) *Handbuch der physiologischen Optik*, 3rd edn, Vol. 3 (trans. J. P. C. Southall). (1962) pp. 313–14. New York: Dover.

Horn, B. K. P. (1974) Determining lightness from an image. *Comput. Vision, Graphics and Image Processing*, **3**, 277–99.

Longuet-Higgins, H. C. (1982) The role of the vertical dimension in stereoscopic vision. *Perception*, **11**, 377–86.

Marr, D. & Hildreth, E. (1980) Theory of edge detection. *Proc. Roy. Soc. Lond.*, B**207**, 187–217.

Mayhew, J. E. W. (1982) The interpretation of stereo disparity information: the computation of surface orientation and depth. *Perception*, **11**, 387–403.

Mitchison, G. J. & Westheimer, G. (1984) The perception of depth in simple figures. *Vision Res.*, **24**, 1063–73.

Ogle, K. N. (1950) *Researches in Binocular Vision*. New York: Hafner.

Rogers, B. & Graham, M. (1983) Anisotropies in the perception of three-dimensional surfaces. *Science*, **221**, 1409–11.

Rogers, B. & Koenderink, J. (1986) Monocular aniseikonia: a motion parallax analogue of the disparity-induced effect. *Nature*, **322**, 62–3.

Rogers, B., Cagenello, R. & Rogers, S. (1987) Simultaneous contrast effects in stereoscopic surfaces: the role of tilt, slant and surface discontinuities. *Perception*, **16**, A27.

Stevens, K. A. & Brookes, A. (1987) *Integrating Stereopsis with Monocular Interpretations of Planar Surfaces*. Department of Computer and Information Science reprint CIS-TR-86-05. University of Oregon.

Westheimer, G. (1978) Vertical disparity detection: is there an induced size effect? *Invest. Ophthal. and Vis. Sci.*, **17**, 545–51.

Westheimer, G. (1984) Sensitivity for vertical retinal image differences. *Nature*, **307**, 632–4.

Westheimer, G. (1986) Spatial interaction in the domain of disparity signals in human stereoscopic vision. *J. Physiol.*, **370**, 619–29.

29

Texture discrimination: radiologist, machine, and man

R. F. Wagner, M. F. Insana, D. G. Brown, B. S. Garra and
R. J. Jennings

Introduction

Over the last few years we have developed machine algorithms for detection and discrimination of liver disease from diagnostic ultrasound scans of the liver (Wagner, Insana & Brown, 1986; Insana et al., 1986a; Insana et al., 1986b; Wagner, Insana & Brown, 1987). Several diffuse disease conditions are manifested through very subtle changes in the texture of the image. In these cases the machine algorithms significantly outperform expert clinical readers of the images (Garra et al., 1989). The discrimination of textures by the machine depends principally on an analysis and partitioning of second-order statistical features such as the autocorrelation and power spectral estimators. This finding has prompted us to investigate whether the human visual system might be more limited in its performance of such second-order tasks than it is for the wide range of first-order tasks where it scores so well.

At the beginning of this decade we learned how to use the words 'well or good' and 'poorly or bad' in the context of visual performance. We enjoyed a very fruitful collaboration with Horace Barlow through Arthur Burgess who split his sabbatical at that time between Horace Barlow's lab and ours (Burgess, Wagner, Jennings & Barlow, 1981; Burgess, Jennings & Wagner, 1982). From this collaboration we learned how instructive it is to compare the performance of the human visual system with that of the ideal observer from statistical decision theory. The latter introduces no fluctuations or sources of error beyond those inherent to the data that conveys the scene or image. The comparison of the human to the ideal observer leads to the concept of observer efficiency, a measure of the effective fraction of the information in the a priori and image data used by the observer. We have recently studied the efficiency of the human observer for tasks that have some overlap with the visual task required of an observer of the diagnostic ultrasound scans in our clinical studies. In this paper we review the results of the first year of these studies.

In the first section we shall give a brief review of the clinical studies that led to this work. We next describe the psychophysical study designed to compare the performance of a specific texture discrimination task by a machine algorithm and by man; we include a sketch of the machine algorithm and attempts to find versions that approach the optimal or ideal. Measurements of the machine performance are then presented followed by measurements of human observer performance. We close with an attempt to interpret the results and offer suggestions for further work along these lines. Just as the present project issues naturally from the intersection of the work of Horace Barlow and our own, one can anticipate a number of useful investigations that might flow from the present one. The multiplier effect of Horace Barlow's inspiration has been and remains very great.

Radiologist and machine

A typical ultrasound scan of a normal liver is shown in Fig. 29.1. The speckled appearance is the result of the phase sensitive detection of interfering coherent waves scattered from a large number of very fine diffuse or randomly-positioned scatterers in the organ. However, there is also a quasi-regular architecture in this organ associated with the functional units – the liver lobules – as shown schematically in Fig. 29.2. By analyzing the autocorrelation function or power spectrum of the envelope (the image parameter) of the back-scattered ultrasonic signals we are able to detect the average spacing or dimension of these units and to

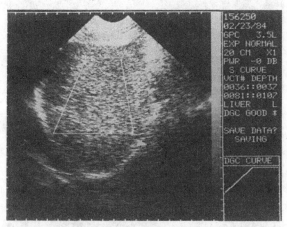

Fig. 29.1. Typical ultrasound scan of a normal liver showing coherent speckle pattern. This image is virtually indistinguishable from a typical heptatitis image.

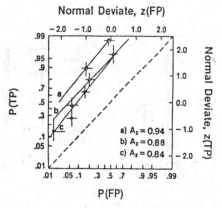

Fig. 29.3. ROC curves for the task of discriminating normals from Gaucher's disease (a), normals from hepatitis (b), and hepatitis from Gaucher's disease (c). Four features were used in a machine analysis of liver scans.

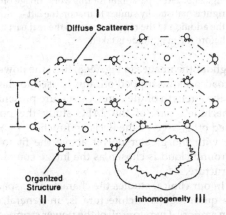

Fig. 29.2. Schematic illustration of human liver parenchyma showing diffuse scatterers, organized structure (portal triads), and inhomogeneity (large blood vessel, which we detect using matched filters and delete from the data to be analyzed).

deduce their contribution to the back-scattered signal relative to that of the diffuse scatterers. These quantities serve as features in a multi-dimensional discriminant analysis that we use to detect, and in some cases to discriminate, disease states of this organ.

A receiver operating characteristic (ROC) curve can be generated by varying the parameter that positions the discriminant surface forming the boundary between normal and abnormal calls in the ultrasonic feature space. The resulting true positive (or 'hit') rate vs. false positive ('false alarm') rate is the desired ROC curve and some examples from our work are shown in Fig. 29.3. The area under the ROC curve, A_z, is a frequently used summary measure of performance. It is effectively the average true positive (TP) rate – with the average taken uniformly over all false positive rates from 0 to 100%. Most of our A_z scores are in the range 0.8–0.98. A score of 1.0 would result from a perfect diagnostic test and a score of 0.5 would result from random guessing. The commonly used Pap smear test that is used to screen for cervical cancer scores an A_z value of 0.87 (Swets, 1984). This indicates that we might have a useful tool for detecting diffuse liver disease, but we do not yet have strong evidence to indicate how well we can discriminate among diseases, except for the cases shown in Fig. 29.3.

Expert clinicians are able to perform well compared to the machine algorithm when the disease markedly affects the organ boundaries but they do not generally get strong cues from the image texture in the case of these diffuse diseases. In particular, we find that for the task of detecting hepatitis the machine dramatically outscores expert clinicians. The ROC curves for this task are shown in Fig. 29.4. Apparently the subtle disruption of the organ architecture that is picked up in the power spectral measurements is not readily appreciated by the human viewer. We shall next describe the most robust features of our machine algorithm – second-order statistical parameters – and indicate how they suggest the psychophysical work that we shall describe in the remainder of this paper.

Tasks and algorithms

We have described elsewhere the details of our statistical analysis of ultrasonic signals (Wagner *et al.*, 1986;

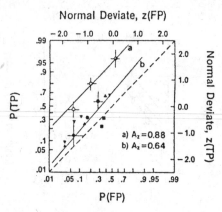

Fig. 29.4. ROC curves for the detection of chronic hepatitis using ultrasound. Curve (a) summarizes the machine performance using linear discriminant analysis. Curve (b) is the average performance of four trained clinicians.

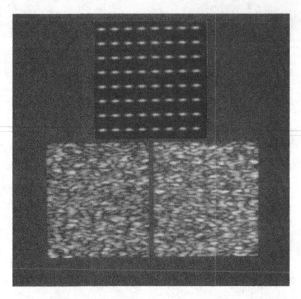

Fig. 29.5. 2AFC paradigm for this work. Image on the right is statistically similar to that on the left – with the addition of the regular lattice to the real part before the magnitude is taken.

Insana *et al.*, 1986a,b; Wagner *et al.*, 1987). The analysis requires both first and second order statistics and allows for a partitioning of the scattering strength into diffuse, specular, and organized specular scattering. Only the organized scattering strength is of interest for our psychophysical studies and we limit ourselves here only to a description of that part of our algorithm.

The psychophysical task that we investigated in the present study follows the paradigm indicated in Fig. 29.5. The bottom two images are speckle fields comparable to those found in ultrasound scans of various abdominal organs. They represent the magnitudes of corresponding complex random variables that derive from radio-frequency signals. Both real and imaginary parts are zero mean Gaussian random variables that are independently distributed; the real and imaginary parts are then independently smoothed to simulate the detector's spread function. In one of the two images – in this case, on the right – a regular lattice-work has been inserted into the real part and similarly smoothed. In all cases the magnitude is what is displayed. The task is the two-alternative forced choice (2AFC) task of selecting the image that has the lattice inserted.

The average one-dimensional (1D) autocorrelation function – pixel-wise along a vertical (or range direction) line – for such an image is shown in Fig. 29.6 (top); the corresponding one-dimensional power spectrum is shown in Fig. 29.6 (bottom). We have developed a curve fiting and stripping routine that first fits the minima of the oscillations in the noisy power spectrum of Fig. 29.6 (bottom) with a Gaussian cloud: this cloud characterizes the speckles seen

throughout the images in Fig. 29.5; then the power in the broad peak is stripped off: this is used to characterize the strength of the regular structure present. In the machine's part of the 2AFC study the power stripped off is used as the decision function; i.e., the image with the greater power above the fit to the background cloud is chosen as the image containing the structure.

In our clinical studies the characteristic spacing of the quasi-regular architecture is, in general, not known a priori. Therefore all of the power stripped off is used as the decision function. We refer to this as the infinite-bandwidth tuning. In the present psychophysical study the mean spacing is specified and observers train themselves to look for it in the images. However, the absolute location of the lattice as a whole, and in most cases the actual location of the individual lattice sites (described below), is randomized. This suggests that the bandwidth over which the machine collects the structured power in the stripping procedure might be subject to optimization depending on the task. In fact, it can be shown (Barrett, Myers & Wagner, 1986; Wagner & Barrett, 1987) that when the actual level of the background signal is indeterminate, the power spectral matched filter approximates the optimum Bayesian receiver for such randomized placements. This receiver is the second-order analog of the linear matched filter discussed in many communications texts (Fukunaga, 1972). In the

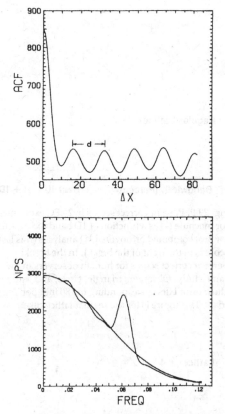

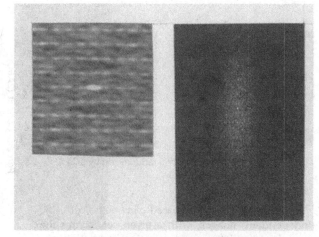

Fig. 29.7. Left: 2D autocorrelation function for speckle pattern with regular lattice in real part. Right: corresponding 2D power spectrum.

Fig. 29.6. Top: autocorrelation function for ideal (large sample) speckle pattern containing regular lattice. Bottom: corresponding 1D power spectrum showing fit to background cloud and signal structure to be collected in stripping procedure.

second-order case both the matched weighting and the data enter quadratically, that is, the measured *power* spectrum is sampled (weighted) by a template constructed from the expected spectrum. We have not yet investigated this optimal tuning. Instead we have used two crude approximations to it by simply narrowing the collection bandwidth first to 33% of the expected frequency, and then to 8%. (When collecting the magnitude of a complex signal, harmonics are generated; these harmonics are also collected, but the fractional bandwith refers to the fundamental.)

Not only would the ideal observer refine its tuning beyond the rough tuning described above, it would also carry out the analysis in two dimensions. The two-dimensional (2D) autocorrelation function corresponding to the structured image of Fig. 29.5 is shown in Fig. 29.7 (left); the corresponding 2D power spectrum is shown in Fig. 29.7 (right). In keeping with the festivity of the occasion of the meeting in Cam-

bridge on which this book is based, we refer to the 2D power spectrum as an ellipsoidal cake with birthday candles inserted. The ideal observer would generate a 2D fit to the cake and strip off the power in the candles. We have not yet developed a 2D fitting and stripping routine for our clinical work because in our first generation digital system the resolution and side-lobes in the cross-range (here, the horizontal) direction are much inferior to the resolution available in the range direction. In the present study in place of a 2D routine we have used two orthogonal 1D routines as described above. That is, we first carry out the above procedure in the range direction with the averaging carried out across range; then we carry out the procedure in the cross-range direction and average over the range direction. This pseudo-2D analysis then uses the combined structured power from both 1D analyses as the decision function. Such a procedure can be seen to be significantly inferior to a true 2D analysis, however. In effect, it only measures the autocorrelation function in Fig. 29.7 (left) along the one horizontal and one vertical line that intersect in the center of the figure. The correlations in diagonal directions are not measured. (Alternatively, the birthday candles in Fig. 29.7 (right) are averaged along strips of the cake before being stripped off.)

In practice these effects are not so profound – although still quite significant – since naturally-occurring structures do not appear on the corners of a rigid lattice. To take the next step, then, toward more realistic structures we have also allowed for a randomization or thermalization of the lattice points by ±25% and by ±50% of the average lattice spacing. Examples of these randomized structures are shown in Fig. 29.8.

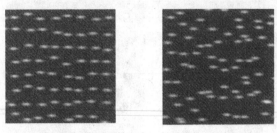

Fig. 29.8. Lattice of Fig. 29.5 randomized by ±25% (left) and by ±50% (right).

Images were prepared in sets of 180 (independent) images, with a given set having the same degree of lattice randomization and lattice contrast. The set containing no lattice contained 200 images. In Figs. 29.9, 29.10, and 29.11 we present the percent correct scores for the case of the regular lattice (lattice point spacing=16 pixels), and the lattice randomized by ±25% and by ±50% respectively, and with the machine working at infinite bandwidth, 33% and 8% bandwidth as indicated. To the far right, beyond the break, we give the best pseudo-2D score obtained by combining two orthogonal 1D analyses. The error bars correspond to our estimate of about 360 independent trials per data point.

We see that narrowing the collection bandwidth indeed improves detectability in the case of machine detection of the regular lattice; it is of questionable utility for the case of the slightly randomized lattice, and degrades performance in the case of the most randomized lattice. In both randomized cases the inclusion of the orthogonal direction represents a great improvement. This would also be expected in the case of the regular lattice if we had started with a weaker signal (this was discovered too late in the study). The 2D effect is then generally expected as argued above and the bandwidth effect is at least qualitatively expected since the thermalization of the lattice broadens the lines in the spectral domain (a melting of the candles).

Machine and man

We started out with three observers. Our best observer (◆) moved to another institution before the mid-point of the current investigations, and so another observer (●) was recruited for the second half of the work. The limited data on the first observer suggest that he had a much greater ability to perform the task of detecting regular and slightly randomized lattices than the other three observers. Unfortunately,

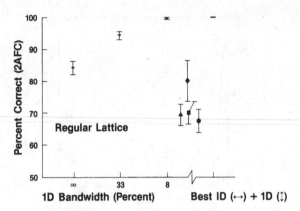

Fig. 29.9. Percent correct scores in 2AFC experiment for machine (–) as a function of 1D bandwidth, and for best combined orthogonal 1D analyses (this last score is to the right of the break). In the break: percent correct scores for human observers in the same study. Observers triangle, circle, and square show error bars corresponding to 180 independent trials. This figure is for the regular lattice case.

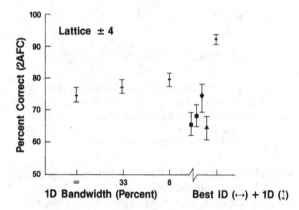

Fig. 29.10. As Fig. 29.9, but for lattice randomized by ±25%.

we shall need to wait for a return visit from the first observer to confirm his results.

The performance of the other three observers tends to cluster as shown by the circles, squares, and triangles in Figs. 29.9 through 29.11. In all three figures we see that human performance is roughly comparable to the crudest level of the 1D machine algorithm. When the machine is allowed to use both dimensions, its performance pulls much farther ahead.

This information is cast in the form of observer efficiency by first inverting the percent correct scores

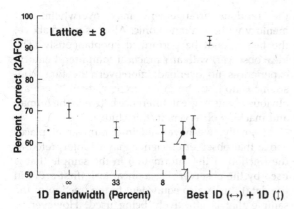

Fig. 29.11. As Figs. 29.9 and 29.10, but for lattice randomized by ±50%.

to obtain the signal-to-noise ratio d (Swets, 1964) – first for the human observers, d_{obs}, and then for the machine, d_{mach}. The efficiency η is then defined (Burgess *et al.*, 1981) as the square of the ratio of these two quantities

$$\eta = (d_{obs}/d_{mach})^2.$$

This fraction may be interpreted as the fraction of the information that is effectively extracted by the observer. A refinement of this will be offered in the section on interpretation below.

The observer efficiencies resulting from the above data – and replications at different signal levels – are given in Fig. 29.12. Three features of these results are apparent. First, there appears to be one observer who performs much better than the others – although in just two tasks and with a smaller number of trials (this was the observer who moved to another institution during the experiment). Second, there appears to be one observer who had more difficulty with the most complex task. Other than these two features, the results have a hint of a trend from an efficiency of roughly 0.05 for the simplest task, up to about 0.10 for the intermediate difficulty task, and back down to about 0.05 for the most difficult task.

We mentioned above that the optimal observer for the tasks studied here – random placement of the signals and indeterminate background level – is the power spectral matched filter (Barrett *et al.*, 1986, 1987), a procedure that is quadratic in the data. This is in fact the paradigm of our experiment since (even for the regular lattice) the placement was at random; and a small bias level was randomly added to one of the two images per trial to discourage the observer from using any first order cues that can enter from the way the

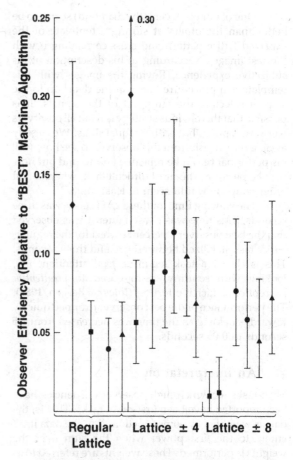

Fig. 29.12. Observer efficiencies for the four observers relative to the best 2D machine performance using percent correct scores from Fig. 29.9–11, and definition of efficiency in text.

structure accumulates in the image. Our 'best' machine algorithms are simple approximations to this observer. But since the human observers did not score well on the scale determined by this quasi-optimal observer, we have the additional negative result that we have found no evidence that the human observer can perform this higher-order nonlinear task. Since the power spectral matched filter is equivalent to using the autocorrelation of the expected signal as a template for sampling the autocorrelation of the data (Barrett *et al.*, 1986, 1987), we have the same negative result with regard to the human observer's ability to carry out this procedure. In an interesting study of the Hotelling trace and its correlation with human-observer performance Fiete *et al.* (1987) found no need to invoke non-linear features to describe their observer results.

One of our observers (the diamond) seems to be better than the others at storing a template of the expected lattice pattern and cross-correlating it with the test images – according to his description of his subjective experience. Roving the images with this template is a procedure linear in the data, up to the step of selecting the strongest of the signals. It is possible that this obvious strategy is what all observers were attempting, but with unequal skills. We eagerly await a return visit from this observer to see how well his performance can be repeated and to find out how well he performs the most difficult task, where a first order template would seem of least utility.

The viewing time for these 2AFC tasks was three seconds. This time was chosen after it was observed that the best observer's percent correct for the regular-lattice task stabilized between two and three seconds. This is clearly a task requiring *focal* attention, i.e., looking with scrutiny, as opposed to *preattentive* perception, which is effortless (Julesz & Bergen, 1983). The performance of the best observer dropped quickly towards guessing as the time was decreased from 0.5 seconds to 0.05 seconds.

An interpretation

Most tasks for which high observer efficiencies have been reported have been first-order tasks. That is, the data is weighted by some function – but the data itself enters to the first power when the sum over the weights is performed. These weights are referred to as a template and Burgess *et al.* (1981, 1982, especially 1984, and also this volume) have argued that given enough a priori information the human observer is capable of performing a cross-correlation with a template corresponding to the expected signal. This template is usually shown to the observer in preparation for and often during the experiment. It is likely that memory plays an important role in the performance of this task: the template is stored and then recalled to perform the weighting (in fact, one wonders if there is an alternative). Now, in the second-order task studied here the optimal performance involves using the data itself as the template, i.e., it requires autocorrelation. It is possible that due to the quite random character of the images, the memory task is formidable. The images in the 2AFC study contained $(128)^2$ pixels, a speckle size of about (2.5×7.5) pixels, or a total of about 900 independent pixels. Some fraction of these are obviously being remembered by the observers – especially when the signal speckles (spaced by 16 pixels, on average) fall more regularly in place – but

the random arrangement may overwhelm the memory without a mnemonic. Also, as noted above, the task cannot be performed spontaneously. The ideal observer, with any practical computer memory, experiences no overload; moreover, the time constraint is no issue for any current system. These are obvious points of great difference between the human and machine observers in this study.

Finally, we have said in a number of places above that observer efficiency may be interpreted as the fraction of the information in the sample that is used by the observer. For a linear task (first-order in the data) this is also equivalent to the fraction of the sample that is effectively being used. However, it follows from Wagner & Barrett (1987) that for a task quadratic in the data – such as the autocorrelation, or power spectral estimates discussed here – the effective fraction of the image sample that is utilized enters the expression for efficiency to the second power. This result allows the nature of the actual task being performed by the observer to be probed further.

Future work

This work involved finding a randomized structure with a well-defined characteristic dimension. The textures described by Mandelbrot (1982) have no characteristic dimension – they are referred to as 'scaling': the same texture is seen at any scale (coastlines, mountains, craters, etc.). Barrett and colleagues (1987) have used this concept to discriminate textures in nuclear medicine images and to screen for disease using machine algorithms. Their pilot study yields A_z scores comparable to those reported here. It will be of interest to compare their machine scores with human observer performance. One has the impression of being able to discriminate among the various members of the texture families given in Mandelbrot's book (1982), and one has the experience of autocorrelating the images at many different scales simultaneously. However, it is very possible that a machine could distinguish these textures at a much finer level. It is of considerable interest to know how man and machine fare in such discrimination tasks. We believe that these higher order tasks are worthy of study and may indicate an area in which signal processing of images might be most fruitful (Wagner, Insana & Brown, 1985).

Conclusions

When human observers' performance of a second-order detection task – detecting a randomized lattice in speckle noise – is compared with our 1D machine algorithm, they fare well. However, when the machine algorithm includes weighting and the inclusion of two orthogonal 1D analyses, the machine pulls far ahead. On this scale, human observers score in the range of 5% to 10% efficiency for the most random task. Since this is intrinsically a second-order task we have the negative finding that human observers give only faint evidence of being able to use this kind of second-order information.

Our machine algorithm here did not use the optimal weighting, nor did it use a true 2D analysis. When these two effects are correctly accounted for, the human observer efficiency will be significantly reduced.

An interpretation of the poor human performance was offered in terms of the difficulty of storing and recalling the template required for optimal performance of this second-order task. Here the required template is the image itself which, in the present study, consisted of a great number of independent pixel groups (~900) with random intensity levels.

It is of great interest to see how this paradigm works out in the context of images that exhibit scaling, i.e., that have no characteristic dimension, as in the many examples of fractals discussed by Mandelbrot and others.

Acknowledgements

This work has been motivated by the crossing of paths of a number of lines of research, especially those of Horace Barlow and our own. It would probably not have reached the present point anytime in this decade had it not been for the special occasion of the Cambridge meeting and this volume. We are grateful to Horace Barlow and to the conference organizers for the opportunity of finding the present results. It is also clear that this work is now a factor that drives our efforts to optimize our machine pattern recognition algorithms. Professor Barlow's influence is more far-reaching in this case than any of us had anticipated. Finding 'what the eye does best' helps us to understand what the eye-brain is trying to do. Finding 'what the eye does worst' should help us to understand what the machines should be trying to do.

We are grateful to Diane T. Crean for filling in for our star peregrine observer (MFI). Finally, we are also grateful to Harry Barrett and Kyle Myers for helpful discussions in the course of this work.

References

Barrett, H. H., Myers, K. J. & Wagner, R. F. (1986) Beyond signal-detection theory. *Proceedings of the Society of Photo-Optical Instrumentation Engineers (SPIE)*, **626**, 231–9.

Barrett, H. H., Aarsvold, J. N., Barber, H. B., Cargill, E. B., Fiete, R. D., Hickernell, T. S., Milster, T. D., Myers, K. J., Patton, D. D., Rowe, R. K., Seacat, R. H., Smith, W. E. & Woolfenden, J. M. (1987) Applications of statistical decision theory in nuclear medicine. In *Information Processing in Medical Imaging: Proceedings of the Tenth Conference*. The Hague: Martinus Nijhoff (to be published).

Burgess, A. E., Wagner, R. F., Jennings, R. J. & Barlow, H. B. (1981) Efficiency of human visual signal discrimination. *Science*, **214**, 93–4.

Burgess, A. E., Jennings, R. J. & Wagner, R. F. (1982) Statistical efficiency: a measure of human visual signal-detection performance. *J. Appl. Photog. Engineering*, **8**, 76–8.

Burgess, A. E. & Ghandeharian, H. (1984) Visual signal detection I: phase sensitive detection. *J. Opt. Soc. Am. A*, **1**, 900–5.

Fiete, R. D., Barrett, H. H., Smith, W. E. & Myers, K. J. (1987) Hotelling trace criterion and its correlation with human-observer performance. *J. Opt. Soc. Am. A*, **4**, 945–53.

Fukunaga, K. (1972) *Introduction to Statistical Pattern Recognition*. New York: Academic Press.

Garra, B. S., Insana, M. F., Shawker, T. H., Wagner, R. F., Bradford, M. & Russell, M. A. (1989) Quantitative ultrasonic detection and classification of liver disease: Comparison with human observer performance. *Investigative Radiology*, **24**, 196–203.

Insana, M. F., Wagner, R. F., Garra, B. S., Brown, D. G. & Shawker, T. H. (1986a) Analysis of ultrasound image texture via generalized Rician statistics. *Optical Engineering*, **25**, 743–8.

Insana, M. F., Wagner, R. F., Garra, B. S., Momenan, R. & Shawker, T. H. (1986b) Pattern recognition methods for optimizing multivariate tissue signatures in diagnostic ultrasound. *Ultrasonic Imaging*, **8**, 165–80.

Julesz, B. & Bergen, J. R. (1983) Textons, The fundamental elements in preattentive vision and perception of textures. *The Bell System Technical Journal*, **62**, 1619–45.

Mandelbrot, B. B. (1982) *The Fractal Geometry of Nature*. New York: W. H. Freeman.

Swets, J. A. (Ed. 1964) *Signal Detection and Recognition by Human Observers: Contemporary Readings*. New York: John Wiley.

Wagner, R. F., Insana, M. F. & Brown, D. G. (1985) Progress in signal and texture discrimination in medical imaging. *Proceedings of the SPIE (see first ref.)*, **535**, 57–64.

Wagner, R. F., Insana, M. F. & Brown, D. G. (1986) Unified

approach to the detection and classification of speckle texture in diagnostic ultrasound. *Optical Engineering*, **25**, 738–42.

Wagner, R. F., Insana, M. F. & Brown, D. G. (1987) Statistical properties of radio-frequency and envelope-detected signals with applications to medical ultrasound. *J. Opt. Soc. Am. A*, **4**, 910–22.

Wagner, R. F. & Barrett, H. H. (1987) Quadratic tasks and the ideal observer. *Proceedings of the SPIE* (see first ref.), **767**, 306–9.

Motion

30

The motion pathways of the visual cortex

S. Zeki

Introduction

One of Horace Barlow's major contributions to neurobiology was the discovery of directionally selective cells in the rabbit retina (Barlow & Levick, 1965) and hence of the neural mechanism for detecting one of the most fundamental and primitive of all visual stimuli, namely motion. It thus seems appropriate that my contribution to this dedicatory volume should be devoted to the same general topic of motion detection, although in the cortex, not the retina, and in the monkey, not the rabbit. My emphasis will be mainly anatomical. Although the occasion may have demanded a more physiological contribution, many of the problems raised by the anatomical facts are themselves physiological and ones in which, as I know, Horace Barlow is deeply interested and to which he continues to make contributions (Barlow, 1981). That I should have allowed myself some speculative asides in the following pages was motivated by the fact that Barlow was never concerned by exposing oneself to possible ridicule (Phillips, Zeki & Barlow, 1984) but welcomed instead informed speculations, particularly when they could be experimentally tested, as many of mine can. Some require simple experiments, others more complex ones. That even the simple ones have not been done, either by myself or others, is really due to nothing more than the exigencies of time, though in writing this article I have often wished, presumably like others, that I had the result of this experiment or that. I can only hope that the results of some of these experiments will be available in the coming years and will come to delight Barlow.

The motion pathways of the primate visual cortex

Area V5 as the pivotal motion area

The 'funnel' for the motion pathways of the visual cortex is area V5, a cytochrome oxidase rich area (Jen & Zeki, 1983) which lies in the upper part of the posterior bank of the superior temporal sulcus (STS) (see Fig. 30.2). All its cells are responsive to motion in the field of view and the overwhelming majority are directionally selective (Zeki, 1974a; Van Essen et al., 1981; Gattas & Gross, 1981; Albright, 1984). The fact that

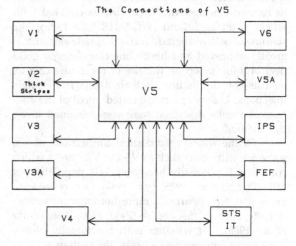

Fig. 30.1. Circuit diagram of the reciprocal connections of area V5, as determined in this laboratory. The density of connections to the various areas differ but this is not indicated in the diagram. For further details see text. IT = infero temporal cortex; FEF = frontal eye fields; IPS = intraparietal sulcus areas; STS = superior temporal sulcus.

none is wavelength selective and the majority are not orientation selective either (Zeki, 1974a, 1983; Maunsell & Van Essen, 1983) led me to propose that it is a cortical visual area specialized for the detection of motion in the field of view (Zeki, 1974a). V5 thus became the cornerstone on which was built the doctrine of functional specialization within the visual cortex (Zeki, 1974b, 1978a). Previous to that, it was commonly supposed that each visual area of the cerebral cortex analyses all the information in the field of view, but at a more complex level than the antecedent area, the areas forming a sort of hierarchical chain (Hubel & Wiesel, 1965).

A glance at a part of the motion pathways of the primate visual cortex, based on V5 and summarized in Fig. 30.1, is enough to convince one of their complexity. The general question that this article addresses itself to is: 'can we learn anything about the rules of cortical connectivity in general from studying the connections of the specialized motion pathways of the visual cortex?' In a broad sense, our main interest here is not what the motion-related visual cortex does, but how it distributes the information it has generated and whether the distribution system that it employs is similar to the distribution system employed by other, even non-visual, cortical areas. A variety of anatomical techniques have been used to study the connections of the cortex. The most recent, and successful, of these is the HRP labelling method, a technique too well known to require description. When HRP is coupled with wheat germ agglutinin (WGA–HRP), a lectin, the staining of both retrograde and orthograde elements is greatly improved and hence one can obtain a good deal of information on the site of projecting cells as well as the destination of their axons from single injections. Unless otherwise stated, most of the anatomical results described here were obtained using this method.

Of the widespread cortical connections of V5, some are with areas such as V1 and V2 – areas which contain a functionally heterogeneous population of cells (Poggio et al., 1975; Zeki, 1983). Others are with areas that are apparently more homogeneous functionally, such as V5A and V6 (Zeki, 1980, 1986; Wurtz et al., 1985). Yet whether with functionally homogeneous or heterogeneous areas, the pattern of cortical connections established by V5, and described briefly below, fall into a limited number of categories. These categories are not mutually exclusive. They are the same everywhere, not just the visual cortex. Hence they amount to rules of cortical connectivity.

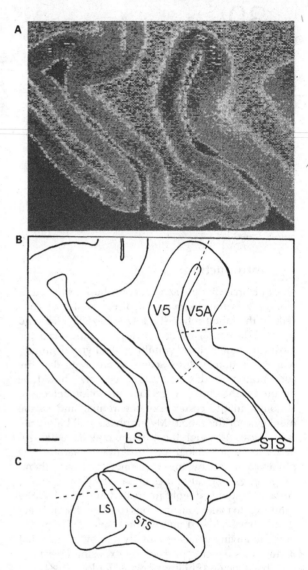

Fig. 30.2. A. Computer contrast enhanced image of a section through the superior temporal sulcus of the macaque monkey, stained for cytochrome oxidase and taken at the level shown in C. The highest density is shown in black. The borders of the V5 complex (V5 and V5A) as determined from anatomical and physiological experiments are shown in B. From this it appears that the V5 complex is a cytochrome oxidase rich area (from Jen & Zeki, 1983). Scale bar represents 2 mm.

Reciprocal connections

Area V5 has reciprocal connections with a number of cortical areas (see also Desimone & Ungerleider, 1986) (Fig. 30.1). A detailed description of the anatomy of these connections would occupy many pages and is beyond the scope of this article. Instead, we review these connections below and discuss their significance for understanding cortical connectivity in general.

Reciprocal connections have been classified in one of two ways, depending upon the cortical distribution of projecting cells and fibres (Rockland & Pandya, 1979; Maunsell & Van Essen, 1983). If two areas, A and B, are interconnected and if the fibres from A to B terminate in layer 4 of area B whereas the majority of the projecting cells in A have their cell bodies in the upper layers, area B is considered to be 'higher' in the hierarchical chain than area A. If, on the other hand, the fibres terminate predominantly in lower and upper layers, particularly layer 1, and largely spare layer 4 and if the projecting cells in A are in both the upper and lower layers, then B is considered to be 'lower' than A. It is important to emphasize that such overall patterns are not necessarily evident from examination of single sections and may require the study of many. Some connections of V5 and of other motion related areas are readily classified using this schema. Others are more awkward to classify. The pattern becomes more variable, and the classification therefore more difficult, when one examines some of the other connections of the motion related areas, such as the visual areas of the intraparietal sulcus or the frontal eye fields (see Figs. 30.3 and 30.9). Even where the anatomical pattern is clear enough, it creates interpretational problems as to whether the sequence inferred from the anatomy corresponds to the temporal order of arrival of signals in these areas. For example, the laminar arrangement of the reciprocal connections between V5 and V3 suggests that V3 is a 'lower' area than V5. Using the same criteria, V5A and V6 would be 'higher' areas than V5, and V5A a 'higher' area than V6. But V2, V3 and V5 all receive direct inputs from the same layer of V1 – layer 4B (Cragg, 1969; Zeki, 1969; Van Essen *et al.*, 1986; Livingstone & Hubel, 1987). The input to V3 and to V5 is through coarse fibres and there is thus no suggestion at present that V3 necessarily receives the signals before V2 or V5. As well, whether the hierarchical interpretation of the anatomical pattern of connections between V5, V5A and V6 reflects accurately the order in which signals proceed between them remains problematical.

What is common in these reciprocal connections is that there is an asymmetry between the distribution of retrograde and orthograde elements. This asymmetry may be classified in a variety of ways (Fig. 30.4). A useful scheme is to classify it under two main

headings, with subdivisions for each. One kind of asymmetry is the *tangential asymmetry*. Here the distribution of the projecting cells and the returning fibres is not coextensive. A good example is to be found in the system connecting V1 with V5. Both the projecting cells and the returning fibres occupy the same layer but are not coextensive within it, in the sense that the territory occupied by the fibres returning from V5 is much more extensive, occupying a greater cortical area than do the projecting cells. However, since both the outward and the returning projection occupy the same layer, we refer to it as *layer symmetric*, though it is *tangentially asymmetric*. Another example of a *tangentially asymmetric* reciprocal connection is found in the system connecting V2 with V5. Here the tangential asymmetry is complemented by a *layer asymmetry*. This is because the cells in V2 projecting to V5 are found to occur predominantly in layers 2 and 3, with some in layers 5 and 6. But the returning fibres, from V5 to V2, terminate most heavily in layers 1 and 6 and are least concentrated in layer 4. It is evident, then, that the two kinds of asymmetry are not mutually exclusive. Layer asymmetry is the more common and is usually accompanied by varying degrees of tangential asymmetry, the significance of which is difficult to gauge. These tangential asymmetries can be classified in a number of ways. For example, the tangential distribution of prograde fibres in layer 4 or in layer 1 may be more extensive, and sometimes a good deal more so, than the tangential spread of labelled cells in upper or lower layers. Alternatively, the lower layer labelled cells may have a more extensive tangential spread than labelled cells and fibres in other layers. In fact, a number of tangential asymmetries are possible and some are illustrated in Fig. 30.3. Although no definite functional significance can be attached to these asymmetries at the present time, their presence and variety suggests a possible role. Thus, remembering the richly organized radial interconnections within the cerebral cortex, a greater tangential spread of fibres than of cells would imply that the returning fibres from B to A are capable of influencing the activity of cells in A projecting to areas other than B, as well as those projecting to B. Conversely, a greater tangential spread of cells compared to fibres in the connections between A and B would imply a system in which some of the cells in A projecting to B are immune from the returning system from B to A.

In one form or another, asymmetries in the ⁻iprocal connections are not unique to the connec- s of motion related visual cortex or indeed to visual

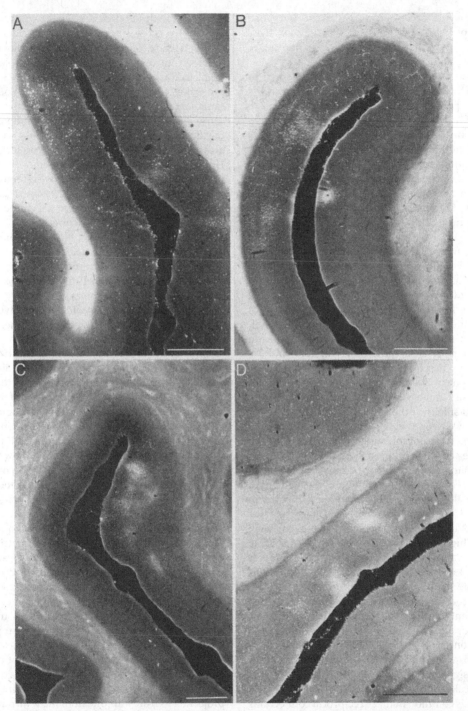

Fig. 30.3. Examples of asymmetries in the distribution of label in motion related visual areas. A, B. Label distribution in the superior temporal sulcus following WGA-HRP injections into V6. C. Label distribution in the posterior bank of the superior temporal sulcus following injections into the V5 complex (the injection site was more ventrally situated). The dense area of label in the upper layers of the anterior bank represent the remnants of the injection site. D. Label distribution in the lateral bank of the intraparietal sulcus following an injection of HRP into area V6. Scale bars represent 2 mm in each case.

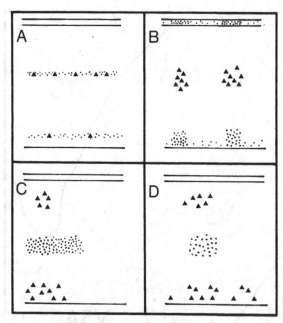

Fig. 30.4. Schematic representation of some asymmetries in the connections of cortical areas. Projecting cells are shown as triangles and input fibres as dots. A. Tangentially asymmetric but layer symmetric connection, as in the example of the V1–V5 connections. B. Tangentially asymmetric and layer asymmetric connections typified by the V2–V5 system. C and D show other, more restricted, types of tangential and layer asymmetry. For further details see text.

grade and retrograde elements, both in terms of region of distribution and in terms of layers.

With injections of label that invade both V5 and V5A, a consistent difference in the laminar distribution of labelled material adjacent to the injection site between V5 and V5A (the V5 complex) is found. The distribution of label in both is radially asymmetric and both share the common feature that there is relatively less label in layer 6 than in the other layers. Whereas the distribution of prograde label in V5A and the anterior bank generally is variable from section to section but is more evenly distributed in all layers, save layer 6, the distribution of label within V5 often displays a pattern that is not readily classifiable. That is, layer 4 is largely empty of labelled material, most of the orthograde label is in the upper layers, especially layer 1, and labelled cells are predominantly distributed in the upper and lower layers (see Fig. 30.3). This pattern presumably reflects the intra-areal connections within V5. (The pattern may reflect the input from V5A to V5, as well as the intra-areal connections of V5. But since the pattern is uniform one would have to assume that at least some of it is due to intra-areal connections within V5.) In fact the two patterns, one more characteristic of V5, the other of V5A, are sometimes juxtaposed, raising the possibility that the boundary between the two may be drawn by observing the laminar distribution of label in the two areas following large injections of HRP label into the V5 complex (see Fig. 30.5).

The V5 complex has widespread connections within the superior temporal sulcus, extending almost to the tip of the temporal lobe. The prograde fibres from the V5 complex are distributed predominantly in layer 4, whereas the returning fibres have their cell bodies distributed in upper and lower layers (see Fig. 30.6). The extent of distribution of label within the temporal lobe is interesting. It is commonly supposed that motion related information is shunted to the dorsal parts of the brain, and in particular to the parietal cortex, and that it spares the temporal cortex which is thought to receive information on colour and form only (see Ungerleider & Mishkin, 1982; Desimone *et al.*, 1985). There is indeed good evidence that motion related information is concentrated dorsally in the cerebral visual cortex. But in our material, we have consistently observed a projection to the temporal lobe from the V5 complex, almost to its very tip. The projection referred to above, largely in the medial bank and depth of the superior temporal sulcus, is hidden from a surface view. There is also a sparse projection to the ventro-medial surface of the temporal lobe, thus suggesting that temporal neo-

cortex in general. They are common in all cortical and many subcortical connections.

The connections of V5

One of the most prominent projections of V5 is to V5A, an area lying immediately adjacent to V5 and extending laterally in the anterior bank of the superior temporal sulcus. It was first described physiologically (Zeki, 1980) and later shown to be directly connected with V5 (Maunsell & Van Essen, 1983). It contains directionally selective cells with very large receptive fields, sparing largely the central 0–5° (Zeki, 1980: Wurtz *et al.*, 1985). The borders of V5A are not yet determined with precision and it may be a composite of more than one area (Tanaka *et al.*, 1986). Its connection with V5 is a reciprocal one. Following injection of HRP–WGA into V5, the orthograde input to V5A is found to be distributed heavily and predominantly in layer 4 with almost equal concentration of retrogradely labelled cells in the upper and lower layers. There is thus an asymmetry between the distribution of pro-

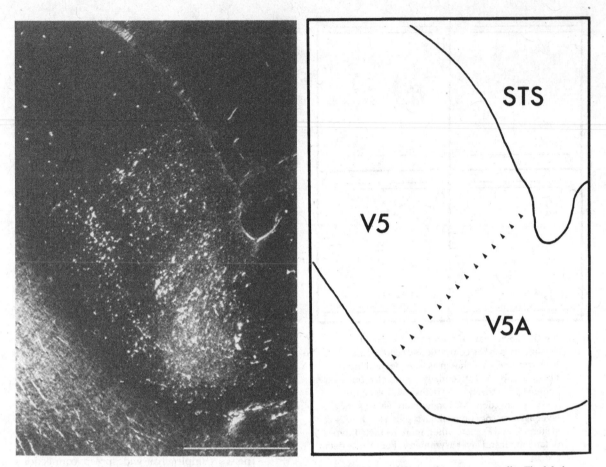

Fig. 30.5. Distribution of HRP label following an injection of WGA-HRP into V5 complex more ventrally. The label so revealed may represent intra-areal connections and the juxtaposition of two different labelling patterns, (i) cells in layers 2 and 3 + layer 5 and (ii) intense prograde label in layers 2, 3 and 4 may represent the functional border between V5 and V5A. Scale bar represents 1 mm.

cortex is also the target of motion related information. How this input relates to the much more prominent input from the V4 complex (Desimone *et al.*, 1980 and author's unpublished results) remains to be determined. The projection from V4 is more to the convexity of the temporal lobe whereas that from the V5 complex is relatively sparse and confined to its ventro-medial surface. Hence any interaction between the inputs from the V4 complex and the V5 complex would presumably be achieved by local connections within temporal cortex. Such connections would form but one of the systems connecting V4 and V5. There are several other anatomical opportunities for the information from the two sources to be brought together. There is the re-entrant input from V5 to V2, discussed below. There is also a direct, though sparse, connection between V4 and V5 (Fries & Zeki, 1983;

Maunsell & Van Essen, 1983; Ungerleider & Desimone, 1986), with labelled cells appearing in both upper and lower layers of V4 following injections of HRP into V5 and with orthograde label occupying all layers. Another region of the visual cortex where colour signals – through the V4 pathway – and motion signals – through the V5 pathway – can be brought together is in the intraparietal sulcus. It is now known that both V4 and V5 project directly to the intraparietal sulcus (Zeki, 1977; Maunsell & Van Essen, 1983), but whether the two inputs overlap there or are merely contiguous to one another remains to be determined. With V5 injections, the label that appears in the intraparietal sulcus is consistent from animal to animal and from section to section – labelled prograde fibres are heavily concentrated in layer 4 and labelled cells appear in both upper and lower layers. There are,

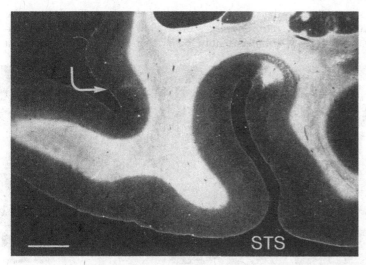

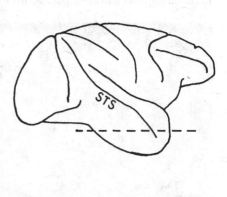

Fig. 30.6. The distribution of label in the temporal lobe, at the level indicated to the right, following an injection of label into the V5 complex. The prograde label in the floor of the superior temporal sulcus is heavily concentrated in layer 4 whereas labelled cells are found predominantly in the lower layers. Two further foci or label, one of which is shown (arrow), occurred medially in the occipito-temporal sulcus. Scale bar represents 2 mm.

however, pronounced asymmetries, discussed below, in the distribution of the two components. Such asymmetries are especially evident following injections of label into V6, another motion related visual area with a prominent projection to the intraparietal sulcus (Zeki, 1986) (see Fig. 30.3).

Other projections of V5 are to areas V3, V3A and V6. The projection to V3 is predominantly characterized by labelled cells (i.e. those projecting to V5) occupying upper layers, and labelled fibres (i.e. those projecting from V5) occupying the upper layers (including layer 1) and lower layers, but largely sparing layer 4. The connection with V3A is more problematic, with the pattern of distribution of prograde and retrograde components being variable from section to section (see also Ungerleider & Desimone, 1986). It is also very limited, suggesting that it may be of the operational kind. The connections between the V5 complex and the V3 complex (V3 & V3A) may help to unite information on motion, form and disparity – a system in which other areas are involved, as discussed below.

The connections with V6 are remarkable for their patchy nature, a system more prominently observed here than in other areas. Indeed the patchiness is observed in all of the connections established by V6, including its intrinsic connections. Just as with V5, and unlike the picture obtained in V5A, the pattern of label distribution within the patches displaying the intrinsic connections of V6 is difficult to classify

and consists of labelled cells occupying upper and lower layers and prograde fibres sparing layer 4 largely and, among other layers, being heavily distributed in layer 1 (see Fig. 30.7). The same kind of patchy connections, though on a more restricted scale, is observed in the connections made by the frontal eye fields with V5 and V6. Here it is common for the patches to take on the shape of two or more elongated stripes running dorso-ventrally (see Fig. 30.8). Following injections into either area, the pattern of label distribution is such as to make classification awkward. Label can, for example, be restricted to layers 2 and 3 after HRP injections into V5 with little or no label, either prograde or retrograde, elsewhere (Fig. 30.9). Or, following an HRP injection into V6, label may appear in two broad patches, one in the upper layers but sparing largely layer 1 and another in the lower layers – with a gap of lower density separating the two (Fig. 30.9).

Perhaps the most interesting connection is the one established between V5 and the cortex of V1 and V2. This is discussed in detail below, under the section on the 're-entrant system'. Here it is sufficient to point out that the cells in V1 projecting to V5 are located in layer 4B and in upper layer 6 only (Lund et al., 1975). This suggests a radial segregation within V1 such that motion related information destined for V5 is concentrated into these two layers and separated from other functional categories of cell, which are concentrated in other layers and project elsewhere. In addition, there is also a tangential segregation whereby cells in these two layers projecting to V5 are grouped together and are separated from other cells in the same layer projecting elsewhere. By contrast, the returning fibres from V5 to V1 are continuously distributed within both layers, thus giving rise to a

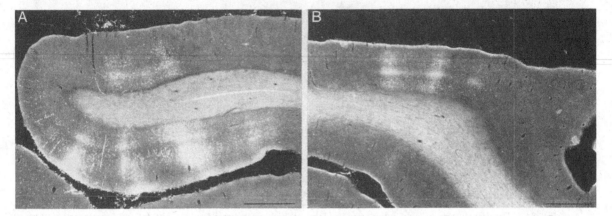

Fig. 30.7. A. Photomicrograph of the distribution of label in area V6 following an injection of HRP label into the same area more dorsally. Four major bands of intrinsic label are seen with a notable paucity of label in layer 4, but with heavy label in upper and lower layers, a pattern that does not conform to ones previously described. This is in contrast to the pattern of label distribution in V8 (a newly defined visual area (Zeki, unpublished results)), on the medial side, shown in greater detail in B. Here the prograde fibres are concentrated predominantly in layer 4, with retrogradely labelled cells occupying upper and lower layers – a pattern characteristic of a 'higher' area. Scale bars represent 2 mm.

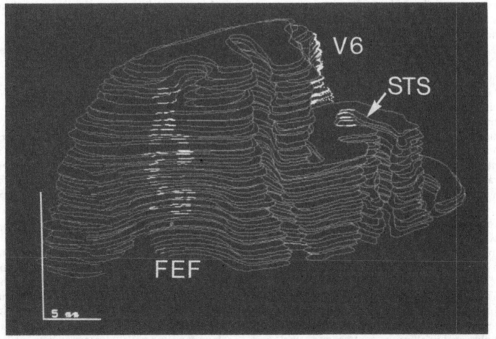

Fig. 30.8. Computer aided three-dimensional reconstruction of the distribution of label in the cerebral cortex following an injection of HRP into area V6. The view shown is that of a left hemisphere rotated so that it is viewed from anterior to posterior. Several regions of the cortex have been 'cut away' so as to reveal the injection site in V6, and the distribution of label in the frontal eye fields. When thus reconstructed, the patchy label in the FEF is seen to consist of dorsoventrally running strips. Scale bars represent 5 mm in both axes.

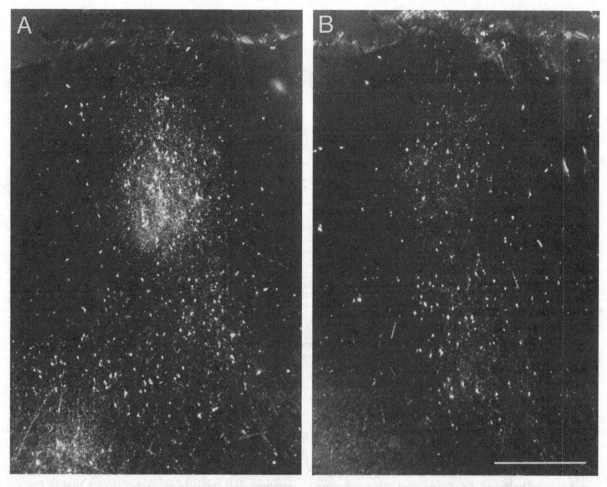

Fig. 30.9. A. Photomicrograph of a section taken through the cortex of the frontal eye fields (FEF) to show the distribution of label following an injection of HRP label into area V5. Note that the label is mainly restricted to layers 2 and 3. B is a photomicrograph taken through the same region in another brain, but following an injection of label into V6. The label is distributed in upper and lower layers, with a gap in between. Though radially asymmetric, in neither case does the pattern of label distribution conform to previously described schemas. Scale bar represents 500 μm.

tangential asymmetric reciprocal connection of profound significance (see below). A similar arrangement prevails for V2, an area known from early anatomical work to project directly to V5 as well as to V4 (Zeki, 1971b, 1976). In V2, the cells projecting to V5 are grouped together and separated from cells projecting to V4, as described in detail below. The returning fibres from V5 to V2, however, do not respect these territories – they are widely distributed within the territory of cells projecting to V5 as well as those projecting elsewhere, including V4 – once again revealing a reciprocal system which is tangentially highly asymmetric.

The anatomical relationship between the motion, form and colour systems

It is now common to speak of two major visual pathways whose cortical destinations differ. One system is dominated by an input from the magnocellular division of the lateral geniculate nucleus (LGN) and is generally considered to be more concerned with motion. A pivotal prestriate area for it is V5. Another system, dominated by an input from the parvocellular layers of the LGN, has V4 as a pivotal prestriate cortical area and is generally considered to be involved with colour. However, in our description of functional specialization in the visual cortex, we were equally impressed by areas V3 and V3A (Zeki, 1978b), a system that is rarely considered to be of equal status to the others, even when it is considered at all. The most detailed studies of V3 and V3A show them to contain predominantly orientation selective cells, with wavelength being an unimportant parameter (Zeki, 1978a,b; Baizer, 1982; Felleman & Van Essen, 1987). There is evidence that many cells in V3 and V3A are strongly disparity tuned (Zeki, 1978; Poggio, 1985; Felleman & Van Essen, 1987) and that the response of a large proportion of cells in both areas may be a function of the angle of gaze (Aicardi *et al.*, 1987). It is thus likely that the V3 complex of areas may play a critical role in form perception, without excluding a role in depth perception which, indeed, may be a role common to many visual areas. Here it is important to emphasize that while the presence of orientation selective cells in V4 (Zeki, 1975, 1983; Desimone *et al.*, 1985; Desimone & Schein, 1987) would argue for a role of V4 in form vision, the case that it is involved in the analysis of form, *independently of colour*, has yet to be made. At any rate, it would be surprising if V4 and the areas of the V3 complex play identical roles in form perception – the information on orientation selectivity reaching these two groups of areas must either be different or be utilized differently. We thus suggest, not less but not more tentatively than before, that V3 and V3A are important in form analysis, without excluding their involvement in other attributes of vision. And we suggest further that they are pivotal areas in a third major cortical pathway, which may receive both a parvo- and a magnocellular input. It is, of course, likely that further subdivisions within these systems will be found. For the present, it is interesting to ask how and where these three systems interact with each other in the cerebral cortex. Put differently, how does the motion system, based on V5, communicate with the V4 and the V3 systems.

Figure 30.10 is a summary diagram of the connections between V1 and V2 and the visual areas of the prestriate cortex to show the separate connections between the functionally segregated components in the visual cortex. The sections shown are taken from small regions of V1 and V2, stained for the metabolic enzyme cytochrome oxidase, which shows the characteristic pattern of blobs in layers 2 and 3 of V1 and the thick and thin stripes, separated by interstripe zones of lower cytochrome oxidase content, in V2. The magnocellular input to the striate cortex is to layer 4C (Hubel & Wiesel, 1974; Hendrickson *et al.*, 1978), which in turn inputs strongly into layer 4B (Lund & Boothe, 1975; Fitzpatrick *et al.*, 1985; Blasdel *et al.*, 1985). Layer 4B projects to areas V5, V3 and to the thick stripes of V2 (see below) (Lund *et al.*, 1975; Maunsell & Van Essen, 1983; Burkhalter *et al.*, 1986; Livingstone &

Hubel, 1987). V3 and V5 both receive an input from the thick stripes of V2 (Shipp & Zeki, 1985); V3 projects to V3A, which may also receive an input from V2 (Zeki, 1978b). The parvocellular input is to layer 4C, which communicates with layers 2 and 3 via layer 4A (Lund & Boothe, 1975; Fitzpatrick *et al.*, 1985; Blasdel *et al.*, 1985). Layers 2 and 3 project directly to V4 from the foveal part of V1 (Zeki, 1975; Yukie & Iwai, 1985) and, more prominently, to the thin stripes and interstripes of V2 (Livingstone & Hubel, 1984) which, in turn, project to V4 (Shipp & Zeki, 1985; De Yoe & Van Essen, 1985). Although the separation between the two systems at these levels is impressive, it is not absolute. In particular, layer 4B projects strongly to layers 2 and 3, thus implying that the latter are not purely parvocellular input layers and layer 6 has some direct input from other layers of V1, suggesting a possible mixture of parvo- and magnocellular inputs there (Lund & Boothe, 1975; Fitzpatrick *et al.*, 1985; Blasdel *et al.*, 1985). Figure 30.11 is a summary diagram of the probable sites of interaction between the three systems referred to above, and is discussed in greater detail later.

The functional logic of cortical connections

The projections described above conform to certain patterns which are not restricted to these motion pathways but are so common that they amount to rules of cortical connectivity. These rules revolve around one apparently overridingly important strategy that the cerebral cortex uses – that of functional segregation, itself a problem of very deep interest. Functional segregation demands that cells with common functional properties be grouped together, either in areas or in subregions within an area. This, in turn, necessitates (a) *convergence* of connections and its reciprocal, (b) *divergence*. It also requires that within both divergent and convergent systems, functionally distinct groupings be maintained separate, a phenomenon manifested anatomically in the system of (c) *patchy connections*. Inevitably, the functionally segregated groups of cells must communicate with each other and this occurs through (d) *direct* and *reentrant* connections. Of these, the speculative *operational connection* (e) is perhaps the most difficult to establish experimentally.

Convergence
It is inevitable that where particular, functionally distinct, sets of signals, distributed in one area which is itself functionally heterogeneous, are to be assembled in another area, a process of anatomical convergence

would be used (Fig. 30.12). One of the most prominent connections of V5 is with the striate cortex, V1 (Cragg, 1969; Zeki, 1969), an area which contains a function-ally heterogeneous population of cells (Poggio *et al.*, 1975; Zeki, 1983; Livingstone & Hubel, 1984). It is a highly convergent projection (Zeki, 1971a). From this

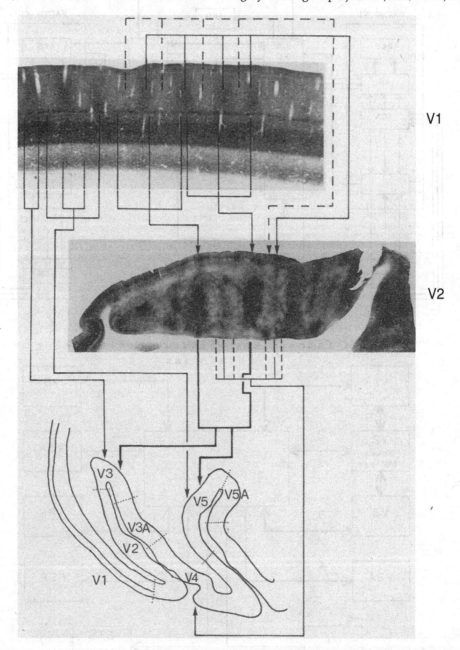

Fig. 30.10. Diagrams to illustrate the segregated pathways from V1 (top) and V2 (middle) to the specialized areas of the prestriate visual cortex. V1 acts as a segregator of signals, sending divergent outputs to V2, V3 and V5. The input to each area is organized in a convergent manner (see text). In particular, signals from the cytochrome oxidase rich blobs of V1 are directed to the thin cytochrome oxidase stripes of V2 whereas the interblobs of layers 2 and 3 of V1 project to the interstripes of V2. The thick strips of the latter receive their inputs from cells in layer 4B of V1. This process of segregation, coupled to convergence, is at work again in the specific connections that the thin stripes and interstripes establish with V4 and that the thick stripes establish with V5 and V3.

A

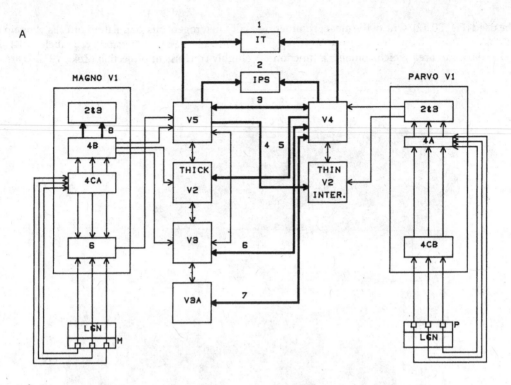

B

The Connections Between Motion and Form Areas

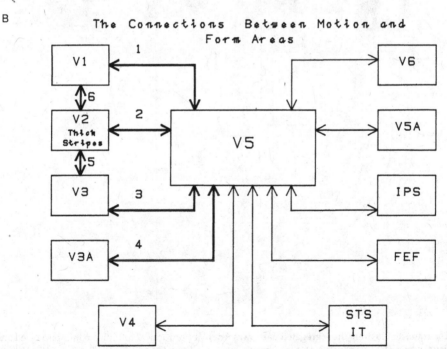

Fig. 30.11. A. Summary diagram to illustrate the flow of information through two of the three major visual pathways – the magnocellular (motion) system and the parvocellular (colour) system. Signals from the magnocellular layers of the LGN are directed predominantly at layer 4CA of V1 which then connects with layers 4B and 6 – the latter also receiving a direct geniculate input. These two layers project directly to V5 and layer 4B projects, in addition, to the thick stripes of

somewhat simple anatomical observation, two powerful conclusions follow. One is that V5 is a much smaller visual area than V1 and, following from this, that its cells must consequently have much larger receptive fields. Both conclusions have been confirmed by subsequent studies (Zeki, 1974a; Van Essen *et al.*, 1981). In a similar way, V2 also has a convergent projection to V5 (Zeki, 1971b; 1976). Since V2 also has a functionally heterogeneous population of cells (Baizer *et al.*, 1977; Zeki, 1978a), it follows that the same principle of anatomical convergence is being used to assemble a particular kind of visual signal, distributed throughout V1 and V2, into a single area, V5. There are many other examples of convergence in the visual cortex, including the pathways connecting V1 with V3 and V2 with V4. On an anatomically smaller scale, the same process of convergence, designed to assemble the same signals into a single subregion, can be found in the connections between V1 and V2. Thus there is a convergent input from the blobs of V1 (in which low spatial frequencies and wavelength selectivity are represented), to the thin stripes of V2, in which cells have similar properties but with larger receptive fields (Livingstone & Hubel, 1984). Equally, there is a convergent input from the interblobs of V1 to the interstripes of V2, with similar consequences. Indeed, the generation of cells with larger receptive fields is one of the principal by-products of anatomical convergence (Fig. 30.12). But what particular advantage cells with larger receptive fields confer is not a question that has ever been satisfactorily answered.

Convergence also occurs in the projections of distinct motion-related areas of the visual cortex. An interesting example is to be found with the connections of V6*. This area lies medially in the brain on the medial bank of the parieto-occipital sulcus, bordering area V3A medially (Zeki, 1986). It has extensive connections, summarized in Fig. 30.13. What is of particular interest in the connections of V6 is the extent to which it connects with areas which V5 and V5A also connect with, given that V6 itself has connections with the latter two areas. Thus inputs from V6 and the V5 complex converge onto V3A, the areas of the intraparietal sulcus as well as the frontal eye fields.

*The relationship of area V6 to area PO described by Covey *et al.*, 1982 is not clear.

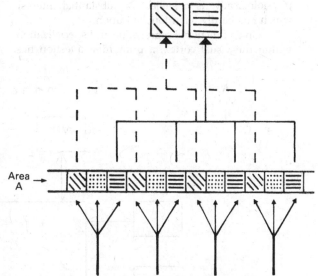

Area A →

Fig. 30.12. Diagrammatic representation of the convergent–divergent system of connections. In an area A, signals relating to different submodalities but referable to the same retinal position are maintained segregated. The divergent connections from A allow signals relating to the same submodality to be assembled in one area through the process of convergence and those relating to another submodality to be assembled in another area. Each divergent pathway from A entails a convergent input to the relevant area, with larger receptive fields in the latter being one consequence.

While we do not know whether the inputs to these areas from V6 and the V5 complex are overlapping, it is nevertheless interesting to note the extent of convergence onto third areas of areas which are themselves interconnected. The functional conclusion seems inescapable that in these areas new categories are generated which are collectively of importance for a given third area and are thus assembled there through the process of convergence. Thus, V5, V5A and V6 would each appear to generate new signal patterns which are of importance to, for example, the frontal eye fields. What common categories are generated in these individual areas, necessitating their convergence onto a third area, and how this information is handled in the third area, both anatomically and

V2 and to V3. The thick stripes project in turn to V3 and V5. Signals from the parvocellular layers of the LGN are directed mainly to layers 4CB and 4A, themselves interconnected. The signals are then communicated to layers 2 and 3 which project to V4 directly (from the foveal region of V1) and indirectly through the thin stripes and interstripes of V2. Heavy lines show possible sites of interaction between these two systems. B. Summary diagram of possible sites of interaction between the form and motion systems. For further details see text.

physiologically, is a subject of substantial interest which has hardly been touched upon.

Given functional segregation and specialization within the visual cortex, a primordial question has

always been, and remains, how the segregated information is re-united to give us our unitary perception of the visual world. Much hope was pinned on the convergent type of connection as a means, not of

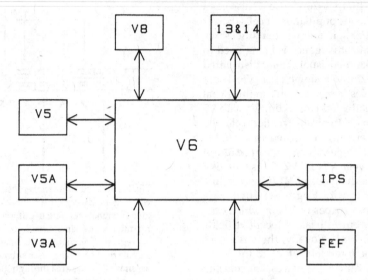

A   The Connections of V6

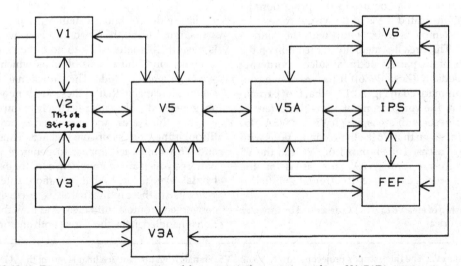

B   Convergent Projections Within Motion Pathways

Fig. 30.13. A. Diagrammatic representation of the anatomical connections of area V6. B. Diagrammatic representation of the convergent anatomical pathways between motion related areas. Of especial note are the convergent pathways to V6 from areas V5, V5A and IPS. There are also convergent pathways leading to FEF from areas V5, V5A, V6 and the visual areas of the intraparietal sulcus (IPS). Examination of the figure reveals other interesting convergent pathways.

concentrating the same kind of signal into a single area, but of assembling disparate kinds of information from different areas into a single area. Early anatomical evidence (Jones & Powell, 1970), antedating the physiological evidence on functional specialization and showing that convergence within systems precedes that between them, offered hope that convergence might be just the mechanism for uniting signals belonging to different modalities or submodalities in one or a few areas of the cerebral cortex. Yet this latter kind of convergence appears to be constrained by the overriding need to maintain functional segregation. Thus, where two functionally distinct areas converge in their projections upon a third, each area nevertheless maintains its own territory within the third. For example, in the convergent projection from the frontal and parietal cortex to the superior temporal sulcus the inputs are organized either into alternating patches tangentially or interlaced in alternating layers (Goldman-Rakic, 1984). While either mode of termination allows inputs from the two different sources to terminate on the same cells (though there is no direct physiological evidence that they actually do so), the fact remains that each input maintains its own territory within the third. The reason why functional segregation is maintained even in territory where modality or submodality convergence might occur remains a central, unsolved problem.

In the visual cortex, inter submodal convergence does not occur at early levels. Such an example may be found at the level of the intraparietal sulcus, where the convergent input from V5 (representing motion information), and V4 (representing colour information among other possible attributes) may constitute one anatomical means of submodality integration. But it is not yet clear whether the two inputs are overlapping or are contiguous. Another kind of submodality convergence may be found in the input to infero-temporal cortex from the motion and colour systems but, once again, how these two inputs relate to each other there remains unknown.

Divergence

Divergent projections from an area such as V1, with its functionally heterogeneous population of cells, is really a means – the reciprocal of convergence – of distributing functionally distinct signals to different areas or sub-areas (see Fig. 30.12). Divergent projections give powerful hints to the organization of an area, especially if it is known that the area is functionally heterogeneous. Thus, long before the anatomical demonstration of functional segregation in the striate

cortex (Livingstone & Hubel, 1984), it was argued, from the anatomical evidence showing it to have multiple and divergent projections to the visual areas of the prestriate cortex, that V1 must act as a functional segregator, parcelling out different signals to different areas for further processing (Zeki, 1975). This was in spite of the impressive physiological evidence of the time, which had shown it to be a uniform cortical area (Hubel & Wiesel, 1974) without any of the functional inhomogeneities which were later discovered, in particular by use of the cytochrome oxidase staining technique (Wong-Riley, 1979) and its correlation with physiological recordings (Livingstone & Hubel, 1984). The logic behind this is simple. Each millimetre of V1 receives its input from a particular part of the retina and thus contains all the visual information destined for the cortex from that retinal point. In addition, each millimetre of V1 cortex has multiple and divergent projections to different areas of the prestriate visual cortex. Since it would be difficult to imagine that each millimetre of V1 would send the same signals to the different prestriate areas in these divergent and parallel pathways, it follows that it must be sending different signals to different areas. It must thus act as a functional segregator, a supposition since amply proven. A glance at the projections of the functionally more homogeneous areas of V5 or V6 shows that they too have multiple projections (Figs. 30.1 and 30.13). Once again, one's initial supposition would be that V5 sends different signals to these different areas, for it is difficult to imagine that each part would relay the same message to the different areas in these independent and parallel pathways. But here the conclusion, derived from the anatomical evidence alone, is less certain. All the physiological evidence suggests that V5 is a homogeneous visual area, in which motion alone is mapped (Zeki, 1974a; Maunsell & Van Essen, 1983; Albright, 1984). Although several different kinds of directionally selective cell have been found in V5, there is no obvious segregation of functional categories within it, as in V1, apart from the groupings of cells with common directional preferences. The possibility remains therefore that the multiple projections of V5 may reflect a different kind of distribution system – one in which the same signal is relayed to the different target areas of V5, which then use this information in different ways, according to their specializations. In general, a *prima facie* case may be made for two areas, A and B, receiving the same signal pattern from area C if it can be shown by some double-labelling anatomical technique that the same cells project to two or more areas by means of bifurcating axons. Such a projection has been demonstrated for the Meynert cells of layer 6 in V1. They have been shown to project through bifurcating axons to both V5 and the superior colliculus (Fries *et al.*, 1985). Even here, however, it does not necessarily follow that identical signals are relayed to the two areas. There might be small, but significant, differences in the timing of arrival of impulses in the two areas. These, when taken in conjunction with the other impulses arriving in the two areas, may render the signals different. Another possibility, however, is that new categories, not so far hinted at by the physiological evidence, may be generated in V5 and that signals related to different categories are distributed to the different areas to which V5 projects. For example, Movshon (personal communication) has found direction invariant and speed invariant cells in V5. One can suggest speculatively that these two groups of cell have different destinations. Others, as yet undiscovered, categories may have still different destinations.

It is a significant fact about cortical connectivity that no area of the cerebral cortex connects with one other area only. This suggests that the distribution and re-distribution of information is a key role of almost all cortical areas, with the important consequence that any function becomes distributed among several cortical areas. At one level, vision as a process is seen to be distributed in several areas. At another, the same distributive process ensures that a submodality of vision, e.g. motion, is also distributed between a number of areas. Detailed anatomical studies of somatosensory, auditory, parietal and frontal cortex show that the same distributive process, implied by the multiple projections of these other cortical areas, is also at work there.

Submodality segregation and its anatomical manifestation in patchy, striped, connections

When the connections between two areas of the cerebral cortex are examined in detail, they are found not to be continuous but to occur in patches or clusters when examined in individual sections. When reconstructed from section to section they are found to take on the shape of elongated stripes, with a periodicity that varies between one set of connections and another. Patchy connections were first observed in the visual cortex (Gilbert & Kelly, 1975; Zeki, 1976) and have since been found to be a characteristic of so many cortical connections (e.g. Jones, 1984; Imig & Reale, 1981) that it is difficult to believe that they are not the anatomical manifestation of a fundamental cortical strategy, operating repetitively throughout the cerebral cortex. In general terms, we suppose it to be the visible manifestation of the cortical strategy of separating groups of cells with a common function from other functional groupings or, more simply, the strategy of functional segregation. Perhaps one of the best examples of how patchy connections relate to submodality segregation is to be found in the connections between V2 and V5 (see below). Area V2 of the macaque monkey has connections with several other visual areas, among them V4 and V5 (Zeki, 1971a,b). It also has a distinctive cytochrome oxidase architecture, consisting of thick stripes, thin stripes and interstripes (see Fig. 30.14). When anatomically identified recordings, in which recording sites can be correlated with the cytochrome oxidase pattern, are made in V2, it is found that directionally selective cells, although small in percentage numbers, are distributed exclusively in the thick stripes. Significantly, there are no wavelength or colour selective cells in the thick stripes (Shipp & Zeki, 1985; Hubel & Livingstone, 1985; De Yoe & Van Essen, 1985). When HRP is injected into V5, the label that appears in V2 occurs in patches. When reconstructed to obtain a tangential view of the cortex of V2, the patches take on the form of elongated stripes running orthogonal to the long axis of V2. Detailed studies in which the distribution of HRP label and cytochrome oxidase architecture are correlated from adjacent sections reveal that, following V5 injections, the label in V2 appears only in the territory of the thick stripes, the very ones that contain the directionally selective cells (Fig. 30.14). This constitutes one of the most striking items of evidence in support of the notion that the patchy connection is the anatomical manifestation of the strategy of functional segregation in the visual cortex.

The anatomic segregation of functional groupings in an area of the visual cortex can occur in the tangential direction or in the radial direction, or both. Good examples are to be found in the projections from V1 to V5. Cells in V1 projecting to V5 are not distributed in all layers but are radially segregated into layer 4B and layer 6 (Lund *et al.*, 1975; Maunsell & Van Essen, 1983) (Fig. 30.15). When one examines either layer after massive injections of HRP label into V5, one finds that labelled cells occur singly or in small groupings of two to three and are separated from each other by unlabelled cells and therefore cells projecting to areas other than V5. This is especially so in upper layer 6, where the number of labelled cells is much smaller than those in layer 4B after the same injections, the latter outnumbering the former by 10 to 1. Thus cells in either layer projecting to V5 are tangentially segregated from cells in the same layers projecting elsewhere. This is well seen in tangential sections

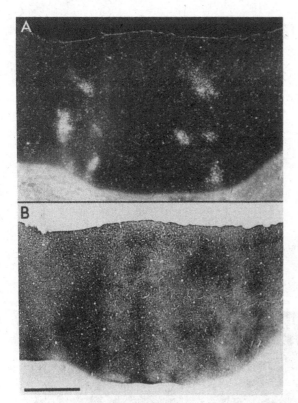

Fig. 30.14. A. Dark field photomicrograph of a small region from a section through area V2, reacted for label following an injection of HRP into area V5. B. Bright field photomicrograph of section adjacent to the one shown in A, stained for the mitochondrial enzyme cytochrome oxidase. Comparison of the two reveals that the label following an injection into V5 is restricted to the thick stripes where it occurs in the form of discontinuous patches, hinting at the possibility of further differentiation within the territory of the thick stripes, which also project to V3 (Shipp & Zeki, 1985). Scale bar represents 2 mm.

taken through layer 4B after HRP injections into V5 (Fig. 30.15). Here labelled material (cells plus their immediate processes) are seen to occur in patches – dramatically illustrating in morphological terms the strategy of functional segregation that is so commonly employed by the cortex.

The patchy pattern of projections is also observed in the prograde projection from V1 to V5 – indeed in monkey visual cortex, it was first observed there (Zeki, 1976). When injections of ³H-proline are made into V1, the distribution of label in V5 is found not to be continuous. Instead it occurs in patches or clusters (Zeki, 1976; Montero, 1980). By analogy with

other connections in visual cortex, this suggests a degree of functional segregation in the projection from V1 to V5 – and hence a functional compartmentalization within the context of motion specificity in V5 – for which the physiological evidence has yet to be adduced. For example, the projections from V1 to V2 are patchy (Van Essen et al., 1986; Zeki, unpublished evidence) and the detailed anatomical studies of Livingstone & Hubel (1984) have shown that a remarkable degree of functional segregation is maintained in the connections between these two areas. The blobs (containing wavelength selective and low spatial frequency tuning cells) connect specifically with the thin stripes, whereas the interblobs (containing cells which are predominantly orientation but not wavelength selective) connect specifically with the interstripes. As well, the radially segregated cells of layer 4B connect specifically with the thick stripes.

While the functional segregation behind these patchy connections is perhaps best understood in the visual system, it is becoming increasingly evident that the same overall process is repetitively used in the cerebral cortex. Thus the connections of the various subdivisions of the somato-sensory cortex and their connections with the motor cortex are patchy (Jones, 1984). Equally, the remarkable combined anatomical–physiological studies of Imig & Reale (1981) show that the connections between the various auditory areas are patchy, the patchiness here reflecting a preferential connection of the representation of the best frequencies in one area with their counterparts in another.

So important does the strategy of functional segregation in the cerebral cortex appear to be that even relatively subtle functional differences are reflected anatomically in patchy connectivity. The callosal connections of the frontal eye fields, which receive inputs from several motion related areas, illustrate this. These callosal connections are not distributed continuously but occur in stripes when the cortex is viewed tangentially. Here the anatomical patchiness reflects the functional segregation of two types of saccade related cells. Vertical saccade related cells are concentrated within the callosally connected patches whereas horizontal saccade related cells are grouped together and situated outside the callosally connected patches, the two groupings alternating repetitively (Goldman-Rakic, 1984).

In summary, it would seem that even where no functional significance can be presently attached to the patchy pattern in some areas, their mere presence would indicate the presence of functional groupings which physiological evidence must ascertain.

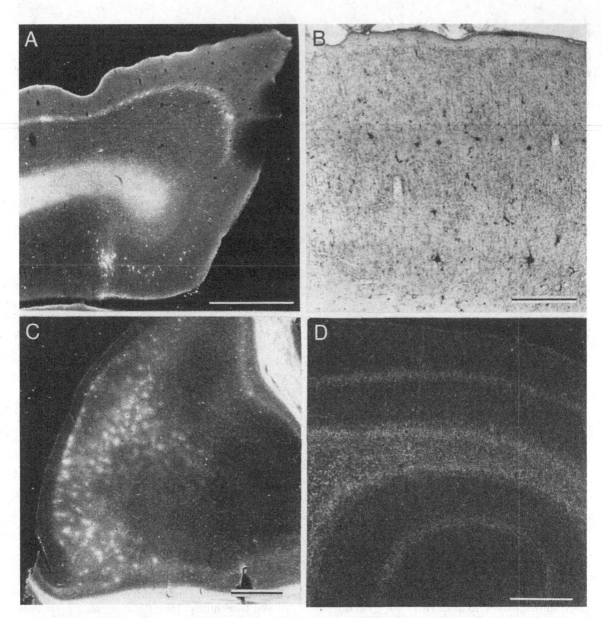

Fig. 30.15. The segregated order in the arrangement of connections between V1 and V5. A shows a dark field photomicrograph of a section passing through V1 and V2 and reacted for label following an HRP injection into V5. The label in V1 is found to be largely confined to layer 4B and, less densely, layer 6. B. Examination at higher magnification of a radial section, counterstained for Nissl substance, taken through V1 in another animal with a V5 injection shows, however, that not every cell in either layer is labelled following a V5 injection, the labelled cells occurring singly or in clusters. The patchy nature of this connection is better seen in a dark field photomicrograph (C) of a low power view of a tangential section through layer 4B, reacted for label following an injection of HRP into V5. By contrast, the re-entrant input from V5 to layers 4 and 6 is continuous, thus engulfing the territory of all cells in either layer, not just the ones projecting to V5. This is seen in D which is a darkfield photomicrograph of a section taken through V1 in an animal whose V5 was injected with a cocktail of ^{3}H-Proline and ^{3}H-Leucine. The section from which D was taken was given by Drs Squattrito and Galetti, University of Bologna. Scale bars represent 2 mm in A, C, D and 500 μm in B.

The re-entrant system and the integration of information

The presence of functional specialization within visual cortex, evident both in the areal specializations as well as in the discrete functional subgroupings within areas such as V1 and V2, naturally raises the question of how the segregated information is re-integrated to give us our unitary perception of the visual world. To put it briefly, how does the visual system achieve the remarkable feat of putting in registration the form, colour and direction and speed of motion of an object, so that the whole can be perceived simultaneously. There is no ready anatomical answer to how such percepts are generated by the cortex but anatomical connections between areas representing different submodalities would obviously be a prerequisite. One theoretical possibility would be that all these areas would eventually communicate their signals in a convergent manner to a single area. This possibility can be easily discounted by the observation that there is no single area to which all the visual areas project. A more plausible means would be for the areas to communicate with each other directly. There is good anatomical evidence that such contacts between areas subserving different submodalities exist. For example, there is a definite, though small, anatomical connection between V4 and V5 (Fries & Zeki, 1983; Maunsell & Van Essen, 1983; Ungerleider & Desimone, 1986). There are also direct connections between V5 and V3, and V5 and V3A (Maunsell & Van Essen, 1983; Ungerleider & Desimone, 1986; Zeki, unpublished results). Such connections are considered under the heading of operational connections below. But another means of combining information is through the re-entrant system, a vast network which has been much overlooked, both anatomically and physiologically. The theoretical need for a re-entrant system is discussed in detail by Edelman (1978). Here I restrict myself to the possible anatomical basis of such a system.

A very good example of a re-entrant system is found in the projections from V5 to V1 and V2 – two antecedent areas from which it receives a direct input. As mentioned earlier, the input from V1 to V5 is patchy in nature, the projecting cells being confined to layer 4B and upper layer 6 (the solitary cells of Meynert). The projection from V2 to V5 is also patchy, the projecting cells being restricted to the territory of the thick stripes. When wheat germ agglutinin HRP is injected into V5, it labels both the cells projecting to V5 as well as the orthograde fibres emanating from V5.

One remarkable observation following such injections into V5 is that the projection from it to layer 4B and layer 6 of V1 is tangentially highly asymmetric with respect to the forward projection and not restricted to the territory of the cells in these two layers projecting to V5. Instead, the back projection is continuously distributed in both layers and thus includes not only the territory of cells projecting to V5 but also the territory of cells projecting elsewhere (see Figs. 30.15 and 30.16). Similar results are obtained when, instead of injecting WGA–HRP into V5, one injects a cocktail of labelled amino acids. The latter are taken up by the cell bodies and incorporated into proteins which are then transported orthogradely, to the axon terminals. The method thus labels orthograde projections alone and is not open to the criticism that some, at least, of the axonal label seen in WGA–HRP injections may be due to labelling of the axonal collaterals of the retrogradely labelled cells. When such injections are made into V5, the label is found to be continuously distributed in layer 4B and in layer 6 (Fig. 30.15). Even more striking is the V5–V2 re-entrant system. Here, as Fig. 30.15 shows, the fibres projecting from V5 to V2 are not restricted to the territory of the thick stripes in V2 but are also distributed in the thin stripes and the interstripes. In other words, the re-entrant projection from V5 to V2 is more divergent than that from V2 to V5 and can therefore influence the other submodalities, besides what is represented in the thick stripes. Double labelling studies on axonal bifurcation show that, in general return projections may be less submodality specific than the outward projections (Bullier & Kennedy, 1987).

Thus in V1, the distribution of the reverse projection from V5 (the re-entrant system) is tangentially asymmetric with respect to the forward projection, though restricted to the same layers. The re-entrant system into V2 has a more complex distribution. Whereas cells in V2 projecting to V5 are found predominantly in layers 2–3, with some in layer 5, the re-entrant system from V5 to V2 terminates most heavily in layers 1 and 6 and is least dense in layer 4. We thus refer to it as being layer and tangentially asymmetric. From which it follows that a re-entrant system may be asymmetric in more than one dimension. In fact, even within a given region, there may be profound asymmetries. For example, the re-entrant fibres from V5 to the thick stripes of V2 are not necessarily co-extensive with the distribution of labelled cells but are more widespread, thus being *zonally asymmetric*.

Such asymmetries have profound conse-

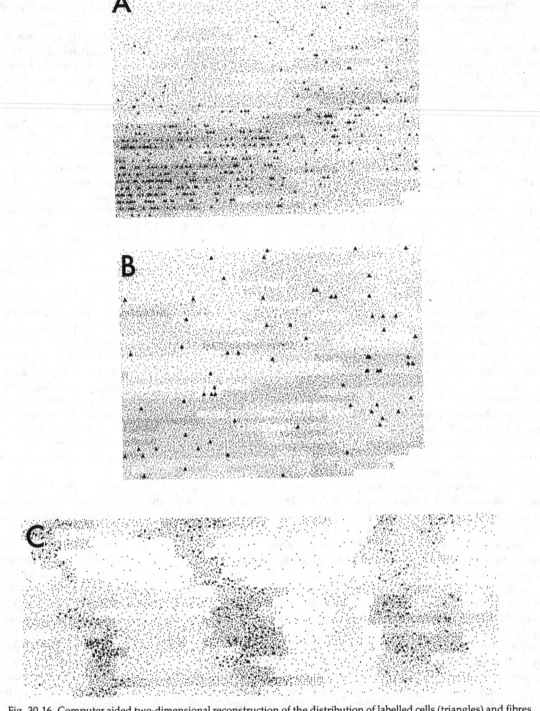

Fig. 30.16. Computer aided two-dimensional reconstruction of the distribution of labelled cells (triangles) and fibres (stipple) in areas V1 and V2 following an injection of HRP into area V5. The reconstructions are limited to small regions of the labelled zone of either area. A and B are reconstructions through layers 4B and 6 of V1, while C is a reconstruction of a small portion of V2 in the lunate sulcus. Note that in all three, the distribution of the prograde label is much wider than that of the orthograde label. Scale bar represents 2 mm.

quences. The tangential asymmetry of the V5–V1 re-entrant system enables V5 to communicate (a) with cells in layer 4B and layer 6 of V1 projecting to it and could thus satisfy, anatomically, the requirement that 'an internally generated signal is re-entered *as if it were an external signal*' (Edelman, 1978). We note here that the re-entrant system is a divergent one, onto an area (V1) with a high topographic precision (Daniel & Whitteridge, 1961), thus possibly enabling the re-entered signals to be referred to a correct spatial (topographic) distribution. However, this re-entrant system also enables V5 to communicate (b) with cells in layer 4B and layer 6 projecting elsewhere. It is known, for example, that layer 4B of V1 projects to V2 and V3, in addition to its projection to V5 (Rockland & Pandya, 1979; Lund *et al.*, 1975; Burkhalter *et al.*, 1986; Zeki, unpublished results). It follows that, at least anatomically, the re-entrant input from V5 can influence the signals from V1 to V3 *before the signals get there*. And given the divergent nature of the back projection, upon a cortical area with a precise topographic map, *it follows that internally generated motion signals can be re-entered onto another subdivision, based on the V3 complex, as if they were external signals*. Equally, the signals from V1 to V2 can also be influenced, or even modified, before they reach their destination in V2. We note that this mode of communication is in addition to the direct reciprocal mode existing between V3 and V5 and V2 and V5. But the V5–V2 re-entrant system also serves to unite the motion system with the parvocellular, chromatic system. Thus in addition to the thick stripes, the re-entrant input from V5 to V2 is also distributed to the thin stripes and the interstripes, the very ones projecting to V4 and containing the wavelength selective cells.

The above are but two, not very common but highly significant, examples of divergent re-entry. Much more common is the kind of reciprocal connection in which one area projects to another and receives a reciprocal input from it. But the forward and backward projections are usually not symmetrical in the sense of occupying the identical parts of the cortex. In general, the reciprocal connections are often so arranged as to exert minimal interference with the input to an area and a maximal influence on the results of its operations. Thus the input is separated from the output radially across the thickness of the cortex, or tangentially or both. A good example is the projection from V2 to V5 and the return projection. Here the return projection avoids layer 4, the layers that receive an input from V1, whereas the outward projection – which sends signals to V5 – is from upper and lower layers, the very ones that receive a re-entrant input

from V5. Although such asymmetries are common, it is notable that in many other instances, e.g. in the reciprocal projections between V5 and the frontal eye fields, the two sets of projections do coincide although there may be zonal asymmetries. Such re-entrant systems may have other functions, e.g. that of correcting eye positions continuously in pursuit of targets.

Re-entry turns out to be a neat device to solve several problems simultaneously, given the overriding importance of maintaining functional segregation in the cerebral cortex. It solves the difficult problem of the pyramid, inherent in repeated convergence leading to an executive area. It can unite information across submodalities, or sub-submodalities, as in the case of the regionally asymmetric V5–V2 re-entrant system, which goes across submodality divisions, or the V5–V1 re-entrant system. Thus functional groupings can be maintained indefinitely separate. It can, together with the operational system (see below), which is itself re-entrant, bring about a certain degree of functional integration, whereas the convergent system, as we have seen, seems not to achieve this and in any case could only do so by eradicating functional segregation at the site of convergence. Finally, it needs to be emphasized that re-entrant circuits, by allowing internally generated signals to be distributed into an area as if they were external signals, would be a powerful anatomical substratum for memory processes.

The operational connection

At early levels of the visual cortex, connections are 'point-to-point' and topographic. Notable examples are the projections from V1 to V2 and V3 (Zeki, 1969; Cragg, 1969). Although the projection from V1 to V5 is highly convergent (Zeki, 1971a), it is nevertheless topographic although the topography within V5 is much eroded compared to that in V1 or V2 (Zeki, 1974a; Ungerleider & Mishkin, 1980). In fact the projections from V1 to V2 are *functionally* topographic, in the sense that functional subgroups in V1 project specifically, and topographically, to their counterparts in V2. This has been shown by detailed anatomical studies, such as the ones of Livingstone & Hubel (1984).

If one were to make a large injection of WGA–HRP into V5, one would find considerable extents of the topographically equivalent regions of V1 or V2 labelled. By contrast, only a very narrow zone of V4 is labelled and this does not conform to a topographic or 'point-to-point' connection. Similarly, following injections of label into V6, only narrow zones of V3A or V5A are labelled, as if only small segments of the latter

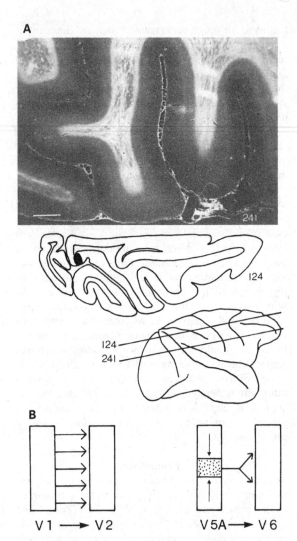

A

B

V 1 ⟶ V 2

V 5A ⟶ V 6

Fig. 30.17. A. Dark field photograph of the distribution of HRP in V5A (anterior bank of superior temporal sulcus) following an injection of WGA-HRP into area V6. In this case the distribution of label in some areas (e.g. V5 and FEF – see Fig. 30.8) was quite extensive while in V5A only a discrete projection zone was seen. Such a zonal connection may be an example of an operational connection – see below. Scale bar represents 2 mm. B. At early levels of the visual system connections are topographic. An example is the connection between V1 and V2, shown to the left. In the example, shown to the right, only a small portion of V5A is seen to connect with V6. Such a restricted pathway may form the basis of an operational connection whereby the results of operations performed by an area may be communicated to a small portion of it (perhaps by lateral connections) which then alone connects with another area.

are connected to V6. This leads us to the entirely speculative concept of an *operational connection* (Fig. 30.17). Here we suppose that although the integrity of the whole of V5 is necessary for it to execute its functions, not all the activity in V5 needs to be communicated to V4. Rather the results of activity in V5 may be internally communicated to one small region and it is this region alone which needs to communicate with V4, thus forming an operational rather than a topographic connection. Of course, in its distributive role, V5 may be sending different types of information to, say V4 and V6 and the results of different sets of operations, performed by the same area, may have different operational outputs. The fact that the outward and re-entrant projection from V5 to V4 are centred on the same geographic locality, although being asymmetric radially, merely serves to emphasize the fact that a re-entrant system is designed to have the maximal opportunity of (a) influencing the results of the operations performed by an area and (b) re-entering internally generated information as if it were an external signal.

The above is, of course, entirely speculative and would need to be rigorously tested experimentally. Indeed, the operational interpretation I have given above to the connections between V4 and V5 is not the only one. Another interpretation is given by Ungerleider & Desimone (1986). They suppose that the limited connections of V4 with V5 reflect the fact that only the relatively few directionally selective cells in the former (Zeki, 1977, 1978a; Desimone & Schein, 1987) need to be connected with the latter area. If that were so, one would still need to ask whether the V4–V5 connection is not of the operational variety. This is because some kind of activity in V4 – relevant to motion – must be channelled to the small regions of it containing directionally selective cells, which alone need to communicate with V5.

The concept of an operational output is, in fact, more general than the specific examples given above would imply. In a more general sense, let us suppose that a radial extent of cortex of diameter m receives an input into its layer 4 from area X and sends an output via its upper and lower layers to area Y. Area Y in turn sends a re-entrant input to the upper and lower layers of area X. Given the pronounced system of radial connections in the cortex, we suppose further that m acts as a 'unit' in the sense that whatever operation occurs in m depends upon the activity of all its layers. Yet the output is not from all layers. This is not a speculative example, but based upon the kind of connectivity shown by, for example, V1. It is far from clear how well the concept of an operational connection will withstand the experimental test. But it is intuitively appealing and there is some hint from the anatomy that such a system may be used by the cortex.

The nature of the anatomical connections between the motion, colour and form systems

With these categorizations in mind, we may now proceed to classify the anatomical connections between the form and motion and colour and motion systems (see Figs. 30.10 and 30.11). We use the terms form, motion and colour somewhat loosely. No area is quite pure in the sense of containing exclusively a single category of cell, a fact reflected in our choice of the term functional specialization rather than functional localization (Zeki, 1978a).

(A) *Direct.* Direct connections between V4 and V5 are one route for interactions between the colour and motion system (Fig. 30.10). Direct connections between the form and motion systems are found in the connections between V3 and V5, and V3A and V5 as well as in the connections between V3A and V6 (Fig. 30.11). The connections between V4 and V5 and V3A and V6 are not widespread and may be of the *operational variety*.

(B) *Convergent.* These are found in the common connections that V4 and V5 have to the intraparietal sulcus and, less prominently, to the inferior temporal cortex. The input to the former may be overlapping, but this is not known. The input to the latter from the two systems is not overlapping. Between the motion and form systems, *convergent* connections are found in the common inputs that V5, V5A and V3A have onto V6. There is also a common input from V3 and V3A on the one hand and V5, V5A and V6 on the other to the frontal eye fields (see Fig. 30.11).

(C) *Re-entrant connections* between the form and motion systems comprise (a) the re-entrant input from V5 to layer 4B of V1, which also projects to V3; (b) the re-entrant input from V5 to V2, which terminates mainly, but not exclusively, in the thick stripes, which also project to V3. The remaining connections of V5, V5A and V6 with V3 and V3A are reciprocal. Most of these connections are *patchy*, but some, consisting of one or two patches, may be of the *operational* variety. Re-entrant connections between the colour and motion systems are found in the prograde input from V5 to the thin stripes of V2.

Conclusion

The simple rules that I have enumerated above are almost certainly not the only ones of cortical connectivity and many other rules will be found in the future. Their significance lies in the fact that they are general rules of cortical connectivity, applicable to the areas of visual cortex dealing with motion just as much as to somato-sensory or auditory cortex. The presence of patchy, divergent and convergent connections, as well as re-entry, is a hallmark of most of cortex just as it is of visual cortex. There are exceptions which merit particular study precisely because they are so unique. Notable are the one way connections between SI and area 5 of parietal cortex and the supplementary motor area and the one way connection between SII and area 4 (Jones, 1984). But, in general, the fact that one can generalize those simple rules of connectivity, derived from a study of motion related visual cortex, to the cortex at large implies that the cortex uses a few versatile connectionist strategies repetitively to generate the infinite number of categories and repertoires of which it is capable.

Note

This article was completed in 1987 and has not been revised since. The attention of the reader is drawn to three papers published since then. Two of these contain a more detailed account of the connections of V5 with V1 and V2. They are S. Shipp & S. Zeki, 'The organization of connections between areas V5 and V1 in macaque monkey visual cortex', *Eur. J. Neurosci.*, **1**, 309–32 (1989) and 'The organization of connections between areas V5 and V2 in macaque monkey visual cortex', *Eur. J. Neurosci.*, **1**, 333–54 (1989). In addition, the classification of anatomical convergence has been altered slightly and this is described in greater detail in S. Zeki & S. Shipp, 'The functional logic of cortical connections', *Nature*, **335**, 311–16 (1988).

Acknowledgements

The author's work reported was supported by grants from The Science and Engineering Research Council and from the Wellcome Trust.

I thank Ray Guillery for his criticisms and improvements of an earlier version of the manuscript.

344   S. Zeki

References

Aicardi, G., Battaglini, P. P. & Galletti, C. (1987) The angle of gaze influences the responses to visual stimulation of cells in the V3-complex of macaque monkey visual cortex. *J. Physiol.*, **390**, 27P.

Albright, T. D. (1984) Direction and orientation selectivity of neurons in visual area MT of the macaque. *J. Neurophysiol.*, **52**, 1106–30.

Baizer, J. S. (1982) Receptive field properties of V3 neurons in monkey. *Invest Ophthal.*, **23**, 87–95.

Baizer, J. S., Robinson, D. L. & Dow, B. M. (1977) Visual responses of area 18 neurons in awake, behaving monkey. *J. Neurophysiol.*, **40**, 1024–37.

Barlow, H. B. (1981) The Ferrier Lecture. Critical limiting factors in the design of the eye and visual cortex. *Proc. Roy. Soc. Lond.*, **B212**, 1–34.

Barlow, H. B. & Levick, W. R. (1965) The mechanism of directionally selective units in rabbit retina. *J. Physiol. (Lond.)*, **178**, 477–504.

Blasdel, G. G. & Lund, J. S. (1983) Termination of afferent axons in macaque striate cortex. *J. Neurosci.*, **3**, 1389–413.

Blasdel, G. G., Lund, J. S. & Fitzpatrick, D. (1985) Intrinsic connections of macaque striate cortex: axonal projections of cells outside lamina 4C. *J. Neurosci.*, **5**, 3350–69.

Bullier, J. & Kennedy, H. (1987) Axonal bifurcation in the visual system. *T.I.N.S.*, **10**, 205–10.

Burkhalter, A., Felleman, D. J., Newsome, W. T. & Van Essen, D. C. (1986) Anatomical and physiological asymmetries related to visual area V3 and VP in macaque extrastriate cortex. *Vision Res.*, **26**, 63–80.

Covey, E., Gattass, R. & Gross, C. G. (1982) A new visual area in the parieto-occipital sulcus of the macaque. *Soc. Neurosci. Abs.*, **8**, 681.

Cragg, B. G. (1969) The topography of the afferent projections in circumstriate visual cortex of the monkey studied by the Nauta method. *Vision Res.*, **9**, 733–47.

Daniel, P. M. & Whitteridge, D. (1961) The representation of the visual field on the cerebral cortex in monkeys. *J. Physiol.*, **159**, 203–21.

Desimone, R., Fleming, J. & Gross, C. G. (1980) Prestriate afferents to inferior temporal cortex: an HRP study. *Brain Res.*, **184**, 41–55.

Desimone, R. & Schein, S. J. (1987) Visual properties of neurons in area V4 of the macaque: sensitivity to stimulus form. *J. Neurophysiol.*, **57**, 835–68.

Desimone, R., Schein, S. J., Moran, J. & Ungerleider, L. G. (1985) Contour, colour and shape analysis beyond the striate cortex. *Vision Res.*, **25**, 41–452.

Desimone, R. & Ungerleider, L. G. (1986). Multiple visual areas in the caudal superior temporal sulcus of the macaque. *J. Comp. Neurol.*, **248**, 164–89.

De Yoe, E. A. & Van Essen, D. C. (1985) Segregation of efferent connections and receptive field properties in visual area V2 of the macaque. *Nature*, **317**, 58–61.

Edelman, G. M. (1978) Group selection and phasic reentrant signalling: a theory of higher brain function. In *The Mindful Brain*, ed. G. M. Edelman & V. B. Mountcastle, pp. 55–100. Cambridge, Mass.: MIT Press.

Felleman, D. J. & Van Essen, D. C. (1987) Receptive field properties of neurons in area V3 of macaque monkey extrastriate cortex. *J. Neurophysiol.*, **57**, 889–920.

Fitzpatrick, D., Lund, J. S. & Blasdel, G. G. (1985) Intrinsic connections of macaque striate cortex: afferent and efferent connections of lamina 4C. *J. Neurosci.*, **5**, 3329–49.

Fries, W., Keizer, K. & Kuypers, H. G. J. M. (1985) Large layer VI cells in macaque striate cortex (Meynert cells) project to both superior colliculus and prestriate visual area V5. *Exp. Brain Res.*, **58**, 613–16.

Fries, W. & Zeki, S. (1983) The laminar origin of the cortical inputs to the fourth visual complex of macaque monkey cortex. *J. Physiol. (Lond.)*, **340**, S1P.

Gattass, R. & Gross, C. G. (1981) Visual topography of striate projection zone (MT) in posterior temporal sulcus. *J. Neurophysiol.*, **46**, 621–38.

Gilbert, C. D. & Kelly, J. P. (1975) The projections of cells in different layers of the cat's visual cortex. *J. Comp. Neurol.*, **163**, 81–106.

Goldmann-Rakic, P. S. (1984) Modular organisation of prefrontal cortex. *T.I.N.S.*, **7**, 419–29.

Hendrickson, A. E., Wilson, J. R. & Ogren, M. P. (1978) The neuroanatomical organisation of pathways between the dorsal lateral geniculate nucleus and visual cortex in old world and new world primates. *J. Comp. Neurol.*, **182**, 123–36.

Hubel, D. H. & Livingstone, M. S. (1985) Complex unoriented cells in a subregion of primate area 18. *Nature*, **315**, 325–7.

Hubel, D. H. & Wiesel, T. N. (1965) Receptive fields and functional architecture in two non-striate visual areas (18 and 19) of the cat. *J. Neurophysiol.*, **26**, 994–1002.

Hubel, D. H. & Wiesel, T. N. (1974) The Ferrier Lecture 1972. Functional architecture of macaque monkey visual cortex. *Proc. Roy. Soc. Lond.*, **B198**, 1–59.

Imig, T. J. & Reale, R. A. (1981) Patterns of cortico-cortical connections related to tonotopic maps in cat auditory cortex. *J. Comp. Neurol.*, **192**, 293–332.

Jen, L. S. & Zeki, S. (1983) High cytochrome oxidase content of the V5 complex of macaque monkey visual cortex. *J. Physiol.*, **348**, 23P.

Jones, E. G. (1984) Connectivity of the primate sensory motor cortex. In *Cerebral Cortex*, vol. 5, Sensory motor areas and aspects of cerebral connectivity, ed. E. G. Jones & A. Peters, pp. 113–83. New York: Plenum Press.

Jones, E. G. & Powell, T. P. S. (1970) An anatomical study of converging sensory pathways within the cerebral cortex of monkey. *Brain*, **14**, 793–820.

Livingstone, M. S. & Hubel, D. H. (1984) Anatomy and physiology of a color system in the primate visual cortex. *J. Neurosci.*, **4**, 309–56.

Livingstone, M. S. & Hubel, D. H. (1987) Connections

between layer 4B of area 17 and thick cytochrome oxidase strips of area 18 in the squirrel monkey. *J. Neurosci.*, **7**, 3371–7.

Lund, J. S. & Boothe, R. G. (1975) Interlaminar connections and pyramidal neuron organisation in the visual cortex, area 17 of the macaque monkey. *J. Comp. Neurol.*, **159**, 305–34.

Lund, J. S., Hendrickson, A. E., Ogren, M. P. & Tobin, E. A. (1981) Anatomical organization of primate visual cortex area VII. *J. Comp. Neurol.*, **202**, 19–45.

Lund, J. S., Lund, R. D., Hendrickson, A. E., Bunt, A. H. & Fuchs, A. F. (1975) The origin of efferent pathways from primary visual cortex (area 17) of the macaque monkey as shown by retrograde transport of horseradish peroxidase. *J. Comp. Neurol.*, **164**, 287–304.

Maunsell, J. H. R. & Van Essen, B. C. (1983) Connections of the middle temporal visual area (MT) and their relationship to a cortical hierarchy in the macaque monkey. *J. Neurosci.*, **3**, 2563–86.

Montero, V. M. (1980) Patterns of connections from the striate cortex to cortical visual areas in superior temporal sulcus of macaque and middle temporal gyrus of owl monkey. *J. Comp. Neurol.*, **189**, 45–59.

Phillips, C. G., Zeki, S. & Barlow, H. B. (1984) Localisation of function in the cerebral cortex. *Brain*, **107**, 327–61.

Poggio, G. F. (1985) Processing of stereoscopic information in primate visual cortex. In *Dynamic Aspects of Neocortical Function*, ed. G. M. Edelman, W. E. Gall & W. M. Cowan, pp. 613–36. New York: Wiley.

Poggio, G. F., Baker, F. H., Mansfield, R. J. W., Sillito, A. & Grigg, P. (1975) Spatial and chromatic properties of neurons subserving foveal and parafoveal vision in rhesus monkey. *Brain Res.*, **100**, 25–9.

Rockland, K. S. & Pandya, D. N. (1979) Laminar origins and terminations of cortical connections of the occipital lobe in the rhesus monkey. *Brain Res.*, **179**, 3–20.

Shipp, S. D. & Zeki, S. (1985) Segregation of pathways leading from area V2 to areas V4 and V5 of macaque monkey visual cortex. *Nature*, **315**, 322–5.

Tanaka, M., Hikosaka, K., Saito, H., Yukie, M., Fukada, Y. & Iwai, E. (1986) Analysis of local and wide-field movements in two superior temporal visual areas of the macaque monkey. *J. Neurosci.*, **6**, 134–44.

Ungerleider, L. G. & Desimone, R. (1986) Cortical connections of visual area MT in the macaque. *J. Comp. Neurol.*, **248**, 190–222.

Ungerleider, L. G. & Mishkin, M. (1980) The striate projection zone in the superior temporal sulcus of Macaca mulatta: location and topographic organisation. *J. Comp. Neurol.*, **188**, 347–66.

Ungerleider, L. G. & Mishkin, M. (1982) Two cortical visual systems. In *Analysis of Visual Behaviour*, ed. D. J. Ingle, M. A. Goodale & R. J. W. Mansfield, pp. 249–68. Cambridge, Mass: MIT Press.

Van Essen, D. C., Maunsell, J. H. R. & Bixby, J. L. (1981) The middle temporal visual area in the macaque: myeloarchitecture, connections, functional properties and topographic organisation. *J. Comp. Neurol.*, **199**, 293–326.

Van Essen, D. C., Newsome, W. T., Maunsell, J. H. R. & Bixby, J. L. (1986) The projections from striate cortex (V1) to areas V2 and V3 in the macaque monkey: asymmetries, areal boundaries and patchy connections. *J. Comp. Neurol.*, **244**, 451–80.

Wong-Riley, M. T. T. (1979) Changes in the visual system of monocularly sutured or enucleated cats demonstrable with cytochrome oxidase histochemistry. *Brain Res.*, **171**, 11–28.

Wurtz, R. H., Richmond, B. J. and Newsome, W. T. (1985) Modulation of cortical visual processing by attention, perception and movement. In *Dynamic Aspects of Neocortical Functions*, ed. G. M. Edelman, W. E. Gall & W. M. Cowan, pp. 195–217. New York: Wiley.

Yukie, M. & Iwai, E. (1985) Laminar origin of direct projection from cortex area V1 to V4 in the rhesus monkey. *Brain Res.*, **346**, 383–6.

Zeki, S. (1969) Representation of central visual fields in prestriate cortex of monkeys. *Brain Res.*, **14**, 271–91.

Zeki, S. (1971a) Convergent input from the striate cortex (area 17) to the cortex of the superior temporal sulcus in the rhesus monkey. *Brain Res.*, **28**, 338–40.

Zeki, S. (1971b) Cortical projections from two prestriate areas in the monkey. *Brain Res.*, **34**, 19–35.

Zeki, S. M. (1974a) Functional organisation of a visual area in the posterior bank of the superior temporal sulcus in the rhesus monkey. *J. Physiol. (Lond.)*, **236**, 549–73.

Zeki, S. M. (1974b) The mosaic organization of the visual cortex in the monkey. In *Essays on the Nervous System*: A Fetschrift for Professor J. Z. Young, ed. R. Bellairs & E. G. Gray. Oxford: Clarendon Press.

Zeki, S. M. (1975) The functional organisation of projections from striate to prestriate visual cortex in the rhesus monkey. *Cold Spring Harb. Symp. quant. Biol.*, **40**, 591–600.

Zeki, S. (1976) The projections to the superior temporal sulcus from areas 17 and 18 in the rhesus monkey. *Proc. Roy. Soc. Lond.*, B**193**, 199–207.

Zeki, S. (1977) Colour coding in the superior temporal sulcus of rhesus monkey visual cortex. *Proc. Roy. Soc. Lond.* B**197**, 195–223.

Zeki, S. (1978a) Uniformity and diversity of structure and function in rhesus monkey prestriate visual cortex. *J. Physiol. (Lond.)*, **277**, 273–90.

Zeki, S. (1978b) The third visual complex of rhesus monkey prestriate cortex. *J. Physiol. (Lond.)*, **277**, 245–72.

Zeki, S. (1980) The response of cells in the anterior bank of the superior temporal sulcus in macaque monkeys. *J. Physiol.*, **308**, 85P.

Zeki, S. (1983) The distribution of wavelength and orientation selective cells in different areas of monkey visual cortex. *Proc. Roy. Soc. Lond.*, B**217**, 449–90.

Zeki, S. (1986) The anatomy and physiology of area V6 of macaque monkey visual cortex. *J. Physiol.*, **381**, 62P.

31

Interactions between motion, depth, color and form: the utilitarian theory of perception

God is a hacker
Francis Crick (1987)

V. S. Ramachandran

Introduction: theories of perception

If you examine the history of ideas on perception during the last century or so you will notice that there have been three major trends in thinking:

(1) Perception as unconscious inference. This view emphasizes that the visual image is inherently ambiguous and that the perceptual apparatus resolves ambiguities by using 'intelligent' processes that *resemble* conscious reasoning. The idea was originally put forward by Helmholtz (1867) and has more recently been revived by Gregory (1970) and Rock (1983).

(2) Direct perception. Emphasizes the richness of the visual input and argues that ambiguity exists only in contrived laboratory situations but not in the 'real world'. A vast amount of information is implicit in the visual image and perception is achieved not by making this information explicit but by direct 'resonance'. Unfortunately, it is never clearly specified how or where in the brain this resonance is supposed to occur.

(3) Natural computation – or the AI approach: is an attempt to bridge (1) and (2) through formal modelling. One begins by rigorously specifying the computational problem that confronts the organism and then one develops a computational theory and a set of algorithms to tackle the problem. Information that is only *implicit* in the retinal image is transformed (through computation) into *representations* that make certain aspects of the information more explicit and accessible for further computation. This view is similar to (1) in that it argues that a knowledge of the statistics of the natural world is indispensable for computing representations and it is also similar to (2) in emphasiz-ing the richness of the visual input. However, it is different from (1) in that it takes advantage of constraints that incorporate general properties of the world rather than 'top-down' influences that depend on high-level semantic knowledge of specific objects. Thus the visual system may have built-in knowledge about surfaces, depth, movement, etc., but not about umbrellas, chairs and dalmation dogs.

Problems with the computational approach

The main strength of the computational approach to vision is that it leads to a much more rigorous formulation of perceptual problems than does psychophysics or physiology alone (Marr, 1982; Ullman, 1979). However, one must beware of three major pitfalls and I shall consider each of these in turn. First, as any biologist knows, simulation of a complex biological system does not guarantee a complete understanding of how the system actually works. As an example, consider the many different kinds of devices that can be used to measure the passage of time. One can use pulse beats, hour glasses, sundials, clepsydras, pendulums, and these days, even digital watches and atomic clocks. All these gadgets are solving the same 'computational' problem – measuring time – yet even the principles underlying their operation are very different from each other. Furthermore, the biological clock inside our brains that allows us to measure the passage of time probably does not even remotely resemble any of these devices! This is something we have to bear in mind constantly when studying biological systems – that they may in fact use mechanisms that are quite different from the ones envisaged by theoreticians.

A second, less obvious problem with the computational approach to vision is that it ignores the evolutionary history of biological systems. Nature is inherently opportunistic and will often adopt some very curious – even bizarre – solutions to its problems, especially when it has to make use of pre-existing hardware. To appreciate this point, consider the three tiny bones in our middle ear which are used to amplify sounds. In the reptilian antecedents of mammals these same three bones constitute part of the hinge mechanism of the lower jaw, used for chewing food. Thus what was originally part of the reptilian lower jaw used for mastication, has now been incorporated into the mammalian middle ear to be used in hearing! No engineer in his right mind would have come up with such an inelegant solution. The only reason Nature adopted it was because it was available and it worked. It is perhaps not inconceivable that the same sort of thing may have happened time and again in the evolution of visual mechanisms in the neocortex.

The third major dogma of AI has been that the neural hardware that mediates perception is not especially relevant or important. One recalls, especially, Marr's point that any complex information processing system can be studied at three different levels: the level of the 'computational problem', the level of algorithms and the level of hardware implementation. According to Marr, since any given computational problem can be tackled by many different algorithms and any given algorithm can by implemented in different kinds of hardware, these different levels of description must be kept quite separate and we must be very careful not to get confused between them.

While I do not disagree with Marr's basic argument, I would like to suggest that when dealing with complex *biological* systems the only sure way to progress is to deliberately get 'confused' between these different levels of analysis, i.e. one must deliberately make what orthodox philosophers would call 'category mistakes' (Ryle, 1949). The reason for this is that the organization of biological systems is dictated just as much by constraints of hardware (and by the organism's evolutionary history) as by the 'computational problem'. For example, consider the manner in which the elucidation of the double-helix structure of DNA led to the subsequent understanding both of heredity (through gene duplication) and of the specification of an organism's phenotype (through gene expression by transcription and translation), even though molecules and heredity obviously belong to very different conceptual (and semantic) categories. It is also worth reflecting on the fact that in this case knowledge of function *followed* naturally from knowledge of structure and not the other way around (resulting in Francis

Crick's famous dictum that if you do not make headway understanding the functions of a complex system, then study its structure, and knowledge of function will follow automatically!).

Perception as a 'bag of tricks:' the Utilitarian Theory of perception

Based on these considerations I would like to replace the three theories of perception I outlined earlier with a fourth theory of perception which I call the 'Utilitarian Theory'. According to this view perception does not involve intelligent reasoning as implied by some psychologists; does not involve resonance with the world as suggested by Gibsonians; and does not require creating elaborate internal representation or solving equations as implied by AI researchers. One could argue, instead, that perception is essentially a 'bag of tricks'; that through millions of years of trial and error the visual system has evolved numerous short-cuts, rules-of-thumb and heuristics which were adopted not for their aesthetic appeal or mathematical elegance but simply because they *worked* (hence the 'utilitarian' theory). This is a familiar idea in biology but for some reason it seems to have escaped the notice of psychologists who seem to forget that the brain is a biological organ just like the pancreas, the liver, or any other specialized organ. The digestion of food, for example, is not brought about by computation, by intelligent deduction, nor even by resonance. The system uses an arbitrary set of special-purpose tricks (e.g. mastication, peristalsis, sequential cleavage by enzymes, specific satiety signals, etc.) that are tailor-made for achieving a step-by-step denudation of food into easily absorbed constituents. Further, the strategies used are different for different kinds of food and at different points along the gastrointestinal tract (and in different animals). It may not be too farfetched to suggest that the visual system also uses an equally bewildering array of special-purpose tailor-made tricks and heuristics to solve its problems. If this pessimistic view of perception is correct, then the task of vision researchers ought to be to uncover these rules rather than to attribute to the system a degree of sophistication that it simply does not possess. Seeking overarching principles may be an exercise in futility.

One example of such a 'trick' is the use of ethological releasers or trigger-features for mediating certain types of visual behavior. Consider, for instance, the food begging behavior of newly hatched herring gull chicks when they encounter their mother. This behavior is elicited by specific releasing stimuli; the chick will not peck at (say) a pig or a peacock. Now an AI researcher watching this behavior might conclude that the way in which the chick's visual system goes about distinguishing its mother from pigs and peacocks is by creating eleborate internal representations for these creatures. Yet if he were to simply remove an adult seagull beak and wave it in front of the chick while holding it vertically the chick will peck quite vigorously – *more* vigorously than it would to a complete adult seagull with its beak painted (say) white. In fact, even a beak is not necessary – a narrow strip of cardboard with a yellow band will suffice. (The band mimics the yellow spot found on the lower bill of the mother bird.) Thus the chick distinguishes its mother from pigs by the mere presence of 'a yellow spot on an oblong vertical object'. This, of course, makes it very easy to fool the chick in the laboratory; it will respond even to a pig if a stick with a yellow spot is simply attached to the animal's snout. But it also makes the chick's visual system nearly infallible *in nature* since oblong objects with yellow spots almost always occur in conjunction with mother seagulls; the chick is highly unlikely to encounter mutant pigs with beaks!

I have used this analogy to illustrate the point that the visual system will often discard vast amounts of information and will use only what is absolutely essential for the job at hand. Notice that in this example it would be highly misleading to say that the chick's visual system was creating representations of gulls and pigs. A much more accurate statement would be that the system uses a simple diagnostic sign (the yellow spot) to identify its mother. The central claim of the utilitarian theory of perception is, quite simply, that *all* of perception is based on this general principle. At the risk of seeming frivolous, I will suggest that one could even think of the various extrastriate visual areas as being analogous to several gull chicks each of which generates the appropriate behavior or percept in response to a set of diagnostic signs in the visual image.

But can all the richness and clarity of human vision be explained by a set of relatively simple mechanisms of the kind used by the gull chick? In trying to answer this question we must bear two things in mind. First, much of vision seems to be concerned only with determining the general spatial layout of objects in the world and, consequently, what is needed most of the time is a qualitative rather than detailed quantitative description of the visual scene. And second, for any given perceptual task the system probably uses not one, but a whole repertoire of gimmicks. Each of these is relatively crude and, consequently, easily fooled in the laboratory. In the natural world, however, they are always used collectively and this enables the visual system to achieve the same high level of apparent sophistication that it could by using a single sophisticated algorithm. What I will try to do in the rest of this article is to provide some empirical evidence for this view by considering two problems: the correspondence problem in motion perception and the problem of recovering the three-dimensional structure of moving objects.

The correspondence problem

How does the visual system match successive views of a moving object to generate an impression of smooth continuous movement? Consider a leopard leaping from branch to branch while chasing one of our arboreal ancestors. How does the visual system know which spot in any given 'view' or 'snapshot' of the leopard corresponds to which spot in the immediately succeeding view?

There have been several approaches to this problem in the past and a particularly ingenious one was introduced by Ullman (1979). He suggests that the visual system tries all possible combinations of matches between the dots and, through successive iterations, arrives at the match which yields the *minimum* total distance. This match is chosen as the solution to the correspondence problem.

Contrary to this view, I would like to suggest that in solving the correspondence problem the visual system actually throws away all the information about the individual dots and resorts to the use of a short-cut or 'trick' which I call 'motion capture'. Figure 31.1 illustrates this effect. Two sparse, uncorrelated random dot patterns were alternated to generate random incoherent noise or 'snowfall' (as in a detuned TV set). A sine-wave grating of low frequency and low contrast was then optically superimposed on this display. Notice that the grating is displaced horizontally in frame 2 in relation to frame 1. When the two frames were alternated the grating appeared to jump left and right as one would expect. But to our surprise we found that all the dots in the display also appeared to jump horizontally along with the grating – as though they were 'captured' by it. Motion capture was not seen if (a) the spatial frequency of the grating was too high (Ramachandran & Inada, 1985) or (b) if the excursion of the grating was small in relation to dot density (Ramachandran & Cavanagh, 1987).

We attempted to measure these effects by using two displays similar to Fig. 31.1 presented simultaneously, one below the other. The top panel was identical to Fig. 31.1 but in the bottom panel the

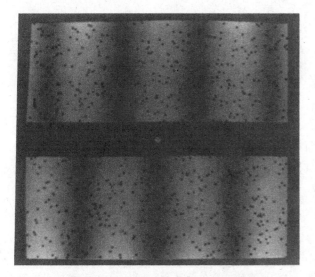

Fig. 31.1. Two frames of an apparent motion sequence. The frames are shown one below the other for clarity but in the original experiment they were optically superimposed and alternated. Even though the dots are uncorrelated in successive frames, they are seen to 'adhere' to the grating and to move with it as a single sheet. In the absence of the grating the dots are simply seen to swirl around incoherently.

dots in the 2 frames were *correlated* in successive frames and they were made to jump horizontally along with the grating. The subjects' task was to gradually reduce the excursion of both gratings until he could just discriminate the two panels (Fig. 31.2). We found that, over a surprisingly wide range of displacement, subjects could not see the difference between the two panels, i.e. they could not discriminate dots which were *captured* by the grating from dots which actually moved physically along with the grating.

These results suggest that unambiguous motion signals derived from certain coarse image features mask or *inhibit* the signals from the finer image features – a process that serves to eliminate spurious motion signals. However, the inhibition of motion signals from the finer features does not cause them to appear stationary; they are in fact seen to jump along with the coarse features. This suggests that when there are no motion signals from some frequency bands and strong signals from another (lower frequency) band, the signal from the latter is spontaneously attributed to the former.

Motion capture with illusory contours

Our next experiment shows that other types of 'features' can also generate motion capture. We began with two illusory squares presented in an appropriately timed sequence to generate apparent motion of an illusory surface (Fig. 31.3; note that the discs themselves do not move). In this motion sequence most subjects perceive an opaque oscillating square that occludes and disoccludes the discs in the background; they never report seeing 'pacmen' opening and closing their mouths or two illusory squares flashing on and off. When a template of this movie was then projected on a regular grid of dots, the dots appeared to move with the illusory surface even though they were physically stationary (Fig. 31.4). Since there is no evidence that the dots have not moved, the brain assumes, by default, that they have jumped with the illusory square (Ramachandran, 1985a, 1986).

These results suggest a simple solution to the correspondence problem. The question posed by AI researchers is: how does the visual system 'know' which spot in any given snapshot of the leopard belongs to which spot in the succeeding snapshot? Our answer is that the visual system simply does not *care*. It extracts motion signals from certain conspicuous features (e.g. the leopard's outline) and these signals are blindly attributed to the spots themselves so that they appear to move with the leopard. In doing this the visual system discards enormous amounts of information about the positions of the individual spots – just as the gull chick throws away information about all features on its mother except the beak. The advantage with this strategy is that it reduces the computational burden on the visual system by eliminating the need to keep track of individual spots on the leopard. The disadvantage is that the system would be 'blind' to small local excursions of the dots. For instance, if the leopard were to smile as he jumped on you, you probably would not notice this but this is a small price to pay if you are trying to run away from him!

Notice that the visual system can afford to use this trick or 'short-cut' only because in the real world spots do not usually fly off leopards. But my point is that although the visual system *takes advantage* of this 'constraint' it does not make very specific or sophisticated use of it. In general, it looks as though the human visual system will do as little processing as it can get away with *for the job on hand* – and in this respect it is no different from the seagull chick. There may, of course, be other visual functions which do require the use of individual dot motions – e.g. motion hyper-acuity or image segmentation from motion –

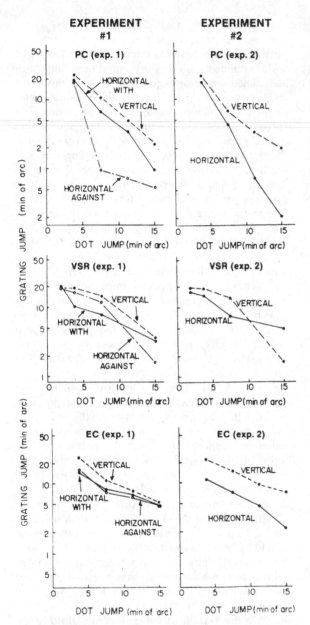

EXPERIMENT #1

EXPERIMENT #2

PC (exp. 1)

HORIZONTAL WITH

VERTICAL

HORIZONTAL AGAINST

PC (exp. 2)

VERTICAL

HORIZONTAL

VSR (exp. 1)

VERTICAL

HORIZONTAL WITH

HORIZONTAL AGAINST

VSR (exp. 2)

VERTICAL

HORIZONTAL

EC (exp. 1)

VERTICAL

HORIZONTAL WITH

HORIZONTAL AGAINST

EC (exp. 2)

VERTICAL

HORIZONTAL

GRATING JUMP (min of arc)

DOT JUMP (min of arc)

Fig. 31.2. Results of two experiments on motion capture (Ramachandran & Cavanagh, 1987). In Experiment 1, dots in one field were uncorrelated in successive frames and in the other field they were correlated and displaced horizontally (solid line) or vertically (dotted line). A vertical sine-wave grating of 1 c/deg and 40% contrast was superimposed on both fields. Subject's task was to gradually reduce the displacement of the grating until the dots were released from capture so that the two fields became discriminable. Above and to the right of the graph the dots were captured and the two fields were

but those systems, in their turn, would be insensitive to the overall direction of motion of the whole object; a function mediated by the long-range motion system. Which system is dominant at any given instant is dictated by the velocity of the moving object and by the immediate behavioral demands on the organism. When the leopard is standing still the visual system

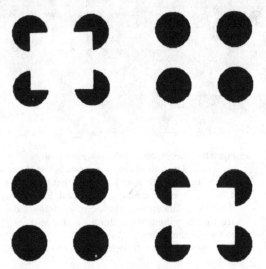

Fig. 31.3. Apparent motion of an illusory square (Ramachandran, 1985a). The two frames of the movie are shown one below the other for clarity, but in the original experiment they were optically superimposed so that the discs were in perfect registration. One has the vivid impression of an opaque illusory surface that jumps left and right while covering (and uncovering) the black discs in the background. Note that all eight discs are present in each frame so that the discs themselves do not move.

indiscriminable. (Each datum point is the mean of four readings.) Note that vertical dot motion is more difficult to capture. Horizontal motion of the correlated dot field in the same direction as the grating (WITH) does not appear to be either easier or harder to capture than motion in the opposite direction (AGAINST). In Experiment 2 the dots were always correlated in successive frames both above and below the central divider. The grating moved in the same direction in both fields but the dots moved in opposite directions. For instance, for vertical dot motion (evenly interrupted line) the dots in the two fields moved either simultaneously towards or away from the central dividing strip. As in Experiment 1, subjects reduced the grating displacement until they could just discriminate the two fields.

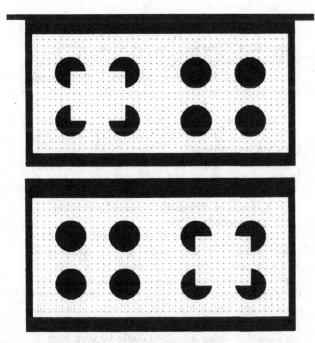

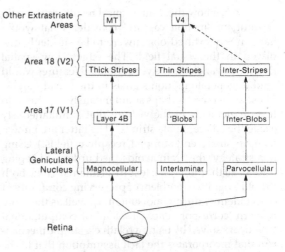

Fig. 31.5. Three parallel channels in the primate geniculo-cortical pathway (after Ramachandran, 1987a). This diagram summarizes information from many sources including Van Essen (1985) and Hubel & Livingstone (1985). For clarity we have left out the relay through layer 4C. Also, the degree of segregation between the channels is somewhat controversial (Schiller, Logothetis & Charles, 1990).

Fig. 31.4. A 'template' of the movie described in Fig. 31.3 is superimposed on vertical rows of dots. The dots are present in both frames and are exactly superimposed on each other so that they can generate no movement signals of their own. However, when the illusory square jumps, all the dots corresponding to its surface appear to jump with it as a single solid sheet – an example of a class of illusions that we call motion capture (Ramachandran, 1985a; Ramachandran & Inada, 1985). The motion of the illusory surface spontaneously generalizes to the dots contained within its boundaries. The reader can view this illusion by using computer software (Apple floppy disc), provided with the recent special issue of the journal *Perception* (London) 1985; Vol. 14 on human motion perception. The disc is included inside the back cover of that journal.

can afford a leisurely inspection of the local movements that define his smile but if he decides to leap at you; the long range system takes over to signal the overall direction of movement (and velocity) of the animal as he approaches you.

Physiological considerations

Are there any specific physiological mechanisms that might help account for 'motion capture'?

Figure 31.5 illustrates the flow of information in the primate visual system. It is a summary of the anatomical and electrophysiological work of Hubel & Livingstone (1985), DeYoe & Van Essen (1985) and Shipp & Zeki (1985). To simplify the diagram we have deliberately left out some of the relays in layer 4. Notice that there are three parallel pathways or 'streams' which are segregated all the way from the lateral geniculate nucleus (LGN) to the visual areas beyond area 18. Physiological recodings from the cells at various points along these pathways reveal that they have very different stimulus requirements. The magnocellular stream, which relays through layer 4B in area 17 and terminates in the broad stripes of area 18 (as well as area MT) is dominated by cells tuned to stereoscopic disparity as well as direction of movement. These cells will respond only to contours defined by luminance contrast and are insensitive to chromatic borders at equiluminance. Cells in the thin stripes of area 18, on the other hand, respond well to chromatic borders. Unlike the broad stripe cells, however, they have circular receptive fields and are insensitive to direction, disparity, and orientation. And, lastly, cells in the 'pale stripes' or interstripes of area 18 are found to be indifferent to disparity and direction of movement but are sharply tuned to *line-length*; i.e. they will respond only to line segments of finite length. Their exact role in vision is unclear but it has been suggested that they may be involved in the early stages of shape, curvature or 'form' recognition (Hubel & Livingstone, 1985) or in the perception of visual *texture* (Ramachandran, 1987a).

To see how these anatomical results might help account for 'motion capture' consider what would happen if a textured object were to be suddenly displaced in the visual field. The edges, low spatial frequencies and other as yet undefined features would tend to generate motion signals in the broad stripes. These signals are perhaps spontaneously attributed to texture elements in the vicinity that simultaneously excite the adjacent pale stripes. (The latter are known to have small, end-stopped receptive fields.) Using this strategy, the brain avoids the burden of keeping track of all the individual texture elements. Thus, both the old 'cognitive' problem of preserving continuity of object identity during movement, as well as the more modern 'correspondence problem' of computational vision, are solved by using a relatively simple mechanism that incorporates the tacit assumption that in the real world textures tend to adhere to objects.

Reduction of motion perception at equiluminance

The anatomical scheme presented above also leads to several other counter-intuitive predictions. Consider a red object moving against a green background. If one were to carefully match the luminance of red and green areas, the moving red-green border would no longer be able to excite the direction selection cells in the broad bands and consequently one should no longer be able to see the object moving! We had originally intended to use 'real' movement of a red object on a green background to test this prediction directly but decided that this would not work because even if the sensation of movement disappeared one might still be able to 'infer' movement at some higher level. Since the object was changing position from moment to moment one might be able to *deduce* that it had moved even if one did not actually experience movement directly. To circumvent this problem we used random-dot kinematograms which eliminate positional cues. We began with two random-dot patterns which were identical (point-to-point) except for a central square shaped matrix which was shifted in the second pattern in relation to the first. We then superimposed the two patterns so that the background dots were in exact registration and then presented them in rapid alternation. The central square was seen to oscillate horizontally as a result of apparent motion. Next, we repeated the experiment using red dots on a green background (instead of black on white) and found that at equiluminance the impression of movement disappeared. This suggests that the motion-perception is at least partially 'color-blind' as predicted from the neuroanatomy (Ramachandran & Gregory, 1978).

These results raise an interesting question. In the real world when a red object moves across a green background we do see it moving – not standing still. Presumably motion signals are extracted mainly from the incidental luminance differences that usually accompany the chromatic border but if this is true why does one also see the *chromatic* border moving? Or, to put it differently, when a colored object moves, how is such perfect perceptual synchrony maintained between the chromatic and luminance borders if it is indeed here that they are being extracted separately? Our next experiment addresses this issue.

Capture of chromatic borders by moving luminance borders

A red square subtending 1° was displayed against an equiluminous homogeneous green background. When a sparse pattern of small black dots was superimposed on the square and moved up and down the square appeared to move in the same direction even though it was physically stationary. The illusion was especially pronounced on eccentric fixation; when we fixated 3° away the effect could be seen even for excursions up to one degree (Ramachandran, 1987b).

This result suggests that chromatic borders can be 'captured' by moving luminance contours in a manner analogous to the capture of texture elements. The curious implication is that if you were to superimpose two identical motion pictures on the screen, one of which had moving luminance edges alone and the other had only equiluminous chromatic edges, then if a deliberate time lag was introduced between the two movies, the visual system would not notice the difference! Figure 31.6 shows that although the illusion can be seen to some extent even when the two regions are not exactly equiluminous, optimum capture does in fact occur at equiluminance. We may conclude that, whenever a colored object is displaced in the visual field, motion signals are extracted primarily from the luminance borders (by the magnocellular pathway) and then blindly applied to chromatic borders that happen to excite the adjacent thin stripes. This ensures perfect perceptual synchrony of color and 'form' as the object moves through space.

Perceptual coupling of motion and stereoscopic disparity

In the previous section we noted that motion detecting cells in the visual pathways of primates are clearly segregated from cells which respond to chromatic borders. The separation of movement sensitive cells from cells turned to stereoscopic disparity, on the other hand, is not quite as clear cut; in fact, MT contains cells which are tuned to both these dimen-

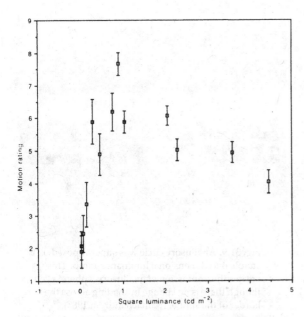

Fig. 31.6. Optimum capture occurs when the red square is approximately equiluminous with the surround. Note however that some illusory movement was seen even when luminance-contrast was present (especially when the red square was brighter). Each datum point is based on 800 readings (11 subjects). Background luminance, 0.87 cd m^{-2}. In this experiment we used motion of an illusory square (rather than motion of random dots) to generate capture (Ramachandran, 1987b).

sions. One perceptual consequence of this might be the close coupling between stereopsis and motion observed by Ramachandran & Anstis (1986). They presented two vertically aligned spots in Frame 1 of an apparent motion sequence followed by two spots shifted horizontally (Fig. 31.7). The spots were always seen to jump horizontally and were never seen to cross paths (Kolers, 1972; Ullman, 1979) even if diagonally opposite pairs were made similar in color or 'form'. However, if two diagonally opposite corner dots were in a separate stereoscopic plane from the other two the dots did cross paths (Ramachandran & Anstis, 1986; Ramachandran, Anstis & Rogers, 1987) (Fig. 31.8A). This was especially true if several such displays were viewed simultaneously (Fig. 31.8B). We may conclude from this result that there is a close linkage in the brain between motion and stereoscopic disparity but not between motion and other stimulus features such as color and 'form' – a conclusion that is consistent with the anatomical results of Hubel & Livingstone (1985).

Unfortunately, not all psychophysical results support this simple scheme. For example, Ramachan-

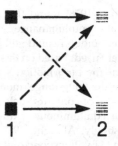

Fig. 31.7. Two vertically aligned dots are flashed in Frame 1 (solid black dots) and followed by two spots shifted horizontally in Frame 2 (grey cross-hatched dots). Horizontal distance between dots was 0.6°. The spots never cross each other's paths (dotted lines) but always move horizontally (solid arrows). Even if diagonally opposite pairs are made similar in color or 'form' crossing never occurs.

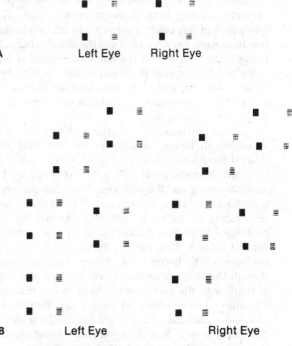

Fig. 31.8. A. A stereogram constructed using two displays similar to Fig. 31.7. Diagonally opposite pairs now occupy slightly different depth planes and this permits the dots to cross each other's trajectories. Grey (cross-hatched) dots appear in Frame 2. B. The tendency to cross can be greatly enhanced by simply viewing multiple displays such as Fig. 31.8A simultaneously. The use of multiple displays seems to amplify small pre-attentive affinities in apparent motion (Ramachandran, Anstis & Rogers, 1987). Subjects now report seeing two lacy planes of dots 'crossing' each other.

dran & Gregory (1978) found that although motion was lost at equiluminance in random-dot kinematograms, motion could still be seen if simple line targets were used. Based on this observation they suggested that the *early* motion system was 'color-blind' but that the 'long-range' motion system can in fact use any type of contours such as chromatic contours or even equiluminous texture borders as an input. Interestingly, Albright (1987) has shown that certain cells in MT will respond quite well to apparent motion of equiluminous texture borders of the kind used by Ramachandran *et al.* (1973) in their psychophysical experiments. It might be interesting to see if these cells would also respond to apparent motion that is based on chromatic borders.

Derivation of shape-from-shading

Consider a ping-pong ball (or any other spherical Lambertian surface) illuminated on one side by parallel rays arising from a single light source. The luminance of this object's surface falls off as a cosine function as one moves away from the illuminated pole towards the 'equator'. If the illumination and reflectance are held constant, it is possible to calculate surface slant by using the variations in luminance alone and various computer algorithms have been proposed for doing this.

Does the human visual system also make use of variations in image intensity in this manner? We created the display shown in Fig. 31.9 to answer this question (Ramachandran, 1988). It was produced by superimposing an 'illusory' circle on a simple one-dimensional luminance-ramp. The region corresponding to the circle initially looks flat but on prolonged inspection it takes on the appearance of a distinct bulge and may even pinch itself off from the background to become an illusory 'sphere' even though the shading in this region is physically continuous with the background! Also, notice that the curvature is seen along all axes even though the luminance gradient exists along the vertical axis alone. The implication is that the *segmentation boundary* that delineates an object from its background can powerfully influence the processing of shading information. If the visual system were making detailed measurements of shading to recover surface orientation there would be no basis for seeing a 'sphere' in this image since the shading does not change abruptly across the border of the sphere. What the system seems to arrive at is merely a *qualitative* description of a sphere and this is quite different from saying that it computes surface orientation by using variations in luminance. Later we

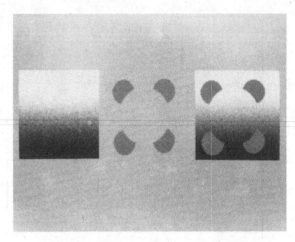

Fig. 31.9. An illusory circle was superimposed on a simple one-dimensional luminance-ramp. This creates the impression of an illusory 'sphere' even though there is no change in shading across the border of the sphere (Ramachandran, 1988).

shall see how these principles may also apply to the problem of recovering the three-dimensional (3-D) structure-from-motion.

The aperture problem

A question of considerable theoretical interest is the so-called 'aperture problem' which arises when a grating (or even a single line) is moved behind a circular aperture so that its ends are not visible (Adelson & Movshon, 1982; Hildreth, 1984). The retinal image motion produced by the line is in fact compatible with a whole family of velocities and directions; a local motion detector (or a human observer) has no way of distinguishing between motions in the directions A, B and C in Fig. 31.10. In the absence of other information observers usually see motion in a direction orthogonal to the grating (arrow B in Fig. 31.10).

If the circular path of grating shown in Fig. 31.11 is viewed through a narrow rectangular window, however, one always sees the grating moving horizontally instead of obliquely (Fig. 31.11A). The 'terminators' of the lines now move unambiguously in the horizontal direction and perhaps the motion signals derived from these are used to resolve ambiguities in the rest of the image. (This would be analogous to motion capture.) This is the usual explanation given for the so-called 'barber pole' illusion – the tendency to see the stripes of a barber pole moving vertically instead of horizontally.

What would happen if the occluder looked

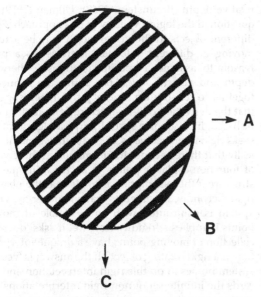

Fig. 31.10. The 'aperture problem' which arises when
a grating moves behind a circular aperture. The
retinal image motion, produced by this stimulus, is
compatible with a whole family of different directions
and velocities (e.g. arrows A, B, and C). Observers
usually see motion at right angles to the grating; i.e.
the percept corresponding to arrow B.

transparent instead of opaque (Fig. 31.11B)? The entire
circular patch of grating was now visible through the
occluder which was made to look transparent by
adjusting luminance ratios within different regions of
the display. The display conveyed the distinct
impression of a circular transluscent glass plate from
which a horizontal window has been removed. The
grating now appeared to move obliquely again and
horizontal motion was no longer visible (Ramachandran & Rogers-Ramachandran, 1989). Perhaps the
visual system no longer regards the ends of the lines
inside the window as 'terminators' since they appear
perceptually continuous with the lines behind the
transparent occluder.

Previous research on stationary stimuli has
revealed that the perception of transparency mimics
the *physics* transparency to a remarkable extent;
transparency is seen only if the luminance ratios of
different regions within the display are adjusted so as
to be compatible with a physically transparent surface
(Beck, 1986). We therefore varied the luminance contrast of the grating outside the aperture so that the
'occluder' no longer looked transparent (Fig. 31.11C).
Remarkably this procedure once again restored the
impression of unambiguous horizontal motion. The

observation suggests that the motion mechanism
must have access to a great deal of tacit 'knowledge'
about the physics of transparency. It strains the
imagination to think of why (or how) such a sophisticated mechanism could have evolved given that
transparent objects are not a very common occurrence
in nature.

These findings also suggest an obvious physiological experiment. Certain cells in the middle
temporal area (MT) of primates are known to show
strong direction selective responses to moving gratings. Would these cells also display a sensitivity to
transparency? If the cells 'classical' receptive fixed
were to fall entirely within the central rectangular
aperture, would it respond differently to Figs. 31.10,
31.11A and 31.11B? Indeed, the same question could
even by asked of an 'end stopped' hypercomplex-type
cell in V1 or V2. Would such a cell be inhibited by the
long lines in Fig. 31.11B but respond vigorously to the
short lines in Fig. 31.11C?

Recovering 3-D structure-from-motion (SFM): some new constraints

A topic that has received a great deal of attention
recently is the problem of how we recover the 3-D
structure of moving objects. Consider the two-dimensional parallel projection of a rotating transparent 3-D
cylinder with dots on its surface. The dots describe
parallel horizontal paths and the velocity of each dot
varies sinusoidally as it moves from one side of the
cylinder to the other and reverses direction. Although
this changing pattern of dots is compatible with an
infinite set of *non-rigid* interpretations (including that
of a single plane of sinusoidally moving dots)
observers always report seeing a rigid rotating 3-D
cylinder; an effect that is often called the kinetic depth
effect (Wallach & O'Connell, 1953) or 'structure-from-
motion' (Ullman, 1979).

One approach to this problem originated with
Helmholtz (1867) and is based on the assumption that
motion parallax and stereopsis are analogous, i.e. 3-D
structure from motion is recovered from velocity
gradients in much the same way that stereopsis is
recovered from disparity gradients (Braunstein, 1962).
When an observer fixates any point in the world and
moves sideways, then objects nearer than the plane of
fixation will appear to move in the opposite direction
while objects further away will move in the same
direction as the observer. Furthermore, the velocities
of the objects will be directly proportional to their
distance from the plane of fixation which implies that
velocity gradients can potentially be used to determine

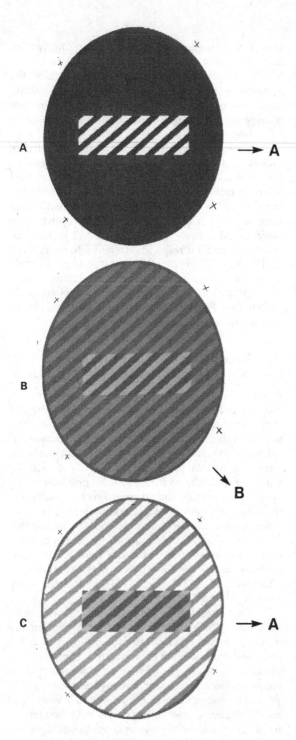

relative depth (Braunstein, 1962). Ullman (1979) has questioned the logical validity of this approach. Since different objects in the visual world may be actually moving at different velocities there is no a priori reason to assume a specific relationship between depth and velocity *unless* the points are connected together to constitute a rigid object. Ullman suggests that the derivation of 3-D structure-from-motion may be based, instead, on a special-purpose algorithm that seeks rigid interpretations. First, he shows mathematically that there is enough information in three views of four non-coplanar points to derive a unique 3-D structure *if* the assumption is made that the object is rigid. Secondly, he suggests that whenever the visual system is confronted with an ensemble of moving points it applies a 'rigidity test', i.e. it asks 'does this collection of moving points have a unique interpretation as a rigid rotating object'. If the answer is 'yes' the system homes in on this rigid interpretation and discards the infinite set of non-rigid interpretations that are theoretically compatible with the same changing pattern.

The computational approach to vision often leads to a clearer understanding of perceptual problems than what would be possible with psychophysics or neurophysiology alone. Ullman's elegant formulation of the structure-from-motion problem is a case in point. Before Ullman, there was a great deal of vague talk about how the visual system had a built-in 'propensity' for seeing things rigid; it was assumed that we usually see things rigid because we *expect* them to be rigid. It was Ullman who first showed clearly that far from being merely a vague propensity built into visual processing, rigidity powerfully constraints the solution to the SFM problem. In fact his argument implies that without the rigidity assumption the problem may be unconstrained and insoluble.

One of our objectives has been to design experiments that would serve to distinguish between velocity-based and rigidity-based schemes for recovering 3-D SFM. Unfortunately this has proved to be notoriously difficult in the past. For any rigid rotating object the velocity of points in a parallel projection will vary with their distance from the observer and consequently in most cases both types of mechanisms would yield the same solution. A critical test,

Fig. 31.11. A. When the grating is viewed through a horizontal rectangular aperture it is seen to move horizontally (arrow A) independent of its true direction of motion. The motion of the tips of the lines is now unambiguously horizontal and perhaps

this 'captures' the motion of the rest of the grating. B. If the occluder is made transparent oblique motion is seen as in Fig. 31.10. C. If the luminance ratios are adjusted so that transparency is destroyed, the impression of horizontal motion (arrow A) is restored once again.

however, would be to confront the observer with two co-axial cylinders of identical diameter spinning at different speeds (Ramachandran, 1985b). The velocity based scheme would make the counter-intuitive prediction that the faster cylinder should look more convex (since the velocity gradient is steeper) whereas the rigidity-based scheme would predict that they should look identical. What do people actually see when confronted with such a display? I shall now describe several demonstrations which were designed to answer this question and to investigate the mechanisms which the human visual system uses for recovering 3-D structure-from-motion.

Demonstration 1: motion parallax: multiple co-axial cylinders

In this experiment we displayed two co-axial cylinders of identical diameter superimposed on each other and spinning at two different speeds – 5 rpm and 10 rpm, respectively. Can the visual system unscramble the two planes of dots and perceive two rotating cylinders? Is the derivation of structure-from-motion (SFM) possible under these conditions?

We found that in this display it was extremely difficult to perceive two cylinders of identical diameter spinning at different velocities (Ramachandran, 1985b; Ramachandran, Cobb & Rogers-Ramachandran, 1987). Instead of seeing the dots occupy only the external surface of the cylinder, what we usually perceived was dots occupying two different depth planes and rotating with identical *angular* velocities; as though there was a small cylinder inside a large outer cylinder. The percept was a curious one since on careful inspection it was obvious that all the dots were in fact making identical horizontal excursions!

We believe that this illusion arises because the brain has a strong propensity to translate velocity gradients into gradients of depth as originally suggested by Helmholtz. In fact, there may be a built-in assumption that if neighboring points have different velocities then the slower ones must be nearer to the axis of rotation even though the ensemble of points has no rigid solution.[1] This interpretation is somewhat at odds with Ullman's contention that velocity gradients cannot directly specify gradients of depth or SFM. In this example, even though the visual system is given the *opportunity* for 'recovering' a rigid solution, it actually rejects this interpretation and prefers to respond directly to velocity gradients.

[1] This implies that for the front surface of the cylinder the faster dots are nearer to the observer whereas for the back surface the faster dots are further away from the observer.

Demonstration 2: coaxial cylinders of dissimilar diameters rotating at different speeds

This display was similar to the previous one except that one of the cylinders was half the diameter of the other. Also the smaller cylinder was made to spin at twice the *angular* (18 rpm) velocity of the larger one (9 rpm).

SFM could be easily recovered from this display and we usually saw two co-axial cylinders. As in the previous demonstration, however, the cylinders appeared to have the same angular velocity. When the dots on the smaller cylinder approached the middle of their excursion they were seen to occupy almost the *same* depth as the dots in the outer cylinder. This is the converse of the result reported above and it supports our contention that the visual systems will assign identical depth values to dots which move at similar linear velocity even if they belong to different cylinders. Notice that this would require a non-rigid deformation of the cylinders which implies that, as in the previous experiment, the visual system will actually *overcome* rigidity in order to utilize velocity cues.

A formal experiment along these lines was conducted on six naive subjects who were unaware of the purpose of the experiment. They were shown two concentric coaxial cylinders of which the inner one was ⅔ the diameter of the outer one. (Their diameters were 2° and 3° respectively.) The angular velocity of the outer cylinder was initially set by the experimenter at some randomly chosen value and the subject's task was to vary the angular speed of the inner cylinder until its surface appeared to bulge out and touch the outer one. We found that subjects could easily make this adjustment (Fig. 31.12). They usually set the angular velocity of the smaller cylinder to be much higher than that of the larger one, confirming our initial impression that the visual system almost directly translates relative velocity into relative depth even if this requires a considerable non-rigid deformation of the cylinders.

Demonstration 3: 'cylinder' of dots moving at linear instead of sinusoidal velocity

In this display we had two transparent planes of dots superimposed on each other and moving in opposite directions at a constant linear velocity. As each dot reached one of the vertical borders it simply reversed direction and retraced its path. Although this display is physically compatible with two flat *co-planar* sheets of dots moving in opposite directions, what we actually observed was a rotating 3-D cylinder. It was as though the mere reversal of direction at the border was

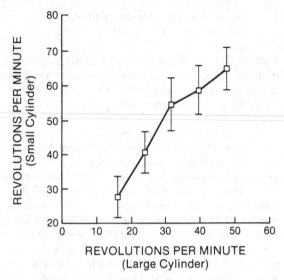

Fig. 31.12. Data obtained from two concentric coaxial cylinders. The angular velocity (RPM) of the inner cylinder was adjusted by the observer until its surface appeared to bulge out and touch the surface of the other cylinder. Each datum point represents the mean of 240 readings (6 subjects × 40 readings each). Vertical lines indicate standard deviation from the mean.

sufficient basis for the brain to perceive a depth separation (and a curved motion path), even though the dots were actually moving at a constant linear velocity. The illusion was especially pronounced at high speeds of rotation (>30 rpm). Notice that no rigid interpretation is theoretically possible in this stimulus and yet the visual system recovers a 3-D shape that *looks* approximately rigid!

Demonstration 4: the role of segmentation boundaries: cylinder viewed through a triangular aperture

We began with a transparent 3-D cylinder and viewed it through a triangular 'window' or aperture so that only a triangular patch of moving dots was visible (the horizontal base of the triangle was exactly equal in width to the diameter of the cylinder). The display was viewed in complete darkness so that the occluder was not visible. To our astonishment, this display looked very much like a solid three-dimensional cone rather than part of a cylinder. Even though there was no velocity gradient along the vertical axis, the dots near the base of the cone were perceived as being further from the axis of rotation than the dots near the apex at the top. This observation implies that although velocity gradients are often sufficient to specify 3-D SFM,

they are not necessary. Furthermore, the *segmentation boundaries* that delineate the object in motion (i.e. the edges of the triangular window) seem to have a strong influence on the magnitude of perceived depth.

Similar results were obtained when the cylinder was viewed through a vertical rectangular window whose width was about half that of the cylinder. This display looked like a much smaller cylinder suggesting, again, that the magnitude of depth perceived for any given velocity gradient is strongly influenced by the total horizontal width of the object.

Using multiple strategies for recovering structure-from-motion

Ullman has shown that 3-D structure-from-motion (SFM) can in principle be recovered from the changing shadow *if* the assumption is made that the object producing the shadow is rigid. Given the rigidity assumption, Ullman's SFM theorem proves that there is enough information available in three views of four non-coplanar points to uniquely specify their 3-D structure. However, our results imply that the particular algorithms suggested by directly applying the methods used in mathematical proof of the theorem are unlikely to be the ones actually used by the human visual system. Demonstrations 1 and 2 are two examples where velocity cues and rigidity are pitted against each other and in both situations velocity seems to win. In fact the system seems to be quite willing to overcome rigidity in order to adhere to the velocity=depth rule.

Our results suggest that the recovery of 3-D structure-from-motion may be analogous to the perception of shape-from-shading (Ramachandran, 1987) in that it relies on the *combined* use of velocity gradients and segmentation boundaries. It does not follow from this, however, that the system *never* uses a rigidity-based algorithm of the kind suggested by Ullman. For example, consider the case of just a small number of widely separated dots spinning (or 'rocking') around a single axis. If the display is very large (e.g. subtending 20° or 30°) it strains the imagination to think of 'segmentation boundaries' in the usual sense and perhaps one would have to resort to the use of a rigidity-based scheme. In our experience, however, such displays usually look very non-rigid and it is difficult to see depth in them. So the question of whether the visual system can actually recover 3-D structure from such displays is still an open one that needs to be tackled empirically.

The velocity scheme leaves one important question unanswered. How does the visual system know what scaling-factor is to be used in translating relative velocities into relative depth? Ullman (1983) has shown that any given velocity gradient is in fact compatible with a whole family of surfaces. How would the visual system know which one to pick? One possibility is that the system sets the scale by simply using the object's outline, i.e. it may use the total horizontal width of the object to adjust the gain of the mechanism that translates velocity gradients into depth gradients. This would explain the critical role played by segmentation boundaries in Demonstration 4.

In addition to velocity gradients and segmentation boundaries, other factors are also undoubtedly involved in the recovery of 3-D SFM. For example, in the displays we have considered so far, the axis of the cylinder was always vertical so that the dots described strictly horizontal excursions. What would happen if the axis were tilted towards the observer in the parasagittal plane? We found that this simple procedure produced a considerable increase in perceived depth. The motion paths now look elliptical rather than horizontal and this seems to enhance the magnitude of perceived depth even though obviously the 3-D structure signalled by the rigidity-algorithm remains unchanged.

Conclusions

Taken collectively our observations suggest that any perceptual process such as the derivation of 3-D SFM or shape-from-shading, is unlikely to be based on a single algorithm or a single constraint. Instead, the brain appears to bring to bear a whole repertoire of strategies which exploit many different regularities in the natural world. And for each perceptual task, the simultaneous use of a wide range of such short-cuts allows the system to achieve the same biological goal as it could with a single sophisticated algorithm.

Ullman (1979) showed that 3-D structure-from-motion can be accurately recovered from a changing shadow if it is assumed that the object producing the shadow is rigid. His theorem proves that there is enough information available in three views of such an object to uniquely specify its 3-D structure. This argument has two important implications: (1) without rigidity the problem may be insoluble; and (2) if you assume rigidity then 3-D structure can *in principle* be recovered without making any other assumptions.

Yet paradoxically, our results suggest that instead of a single rigidity-seeking algorithm of the kind described by Ullman the visual system uses a wide variety of mechanisms to recover 3-D SFM. These include (a) velocity gradients, (b) segmentation boundaries, (c) segregation of dots moving in opposite directions into different depth planes. Why does the system resort to using so many strategies if a rigidity based algorithm alone will suffice, theoretically, to recover 3-D structure? There are at least three answers. First, since evolution has no 'foresight' it may be much easier to evolve multiple parallel gimmicks than a single sophisticated mechanism. Second, by using multiple parallel strategies the system can get away with each of them being relatively crude and, therefore, easy to implement in real neural hardware. And lastly, the use of multiple parallel mechanisms allows the visual system to achieve a high degree of tolerance for 'noisy' images of the kind it would encounter in the natural world. It is this remarkable tolerance for noisy images that characterizes biological vision and sets it apart from machine vision.

The idea that the visual system may use short-cuts to solve perceptual problems is not entirely new and in fact similar ideas have been previously proposed by Gibson (1966) and Runeson (1977). There are, however, several important differences between these earlier approaches and ours. First, Gibson spoke of perception as being direct 'pick up' of information and denied the need for intermediate stages of processing whereas the Utilitarian Theory explicitly acknowledges the need for such stages. For instance, the specific mechanism we propose for solving the correspondence problem – the inhibition of short-range by long-range motion signals – is very different from the 'resonance' that Gibson would have envisaged. Second, contrary to many psychological theories which emphasize the flexibility and intelligence of perception we would argue that the mechanisms of perception are often relatively 'crude' although always *adequate* for the job on hand. What makes vision so efficient and reliable in our scheme is the use of multiple parallel mechanisms for each perceptual task. And lastly, although the idea of using short-cuts in vision is a plausible one, there have been very few attempts to devise critical empirical tests that would serve to distinguish this view from computational approaches to vision. Our purpose in this paper has been to provide examples of such experiments.

Acknowledgements

We thank Francis Crick, Dorothy Kleffner and Chandramani Ramachandran for helpful discussions. V. S. Ramachandran was supported by grant 89–0414 from the US Air Force Office of Scientific Research.

References

Adelson, E. H. & Movshon, J. A. (1982) Phenomenal coherence of moving visual patterns. *Nature*, **300**, 523–5.

Albright, T. (1987) Isoluminant motion processing in area MT. *Soc. Neurosci. Abstr.*

Beck, J. (1986) Perception of transparency in man and machine. In *Human and Machine Vision II*, ed. A. Rosenfeld. New York: Academic Press.

Braunstein, M. (1962) Depth perception in rotation dot patterns: effects of numerosity and perspective. *J. Exp. Psychol.*, **64**, 415–20.

DeYoe, E. A. & Van Essen, D. C. (1985) Segregation of efferent connections and receptive field properties in visual area V2 of the Macaque. *Nature*, **317**, 58–61.

Gibson, J. J. (1966) *The Senses Considered as Perceptual Systems*. Boston: Houghton Mifflin.

Gregory, R. L. (1970) *The Intelligent Eye*. London: Weidenfeld and Nicholson.

Helmholtz, H. L. F. Von (1867) *Handbuch der Physiologischen Optik*. Leipzig: Voss.

Hildreth, E. C. (1984) *The Measurement of Visual Motion*. Cambridge: The MIT Press.

Hubel, D. H. & Livingston, M. S. (1985) Complex unoriented cells in a subregion of primate area 18. *Nature*, **315**, 325–7.

Kolers, P. (1972) *Aspects of Motion Perception*. New York: Academic Press.

Marr, D. (1982) *Vision*. San Francisco: Freeman.

Ramachandran, V. S. (1985a) Apparent motion of subjective surfaces. *Perception*, **14**, 127–34.

Ramachandran, V. S. (1985b) Inertia of moving visual textures. *Invest. Ophthal and Visual Sci. (Suppl.)*, *ARVO abstract*. **26**, (3), 56.

Ramachandran, V. S. (1986) Capture of stereopsis and apparent motion by illusory contours. *Perception & Psychophysics*, **39**(5), 361–73.

Ramachandran, V. S. (1987a) A visual perception of surfaces: a biological theory. In *The Perception of Illusory Contours*, ed. S. Petry & G. Myers, pp. 93–108. Berlin: Springer-Verlag.

Ramachandran, V. S. (1987b) Interaction between color and motion in human vision. *Nature (Lond.)*, **328**, 645–7.

Ramachandran, V. S. (1988) Perceiving shape-from-shading. *Sci. Am.*, **259**, 76–83.

Ramachandran, V. S. & Anstis, S. M. (1986) The perception of apparent motion. *Sci. Am.*, **254**, 102–7.

Ramachandran, V. S., Anstis, S. M. & Rogers, D. R. (1987) Correspondence strength in apparent motion is amplified in multiple ambiguous displays. *Invest. Ophthal and Vis. Sci. (Suppl.)*, *ARVO* **28**, (3), 297.

Ramachandran, V. S. & Cavanagh, P. (1987) Motion capture anisotropy. *Vision Res.*, **27**, 97–106.

Ramachandran, V. S., Cobb, S., & Rogers-Ramachandran, D. R. (1987) Deriving 3-D structure from motion: some new constraints. *Soc. Neurosci. Abstr.*

Ramachandran, V. S. & Gregory, R. L. (1978) Does colour provide an input to human motion perception. *Nature*, **275**, 55–6.

Ramachandran, V. S. & Inada, V. (1985) Spatial phase and frequency in motion capture of random-dot patterns. *Spatial Vision*, **1**, 57–67.

Ramachandran, V. S., Rao, V. M. & Vidyasagar, T. R. (1973) Apparent motion with subjective contours. *Vision Res.*, **13**, 1399–401.

Ramachandran, V. S. & Rogers-Ramachandran, D. R. (1989) Occlusion and transparency in human motion perception. *Soc. Neurosci. Abstr.*

Rock, I. (1983) *The Logic of Perception*. Cambridge: The MIT Press.

Runeson, S. (1977) On the possibility of 'smart' perceptual mechanisms. *Scandanavian Journal of Psychology*, **18**, 172–9.

Ryle, G. (1949) *The Concept of Mind*. Harmondsworth, Middx: Penguin Books (reprinted 1963).

Schiller, P. H., Logothetis, N. K. & Charles, E. R. (1990) Functions of the colour-opponent and broad-band channels of the visual system. *Nature*, **343**, 68–71.

Shipp, S. & Zeki, S. M. (1985) Segregation of pathways leading from area V2 to areas V4 and V5 of macaque monkey visual cortex. *Nature*, **315**, 322–4.

Ullman, S. (1979) *The Interpretation of Visual Motion*. Cambridge, Mass: MIT Press.

Ullman, S. (1983) Recent computational studies in the interpretation of structure from motion. In *Human and Machine Vision*, ed. J. Beck, B. Hope & A. Rosenfeld. New York and London: Academic Press.

Van Essen, D. C. (1985) Functional organization of primate visual cortex. In *Central Cortex*, ed. A. Peters & E. G. Jones. New York: Plenum.

Wallach, H. & O'Connell (1953) The kinetic depth effect. *J. Exp. Psych.*, **45**, 205–17.

From image to
object

32

A theory about the functional role and synaptic mechanism of visual after-effects

H. B. Barlow

Many striking visual illusions are caused by disturbances to the equilibrium of the visual system resulting from relatively short periods of intense activation; after-images fall into this category, as do motion and tilt after-effects. I am going to suggest a goal, or computational theory, for the equilibration mechanisms that are revealed by some of these illusions: I think they take account of the correlational structure of sensory messages, thereby making the system specially sensitive to new associations. The suspicious coincidences thus discovered are likely to signal new causal factors in the environment, so adaptation mechanisms of the kind suggested could provide the major advantageous feature of the sensory representations formed in the cortex.

Visual adaptation

The visual system changes its characteristics when the image it is handling alters. The simplest and best understood example is the change in sensitivity that occurs when the mean luminance increases or decreases, and it is now well recognised that this parallels the electronic engineer's automatic gain control. The idea was formulated by Craik (1938) and recordings from photoreceptors and bipolars in the retina show the system in operation (e.g. Werblin, 1973), though the exact parts played by the different elements are not yet clear. What is obvious, however, is that the retinal ganglion cells could not possibly be so sensitive to small increments and decrements of light if they had to signal the whole range of luminances the eye is exposed to without changing their response characteristics. This is because spike trains in optic nerve fibres are a somewhat crude method of signalling a metrical quantity; the number of reliably distinguishable levels of activity in a small time interval is very limited, so the distinguishable steps of luminance would be very large without the adaptive mechanisms of the receptors and bipolars to adjust the ganglion cell's gain and range of responsiveness.

There are also maladaptive aspects of light adaptation. When the rods have been strongly illuminated and contain bleached photopigment they give responses as if they were being illuminated, even in darkness (Barlow, 1964; Barlow & Sparrock, 1964; Lamb, 1980 and this volume), and this is what causes the well-known positive after-image; the gain-control mechanism described above cannot distinguish between the spurious light signals from the receptors and real ones, so sensitivity is reduced and this is what causes both the high threshold early in dark adaptation, and the negative after-image. It is not certain how much of this applies to cones, but if it does most of the changes due simply to exposure to bright light can be explained.

The properties of the visual system also change in response to other aspects of recent visual experience. The waterfall phenomenon – the after-effect of exposure to motion in one direction – was apparently known to Aristotle, and was very thoroughly investigated by Wohlegemuth (1911). Gibson (1933) described the after-effects both of viewing curved lines and of seeing chromatic fringes when wearing prismatic spectacles, and Kohler & Wallach (1944) studied the distortions in apparent position and size that follow lengthy exposure to a figure in one position in the visual field. A number of after-effects have been discovered more recently, for instance the loss of contrast sensitivity to a particular spatial frequency following exposure to high contrast gratings of that frequency (Gilinsky, 1968; Pantle & Sekuler, 1968; Blakemore & Campbell, 1969), the changes in apparent size following similar adaptation (Blakemore & Sutton, 1969), and the colour contingent after-effects described by McCollough (1965).

Pronounced after-effects from more drastic procedures such as wearing inverting spectacles have been well known since Stratton's work (1897), followed up by Kohler (1964). Held (1980) and Harris (1980) have written thoughtful and thought-provoking reviews which show that the relationship between seen position and the body's sensed position is involved in the experiments with inverted vision or laterally displacing prisms. But as a result of their discussions I think it is reasonable to distinguish a group of adaptive effects that are truly perceptual and lie at the next level of complexity above straightforward adaptation to luminance. These are the ones considered here, and a new interpretation will be offered. It is suggested that the after-effects result from adaptation to the *relationships* between input variables, rather than to changes in the mean value of a single feature, and this is thought to achieve the same end for two variables that automatic gain control achieves for a single one; adjustments to the coordinate frame in two or more dimensions are needed, rather than simple scaling along one dimension. A brief description of the after-effects themselves and of the ideas that have been held about them will first be given.

After-effects of motion, gratings, tilt and size

I do not see how anyone can fail to be intrigued by the after-effect of motion, and it was one of the phenomena that attracted me into vision research when William Rushton demonstrated it to us in his second year lectures on special senses about 45 years ago. If you look at the centre of a disk such as that shown in Fig. 32.1 while it is rotated anti-clockwise for about a minute, then when it stops you will experience a vivid and unpreventable sensation of expansion in the region that has been exposed to the motion.

Figure 32.2 shows an after-effect notable for its simplicity. It was discovered independently by Gilinsky (1968), Pantle & Sekuler (1968), and Blakemore & Campbell (1969). Note that in this case there is simply a loss of sensitivity to the stimulus following adaptation, whereas in the other cases considered here there is a perceptually detectable negative after-effect: one perceives the weakened opposite of the adapting stimulus.

That is only one of a large class of perceptual effects. Figure 32.3, from Blakemore (1973), shows two

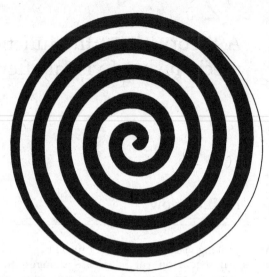

Fig. 32.1. Plateau's spiral. Gaze at the centre of such a disk for about one minute while it is rotated anti-clockwise. When it stops rotating one has a very definite impression, lasting 10–15 seconds, that it is expanding. A change in the pattern of eye movements has been advanced as an explanation for the similar after-effects obtained with linear movements, but this could not explain the result with a contracting spiral. It is easy to show that: (a) the after-effect transfers to other objects viewed in the part of the visual field that was adapted; (b) if one eye is adapted, stationary objects viewed with the other eye expand, though less distinctly than when seen with the adapted eye.

more. If you look for about a minute at the bar between the tilted lines and then transfer your gaze to the dot between the central gratings you will see the upper ones tilted to the right and the lower to the left. Similarly gazing between the fine and coarse gratings on the right and then looking at the centre pair makes their apparent sizes change in the opposite direction to the size of the grating you have just been seeing with that part of your retinotopic visual field.

A major change in the explanations offered for these after-effects occurred when it was realised that extensive coding of images takes place in the retina and primary visual cortex (Barlow, 1953; Lettvin, Maturana, McCulloch & Pitts, 1959; Hubel & Wiesel, 1959). Before then Kohler and Wallach's explanation in terms of electrical fields which distorted the map were much discussed, but this failed to account for many of the phenomena, and there is absolutely no physiological evidence for the postulated fields. Sutherland (1961) was probably the first to point out

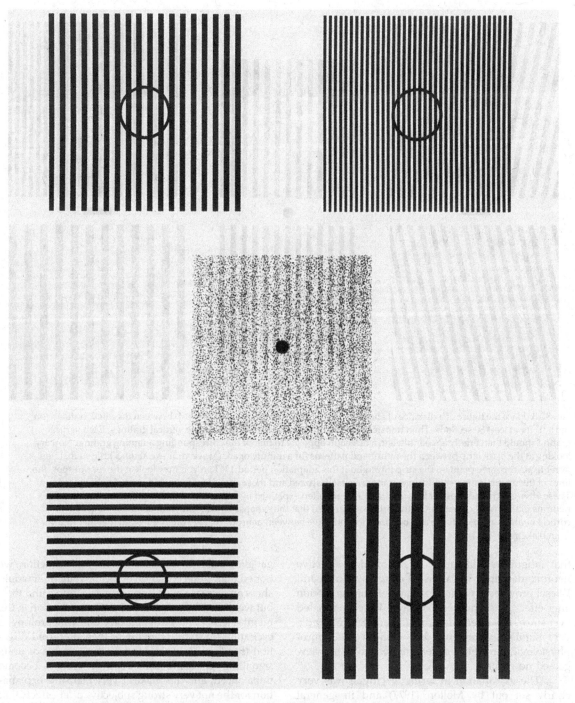

Fig. 32.2. The after-effect of viewing a high contrast grating. Gaze at the top left grating, held at arm's length, for about a minute, allowing your eyes to fixate points within the circle but not outside it. Then transfer your gaze to the central patch, fixating on the spot at the middle of it. Initially the faint grating that is normally visible will not be seen, but it will become visible in about 5 to 10 seconds. Repeat the experiment by fixating on the other three gratings: you should obtain negative results for these indicating that exposure to a grating of a particular orientation and spatial frequency only desensitises the system for similar orientations and frequencies (see Blakemore & Campbell, 1969).

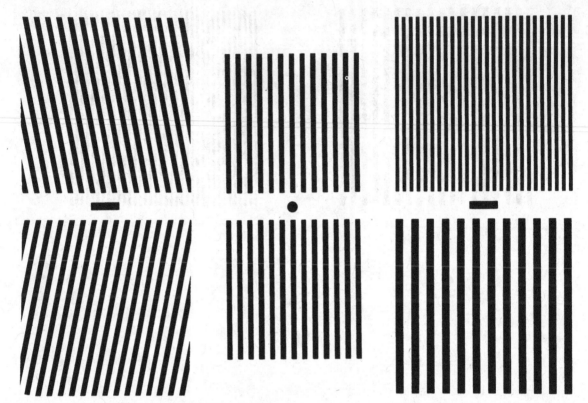

Fig. 32.3. Place the figure at a distance of about 50 cm and fix your eye on the black strip between the tilted gratings (on the left) for at least 30 seconds. Then transfer your gaze to the round dot between the vertical gratings. Each vertical grating should then briefly appear tilted in a direction opposite to that of the corresponding adapting grating. Now try looking at the black strip between the right-hand patterns for a minute or so. (Move your eye about a little so that you don't fixate the same point on the strip throughout this adaptation period.) When you now look at the central spot, the lines of the upper grating should appear more coarsely spaced and those of the lower grating, more finely spaced. These after-effects and those of Figs. 32.1 and 32.2 are often explained by fatigue or adaptation of pattern selective neurons in the visual cortex, but in this article it is argued that the synapses mediating mutual inhibition between cortical neurons are modifiable and become more effective between neurons that are often activated together (figure from Blakemore, 1973).

that fatigue or adaptation of the motion selective neurons described in cat visual cortex by Hubel and Wiesel provided a natural explanation for the motion after-effect, and such explanations have dominated ever since. It is interesting that Exner (1894) offered a very similar explanation, but without the neuro-physiological evidence of feature detectors this view gained no ground.

The explanation in terms of fatigue was very clearly set out by Mollon (1977) and its general acceptance is obvious in the reviews by Held and Harris already quoted, though both of them also express reservations. There is, however, direct neuro-physiological support. When Hill and I looked at directionally selective units in the rabbit retina we hoped to find 'rebound excitation'; after stimulating a

ganglion cell with movement in its 'null' direction, we hoped that, upon cessation of the movement, it would show an increase in its firing rate. We didn't find that, but we did find (Barlow & Hill 1963) a reduction in the maintained discharge of neurons following prolonged excitation by stimuli moving in their preferred direction (see Fig. 32.4); thus the discharge rates of units signalling opposing directions of motion become unbalanced, and this makes a very plausible explanation for the not very strong subjective after-effects that are experienced. The situation may be different in the 'on' type of directionally selective ganglion cell, where rebound excitation can occur (Oyster, personal communication).

Probably more relevant to after-effects in humans are the results obtained on direction selective

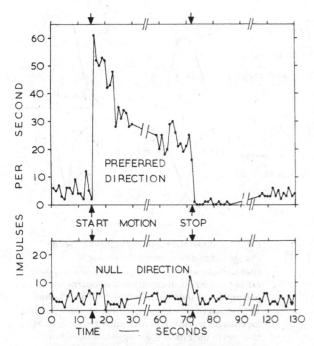

Fig. 32.4. Effects of stimulating a directionally selective unit in the rabbit retina for 1 min by motion in the preferred and null directions. Impulses/second are plotted vertically, time horizontally. The maintained activity is suppressed following 1 min of excitation by motion in the preferred direction. Motion in the null direction has no significant effect, the peak at 70 s being an artefact. Such changes may underlie visual after-effects, but they may be caused by increased mutual inhibition rather than fatigue (figure from Barlow & Hill, 1963).

neurons in primary visual cortex by Maffei, Fiorentini & Bisti (1973), Vautin & Berkeley (1977) and Ohzawa, Sclar & Freeman (1985); these provide strong and direct evidence for modifications in the responsiveness of cortical neurons, but the results of Movshon & Lennie (1979) suggest that something more than the simple loss of sensitivity of a pattern selective element is involved. They measured the loss of contrast sensitivity of neurons at two spatial frequencies, one on either side of the peak, following adaptation to one or other of these same two frequencies; their results show that the losses of sensitivity are not equal, but greater at the adapting frequency. Thus the contrast sensitivity functions of frequency selective channels are not fixed, but their shapes can be modified by adaptation. This suggests that simple fatigue of the neuron cannot be responsible.

It is hard to believe that effects like those shown

in Figs. 32.1, 32.2 & 32.3 are the accidental result of physiological processes, and if we could discover their functional role this should tell us something important about the organisation of perception and the relation between the subjective sensations of motion, tilt, and size, and the physical stimuli that cause them. Are they advantageous in the way that reduction of sensitivity is advantageous in light adaptation? Our own attempts to show improvements in contrast sensitivity at high contrasts following adaptation were a dismal failure (Barlow, MacLeod & Van Meeteren, 1976), but others have been more successful (De Valois, 1977; Tolhurst & Barfield, 1978; Greenlee & Heitger, 1988). I suspect, however, that there is more behind these after-effects than the marginal improvements that have been reported, and that the clue is provided by the contingent nature of the adaptation effect described by McCollough (1965).

The McCollough effect

This is such a striking effect that most books on vision demonstrate it (e.g. Barlow & Mollon, 1982). You gaze for a few seconds at a red vertical grating, then switch your gaze to a green horizontal grating, and continue alternating between red and green for a minute or two. You then look at a set of black and white gratings and see that the vertical one is tinged with the complementary colour of the vertical grating you looked at previously, that is it is tinged with green, while the horizontal one is tinged with red, the complement to the colour of the horizontal adapting grating.

McCollough's work was inspired partly by the reports of coloured fringes following adaptation to displacing prisms (Gibson, 1933), partly by the discovery (Hubel & Wiesel, 1959) of orientation selective neurons. Later a few neurons were described with the combined orientation and colour selectivity that McCollough's results seemed to require (Hubel & Wiesel, 1968; see also Michael, 1978), but the idea that a contingent after-effect necessarily implies the existence of neurons specifically tuned to that contingency has lost its appeal for two reasons. First, the review by Stromeyer (1978) tends to support Harris's contention that wherever one looks for a contingent after-effect, one finds it. Harris went on to advance the 'yellow Volkswagen' argument, a *reductio ad absurdum* which suggests that, although one might perhaps have selective neurons for every noun species, that would not be possible for every adjective–noun combination. Second, both Shipp & Zeki (1985) and Hubel & Livingstone (1985) agree that colour and form are kept rather well segregated even in V1. Thus one should be cautious in attributing after-effects to simple adaptation or fatigue of cells with specific selectivity for the contingency embodied in the adapting stimulus.

At this point the functional role of contingent after-effects is far from obvious. The McCollough effect, which is the easiest to elicit, might possibly be a means of concealing the coloured fringes resulting from chromatic differences of magnification and the small displacements due to off-axis imaging that are normally present in retinal images. It has also been pointed out that contingent effects are in many ways like simple conditioning, so they might be a by-product of learning mechanisms (see Mollon, 1977, Harris, 1980, Skowbo, 1984, Brand Holding & Jones, 1987). The argument pursued here does not contradict these suggestions, but I shall approach the problem from a different angle, through the notion of automatic gain control. I shall ask what one would expect of a mechanism designed to take account of *contingencies* in the same way that light adaptation adjusts the range and sensitivity of retinal ganglion cells when mean luminance changes.

A law of repulsion between habitually associated events

Let us start with the analogy of light adaptation. When the mean luminance increases we judge brightness and dimness by a new standard; it is as if we take the raised mean luminance for granted and judge brightnesses by reference to it. By analogy, when vertical stripes and redness habitually occur together their association comes to be taken for granted; the expected colour for vertical gratings has been shifted towards the red, so if uncoloured vertical stripes are presented we experience the lack of red, i.e. green. This shifting of the reference point is in fact very similar to the explanation formulated by Gibson (1937) for the after-effect of viewing curved lines, tilted lines, motion, and so on, but the important point about the McCollough effect is that the adaptation occurs in response to an association, not to a change in the amount of a unidimensional variable.

In the simple case, the stimulus to adaptation is a shift in the distribution of some variable along one axis, as shown diagrammatically at the top of Fig. 32.5, and the adaptive response is simply a shift of the response characteristic along the same axis, as shown in the lower part of the figure; if the response range of the neurons is not adjusted to match the range of intensities that actually occur, then the intensities in the image will not be transmitted and will be indis-

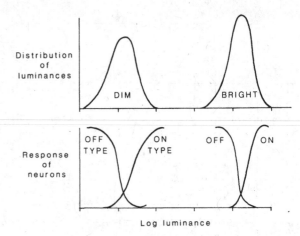

Fig. 32.5. When the mean luminance of a scene changes from dim to bright the response characteristic of a neuron shifts so that its response range fits the new distribution of luminances (examples are shown in Werblin, 1973 and Barlow, 1969). Such adaptation in one dimension might cater for changes in the width of distributions as well as changes in their means, as suggested here, but cannot deal with changes in the correlation between variables illustrated in Fig. 32.6.

tinguishable. For contingent adaptation the stimulus is a change in the joint distribution of the magnitudes of two variables, as shown diagrammatically at the top of Fig. 32.6. Such a change in the joint distribution can occur without any change at all in the distribution of values of either of the variables considered separately, so unidimensional adaptation of the type illustrated in Fig. 32.5 cannot help. What is needed is a change in the axes of representation.

Figure 32.6a shows scatter diagrams of two variables each of which has only 4 distinguishable values; if the scatter diagram shows no correlation, as in Fig. 32.6a, the two variables can jointly signal almost the full 16 possibilities, but if they are strongly correlated as in Fig. 32.6b, only 7 distinguishable possibilities actually occur. For these two variables to be useful it is at least as important to ensure that they occur independently as it is to ensure that they respond over the appropriate range. The two variables can be made independent in the manner shown in Fig. 32.6c & d.

The coordinates in Fig. 32.6a & b were the physical stimuli, and it was assumed that the perceptual variables would be proportional to them so that the axes for the perceptions would be parallel to the physical axes. Suppose that the directions of the perceptual axes are changed in response to the correlated activity shown in Fig. 32.6b, so that they come

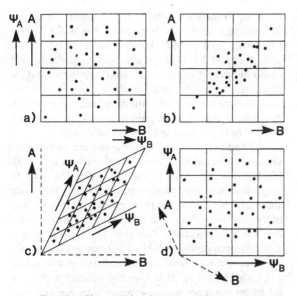

Fig. 32.6. The need for oblique coordinates when adapting to contingencies. Two perceptual variables Ψ_A and Ψ_B, each only capable of discriminating four levels, depend principally on two physical variables A and B. At top left the physical variables are uncorrelated and a scatter diagram of joint occurrences shows that they fill the whole plane. The variables Ψ_A and Ψ_B can represent all 16 different joint values. At top right the physical variables are correlated; perceptual variables simply proportional to A and B would represent this ineffectively because only 7 of the 16 possible joint values occur. The solution, shown at bottom left, is to make the perceptual axes oblique; the grid now fits the joint values of the physical values that actually occur, and all 16 joint values of the perceptual variables are utilised. At bottom right the scatter diagram is plotted with Ψ_A and Ψ_B as orthogonal axes instead of A and B; this perceptual plane is properly covered and all 16 joint values are used. The oblique axes for Ψ_A and Ψ_B are obtained if repulsion develops between them, so that $\Psi_A = A - k\Psi_B$ and $\Psi_B = B - k\Psi_A$ (see Fig. 32.7). Note that the axes for the physical variables are now oblique; A is tilted backwards and has a negative component on the perception Ψ_B, as implied by contingent after-effects such as McCollough's.

to lie in the positions shown by the continuous lines in Fig. 32.6c, the physical variables being horizontal and vertical as before. The perceptual coordinate system is indicated by the skewed grid, and it can be seen at once that this grid fits the elongated scatter of points better than the rectangular grid of Fig. 32.6b, and will allow them to be separated better. Fig. 32.6d shows the scatter diagram replotted with the perceptual coor-

dinates as horizontal and vertical; the points occupy most of the space that can be signalled by these two variables, so the number of distinguishable states is increased.

The dotted lines in Fig. 32.6d show the directions of the original physical variables in this new perceptual space. The axis of the physical variable originally plotted vertically upwards now has a backward slant, and hence has a negative component on the perceptual axis plotted horizontally. Thus the white grating comes to be tinged with negative red, or green. Held (1980) and Stromeyer (1978) show that one can obtain some at least of the reverse contingent effects predicted from the downward slope of the horizontal axis of this figure.

One can look at the lesson of the McCollough effect intuitively in the following way. It is telling us that perceptions are intended to occur independently and define independent axes in perceptual space. When the physical stimuli that are presented lead to clustering in this space (e.g. by artificially linking verticality and redness), then a repulsive force develops between the two perceptions which spreads the cluster out in perceptual space. How might the direction of a perceptual variable be changed in this way?

It will be suggested below that this can be done by increasing the mutual inhibition between elements representing the perceptions, but notice that mathematically all that is required is to subtract a fraction of one quantity from the other. Thus if A and B are the physical variables, the rectangular coordinate system corresponds to the perceptual variable ψ_A being proportional to A and likewise for ψ_B; if instead ψ_A is proportional to $A - k\psi_B$, and likewise ψ_B is proportional to $B - k\psi_A$, the axes are made oblique in the manner required. The suggested law of repulsion then says very simply:

The repulsion constant between two perceptual variables increases when the two perceptions frequently occur together.

It is obviously oversimple to suppose that a perception is directly proportional to a physical variable, and one must bear in mind that there are not just two perceptual variables but a large number, many of them supposedly interacting in this way. The box (Fig. 32.7) gives a slightly more complete description and the theory has been extended to the decorrelation of many variables in Barlow & Földiák (1989).

The law obviously accounts for the McCollough and other similar effects, but what about the after-effects of gratings, motion, tilt and size which might

---

The law of repulsion

ψ_A is a perceptual variable directly proportional
to A, which is a function changing with
adaptation (as in Fig. 32.5) of a physical
variable a.
Similarly for ψ_B, B & b.

ψ_A and ψ_B interact through mutual inhibition so
that:
$$\psi_A = A - K\psi_B = (A - KB)/(1 - K^2)$$
$$\psi_B = B - K\psi_A = (B - KA)/(1 - K^2)$$

*The law states that the repulsion constant K
increases when ψ_A and ψ_B are correlated.*

Complications – The repulsion of ψ_A on ψ_B
is not necessarily equal to the repulsion of ψ_B
on ψ_A.
And more than two perceptual variables will
interact simultaneously.

Fig. 32.7. The law of repulsion.

perhaps be explained more simply? These will be
considered below, but the change of coordinate frame
of Fig. 32.6 would be more believable, and also more
testable, if a mechanism could be proposed.

Modifiable inhibitory synapses between cortical neurons

I am not sure how new the following idea is;
Blakemore & Tobin (1972) provide neurophysiological, and Carpenter & Blakemore (1973) psychophysical, evidence for mutual inhibition between cortical
orientation detectors; accumulation or modification of
this inhibition has been suggested previously as a
cause of after-effects (Blakemore, Carpenter &
Georgeson, 1971; Tolhurst, 1972; Dealey & Tolhurst,
1974; Wilson, 1975). Modifiable inhibitory synapses
have been advocated in nerve nets (Dobson, 1985),
there is experimental evidence for modifications of
inhibitory effectiveness (Barlow, Fitzhugh & Kuffler,
1957), and MacKay & MacKay (1974) specifically suggested that the McCollough effect was caused by
changes distributed amongst many synapses.
Whether new or not, the merit of the proposal is that it
explains how a set of neurons can adapt to, and hence
store information about, *contingent* effects without
there being any neurons that are directly sensitive to
those contingencies. This is theoretically important,
for among N elements there are of the order N^2 contingencies, so it would take an awful lot of neurons to
store them all if a different one was required for each
contingency. Of course one cannot suppose that the
mechanism would work for all sensory inputs to a
system because mutual inhibition will not extend to
remote elements, but the gain is considerable even if N
applies only to small subsets of the inputs.

Modifiable excitatory synapses are called Hebb
synapses because they were first discussed in Donald
Hebb's influential book (Hebb, 1949). The rule he
suggested was that presynaptic terminals that were
successful in exciting the postsynaptic neuron became
more effective, while terminals that were unsuccessful
became less effective. The rule I am proposing is
similar in principle to Hebb's, but applies to the synapses mediating lateral inhibition between neurons in
a sensory pathway. It is that the strengths of these
inhibitory synapses increase when they are activated
simultaneously with depolarisation of their post-
synaptic neurons caused by activity of excitatory
presynaptic terminals, while inhibitory terminals that
are active when the postsynaptic neuron is unde-
polarised become less effective.

One can see what would happen if such modifiable inhibitory synapses convey mutual inhibition
between the neurons in a network: those neurons
that, in the absence of mutual inhibition, would often
fire together become strongly mutually inhibitory,
whereas those that have no tendency to fire together
would be free to do so if the appropriate stimuli were
delivered. Notice that it is what actually happens that
determines the strength of the inhibition; the
inhibitory coefficients in the network correspond to
the frequencies of the contingencies that have actually
occurred.

Consider how this explains the McCollough
effect. 'Redness' neurons and 'verticality' neurons are
excited simultaneously, so the strength of mutual
inhibition between them increases. When a vertical
white grating is shown, this inhibits the redness
neurons, so the lack of redness biasses the output of
the colour system towards green. Similar explanations
can be found for other contingent after-effects, but
after-effects for gratings, tilt, motion and size need
further consideration.

The redundancy of adapting stimuli

When eliciting the motion and other after-effects the
stimulus used is usually large enough to cover the
receptive fields of many motion-selective neurons, so

during exposure to sustained motion many neurons will be responding actively; according to the repulsion law the mutual inhibition between them will slowly increase, and as a result their response rates will decrease. The appearance of motion should decrease, which it does, and then when normal viewing of the stationary world is resumed the mutual inhibition will persist, and the pattern of discharge rates for a neutral stimulus will give the appearance of reverse motion. Thus modifiable inhibitory synapses can give rise to these visual after-effects, but notice that the contingency that causes it is *joint activity of a group of motion selective neurons*; it is not simply the result of the individual neurons' activities.

At this point one must consider other contingencies that are necessarily involved in detecting motion, orientation or size. For motion, excitation at two points at successive moments in time is the minimum that must be detected; for orientation, excitation at the two points that define a direction; and for size, two points that define a distance. It is natural to ask if these are the contingencies involved in after-effects to such stimuli. As a specific case, let us look at the possibility that the inhibitory mechanisms that are probably responsible for motion selectivity play a role in the after-effects.

If these synapses were modifiable according to the same rule, the inhibitory strength of the synapses of neurons receiving stimulation in the *null* direction would be strengthened during exposure, and the persistence of this would be expected to *decrease* the responsiveness of this non-responding set of neurons, thus giving rise to the opposite of the observed effect. It is probable that inhibitory mechanisms are involved in other forms of selectivity of cortical neurons, and again their increased effectiveness during an adaptation period would produce quite the wrong results to explain the observed after-effects. These considerations suggest that inhibitory synapses are not all modifiable according to the proposed rule; it seems to apply to those subserving mutual inhibition, but not to the forms of inhibition that are responsible for pattern selectivity itself.

The repulsion law can be justified as an empirical generalisation based on the occurrence of after-effects, but what is its functional role in organising perception? I have already suggested that it improves perception by making the representational variables more nearly orthogonal, and I think one can point to instances of the law operating to produce improvements in our perception of the world and not just bizarre illusions.

The functional role of repulsion

If you are looking at an object and it comes closer to you, several changes take place: first the angle it subtends increases so that its retinal image enlarges; second it goes out of focus and increased accommodative effort is required to refocus; and third you will need to converge your eyes to ensure that the two images fall on corresponding points. The experience of an enlarging image is thus habitually coupled with accommodative and convergence effort, and although these are not 'experiences' they are probably accompanied by neural activity in the cortex, and one might expect the habitual association of the two to be used to determine what is taken for granted. So what would be expected if there was a need for increased accommodation or convergence under conditions when there was no change in retinal image size?

As the law suggests, the apparent size is modified in a direction opposite to the habitual enlargement, that is the object appears smaller. I am of course referring to accommodation and convergence micropsia: if accommodation is paralysed with a mydriatic drug, increased accommodative effort is required even without bringing an object close to the eyes, and the striking diminution in apparent size of a familiar object such as a coin or matchbox will be experienced as a result. The same effect can be produced by placing a negative lens in front of the eye, but in this case there is a real, though small, diminution of the actual image size and this makes the effect less convincing. If convergence is made necessary by slipping a divergent prism in front of one eye, or by adjusting the interpupillary setting of a stereoscope, a familiar object at a known distance appears smaller; the explanation according to the suggested law is the same.

Wheatstone (1852) understood these effects more than 100 years ago, and referred to them as 'corrections' to our perceptions. By setting up a 'prediction' of change of size when convergence changes we tend to compensate for changes of retinal image size, though it must be added that this cannot be the only mechanism for achieving size constancy. For Helmholtz (1925) too they made sense and were evidence for unconscious inductive inference. Thus we can see that predictions based upon habitual associations can play an important and positive role in perception. Another example should bring this home.

Movement and binocular parallax are habitually associated, but they can be dissociated if one views a stereo pair under conditions in which one can move one's head. According to the repulsion law the constants between the neurons signalling equal binocular and motion parallax should have been increased by these past associations, and the subjective results give evidence that they have been. Normally as you move your head to the left close objects move to the right relative to distant objects, but when viewing a stereo pair this motion parallax is absent. The subjective experience when stereoscopic depth is present but motion parallax is absent is what you would expect from the 'repulsion' set up by their habitual association: the scene is modified towards the opposite of the normally associated motion, and one experiences motion in the reverse direction. Hence on moving the head to the left near objects are seen to move to the left. This is of course the only geometrically correct thing one could see, but this geometric fact would not by itself enable one to predict that one would experience a vivid sensation of motion from what is actually the absence of motion!

Here again one can see how the suggested law helps to convert the experiences gained in a three-dimensional world into proper perceptions of that world. The 3-D world determines what habitually happens and this is what defines the normal; in the above case the unusual absence of relative motion modified our perception towards the opposite of the usual motion, and that is what we see.

Finally the McCollough effect may itself provide another example of improved perception through repulsion if one accepts the suggestion that it eliminates the perception of the coloured fringes normally present in retinal images (see p. 368).

The need for habituation to contingencies

The mechanism so far described uses what habitually happens in the visual scene as a definition of what is normal, and presents to our perception the deviations from this expected normality. But what has been habituated to in the visual scene are not just the means and averages of single events, but the rates of the *joint* motions, tilts, separations, contingencies of colour and orientation, contingencies of size with accommodation or convergence, and contingencies between binocular and motion parallax. Apparently our perceptions take for granted these normal associations: we look out at the world through a censoring screen, and the messages that get through to tickle our consciousness are departures from expected rates of occurrence of contingent events, or coincidences.

The way to understand the theoretical need for this rather subtle mechanism is as follows. The prime function for the cortex must be to detect *new* associations, and the existence of complex patterns of *old* associations among sensory stimuli makes this a very difficult task. What the cortex does is to discount old associations by forming a representation in which the elements occur independently, as far as possible, when the animal lives and moves in its normal environment. This requires the setting up of repulsion or mutual inhibition between events that frequently occur together, and this in turn leads to the after-effects I have described.

If this is a correct account of the visual cortex, it is a null instrument for detecting new associations – a Wheatstone bridge for suspicious coincidences – and this fits in very well with views expressed elsewhere (Phillips, Zeki & Barlow, 1984; Barlow, 1985). To see the potential of such a device, remember that these new associations or coincidences result from *new* causal factors in the environment, for the old ones should have been taken care of by the adjustments of the repulsion coefficients outlined above.

You may have seen the trick of illuminating a picture with a projected image of its own negative; everything looks a uniform grey, but the very slightest change, such as a tiny movement of the picture (or any part of it), leads to the dramatic appearance of black and white lines at edges. So it will be with this screen for suspicious coincidences; provided the causal nexus in the scene in front of us is unchanged, all will be dull and uneventful, but as soon as a new causal factor intrudes it will upset the usual pattern of relationships and vigorous extra activity will be aroused.

Of course the suggested mechanism could only work locally because not all parts of the cortex are interconnected, and the effects observed suggest that adaptation is usually far from complete, but the principle of decorrelation is none the less a powerful one. Surely it must be relevant to the representation of our perceptions by elements with the poor dynamic range of neurons.

Conclusions and questions

I hope I have made an adequate case for suspecting that the after-effects discussed here reveal a very interesting and important functional role for interactions between neurons in the cortex. Perhaps this will provoke more thorough physiological investigation, for the implications of the repulsion law and of its suggested mediation through modifiable inhibitory synapses are reasonably unambiguous and should be testable in a variety of experiments.

The most relevant observations at the moment are those already referred to, by Movshon & Lennie (1979) and Ohzawa *et al.* (1985). The former results give quite strong evidence against fatigue of pattern selective neurons as an explanation of after-effects, and would fit the present hypothesis well. The work of Ohzawa, Sclar & Freeman provided evidence for 'contrast gain control' in cortical neurons, and their use of that term implies that they think the reduction in contrast sensitivity following adaptation fulfils the same role as the reduced luminance sensitivity in light adaptation. But the analogy is not a good one because the range of contrasts is so much less than the range of luminances the eye has to handle. The loss of sensitivity they describe could equally well be the result of adaptation contingent on the *pattern* of excitation caused by the adapting stimulus, as suggested here. There is, it is true, one detail in their results that may not fit such an explanation, namely that the effects were as great following adaptation to a grating that just covered the receptive field as they were to a larger, even more redundant stimulus; on the current hypothesis the latter should probably have been more effective, though even their small stimulus must have excited many neurons, so there would have been plenty of opportunity for mutual inhibition to develop. Blakemore & Tobin (1972) showed that inhibition came from outside the excitatory receptive field, and Maffei *et al.* (1973) claim that adaptation in this region is effective; these results point to the need to find out more about the range of mutual interaction in the cortex, and the laws controlling which neurons it operates between.

Four other interesting questions are worth raising.

(1) Would the development of the appropriate pattern of mutually inhibitory connections according to the repulsion law explain improvements in cortical function that have hitherto been explained in other ways? The most striking change that occurs with, and only with, experience is the great increase in contrast sensitivity for gratings that takes place during the sensitive period in kittens and monkeys (Blakemore & Vital-Durand, 1983; Derrington, 1984). At first it may sound preposterous to suggest that the development of inhibition could account for this, but a proper understanding of the role of lateral interactions in the retina leads one to realise that inhibition is essential for the high discriminative ability of retinal ganglion cells (Barlow & Levick, 1976). It achieves this by subtracting out the mean level of illumination, thereby leaving the ganglion cells free to signal small differences; in the same way the detailed pattern of mutual inhibition that results from the repulsion law might enable cortical neurons to be exquisitely sensitive to changes in the patterns of contingent excitation. One obviously cannot dispense with the ontogenic forces so strongly emphasised by Hubel & Wiesel (1970) as factors moulding the cortex, and it is interesting to note that the inhibition that underlies pattern selectivity seems not to follow the modification rule (see p. 371); perhaps these are ontogenetically fixed. The Hebb type synapses postulated, for instance, by Rauschecker & Singer (1981), are probably also required, but the large increases in contrast sensitivity and acuity that do not occur without visual experience might result from the pattern of mutual inhibition brought about by the repulsion law.

(2) It is a surprising fact that the McCollough effect does not transfer readily from one eye to the other, whereas the other after-effects do. One would expect contingent selectivity to be a higher characteristic than simple feature detection, and thus to occur at a higher level where the inputs from the two eyes would be less easily separated so that interocular transfer would be more difficult. The lack of transfer may be related to the suggested role of the mechanism in correcting for the chromatic fringes in the image (see p. 368), since these fringes are in the opposite direction in the two eyes. One should note that this possible functional role does not contradict the idea of repulsion and modifiable inhibitory synapses, for these may provide the mechanism of the correction.

(3) The duration of the after-effects raises another important question, for they can last several days, and the decay is not exponential (McCollough, 1965; MacKay & MacKay, 1974; Shute, 1979). These prolonged effects are well recognised for the McCollough effect, but also occur for others (Harris, 1980).

(4) A final point of interest is the claim made by Shute (1979) about the sensitivity of the McCollough effect to drugs, fatigue and stress. These might provide clues to the pharmacology of the postulated modifiable inhibitory synapses.

One challenging feature of these visual after-effects is the opportunity they give of linking our subjective world with the objective world of nerve impulses and pharmacological actions. But it is even more exciting that they suggest a novel role for the cortex as censor, habituating to established contingencies and thereby giving emphasis to the new contingencies that betray new causal factors in the environment. This idea might be applicable elsewhere in the brain.

References

Barlow, H. B. (1953) Summation and inhibition in the frog's retina. *J. Physiol.*, **119**, 69–88.

Barlow, H. B. (1964) Dark adaptation: a new hypothesis. *Vision Res.*, **4**, 47–58.

Barlow, H. B. (1969) Pattern recognition and the responses of sensory neurons. *Annals of the New York Academy of Sciences*, **156**, 872–81.

Barlow, H. B. (1985) Cerebral cortex as model builder. In *Models of the Visual Cortex*, ed. D. Rose & V. G. Dobson. New York: John Wiley.

Barlow, H. B., Fitzhugh, R. & Kuffler, S. W. (1957) Change in organization in the receptive fields of the cat's retina during dark adaptation. *J. Physiol.*, **137**, 338–54.

Barlow, H. B. & Földiák, P. F. (1989) Adaptation and decorrelation in the cortex. In *The Computing Neuron*, ed. R. Durbin, C. Miall & G. M. Mitchison; Ch. 4 pp. 54–72. New York: Addison-Wesley.

Barlow, H. B. & Hill, R. M. (1963) Evidence for a physiological explanation of the waterfall phenomenon and figural after-effects. *Nature*, **200**, 1345–7.

Barlow, H. B. & Levick, W. R. (1976) Threshold setting by the surround of cat retinal ganglion cells. *J. Physiol.*, **259**, 737–57.

Barlow, H. B., Macleod, D. I. A. & Van Meeteren, A. (1976) Adaptation to gratings: no compensatory advantages found. *Vision Res.*, **16**, 1043–5.

Barlow, H. B. & Mollon, J. D. (eds.) (1982) *The Senses.* Cambridge: Cambridge University Press.

Barlow, H. B. & Sparrock, J. M. B. (1964) The role of after-images in dark adaptation. *Science*, **144**, 1309–14.

Blakemore, C. (1973) The baffled brain. In *Illusion in Nature and Art*, ed. R. L. Gregory & E. H. Gombrich, pp. 8–47. London: Duckworth.

Blakemore, C. & Campbell, F. W. (1969) On the existence of neurons in the human visual system selectivity sensitive to the orientation and size of retinal images. *J. Physiol.*, **203**, 237–60.

Blakemore, C., Carpenter, R. H. S. & Georgeson, M. A. (1971) Lateral thinking about lateral inhibition. *Nature*, **234**, 418–19.

Blakemore, C. & Sutton, P. (1969) Size adaptation: a new after-effect. *Science*, **166**, 245–7.

Blakemore, C. & Tobin, E. A. (1972) Lateral inhibition between orientation detectors in the cat's visual cortex. *Exp. Brain. Res.*, **15**, 439–40.

Blakemore, C. & Vital-Durand, F. (1983) Visual deprivation prevents post-natal maturation of spatial resolution and contrast-sensitivity for neurones of the monkey's striate cortex. *J. Physiol.*, **345**, 40P.

Brand, J. L., Holding, D. H. & Jones, P. D. (1987) Conditioning and blocking of the McCollough effect. *Perception and Psychophysics*, **41**, 313–17.

Carpenter, R. H. S. & Blakemore, C. (1973) Interactions between orientations in human vision. *Exp. Brain Res.*, **18**, 287–303.

Craik, J. K. W. (1938) The effect of adaptation on differential brightness discrimination. *J. Physiol.*, **92**, 406–21.

Dealey, R. S. & Tolhurst, D. J. (1974) Is spatial adaptation an after-effect of prolonged inhibition? *J. Physiol.*, **241**, 261–70.

Derrington, A. M. (1984) Development of spatial frequency selectivity in striate cortex of vision-deprived cats. *Exp. Brain. Res.*, **55**, 431–7.

De Valois, K. K. (1977) Spatial frequency adaptation can enhance contrast sensitivity. *Vision Res.*, **17**, 1057–65.

Dobson, V. G. (1985) Decrementory associative net models of visual cortical development. In *Models of the Visual Cortex*, ed. D. Rose & V. G. Dobson, pp. 182–99. New York: John Wiley.

Exner, S. (1894) *Entwurf zu einer physiologischen erklarung der psychischen ersheinungen.* 1 Theil Leipzig und Wien: Franz Deuticke.

Gibson, J. J. (1933) Adaptation, after-effect and contrast in the perception of curved lines. *J. Exp. Psychol.*, **16**, 1–31.

Gibson, J. J. (1937) Adaptation with negative after-effect. *Psychological Review*, **44**, 222–44.

Gilinsky, A. S. (1968) Orientation-specific effects of patterns of adapting light on visual acuity. *J. Op. Soc. Am.*, **58**, 13–18.

Greenlee, M. W. & Heitger, F. (1988) The functional role of contrast adaptation. *Vision Res.*, **28**, 791–7.

Harris, C. S. (1980) Insight or out of sight? Two examples of perceptual plasticity in the human adult. In *Visual Coding and Adaptability*, ed. C. S. Harris, pp. 95–149. New Jersey: Lawrence Erlbaum Assoc.

Hebb, D. O. (1949) *The Organization of Behaviour.* New York: John Wiley.

Held, R. (1980) The rediscovery of adaptability in the visual system: effects of extrinsic and intrinsic chromatic dispersion. In *Visual Coding and Adaptability*, ed. C. S. Harris. New Jersey: Lawrence Erlbaum Assoc.

Helmholtz, H. von (1925) *Treatise on Physiological Optics. Volume III The Theory of the Perception of Vision.* Translated from 3rd German Edition, ed. J. P. C. Southall. Optical Society of America.

Hubel, D. H. & Livingstone, M. S. (1985) Complex unoriented cells in a sub-region of primate area 18. *Nature*, **315**, 325–7.

Hubel, D. H. & Wiesel, T. N. (1959) Receptive fields of single neurones in the cat's striate cortex. *J. Physiol.*, **148**, 574–91.

Hubel, D. H. & Wiesel, T. N. (1968) Receptive fields and functional architecture of monkey striate cortex. *J. Physiol.*, **195**, 215–43.

Hubel, D. H. & Wiesel, T. N. (1970) The period of susceptibility to the physiological effects of unilateral eye closure in kittens. *J. Physiol.*, **206**, 419–36.

Kohler, I. (1964) The formation and transformation of the perceptual world. *Psychological Issues* **3**, 1–173. (monograph 12). New York: International Universities Press.

Kohler, W. & Wallach, H. (1944) Figural after-effects. An investigation of visual processes. *Proceedings of the American Philosophical Society*, **88**, no. 4, 269–357.

Lamb, T. D. (1980) Spontaneous quantal events induced in toad rods by pigment bleaching. *Nature*, **287**, 349–51.

Lettvin, J. Y., Maturana, H. R., McCulloch, W. S. & Pitts, W. H. (1959) What the frog's eye tells the frog's brain. *Proc. Inst. Rad. Eng.*, **47**, 1940–51.

Maffei, L., Fiorentini, A. & Bisti, S. (1973) Neural correlate of perceptual adaptation to gratings. *Science*, **182**, 1036–8.

McCollough, C. (1965) Color adaptation of edge-detectors in the human visual system. *Science*, **149**, 1115–16.

MacKay, D. M. & MacKay, U. (1974) The time course of the McCollough effect and its physiological implications. *J. Physiol.*, **237**, 38–9.

Michael, C. R. (1978) Color vision mechanisms in monkey striate cortex: simple cells with dual opponent-color receptive fields. *J. Neurophysiol.*, **41**, 1233–49.

Mollon, J. D. (1977) Neural analysis. In *The Perceptual World*, ch. 4, ed. K. Von Fiendt & I. K. Monstgaard. London and New York: Academic Press.

Movshon, J. A. & Lennie, P. (1979) Pattern selective adaptation in visual cortical neurones. *Nature*, **278**, 850–2.

Ohzawa, I., Sclar, G. & Freeman, R. D. (1985) Contrast gain control in the cat's visual system. *J. Neurophysiol.*, **54**, 651–67.

Pantle, A. & Sekuler, R. (1968) Size detecting mechanisms in human vision. *Science*, **162**, 1146–8.

Phillips, C. G., Zeki, S. & Barlow, H. B. (1984) Localization of function in the cerebral cortex: past, present and future. *Brain*, **107**, 327–61.

Rauschecker, J. P. & Singer, W. (1981) The effect of early visual experience on the cat's visual cortex and their possible explanation by Hebb synapses. *J. Physiol.*, **310**, 215–39.

Shipp, S. & Zeki, S. (1985) Segregation of pathways leading from area V2 to areas V4 and V5 of macaque monkey visual cortex. *Nature*, **315**, 322–4.

Shute, C. C. D. (1979) *The McCollough Effect*. Cambridge: Cambridge University Press.

Skowbo, D. (1984) Are McCollough effects conditioned responses? *Psych. Bull.*, **96**, 215–26.

Stratton, G. M. (1897) Vision without inversion of the retina image. *Psychol. Rev.*, **4**, 341–60.

Stromeyer, C. F. III (1978) Form-color after-effects in human vision. In *Handbook of Sensory Physiology*, **8**, ch. 4, ed. R. Held, H. Leibowitz & H. L. Teuber, pp. 97–142. New York: Springer.

Sutherland, N. S. (1961) Figural after-effects and apparent size. *J. Exp. Psychol.*, **13**, 222–8.

Tolhurst, D. J. (1972) Adaptation to square-wave gratings: inhibition between spatial frequency channels in the human visual system. *J. Physiol.*, **226**, 231–48.

Tolhurst, D. J. & Barfield, L. P. (1978) Interactions between spatial frequency channels, *Vision Res.*, **18**, 951–8.

Vautin, R. G. & Berkeley, M. A. (1977) Responses of single cells in cat visual cortex to prolonged stimulus movement: neural correlates of visual after-effects. *J. Neurophysiol.*, **40**, 1051–65.

Werblin, F. S. (1973) The control of sensitivity in the retina. *Sci. Am.*, **228**, 70–9.

Wheatstone, C. (1852) Contributions to the physiology of vision – part the second. On some remarkable, and hitherto unobserved phenomena of binocular vision. *Phil. Trans. Roy. Soc.*, 1852, 1–17.

Wilson, H. R. (1975) A synaptic model for spatial frequency adaptation. *J. Theoret. Biol.*, **50**, 327–52.

Wohlgemuth, A. (1911) On the after-effect of seen movement. *J. Psychol.*, monograph supplements, **1**, 1–117.

33

Spatial and temporal summation in human vision

T. E. Cohn

Symbols used:

$\triangle I$ increment threshold (quanta @ 507 nm)/ (deg squared) (s)

I background intensity (units as for $\triangle I$)

A stimulus area (deg squared)

T stimulus duration (s)

F detective quantum efficiency

d' detectability

t_m minimum summing time

a_m minimum summing area

A_m maximum summing area

T_m maximum summing time

Introduction

The concept of summation in vision is, today, greatly more complex than it was some 100 years ago when first Ricco (1877), then Bloch (1885) and Charpentier (1890) examined the ability of the eye to integrate photons (see also Hallett, 1962). In those early days it seemed natural to draw an analogy between the properties of stimuli at threshold and the properties of chemical reactions as expressed in the Bunsen–Roscoe law. For example, Bloch's law ($\triangle I{=}KT$), sometimes called the Bloch–Charpentier law (Owen, 1972) is still viewed as a manifestation of an integration mechanism, despite paradoxical failures of this law (Zacks, 1970). Equivalent arguments can be made for spatial summation, Ricco's law ($\triangle I{=}KA$) and its paradoxical failures (Sakitt, 1971). Empirically, both laws hold for small values of the independent variable (T or A respectively).

    The summation of quanta by the eye changes as duration or area are increased. Relations were found to take the form $\triangle I{=}kT^p$, where $0{<}p{<}1$ and were discovered just around or after the turn of the century.

Often these laws are associated with the names of their discoverers, Pieron and Piper, respectively.

    Nearly a half century later, the concurrent analytic discoveries of DeVries (1943) and of Rose (1948) that square-root relations ($p{=}0.5$) were to be expected in situations where sensitivity was governed solely by quantum fluctuations breathed new life into this subject matter. Finally, Barlow's elegant work of the late 1950s, showing conditions where the square-root laws existed, brought the matter to its present status (Barlow, 1957, 1958).

    The purpose of this paper is to outline present-day understanding of human temporal and spatial summation and then to explore several aspects of these phenomena that have not been obvious, but which, nonetheless, supply additional insight into the coding of the visual message in the eye and the efficiency with which this task is performed.

Concept of summing area or time

A number of investigators have observed a duality between space and time integration by the eye (Barlow, 1964). That duality allows us to discuss several issues in terms of just space or just time. Consider the 'integrating time' of the eye, the stimulus duration within which quanta are completely and flawlessly summed. Bloch's law, on its face, provides a means of determining, albeit approximately, the value of the summing time under given stimulus conditions. This would be the largest duration for which complete summation (Bloch's law) is observed. Consider the data of Fig. 33.1 which are replotted from Barlow (1958). Each curve of the upper panel is for a particular area and for a particular background. Data in the lower panel are for the analogous area/threshold task. Using the definition above, the integrating time can be seen

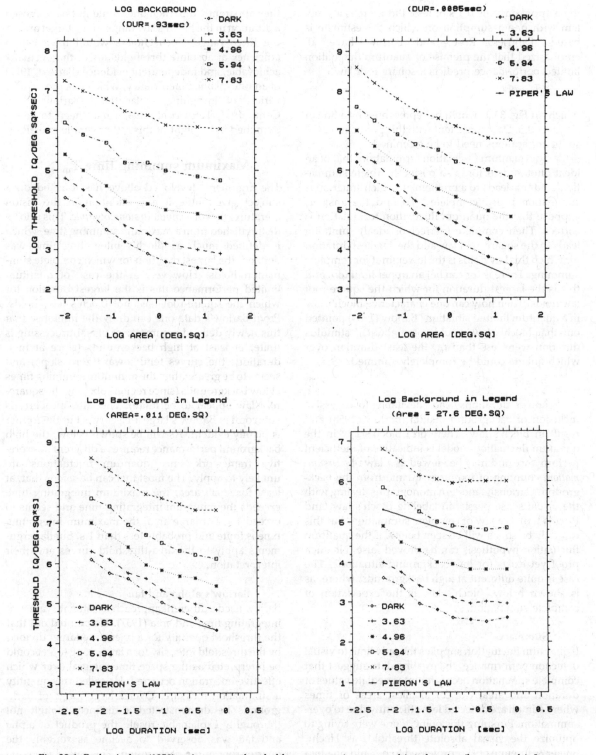

Fig. 33.1. Barlow's data (1958) on increment threshold versus area (upper panels) or duration (lower panels). Log background given in log (quanta/deg sq∗s).

to be approximately 0.1 s or less. But there is a problem with one assumption on which the estimate is based. DeVries, Rose, and Barlow have all emphasized that the premise of quantum fluctuation limited performance predicts a square-root law

$$\triangle I = kT^{0.5} \qquad (1)$$

which, in Fig. 33.1, would be represented by a line of slope = −0.5. Data consistent with this prediction exist so its implications need to be examined.

The quantum fluctuation formulation, that of an ideal photon detector, also posits 'complete summation' and this leads to a problem: in which situation is summation really 'complete'? To find the answer, suppose that the quantum fluctuation formulation is correct. Then complete (perfect or ideal) summing leads to the square-root law and the smallest duration for which this law holds is the lower limit for complete summing. There is (or can be) an upper limit too, and this is the largest duration for which the square-root law holds. Then how can one characterize Bloch's law in a quantum limited situation? Barlow (1964) pointed out that Bloch's law would come about if stimulus duration were less than t_m, the least duration over which quanta could be completely summed.

$$\triangle I = kT^{-1}/t_m{}^{0.5} \qquad (2)$$

Lower durations lead inevitably to excessive inclusion of background quanta (Barlow, 1958) and result in Bloch's law. Therefore, Bloch's law in the quantum fluctuation model is indicative of inefficient performance and may be viewed as a law of *oversummation*, counting of too many quanta from the background. Curiously, modern monographs dealing with the visual sense persist in labeling Bloch's law (and Ricco's too) as a law of complete summation, but this can only be so, as will be seen below, if the quantum fluctuation hypothesis can be proved false. No such proof yet exists for low background situations. The case is quite different at high backgrounds, where, as is shown below, Bloch's law is the expectation of complete summation.

Summary

If quantum fluctuation supplies the only limit to visual detection performance, the existing data suggest that complete summation occurs for intermediate values of duration and area, not for smallest areas or times where stimuli are detected less efficiently due to oversummation. Pursuing this point, if one were trying to optimize the visual absolute threshold, as Hecht, Shlaer & Pirenne (1942) professed to be, and one had adopted the premise of quantum-limited behavior (as

they apparently did) then one would not have chosen a duration in the Bloch's law range, nor a target area in the Ricco range. Such choices would have led to efficiency at absolute thresholds lower than actually achievable, and independent evidence (Barlow, 1977) of an unexplained inefficiency, which has provoked a variety of intriguing explanations (Barlow, 1977; Cohn, 1981; Teich *et al.*, 1982), may need to be re-examined in the light of this rather simple oversight.

Maximum summing time, T_m

The argument developed above has touched on a subject given little if any attention in the vision literature, that of a *minimun summing time*. This is to be distinguished from a maximum summing time, which is defined much as Bloch's integrating time was defined, the largest duration for which complete summation holds. However, in the case of quantum limited performance this is the largest duration for which the square-root law, not Bloch's law, holds. From Barlow's data one can draw the inference that this newly defined parameter of visual processing is finite, at least at high backgrounds (since at high durations the curves tend toward zero slope) and seems to be greater than the minimum summing times at low backgrounds (since regions obeying the square-root law appear to be finite). The latter property is equivocal in Barlow's large area curves but the former is plainly evident. As will be shown below, the high background performance requires a different interpretive framework since quantum fluctuations are unlikely to apply. The most that can be said is that, at least for small area, the maximum integrating time exceeds the minimum integrating time and seems to exceed 1 s. For large area, the maximum integrating time is finite and probably less than 1 s. Similar arguments apply to the area-threshold curves and their interpretation.

Barlow's alpha and tau

Barlow used a different approach to estimate values of integrating time and area (1957). He pointed out that the threshold quantity for a brief, tiny target divided by the threshold intensity for a large, long target could be interpreted as the space time integral over which effective integration occurred. He called this quantity a summation measure. Over a large range of backgrounds he demonstrated a distinct, though not thoroughly explainable result: the product of alpha and tau was observed to decline as roughly the quarter-root of the background. This raised the issue of whether the integrating properties of the visual system might vary with adaptation level. However, as will be discussed below, the matter is more complex, involving a problem of interpretation that is rooted in the model chosen to represent the visual system under a given set of conditions.

Threshold against finite backgrounds

One of the major points of Barlow's 1957–8 papers was the degree to which the now-classical quantum fluctuation predictions (square-root laws for area, time and background) were consistent with measured performance. Each prediction could be demonstrated and in a manner sufficiently robust that the phenomena could not be dismissed as the inevitable transition

region between a region of no variation and a region obeying one of the linear laws (Rushton, 1965). A perplexing development, however, was that all three laws were not found to hold simultaneously under any of the conditions examined (Barlow, 1958). For example, while the DeVries–Rose law provided a good fit at middle backgrounds, this only applied to small, brief targets. For such targets, Bloch's and Ricco's relations were found.

Figure 33.2 displays the totality of the data published by Barlow in his paper on spatial and temporal summation. It thus includes both the area – threshold and the duration – threshold data displayed in Fig. 33.1. The display in Fig. 33.2 is in three dimensions with log area and log duration forming the base

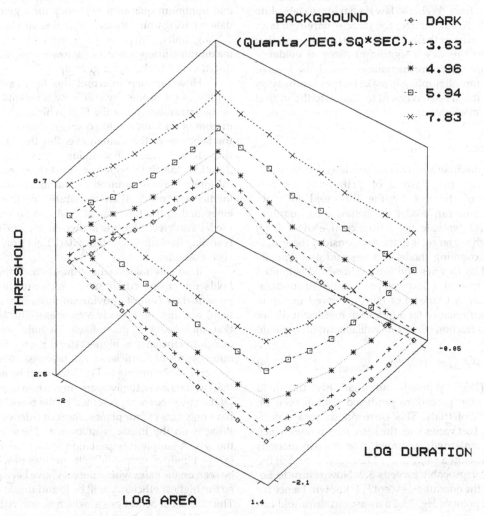

Fig. 33.2. Threshold versus area and duration. Data of Fig. 33.1 replotted in three dimensions. All of the data of Fig. 33.1 are shown here, each face of the cube representing one of the panels of the earlier figure.

plane, log threshold supplying ordinate values and background being the parameter of the several curves. Points along the ordinate, if replotted versus background, obey the DeVries–Rose law over a wide range and it can be seen in both panels of Fig. 33.1 that both Bloch's law and Ricco's law hold in the immediate vicinity. Those points ascending the other three corners of the box essentially follow Weber's law. One set of such points (thresholds for a brief presentation of a large target) were not displayed in the 1957 paper. Increasing target area or duration from the smallest values does lead eventually to the square-root laws for area and duration, but under these conditions it is Weber's law that describes the variation with background, except for perhaps one low background where the curve is less steep, presumably due to a transition from Weber's law behavior to absolute threshold. To summarize, the three square-root laws do not co-exist in these data except trivially, and that remains to this day a significant piece of evidence against the quantum fluctuation model for human vision. Before attempting to make further headway on this issue it will be convenient to digress to the subject of quantum efficiency.

Quantum efficiency

The data discussed above can be viewed from a different perspective. Instead of quantifying the performance of the eye by the threshold intensity achieved, one can model the behavior as quantum limited and estimate the efficiency (DeVries, 1943) with which the target is detected. Consider the simple quantum counting model of threshold as originally described by DeVries and Rose. Threshold is limited solely by quantum fluctuations. In a recent formulation Tanner & Clark-Jones (1960) showed quantum limited performance for a quantum inefficient device catching a fraction, F, of the available quanta, would be

$$d' = F^{0.5} \triangle I A^{0.5} T^{0.5} I^{-0.5} \qquad (3)$$

Barlow (1957) pointed out that his threshold determination procedure produced stimuli seen on about 80% of trials. This corresponds to a detectability, d', that varies with the False Alarm rate (which was not measured) assumed. For the calculations described below a value of $d' = 1$ has been used, but the actual value probably exceeds 3.0. Now return to Eq. 3. Each of the quantities, except F, is known. Hence for each data point of Fig. 33.2 a measured threshold can be used to estimate a measured quantum efficiency, F.

Figure 33.3 displays the results of this computation, again in a three-dimensional format. The ordinate is log F to within an additive constant that depends on false alarm rate. The curves are shaped differently from those of Fig. 33.2 and the backgrounds for best performance (highest F) are the middle backgrounds, not the lowest as they were in Fig. 33.2. The curve for zero background is lowest of all but its placement is arbitrary since, in the model of Eq. 3, there is a term for log background. Quantum efficiency is the same low value at lowest area and duration independent of background, which restates Barlow's (1957) finding that the DeVries–Rose law holds over a large range of backgrounds. Against either area or duration, F may be seen to peak in the middle of the range, not at lowest values. The least difference between maximum and minimum quantum efficiency for a given set of data is 0.6 log units, though typical values lie closer to 1.2 log units. There is a consistent trend for the maximum efficiency to occur at lower areas and lower durations as background goes up.

How can one interpret this behavior? In the context of the model, by efficiency is meant the value of the transmissivity of the filter which, when placed in front of the ideal photon counter, causes it to mimic the behavior of the human eye. But the variation of this inferred value with stimulus parameters, area and duration, forcefully weighs against the purely physical interpretation required by the model. Causes of inefficiency other than quantum inefficiency (as embodied in the filter) must exist and so render the model incorrect. Barlow's own work (1956, 1977) revealing the important role of dark light provides one such example.

If so this raises a new question: if the model holds under any conditions, which are these? The present data cannot provide an answer, as will be seen, but they do provide a compass. The answer is that the model is most likely to hold where the quantum efficiency is highest (for it is only there that other causes of inefficiency can be considered inconsequential). Returning to Fig. 33.3 it can be now seen that the data are actually sparse in relation to our need. Of the entire space represented by the box of data, we have only cuts in four planes, the four sides of the box. What is on the inside is unknown. There are clues though. A simple interpretation is that the box contains a family of unimodal hills, profiles of which can be seen on the sides where the cuts have been made. If so the highest efficiency will be found inside the box. Thus the set of conditions at which non-trivial coexistence of the square-root laws may occur is not dis-

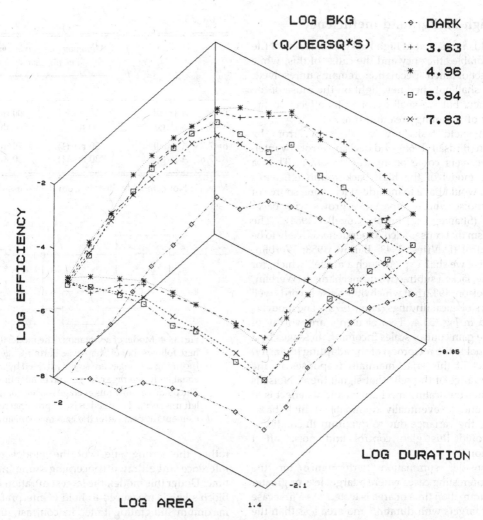

LOG BKG
(Q/DEGSQ*S)

⋄ DARK
+ 3.63
* 4.96
□ 5.94
× 7.83

Fig. 33.3. Log 'quantum efficiency' versus area and duration. Thresholds of Fig. 33.2 have been used to calculate quantum efficiency assuming ideal photon detection (see text and Eq. 3). Threshold is assumed to mean $d' = 1.0$. To the extent that this underestimates actual performance, the curves must be slid upward by $\log(d'^2)$. Quantum efficiency for dark adapted conditions (diamonds) lies below that for other conditions but by an unknown amount. Strictly, since calculated quantum efficiency varies with stimulus parameters, the ideal photondetector model does not hold. Hence, except where it reaches a maximum, the calculated value must be treated as a lower limit.

played above, and possibly has yet to be the subject of a test.

Summary
While Barlow's 1957 and 1958 threshold data did not exhibit square-root behavior simultaneously along all three dimensions of the independent variables, and while such square-root behavior is a critical prediction of the quantum fluctuation hypothesis of visual threshold, it remains possible that conditions exist

where such behavior can be found. Extrapolating from Barlow's data, it is most likely to occur (for targets imaged 7 deg in the periphery) at backgrounds around 4 log (quanta/deg²s), for areas near 0.5 deg² and for durations near 0.1 s. As a final point it may be noted that efficiency under these conditions is expected, in fact is required, to exceed that of any other condition displayed above (including especially the condition of absolute threshold) and to do so by a large fraction of a log unit.

High background inefficiency

Thresholds measured at high backgrounds reveal the least favorable efficiency and the cause of this, while the subject of much speculation, remains unresolved. Here we shall not shed new light on the cause of the inefficiency, but we shall examine its effects on the concepts of summing area and time.

Threshold tasks involve decision errors by definition (Birdsall, 1966), and decision errors by intelligent receivers come about due to noise. Thus a plausible model of the high background efficiency shortfall, would have to include at least one source of internal noise whose importance grows with background (Shapley & Enroth-Cugell, 1984). The mechanism that causes such dependence is likely to be gain control (DeVries, 1943; Barlow 1958; Werblin, 1971). Here we shall explore such a model, which, for simplicity, lacks a subtractive dc mechanism (Werblin, 1971; Adelson, 1982) but which otherwise accords well with physiological findings (Fain, 1975). The model is illustrated in Fig. 33.4. Two elements are worthy of note. The gain control scales incoming messages by a factor equal to the reciprocal of the adapting intensity. The effect of this is to maintain responses in the sensitive range of the cells that signal them. Noise is added after the scaling mechanism and its effect is to add to, and to eventually dominate at high backgrounds, the variance due to quantum fluctuations. How would this gain control and noise affect summation?

Consider summation performance for the several interesting cases where a target less or greater than a summation time or area is tested. As a first case consider targets with duration and area less than the corresponding minimum summing area and time, a_m and t_m. In this case target quanta are all counted but are scaled by I. Thus:

$$d' = \triangle IAT/Ic \qquad (4)$$

where c is a constant dependent upon the noise. If, in the second case, A and T exceed a_m and t_m respectively, the same result holds. Finally, if A and T exceed the maximum summing time and area T_m and A_m, one has:

$$d' = \triangle IA_mT_m/Ic \qquad (5)$$

which is independent of both A and T.

The reader will note that such a model predicts Weber's law, Bloch's law and Ricco's law for small values of A and T, and the familiar non-variation at high A and T. The main point is not the correspondence between model and data however. It is

Table 33.1.

		Minimum and maximum summing times	
		t_m	T_m
$B=0$,	A small	50 ms	1000 ms
$B=0$,	A large	50 ms	200 ms
$B=7.83$,	A small	<50 ms (1)	50 ms
$B=7.83$,	A large	<30 ms (1)	30 ms

Note: (1) Not estimable directly from data. Less than T_m.

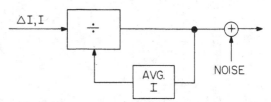

Fig. 33.4. Model of adaptation. The model illustrated here follows that of Shapley & Enroth-Cugell (1984). Incoming messages are scaled (divided by) a factor equal to the average background or adapting level. The details of how this average is itself computed are left unspecified. Added noise of proximal retinal elements appears after the gain mechanism.

rather the strong effect of the model upon the inference to be drawn concerning summing area or time. Under this model, the largest duration for which Bloch's law is measured to hold is interpreted as the maximum integrating time. In contrast, under the quantum fluctuation model, such a value estimates instead the minimum summing time. The same holds for area. Thus, high background thresholds do not directly supply estimates of (minimum) summing area or time. Rather they supply limits on such estimates.

Let us examine Barlow's data in the light of this analysis. In particular, let us examine the difference between the zero background and highest background curves, and how this allows inferences concerning summing properties.

For duration, the values of t_m and T_m at zero background and at high background are indicated in Table 33.1. Note that values of t_m for high background are not determined directly from the data, but rather are bounded by the value of T_m. These results are quite interesting for they show that integration time declines with background, but what has not been fully appreciated is the magnitude of this decline. The maximum summing time decreases by a factor of 7 at large area and by a factor of 20 for small area. Similarly, results for integrating areas show a decline by a factor of 10 at large duration and by a factor of 80 at small duration. Such differences are perhaps larger than others have inferred. Before attempting to explain such effects it is instructive to examine their predicted influence on Barlow's summation measure.

Summation measure

The definition of the summation measure has been given above. This quantity declined markedly with background as shown in Fig. 33.5. Let us examine the meaning of this measure in terms of the two models presented above. At low backgrounds, $\triangle IAT$ for A and T less than a_m and t_m respectively is given by:

$$\triangle IAT = (Ia_m t_m)^{0.5} \tag{6}$$

and the threshold intensity for $A > A_m$ and $T > T_m$ by:

$$\triangle I = (I/A_m T_m)^{0.5} \tag{7}$$

Likewise, at high background the threshold quantity for $A < a_m$ and $T < t_m$ is given by

$$\triangle IAT = cI \tag{8}$$

and the threshold intensity for large A and T by:

$$\triangle I = cI/A_m T_m \tag{9}$$

The quotient is the summation measure, s_m, and equals

$$s_m = (a_m t_m A_m T_m)^{0.5} \tag{10}$$

at low backgrounds and

$$s_m = (A_m T_m) \tag{11}$$

at high backgrounds. Now since A_m and T_m decline markedly at high backgrounds, it follows that the empirical summation measure must decline with background simply because it is defined differently at different backgrounds. At low backgrounds it should be fixed and as given in Eq. 10. At high backgrounds it should be less and also fixed. Allowing for a range of transition, this gives a z-shaped function which supplies a plausible fit to Barlow's data shown in Fig. 33.5.

Why summing areas and times decline with background

There are at least three physiological mechanisms whose properties tend in the direction seen in these data:

(1) Receptor coupling (Fain, 1975)

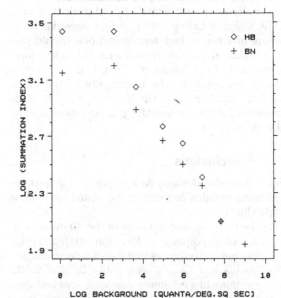

RATIO OF THRESHOLD QUANTITY (SMALL STIM)
TO THRESHOLD INTENSITY FOR LARGE STIM

Fig. 33.5. Barlow's summation measure versus background. These data are replotted from Barlow (1957). The ordinate is the log of the ratio of the threshold quantity for a brief, small stimulus and the threshold intensity for a long, large stimulus. The abscissa is the log of the background level with the exception that values determined in the dark are shown at the origin (log $B = 0$). Data from two subjects are shown. While Barlow observed that the data are well fit by a line of slope $-1/4$, no explanation of the observed behavior has been given. The model advanced in the text predicts a constant high summation measure at low background, a constant low value at high backgrounds, and a region of transition between these.

(2) Ganglion cell surround inaction at low background (Barlow *et al.*, 1957)
(3) Speed of response change with background (Baylor & Hodgkin, 1974)

The first of these might increase a_m at low backgrounds. The second might affect A_m. In the case of the third, changes of only $2-4x$ have been seen. Accordingly, this cannot be the entire story.

We advance here an additional hypothesis for consideration, one that is formulated as an inefficiency which might explain why we do not see as well as we should (Werblin, 1971). It has recently become known that the peripheral retina, where these data were taken, is intrinsically uncertain both for spatial and temporal parameters of the target to be detected (Pelli,

1985). What is less well appreciated is that, at threshold, certain consequences of uncertainty and summation are mathematically equivalent (Cohn, 1978; Cohn & Lasley, 1986). If one does not know where or when to look for a target one should sum (approximately) quanta from the candidate locations. The thrust of this hypothesis then, is that at least at lowest backgrounds, the uncertainty of the visual system is another cause of inefficiency, one that can be minimized if not eliminated, by casting more light on the visual scene.

Conclusions

Some three decades ago, Barlow supplied us with the following insights concerning the visual summation capabilities.

(a) The three square-root laws of the quantum fluctuation hypothesis can be demonstrated to exist, but not altogether as that hypothesis predicts

(b) Bloch's and Ricco's laws could be due to the existence of a minimum summing area and time

(c) The lack of a change of threshold with large area or duration can be explained by the concepts of maximum summing area and time

(d) The product of summation time and area is measured to decline with background

Using his data, and some additional assumptions prompted by the possibility of internal-noise limited performance at high backgrounds, the following additional insights may be derived from his data:

(e) A maximum summing time and area must exist

(f) These too are a function of background

(g) Internal noise leads to Weber's, Bloch's and Ricco's laws at high backgrounds

(h) The summation measure, defined as the quotient of threshold quantity for a small brief target and threshold intensity for a long large one, should thus decline with increases in background

(i) The amount of such declines is quite large and thus cannot be explained with known physiological phenomena

(j) Uncertainty is one factor which could cause an increase of summation with decreased background. This may also depress efficiency at low backgrounds

(k) Conditions may exist where all three square-root laws simultaneously hold

(l) A necessary though not sufficient condition for the quantum fluctuation hypothesis is that where the three laws simultaneously hold the measured quantum efficiency should be maximum

Barlow's work in this area may be likened to the wrapping on a present to his and to future generations of visual scientists. The wrapping itself has supplied important additions to the literature that remain as useful now as when first presented. Additionally, the gift contained therein is rich and remains to be fully explored.

Acknowledgement

The preparation of this chapter was supported by grant EY07606, from the US National Eye Institute.

References

Adelson, E. (1982) Saturation and adaptation in the rod system. *Vis. Res.*, **22**, 1299–312.

Barlow, H. B. (1956) Retinal noise and absolute threshold. *J. Opt. Soc. Am.*, **46**, 634–9.

Barlow, H. B. (1957) Increment thresholds at low intensities considered as signal/noise discriminations, *J. Physiol.*, **136**, 469–88.

Barlow, H. B. (1958) Temporal and spatial summation in human vision at different background intensities. *J. Physiol.*, **141**, 337–59.

Barlow, H. B. (1964) The physical limits of visual discrimination. In *Photophysiology*, ed. A. C. Giese. New York: Academic Press.

Barlow, H. B. (1977) Retinal and central factors in human vision limited by noise. In *Vertebrate Photoreception*, ed. H. B. Barlow and P. Fatt. New York: Academic Press.

Barlow, H. B., Fitzhugh, R. & Kuffler, S. (1957) Changes in the organization of the cat's retina during dark adaptation. *J. Physiol.*

Baylor, D. A. & Hodgkin, A. L. (1974) Changes in time scale and sensitivity in turtle photoreceptors. *J. Physiol.*, **242**, 729–58.

Birdsall, T. G. (1966) The ROC curve and its character. Ph.D. Thesis, University of Michigan. University Microfilms, Ann Arbor No. 70–21630.

Bloch, A. M. (1885) Experiences sur la vision. *C. r. Seanc. Soc. Biol.*, Ii, **8**, 493–5.

Charpentier, A. (1890) Recherches sur la persistance des impressions rétiniennes et sur les excitations lumineuses de courte durée. Paris: Steinheil.

Cohn, T. E. (1978) Detection of 1-of-M orthogonal signals: asymptotic equivalence of likelihood ratio and multiband models. *Optics Letters*, **3**, 22–3.

Cohn, T. E. (1981) Absolute threshold: analysis in terms of uncertainty. *J. Opt. Soc. Am.*, **71**, 783–5.

Cohn, T. E. & Lasley D. J. (1986) Visual sensitivity. *Ann. Rev. Psychol.*, **37**, 495–521.

DeVries, H. (1943) The quantum character of light and its bearing upon the threshold of vision, the differential sensitivity and acuity of the eye. *Physica*, **10**, 553–64.

Fain, G. (1975) The quantum sensitivity of toad rods. *Science*, **187**, 838–41.

Hallett, P. (1962) Spatial summation. *Vision Res.*, **3**, 9–24.

Hecht, S., Shlaer, S. & Pirenne, M. H. (1942) Energy, quanta, and vision. *J. Gen. Physiol.*, **25**, 819–40.

Owen, W. G. (1972) Spatio-temporal integration in the human peripheral retina, *Vision Res.*, **12**, 1011–26.

Pelli, D. G. (1985) Uncertainty explains many aspects of visual contrast detection and discrimination. *J. Opt. Soc. Am.*, A **2**, 1508–32.

Ricco, A. (1877) Relazione fra il minimo angolo visuale et l'intensita luminosa. *Memorie R. Accad. Sci. Lett. Modena*, **17**, 47–160.

Rose, A. (1948) The sensitivity performance of the human eye on an absolute scale. *J. Opt. Soc. Am.*, **38**, 196–208.

Rushton, W. A. H. (1965) The Ferrier Lecture; visual adaptation, *Proc. Roy. Soc. Lond.*, **B152**, 20–45.

Sakitt, B. (1971) Configuration dependence of scotopic spatial summation. *J. Physiol. (Lond.)*, **216**, 513–29.

Shapley, R. & Enroth-Cugell, C. (1984) Visual adaptation and retinal gain controls. *Progress in Retinal Research*, **3**, 263–346. New York: Pergamon.

Tanner, W. P. Jr & Clark-Jones, R. (1960) The ideal sensor system as approached through statistical decision theory and the theory of signal detectability. In *Visual Search Problems*, ed. A. Morris & E. P. Horne. Washington, DC: Armed Forces NRC Committee on Vision (NAS-NRC Publication No. 712).

Teich, M. C., Prucnal, P. R., Vannucci, G., Breton, M. E. & McGill W. J. (1982) Multiplication noise in the human visual system at threshold: I. Quantum fluctuations and minimum detectable energy. *J. Opt. Soc. Am.*, **72**, 419–31.

Werblin, F. S. (1971) Adaptation in a vertebrate retina: intra-cellular recording in *necturus*. *J. Neurophysiol.*, **34**, 228–41.

Zacks, J. (1970) Temporal summation phenomena at threshold: their relation to visual mechanisms. *Science*, **170**, 197–9.

34

The efficiency of pictorial noise suppression in image processing

A. Van Meeteren

Introduction

In many electro-optical displays or photographic recordings visual detection is limited by some kind of pictorial noise. Practically all modern medical and military observation devices suffer from this problem occasionally or regularly. In this paper some psychophysical measurements will be described and discussed in order to evaluate the possible gain of noise cleaning techniques. In textbooks on image processing the justification of the various techniques usually is a matter of face-validity. Pictures are shown before and after image processing and then obviously look much better. However, there is, as far as we know, little experimental evidence of improved visual performance.

The problem of target detection in the presence of visible pictorial noise is the disentanglement of the two. Signal and noise must be separated on the basis of a priori knowledge about their differences. In this respect it is most helpful to analyse the noise into components that can be ordered according to their perceptual distance from the target. Obviously, spatial frequency analysis is attractive in this respect, both, because of its mathematical transparency and because of the present preference in the literature on visual performance. In line with this tradition visual performance is expressed in this paper in terms of contrast sensitivity for sine wave test gratings, measured as a function of spatial frequency in a number of pictorial noise conditions. Sine wave gratings may not be the most natural stimuli for the visual system, and it cannot be claimed beforehand that this angle of approach leads to a clear and complete insight into the interference of pictorial noise with the detection of arbitrary targets. However, the main aspects of visual performance, such as contrast sensitivity, resolution

and spatial integration are all present in the detection of sine wave gratings, so that the results will certainly be representative.

The problem of the separation of the signal from the noise can be attacked in two different ways. One can try to single out the signal by matched filtering, or one can try to remove the noise as far as this is possible without damaging the signal. As will be discussed below the visual system is served best by the removal of the noise. Harmon & Julesz (1973) along this line have demonstrated that face-recognition in the presence of high spatial frequency noise can be improved by deliberate blurring. In their explanation they suppose that the detection of the relevant lower spatial frequencies is masked by nearby higher spatial frequency noise components, which are removed by the blurring operation. In order to further explore the possibilities of simple blurring operations we have measured contrast sensitivity functions for the detection of sine wave gratings against backgrounds of fine grain pictorial noise and coarse grain pictorial noise, such as would be left after blurring fine grain pictorial noise.

Returning to the alternative of singling out the signal by matched filtering, its potential gain can be evaluated by a comparison of actual visual threshold measurements with the expected ideal threshold values. Ideal detection of a sine wave grating would be realized by tuning in exactly to the spatial frequency and orientation of the grating. In that case the effect of the noise would be restricted to the only one possible component that is identical with the target. All other components of the noise would be neglected, i.e. nothing would be known about their presence or absence. Green et al. (1959), Barlow (1978) and Van Meeteren & Barlow (1981) among others have already reported that visual detection is not ideal for a number of visual tasks and noise configurations. More particularly, Stromeyer & Julesz (1972) among others have shown that sine wave test gratings can be masked by noise components as far as one octave above and below the test grating spatial frequency. The main purpose of the measurements presented here has been to determine the gap between actual visual detection and ideal detection in conditions of additive circularly symmetrical lowpass-bands of two-dimensional pictorial noise. Obviously, this gap indicates the potential gain of intelligent image processing if we may assume that the signal, once detected by an ideal detection algorithm, can be made visible. This leads to the highly interesting question whether or not the output of the ideal detector allows a visible reconstruction of the signal.

Methods

Pictures of 180×180 pixels with an 8 bit pixel intensity code C_p were generated by a digital computer and displayed on a video monitor through use of a Ramtek frame store. Pixel luminances L_p on the display screen were made $100(1+C_p)$ cd/m^2 with the aid of a look-up table, where C_p is in the range $-1.000 < C_p < 1.000$. The look-up table was calibrated regularly during the experiments.

Noise pictures of three different spectral classes were used: fine, medium and coarse grain noise as illustrated in Fig. 34.1. Fine grain noise was generated by simply assigning a random intensity value from a uniform distribution to each pixel. Medium and coarse noise pictures were generated in two steps. In the first step, a random value was assigned to only those pixels which lie on a node of a rectangular grid with a spacing E of 5 pixels for medium noise and a spacing of 20 pixels for coarse noise. In the second step a value for all the remaining pixels was calculated by interpolating between the node points using a first order Bessel-function. The corresponding two-dimensional spectral distributions should be flat and radially limited to a bandwidth $W = 1/2E$ cycles per pixel interval (Pratt, 1978).

In the pixel domain the noise pictures are characterized by the standard deviation σ_p of the single pixel values C_p and by the spacing E between uncorrelated pixels. Correspondingly, in the spatial frequency domain the noise pictures are characterized by the amplitude m_n of the spectral components and by the bandwidth W. Table 34.1 presents the values of E, σ_p, W and m_n for the different noise conditions. Note that C_p is limited to values between -1 and 1. As a consequence 0.45 is about the highest possible value

Table 34.1. *Grid spacing* E *(see text) expressed in pixel-intervals, standard deviation* σ_p *of pixel intensity values, bandwidth* W *expressed in cycles per degree, and noise amplitude* m$_n$ *for the different sets of noise pictures as used in the experiments*

Condition	E	σ_p	W	m_n
Fine noise	1	0.45	90	0.0028
Medium noise	5	0.22	18	0.0069
Coarse noise	20	0.22	4.5	0.028

of σ_p. Thus the energy σ_p^2 of the noise per pixel is limited. Note further that this energy is equally distributed over all spectral components ($\sigma_p^2 = \pi W^2 m_n^2$). As a consequence it is impossible to have a broad spectrum with strong spectral components. In order to verify the spectral compositions of the noise pictures produced according to the above procedure, Fourier-spectra were determined afterwards. Figure 34.2 illustrates average amplitudes of Fourier-components in vertical orientation. It appears that the pictures fulfil requirements satisfactorily and that the actual modulations m_n agree quite well with the predicted values given in Table 34.1.

Sine wave test gratings were also generated digitally and specified in terms of pixel intensity values C_p. Due to imperfect imaging the modulation of the sine wave gratings as presented on the display screen in general will be lower than the modulation in the computer-generated pixel-intensity matrix. Figure 34.3 illustrates the modulation transfer function (MTF) of the display device. Low and medium spatial frequency gratings were generated directly in sine wave form. High spatial frequency gratings were generated in square wave form, but practically displayed in sine wave form, as one can conclude from the MTF of the display device.

Series of 96 different noise pictures were generated off line and stored on disk memory. Test gratings were generated on line during the measurements. Noise pictures and test gratings were added in terms of their pixel intensity values C_p prior to display. After addition C_p values below -1.00 and above $+1.00$ were replaced by -1.00 and $+1.00$ respectively. This happened with a small percentage of pixels, depending on conditions, without consequence for the measurements, as followed from a pilot experiment with much stronger 'peak-clipping'.

The observations were made with both eyes in normal free vision from a distance of 3.5 m. The

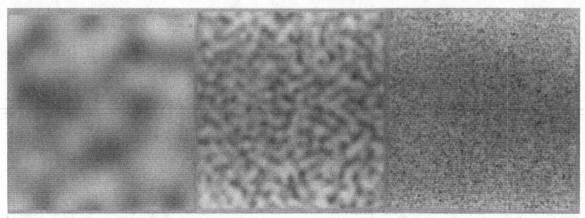

Fig. 34.1. Pictures with fine, medium, and coarse grain pictorial noise. In the experiments the pictures, observed from a distance of 3.5 m, were seen under a visual angle of 1° × 1°.

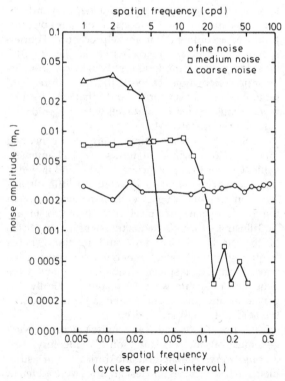

Fig. 34.2. Spectral compositions of the fine, medium, and coarse grain noise pictures used in the experiments.

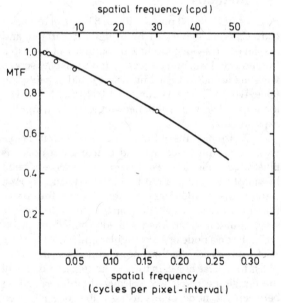

Fig. 34.3. Modulation transfer function (MTF) of the display device. This MTF refers to the transfer of the modulation in the computer-generated pixel-intensity matrix to the modulation presented at the display screen.

pictures were seen under a visual angle of 1°×1°. The size of the pixels was $\frac{1}{3}$ of a minute of arc in this way, too small to be resolved. Pictures were surrounded by a large field with the same uniform luminance. Two subjects participated in the experiments, both with normal visual acuity, using their own spectacle glasses.

The measurements were made in sessions of 96 picture presentations. A vertical sine wave grating was added to half of the pictures randomly. Spatial frequency and modulation depth were held constant within sessions. A 'yes' or 'no' response was requested. The response triggered the next presentation a few seconds later, preceded by a warning tone. The presentation time was 0.2 s. After presentation pictures were replaced by a uniform field with the same luminance.

Each experimental session started with a number of picture presentations for exercise. In this phase the correct answer was revealed to the subject immediately after his response. The subject initiated the real measurements, during which no feedback of correct answers was given, as soon as he felt familiarized.

For each session the sum of the standard scores, corresponding with the correct 'yes' and 'no' responses, was taken as the detection measure Z_d. Note that Z_d is identical to d' when the conditions for d'-analysis are satisfied. Z_d was measured as a function of the modulation depth of the test grating in a number of sessions, as illustrated in Fig. 34.4. Choosing $Z_d=1$ as the threshold criterion the corresponding threshold modulation was determined by linear maximum likelihood curve fitting. This rather elaborate procedure was chosen in view of a possible direct comparison with ideal detection mechanisms (see Discussion). An error of about 20% was obtained, which is no better than for other, more simple, methods.

Results

The main results of the threshold measurements are presented in Fig. 34.5. Contrast sensitivity for sine wave test gratings, defined as the reciprocal of threshold modulation, is plotted here as a function of spatial frequency for pictures with fine, medium and coarse additive noise, and for the no-noise condition. The results obtained with two subjects, AVM and MV, are similar.

The effects of the three different noise spectra upon the detection of target gratings roughly agree with expectations. Coarse noise, according to its spectral composition as illustrated in Fig. 34.2, is expected to mask low spatial frequency target gratings strongly, and not to interfere with the detection of high spatial frequency target gratings. Next, the masking effect of medium noise is expected to be smaller, but to extend over a broader range of spatial frequencies. Finally, fine noise according to Fig. 34.2 is expected to have a small but equal masking effect over the whole range of spatial frequencies. This is all largely confirmed by the results in Fig. 34.5, making allowance for the fact that all contrast sensitivity functions run into the same high frequency decay, so that possible differences are difficult to measure in that region. However, comparing the effects of fine and medium noise it is puzzling that removal of the finest grains results in higher

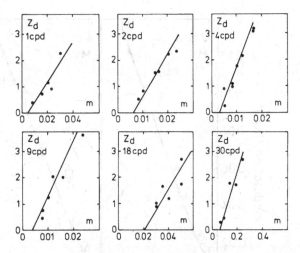

Fig. 34.4. Raw data for one experimental condition and one subject (no noise, AVM). Z_d is the sum of the standard scores (proportion under a unit normal distribution) corresponding with the proportions of correct 'signal' and 'no signal' classification.

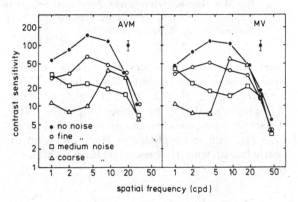

Fig. 34.5. Contrast sensitivity of two subjects as a function of spatial frequency for pictures with fine, medium, and coarse grain noise, compared with the no-noise condition. Contrast sensitivity is defined as the reciprocal of the threshold modulation corresponding with $Z_d = 1$ in Fig. 34.4. Errors expressed in standard deviation were evaluated as a result of the curve-fitting procedure illustrated in Fig. 34.4.

contrast sensitivity at the low end of the spatial frequency range rather than at the high end.

So far the effects of strength and spectral composition have been confounded in the measurements. It is necessary therefore to make additional measurements in order to investigate further how thresholds for test gratings are raised as a function of noise amplitude within at least one of the spectral condi-

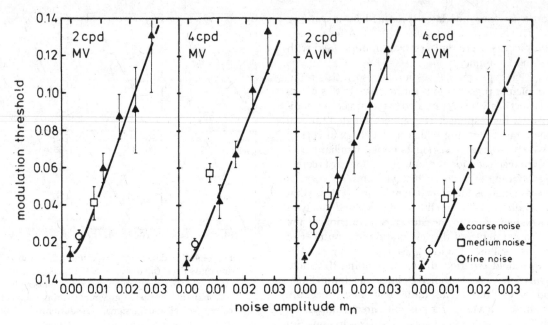

Fig. 34.6. Threshold elevation for 2 and 4 cpd test gratings caused by coarse grain noise with increasing noise amplitude, measured with two subjects. For comparison, the corresponding data points for fine and medium noise (taken from Fig. 34.5) are replotted here.

tions. Figure 34.6 illustrates the results of such measurements made for coarse noise. The thresholds for test grating frequencies of 2 and 4 cpd practically are proportional to the noise amplitude. The thresholds found with fine and medium noise, taken from Fig. 34.5 and replotted in Fig. 34.6, seem to nearly line up with the thresholds found with coarse noise.

Discussion

Separation of the masking effect

For a quantitative evaluation of the masking effect of additive pictorial noise it is necessary to separate the threshold elevation from the original threshold in the no-noise condition. With m as the threshold when pictorial noise is added, and m_i as the threshold in the no-noise condition one can consider $m - m_i$, m/m_i, or $(m^2 - m_i^2)^{1/2}$ as possible measures for the threshold elevation caused by the noise. If it is assumed that the threshold in the no-noise condition is set by an internal noise source, geometrical subtraction according to $m_e = (m^2 - m_i^2)^{1/2}$ must be preferred as most logical. Obviously, it is expected that the threshold elevation m_e will be proportional to the noise amplitude m_n, as introduced in the section on the description of the

noise pictures. This has been demonstrated earlier by Pollehn & Roehrig (1970) in similar experiments. It is also confirmed by the data of Fig. 34.6. This supports the idea of direct masking in the sense that the detection mechanism picks up components of the noise together with the signal, so that the signal-to-noise ratio is reduced proportionally when the strength of the noise is increased. In this line of thought the threshold enhancement m_e should be independent of the spectral composition of the noise in first approximation, after correction for possible differences in the noise amplitude m_n. In order to verify this the ratio of m_e and m_n is plotted in Fig. 34.7 for test grating spatial frequencies below the cut-off frequency of the respective noise conditions. The results for test grating frequencies above 20 cpd have also been omitted in Fig. 34.7 for the fine noise condition, because of their inherent inaccuracy. Figure 34.7 can be interpreted as an illustration of the relative effects of fine, medium and coarse noise, when the corresponding noise amplitudes are made equal. It now appears that adding fine noise causes a higher threshold elevation for low spatial frequency target gratings than adding coarse noise with the same spectral amplitudes. This difference was found to be statistically significant according to an analysis of variance applied to the data

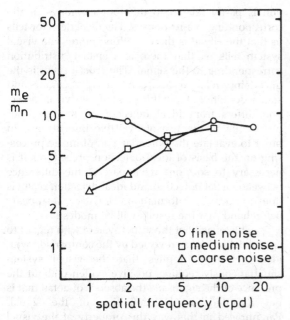

Fig. 34.7. Ratio of the threshold elevation m_e caused by pictorial noise and the noise amplitude m_n. The threshold elevation m_e is derived from the data in Fig. 34.5 as described in the text.

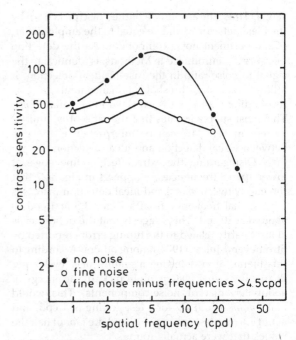

Fig. 34.8. Improvements of contrast sensitivity that can be obtained by removal of spatial frequencies above 4.5 cpd (blurring). The data for no noise are taken from Fig. 34.5. All other data are reconstructed as described in the text, starting from strong fine noise with $\sigma_p = 0.5$ and $m_n = 0.0031$.

of Fig. 34.7, and must be considered as a complication. However, there is no reason to reject masking in the sense as mentioned above, as the primary effect, explaining the greater part of the results shown in Figs. 34.5 and 34.6.

The extra effect of noise components above 18 cpd upon the detection of spatial frequencies more than 3 octaves lower deserves further attention. Undoubtedly more measurements are required in order to first establish and second reconnoitre this interesting phenomenon.

Effect of blurring
Returning to one of the original objectives of the measurements described here, the effect of high spatial freqency noise components upon contrast sensitivity at the lower end of the spatial frequency range confirms the potential profit of deliberate blurring. Figure 34.8 shows the improvement of contrast sensitivity for lower spatial frequencies when all frequencies above 4.5 cpd are removed from strong fine additive noise with $\sigma_p = 0.5$ and $m_n = 0.0031$ (see Methods). The threshold elevations m_e caused by the remaining noise components were derived from the data of Fig. 34.7. The improvement caused by 'deliber-

ate blurring' is not altogether negligible and these results certainly can explain why observers of images with pictorial noise occasionally claim to see better when defocusing, or at distance.

However, the practical value of deliberate blurring appears to be rather meagre when applied to a broad white spectrum of pictorial noise, as the basic effect of such noise is small beforehand. Obviously, the profit will be more substantial when the noise happens to be high frequency noise originally, so that all noise can be removed by blurring. This has been the case in the demonstration by Harmon & Julesz (1973).

Potential gain of ideal detection
As we have seen, the greater part of the threshold enhancement is caused by noise components in the direct vicinity of the signal, which cannot be removed by a simple blurring operation. In this situation the alternative approach of singling out the signal by an ideal detection algorithm may offer better prospects. The effect of the noise ideally is limited to the one and only possible component that is identical with the

signal. Thus, the amplitude of the noise picked up by the ideal detector would be equal to the amplitude m_n of the pertinent noise component. As the detection measure Z_d, introduced in Methods, is identical to the signal-to-noise ratio in the case of ideal detection, it follows that the threshold enhancement m_e corresponding with $Z_d = 1$ is expected to be equal to m_n. This most simply implies that the ratio of m_e and m_n plotted in Fig. 34.7 can be interpreted as the gap between visual detection and ideal detection.

Disregarding the extra effect of fine noise at lower spatial frequencies, it appears in Fig. 34.7 that the gap between visual and ideal detection increases with spatial frequency from a factor 3.5 at 1 cpd to about 8 at 10 cpd. This suggests that the deficiency is at least partly related to the tuning errors reported by Stromeyer & Julesz (1972) among others. According to this literature in detecting a grating of w cycles per degree the visual system might pick up the energy of about $2w$ adjacent noise-components. This would make m_e/m_n about 1.7 for a test grating of 1 cpd, and about 4.6 for a test grating of 10 cpd, i.e. about half the values that were actually found.

Apart from tuning errors the visual system probably fails to completely utilize the whole picture. Mathematically the receptive fields corresponding with the spectral windows are relatively small. As a consequence it appears that the pictures are processed piece-meal by the visual system. This does not necessarily imply that information is wasted, but this certainly cannot be excluded.

The question is to what extent the gap between visual detection and ideal detection can be considered as the potential gain of smart image processing. It is tempting to think that the signal, once detected by an ideal detection algorithm, can be made visible as such. However, coming to think about implementation, we realize that the observer will still require a visual manifestation of the signal, that cannot be delivered by the output of the ideal detection mechanism. The difference between ideal detection and visual detection is partly related to different meanings of the corresponding yes-responses. The ideal detector tells us that the signal is there, nothing more. The visual system tells us that there is a spatial distribution corresponding to the signal. The crucial point is the uncertainty-relation between tuning accuracy and spatial definition. From this point of view visual detection differs from ideal detection in strategy, not necessarily in the use of available information. In order to evaluate the potential gain of image processing on the basis of ideal detection procedures it is necessary to sort out what part of the difference between visual detection and ideal detection really is due to waste of information. However, it appears beforehand that the results will be modest.

The tenacity of the visual system with regard to spatial definition, as revealed by the comparison with ideal detection, implies that the visual system simultaneously requires positive evidence about the presence of the signal *and* the absence of detail that is not included in the definition of the signal. Paraphrased in this way this property of the visual system may also explain the extra effect of fine noise upon the detection of lower spatial frequencies, as mentioned above. More particularly one might wonder whether the difficulty of face recognition in the presence of disturbing high frequency detail, demonstrated by Harmon & Julesz (1973), is related with the threshold elevation of the relevant low frequency detail. An alternative hypothesis is that face recognition simply requires the absence of high frequency detail, because that is the way faces are stored in memory.

Summarizing, the efficiency of pictorial noise suppression in image processing is not spectacular in terms of visual performance. It must be remarked, though, that image processing applied to pictorial noise may be attractive in terms of visual comfort and the reduction of fatigue, and thus may help to improve visual performance in sustained observation tasks indirectly.

References

Barlow, H. B. (1978) The efficiency of detecting changes of density in random dot patterns. *Vision Res.*, **18**, 637–50.

Green, B. F., Wolf, A. K. & White, B. W. (1959) The detection of statistically defined patterns in a matrix of data. *Am. J. Psychol.*, **72**, 503–20.

Harmon, L. D. & Julesz, B. (1973) Masking in visual recognition: effects of two-dimensional filtered noise. *Science*, **180**, 1194–7.

Pollehn, H. & Roehrig, H. (1970) Effect of noise on the modulation transfer function of the visual channel. *J. Opt. Soc. Am.*, **60**, 842–8.

Pratt, W. K. (1978) *Digital Image Processing.* New York: Wiley.

Stromeyer, C. F. & Julesz, B. (1972) Spatial frequency masking in vision: critical bands and spread of masking. *J. Opt. Soc. Am.*, **62**, 1221–32.

Van Meeteren, A. & Barlow, H. B. (1981) The statistical efficiency for detecting sinusoidal modulation of average dot density in random figures. *Vision Res.*, **21**, 765–77.

35
Algotecture of visual cortex

A. B. Watson*

Introduction

Our knowledge of the primary visual pathway is voluminous but fragmentary. We know a great deal about the behavior of cells in the major waystations of this pathway – the retina, lateral geniculate nucleus (LGN), and striate cortex – but know rather little about how they function together to process the visual image. At each level, we know about various classes of cells, and about the spatial, temporal, and chromatic aspects of their receptive fields. But we know rather little about how cells at one level converge upon those at the next, and we know still less about the function of these receptive fields, and why particular receptive fields are employed at each level. An answer to these questions constitutes a theory of the algorithmic architecture (*algotecture*) of the visual pathways. This theory must address data from many sources, and must adhere to numerous mathematical constraints. In what follows, I will enumerate some of the considerations that must guide the attack upon this fundamental problem in vision and brain science. I will then sketch the beginnings of a candidate theory for one part of cortex. The theory raises as many questions as it answers, but that is not necessarily a bad thing, and at least it provides a concrete hypothesis that can be tested, modified, or replaced by a better theory.

I will restrict my focus to one portion of the visual pathway: the oriented simple cells of primate striate cortex. This system, while much less than the whole primary visual pathway, is nonetheless immense and fundamental. It contains a substantial

fraction of the visual cortex, and is the destination of the majority of cells in both retina and LGN. It is the putative basis of detailed form vision. If we could understand it, we would understand much of early visual processing. While my focus is on the cortex, a specific theme of this chapter is that cortical structure and function cannot be understood without reference to the structure and function of its tributaries, notable retina and LGN, so that some discussion of their properties is essential.

In pondering the striate cortex, one cannot help but be struck by the orderly, almost crystalline architecture, by the laminar and columnar organization, and by the properties of orientation and frequency tuning that are the hallmark of so many receptive fields. It is clearly an intricate analytical engine, but what does it compute, and how?

Constraints

The constraints that must guide a theory of visual cortex may be organized into the following categories: functional, mathematical, perceptual, physiological, and anatomical. Each category is reviewed briefly below. These reviews are partial and arguable.

Functional constraints

Functional constraints address the question of why the visual cortex does what it does. A most fundamental function of the cortex is to represent the visual image, to provide a 'sensorium' that subsequent visual processes may query (Koenderink & van Doorn, 1987). We may therefore think of the responses of cells of the cortex as providing a code of the visual image. It is important that the representation be complete, in the sense of not neglecting any information present in the image, at least within its chosen 'window of visibility' (Watson, Ahumada & Farrell, 1986). It has also been argued that an important function of the cortical code is to decorrelate individual elements of the code (Buchsbaum, 1987; Field, 1987; Laughlin, this volume). In the retina, signals from neighboring receptors are highly correlated and hence redundant, while in the cortex, through the construction of more elaborate receptive fields, there is an opportunity to produce cells whose responses are much more nearly independent. This is one aspect of coding efficiency, which we may take as another general functional goal of cortex. Another notable feature of visual cortex is heterogeneity: individual cells differ widely in their receptive field size, shape, and chromatic properties. The functional goal here may be to provide multiple representations of the image suited to various tasks. A specific example is the existence of many sizes of otherwise similar receptive fields, which may permit scale-invariant analysis of the image. Multiple representations may also aid in the segregation of regions within the image by common attributes, such as spatial frequency, orientation, bandwidth, and color and motion (Barlow, 1983). Finally, it is often argued that the cortical code must provide elements that are convenient for subsequent processing. An example is Koenderink's discussion of geometrical measures computed by cortical receptive fields (Koenderink & van Doorn, 1987).

Mathematical constraints

Mathematics cannot dictate physiology, but it can ensure that our theory is sensible and consistent. Furthermore, there is a rich mathematical literature on subjects such as coding, signal processing, and image processing that are of great value in understanding the cortex. Several principles in particular are fundamental.

The first principle is that since cortical information is represented in cell activity, the representation of visual information must be discrete. Each cell holds a *sample* of the visual image, and the receptive field defines the nature of that sample. The sampling process operates over all the dimensions of the input, including spatial, temporal, and chromatic. Sampling theory describes which collections of samples suffice to capture the information in a signal (Shannon, 1949; Jerri, 1977; Dudgeon & Mersereau, 1984). Sampling theory must be the foundation of any theory of the representation of visual information in cell activity (Hughes, 1981; Crick, Marr & Poggio, 1981; Sakitt & Barlow, 1982; Yellott, 1982, 1983; Robson, 1983; Watson, 1983, 1987a,b; Williams, 1985; Geisler & Hamilton, 1986; Maloney & Wandell, 1986; Ahumada

& Poirson, 1987). Since spatial imagery is two-dimensional, both the spatial receptive fields and sampling rules must be specified in two dimensions.

In the preceding section I noted the desirability of a complete representation. Sampling theory is one means of ensuring a complete representation. A closely related but somewhat different approach is exemplified in the theory of coding and reconstruction of images (Chellappa & Sawchuck, 1985). One simple principle from this field is that a complete representation must have a reconstruction algorithm, by which one computes the image from the code. Thus we would like to understand at least in principle, how to get back to the image from the cortical code.

Two different codes may be complete, yet differ in efficiency. Efficiency may be quantified in various ways, for example in terms of the number of coefficients (receptive fields), or in terms of the total entropy of the code (Watson, 1987b), or by yet other code statistics (Field, 1987). The efficiency of a code is closely related to the redundancy among coefficients discussed above. In any case, an understanding of the mathematical principles of coding efficiency is likely to enhance our understanding of the visual code.

I have already mentioned one intriguing aspect of visual cortex, namely the existence of multiple sizes and orientations of otherwise similar receptive fields. This feature is also found in image codes that have a *pyramid* structure, so-called because at each level the number of samples declines exponentially (Tanimoto & Pavlidis, 1975; Burt & Adelson, 1983; Woods & O'Neil, 1986; Watson, 1986, 1987a,b). These codes, also described as 'multi-resolution', or 'sub-band', employ kernels (receptive fields) that are self-similar (identical but for a change of scale or orientation). Since the brain appears to use pyramid coding, the principles that underlie these codes may prove helpful in understanding the cortical code.

Perceptual constraints

In the perceptual category, without meaning to disparage psychophysics, I have only one item: *perceptual completeness*. Earlier I said the code must be complete. But it must be complete only up to the perceptual capacity of the observer – it may lose whatever information the human loses. Psychophysics show us what information is retained and what is lost (Watson, Ahumada & Farrell, 1986). The goal is to construct a code that is as complete as the human or primate observer.

As an illustration, Fig. 35.1A is an image represented by 256^2 pixels, each of 24 bits. Elsewhere I have described a code modeled on visual cortex which

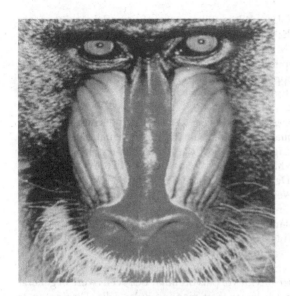

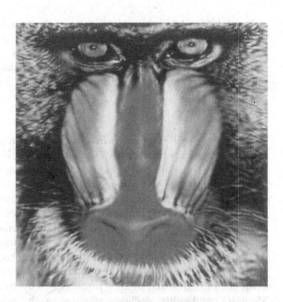

A **24 BITS/PIXEL**   B **0.85 BITS/PIXEL**

Fig. 35.1. A. An image coded at 24 bits/pixel. B. The same image, reconstructed from a code of 0.85 bits/pixel.

employs achromatic oriented frequency tuned cells and chromatic low resolution non-oriented cells (Watson, 1987a,b). The resulting code for this image uses less than 1 bit/pixel, and hence discards masses of information. But as the reconstruction in Fig. 35.1B illustrates, it is nevertheless perceptually almost complete.

One difficulty with applying perceptual constraints to a theory of visual cortex is that we rarely are able to locate with any precision the anatomical site at which perceptual judgements are made, or more precisely, at which visual information is lost. Nevertheless some general statements can be made. For example, if the physiological pathway under consideration is argued to be the site for high-resolution spatial vision, then it should manifest the general limitations of that capacity, in terms of the contrast sensitivity function and the like.

Physiological constraints

This large category primarily describes properties of the receptive fields of simple cortical cells. Space does not permit a detailed review, and I will highlight only what seem to me the most critical points. Excellent reviews are available elsewhere (Lennie, 1980; Shapley & Lennie, 1985).

Oriented, local, frequency-tuned receptive fields. The fundamental work of Hubel and Wiesel (reviewed in Hubel & Wiesel, 1977) and subsequent observations by others (Movshon *et al.*, 1978a,b; De Valois, Albrecht & Thorell, 1982; De Valois, Yund & Hepler, 1982; Schiller *et al.*, 1976; Foster *et al.*, 1985) has shown that most cortical simple receptive fields consist of a small number of parallel elongated regions of alternating excitation and inhibition. As a consequence, they are relatively compact in space, spatial frequency, and orientation: each cell responds over a limited region of space and to a limited band of spatial frequency and orientation. (The latter two restrictions may be described jointly as a compactness in two-dimensional spatial frequency.) To ensure completeness, there must be many cells, tuned to different spatial frequencies, orientations, and locations. Together the collection of cells must cover the visible regions of space, spatial frequency, and orientation. This distribution of cell properties has in fact been observed (De Valois, Albrecht & Thorell, 1982; De Valois, Yund & Hepler, 1982).

Frequency and orientation bandwidths. Within a simple receptive field, the extent in space (size) and in frequency (bandwidth) are inversely related. The median frequency bandwidth is about 1.5 octaves (De Valois, Albrecht & Thorell, 1982; Foster *et al.*, 1985; Hawken & Parker, 1987). The median orientation bandwidth estimate is about 40 degrees (De Valois, Yund & Hepler, 1982).

Heterogeneity. An important property of the population of cortical receptive fields is heterogeneity. This is perhaps best illustrated by the distributions of frequency and orientation bandwidth. The medians are cited above, but the distributions are broad and relatively shallow. A comprehensive theory must account for these ranges.

Bandwidth vs. peak frequency. In spite of the broad range of frequency bandwidths, we can nevertheless consider the covariation of peak frequency and bandwidth. Two simple cases are possible. If receptive fields were of constant size in degrees, then octave bandwidth would be inversely related to peak frequency. If receptive fields were a constant number of cycles of the underlying modulation (constant number of bars), then octave bandwidth would be constant, and independent of peak frequency. Available evidence indicates that neither result is strictly true. Median bandwidth declines slightly with peak frequency, but is much nearer to the constant octave hypothesis (De Valois, Albrecht & Thorell, 1982).

Phase. There is some evidence that cortical receptive fields exist in quadrature pairs, that is, that their spatial phases are 90° apart (Pollen & Ronner, 1981). Examples might be receptive fields with even and odd symmetry (0° and 90° phases, or so-called bar-detectors and edge-detectors), but current evidence suggests that such canonical phases are not the rule (Field & Tolhurst, 1986).

Aspect ratio. Another quantitative measure of receptive field shape is the aspect ratio, which describes the ratio of receptive field length (along the axis of orientation) to width. In linear cells, this is inversely related to the ratio of frequency and orientation bandwidth. For a cell whose two-dimensional frequency support is circular, the aspect ratio is 1. Estimates vary from cell to cell, with no consensus on a mean value different from 1 (De Valois, Albrecht & Thorell, 1982; Daugman, 1985; Webster & De Valois, 1985).

Linearity. Typically about half of the cells recorded in V1 in primate can be classified as 'simple' (Hubel & Wiesel, 1968; De Valois, Albrecht & Thorell, 1982; Hawken & Parker, 1987). These cells may exhibit output non-linearities, but show approximately linear spatial summation, and thus presumably receive input from linear X-like cells of the geniculate and retina. Thus the convergence of retinal and geniculate cells on the simple cortical cell may be modelled by purely linear operations.

Color. While still a matter of some debate, it appears that the majority of simple oriented V1 cells in primate are achromatic (Lennie, personal communication). In spite of the fact that they receive input from color opponent geniculate cells, they show little evidence of chromatic opponency.

Sensitivity and noise. A number of schemes exist for quantifying the sensitivity of visual cells (Enroth-Cugell et al., 1983; Kaplan & Shapley, 1986), some of which take into account the noise in the cell's response (Derrington & Lennie, 1984; Hawken & Parker, 1984). We define sensitivity as the inverse of the signal contrast which produces a response greater than one standard deviation of the noise on 50% of the trials. This corresponds directly to a signal/noise or d' measure (Green & Swets, 1966).

Kaplan & Shapley (1982) observed that peak sensitivities of parvocellular LGN cells were in general much lower than magnocellular cells. Derrington & Lennie (1984) indicate peak parvocellular sensitivities of around 20. Hawken & Parker (1984) have measured sensitivity of cells in layer 4 of primate cortex. They found a wide range of values (from about 1 to about 200). Within sublaminae receiving direct parvocellular input (IVa and IVcβ) sensitivities were generally lower (between about 1 and 60). As I shall show, specific schemes for the construction of cortical receptive fields from geniculate inputs must accommodate these estimates of sensitivity.

Anatomical constraints

Recent years have seen a profusion of results on the anatomical structure of the striate cortex (reviewed in Hubel & Wiesel, 1977; Gilbert, 1983; Livingstone & Hubel, 1984) and of its tributaries in the retina and LGN (Sterling, 1983; Hendrickson, Wilson & Ogren, 1978; Perry, Oehler & Cowey, 1984). Here again I can only highlight the small fraction of this literature that seems fundamental or particularly germane.

Retinal and geniculate inputs. Primate striate cortex receives all of its visual input from the LGN, which in turn is driven by retinal ganglion cells. Thus cortical cell receptive fields must be constructed from LGN receptive fields, which must in turn be constructed from ganglion cell receptive fields.

The most numerous of the various ganglion cell types in the primate retina are the X-type, which show high spatial resolution and linear responses (De Monasterio, 1978; Kaplan & Shapley, 1986). X receptive fields consist of antagonistic center and surround regions, and can be modelled as the difference of two radially-symmetric Gaussians. Receptive field size increases with eccentricity, and only one size appears to exist at a given eccentricity (Perry & Cowey, 1981, 1985).

The primate LGN is divided into six lamina. The two dorsal layers contain magnocellular cells, and the four ventral layers contain parvocellular cells (Hubel & Wiesel, 1972). We confine our attention to the parvocellular cells, which are highly linear, have high spatial resolution, and relatively low peak sensitivity (Blakemore & Vital-Durand, 1981; Kaplan & Shapley, 1982; Derrington & Lennie, 1984). Their receptive fields also have a center-surround receptive field, may also be modelled as a difference-of-Gaussian (DOG), and are in general difficult to distinguish from those of X-type retinal cells (So & Shapley, 1981; Derrington & Lennie, 1984). Parvocellular geniculates appear to be driven by retinal X cells with highly similar receptive fields (Kaplan & Shapley, 1986).

Most of the cells in the parvocellular layers of the LGN are chromatically and spatially opponent, most frequently with a red center and green surround, or green center and red surround (Derrington, Krauskopf & Lennie, 1984).

Parvocellular geniculate afferents terminate in layers IVa and IVcβ of the primate cortex (Hubel & Wiesel, 1972; Hendrickson *et al.*, 1978; Blasdel & Lund, 1983). However, in view of intracortical connections, we cannot say with certainty which layers, if any, receive exclusively parvocellular input (Gilbert, 1983).

Hexagonal input lattice. Since the parvocellular LGN appears to provide a transparent conduit between retina and cortex, we can consider the 'parvocellular' retinal cells (Kaplan & Shapley, 1986) as providing input to the cortex. In this light it is interesting to observe that the foveal receptor lattice is nearly hexagonal (Hirsch & Miller, 1987). Furthermore, available evidence suggests that in the foveal region, each ganglion cell center receives input from a single cone (Boycott & Dowling, 1969). This means that the ganglion cell RF centers also form a hexagonal lattice, and if the geniculate cells are likewise matched one-to-one with ganglion cells, then they too have a hexagonal sample lattice. The cells of the cortex must be constructed from this hexagonal array of retinal ganglion cell samples.

Cortical magnification. While the mapping between retina and cortex is topographic, the amount of cortex devoted to each retinal area declines with eccentricity. This relationship may be quantified by the cortical magnification factor, describing the linear mm of cortex devoted to a degree of visual field (Daniel & Whitteridge, 1961). A recent estimate in macaque is about 15–20 mm/deg for the fovea, with peripheral values about 10 times the inverse of eccentricity (Van Essen *et al.*, 1984). The magnification of the fovea relative to periphery is much greater in cortex than in either retina or LGN, so the spatial transformations among these layers cannot be spatially homogeneous (Perry & Cowey, 1985).

Hypercolumns. Area V1 is organized into hypercolumns of approximately 4 mm² (Hubel & Wiesel, 1977). Each hypercolumn is believed to perform a complete analysis of a local region of the visual field. Cells with the same ocular dominance tend to lie in parallel slabs orthogonal to the cortical surface. Cells with a common orientation preference also form slabs, or perhaps whirls, which intersect the ocular dominance columns. A hypercolumn consists of a portion of cortex with both ocular dominance columns and a complete set of orientation columns. At the center of each ocular dominance column 'blobs' of non-oriented cells have been found in layers 2 and 3, many of which are color selective (Livingstone & Hubel, 1984). Electrode penetrations tangential to the cortical surface often reveal a progressive change in receptive field orientation with penetration depth, covering 360° of orientation in approximately 1 mm of cortex (Hubel & Wiesel, 1977; Livingstone & Hubel, 1984).

Laminar structure. The striate cortex consists of a number of anatomically distinct layers. There is as yet no clear picture of the functional aspects of cells in each layer, but evidence on this matter is accumulating rapidly (Gilbert, 1983; Livingstone & Hubel, 1984; Hawken & Parker, 1984). Models of striate cortex should acknowledge the laminar structure and functional differences among lamina, and ultimately provide a functional explanation for the lamination.

Oversampling. While we have earlier pointed to efficiency as a plausible goal of the cortical code, and have noted that this may translate into a minimum number of cells, we must acknowledge that the striate cortex effects an enormous multiplication in the number of cells, relative to the number of retinal ganglion cells. This multiplication factor may be as high as 1000 (Barlow, 1983). Since the number of ganglion cells absolutely limits the degrees of freedom of the incoming signal, the cortex clearly does not seek to minimize its total number of cells. However, we have already noted the heterogeneity of visual cortex, and it is plausible that this multiplicity of cells reflects a multiplicity of codes, rather than an inefficiency in any one. The laminar structure itself suggests a multiplicity of cell types and perhaps codes.

Retinal disorder. Earlier I noted that the retina may impose its hexagonal structure on the cortex, and in this light it is worth noting that the receptor lattice becomes progressively more disordered with eccentricity (Hirsch & Miller, 1987; Ahumada & Poirson, 1987). This disorder may give rise to some of the heterogeneity at the cortical level, but must at any rate be taken into account in a description of the mapping from retina to cortex.

Receptive field models

There have been attempts to describe detailed receptive field shape with mathematical models. Marr & Hildreth have proposed $\nabla^2 G$, the Laplacian of a Gaussian (Marr & Hildreth, 1980). This is inadequate because it lacks orientation tuning. Young (1985) and Koenderink & van Doorn (1987) have proposed $D_N G$, the successive derivatives of a Gaussian. This is problematic because it predicts a constant linear bandwidth, and because it has no plausible extension into two dimensions. The Gabor function, the product of a Gaussian and a sinusoid, fits simple cell receptive fields well in many respects (Marcelja, 1980; Marcelja & Bishop, 1982; Webster & De Valois, 1985; Daugman, 1985; Field & Tolhurst, 1986). But detailed comparisons with empirical tuning functions show that the Gabor has too much sensitivity at low frequencies (Hawken & Parker, 1987). Put another way, the Gabor is highly asymmetrical in log–log coordinates, whereas actual tuning profiles are more nearly symmetrical. As an alternative Hawken & Parker have proposed the difference-of-separated-DOGs (d-DOG-s) model, describing the one-dimensional receptive field profile as the sum of 3 DOGs, a large positive central one flanked by two smaller negative ones. The fits of this model are generally much better than a Gabor, and are quite good overall. The objections to this model are, first, that it requires nine parameters to get this good fit. Second, it is not specified in the second spatial dimension, which would require still more parameters.

The chexagon model

I turn now to a description of a new model, which attempts to deal with many of the constraints I have described. While many of these constraints guided the design of this model, two were particularly influential. The first was the simple fact that cortical cells must be constructed from retinal inputs with DOG receptive fields. The second was that foveal receptors form an approximately hexagonal lattice. This means that X ganglion cells, and parvocellular cells of the LGN, must likewise have receptive fields forming a hexagonal lattice.

While the direct input to cortex is from the LGN, this input is in turn derived from retinal ganglion cells. Furthermore, there is as yet little evidence regarding how geniculate cells alter the retinal signals. I will therefore speak of the retinal ganglion cells as 'inputs' to the cortex. Accordingly, we begin with a retinal parvocellular receptive field, which we model as a DOG. The center Gaussian has a radius w, and the surround Gaussian a radius qw. The center Gaussian has volume $\varkappa$, and the surround Gaussian $s\varkappa$. Note that when s is 0, the frequency response is low-pass, when it is 1, the response is band-pass with no DC response.

The receptive fields are arranged in a hexagonal lattice with spacing λ. The DOG center radius can be expressed as a proportion of λ,

$$w = r\lambda \qquad (1)$$

A value of $r=1$, illustrated in Fig. 35.2, provides adequate sampling, and is in general agreement with what is known about the coverage factor of primate X parvocellular geniculate cells (the ratio of cell density to receptive field size) (Perry & Cowey, 1985).

In the remainder of this paper I will consider cortical receptive fields constructed from linear com-

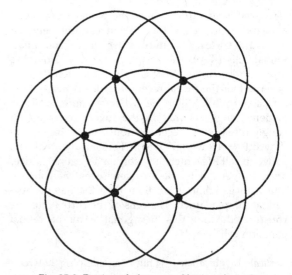

Fig. 35.2. Portion of a hexagonal lattice of ganglion cells. The ganglion cells are modelled by a difference-of-Gaussians (DOG). Circles represent center Gaussians at half height. In this example, the center Gaussian radius is equal to center spacing.

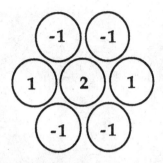

Fig. 35.3. Simple chexagon kernel. The numbers are weights assigned to each ganglion cell in the lattice of Fig. 35.2.

binations of these hexagonally spaced DOG inputs. Each receptive field is defined by the weights assigned to each point in the lattice. I will call this set of weights, and its topographic arrangement, a *kernel*. I will describe two schemes in which the kernels employ only a point and its six neighbors in the lattice, which I will call *chexagons* (cortical hexagon). The name is not to be taken too seriously, but provides a useful shorthand. In the discussion I will consider generalizations to other kernels that may employ larger numbers of weights.

Simple chexagon

Kernel. Our first scheme consists of kernels using a point and its six neighbors. We select weights such that the resulting receptive fields will have no response to uniform illumination (0 DC), will be oriented, and will be band-pass in spatial frequency. A particularly simple arrangement is shown in Fig. 35.3. In other words, we combine the signals from these seven DOG receptive fields, weighting each by the value shown. Two more receptive fields can be constructed by rotating the kernel by angles of 60° and 120°, providing a set of three oriented receptive fields, as shown in Fig. 35.4.

Figure 35.5 shows the 1D spectrum of one receptive field, measured at optimal orientation. Also shown are the spectrum of the underlying DOG, and the spectrum of a Gabor function of the same peak frequency and bandwidth. The 1D bandwidth of the chexagon is about 1.6 octaves, near to the median estimate for primate cortical cells. The chexagon spectrum is considerably narrower than the DOG spectrum, and in effect selects a slice, or sub-band of the DOG spectrum. The chexagon bandshape is much more nearly symmetrical (on log–log coordinates) than the Gabor, and is therefore likely to provide a much better fit to measured 1D spectra of cortical cells (Hawken & Parker, 1987).

Pooling. I have constructed a receptive field tuned to a particular frequency band, and note that it is at the upper end of the pass-band of the DOG spectrum, and thus of the pass-band of the system as a whole. It is, in other words, a high-frequency cell. I will call these the *level* 0 cells. Now we ask: where do we get the lower-frequency cells? We cannot simply increase the separation between geniculate inputs λ, as that will produce severe undersampling and aliasing. Likewise we cannot vary w, since retinal ganglion cell centers do not vary in size at one eccentricity.

The solution is to create *pooling units*, through linear combination of the original retinal inputs. There are various pooling kernels that might be used. For simplicity, we consider a Gaussian function of distance from the central sample point. The pooling units then have individual receptive fields that are the convolution of a DOG and the Gaussian kernel. These will resemble the original DOGs but will be somewhat larger, depending on the size of the Gaussian. These pooling units now provide the input to the next set of kernels, which are identical to those at the previous level except that they are enlarged by a factor of two. In other words, the distance between weights in the kernel is now 2λ. These new kernels generate the receptive fields of cells at level 1. The same procedure may be repeated, successive applications yielding larger and larger pooling units, and lower and lower frequency cells.

Receptive fields and spectra. Figure 35.6 illustrates the receptive fields, and their frequency spectra, at four levels. The figure also shows the spectra of the components used to construct the receptive field: the DOG, the hexagonal kernel, and the pooling kernel. The receptive field spectrum is the product of these three spectra. The receptive fields have a shape that roughly resembles cortical cells. The spectra are smooth, band-pass, and oriented, and generally consistent with what is known about 2D spectra of single cortical cells (De Valois, Albrecht & Thorell, 1982; De Valois, Yund & Hepler, 1982).

Sensitivity. Earlier we noted that the sensitivity of a cell may be expressed in signal/noise terms. Given a signal/noise description of retinal ganglion cell sensitivity, the sensitivity of the computed cortical receptive field can be expressed in the same terms. Specifically, assume that each ganglion cell has identical independent Gaussian noise, and that no additional noise is introduced at geniculate or cortical levels (this assumption can be relaxed in a more elaborate formulation). Then the noise at the cortical

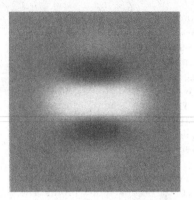
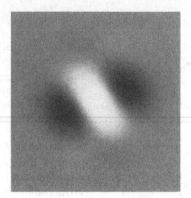
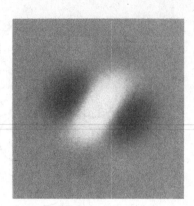

Fig. 35.4. Receptive fields of the simple chexagon model. The three orientations are produced by rotating the kernel of weights by 0°, 60°, and 120°. The dimensions of each image are 8λ. Parameters are $r = 1, q = 6, s = 0.5$.

cell will have a variance equal to the sum of the squared kernel weights times the retinal variance. To express sensitivities in signal/noise terms, the kernel must be normalized, so that the sum of the squared kernel weights is 1 (the kernel has a unit norm). For the higher order cells, this unit norm applies to the convolution of the pooling function and the chexagon kernel.

Figure 35.7 shows the 1D spectra at four levels, as well as the spectrum of the retinal DOG. The curves are correctly placed on the vertical axis. Note that the cortical sensitivity can be substantially above that of the ganglion cells, because of spatial pooling. At each level the spectra are similar in shape, but displaced downwards on the frequency axis by approximate factors of two. The spectra have approximately constant log bandwidth, consistent with the data cited earlier.

Subsampling. The centers of the kernels of the level 0 cells are coincident with the centers of the retinal inputs. Since there are three orientations, there are therefore three times as many of these level 0 cells as there are retinal inputs. The size of the pooling Gaussian may be chosen so as to permit subsampling at each level without substantial aliasing. By subsampling we mean the construction of receptive fields at a subset of the locations in the input sample lattice. As an example, we consider subsampling by a factor of two in each dimension at each level. The distance between receptive field centers at level n is then $\lambda 2^n$. This results in a total number of cortical cells equal to four times the number of retinal inputs. The various levels of cells together form a pyramid structure as discussed above. Figure 35.8 illustrates several levels of this pyramid.

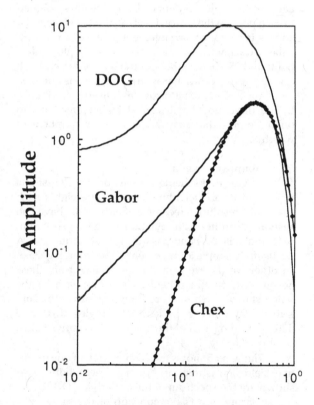

Spatial Frequency

Fig. 35.5. 1D spectrum of the chexagon receptive field at optimal orientation. Also shown are the spectrum of the retinal DOG receptive field and of a Gabor function of similar frequency and log bandwidth. Parameters are $\varkappa = 15, \lambda = 0.5, r = 1.15, q = 3, s = 0.95$.

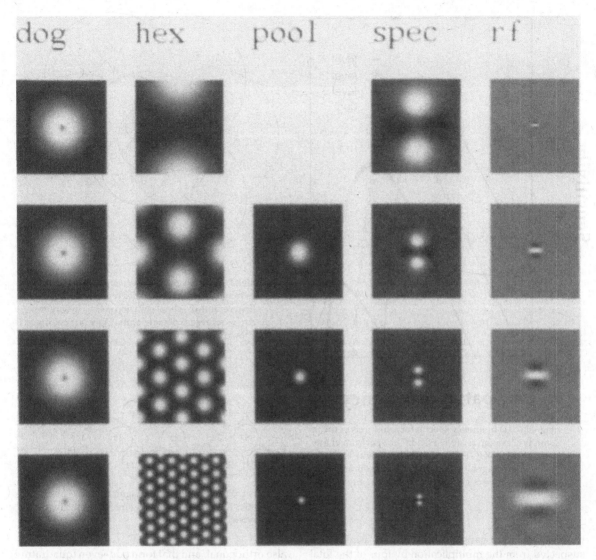

Fig. 35.6. Receptive fields and frequency transforms for four levels of the simple chexagon pyramid. Only the even receptive field at one orientation is shown. From left to right, the columns show the spectrum of the retinal inputs (DOG), the spectrum of kernel of weights, the spectrum of the pooling kernel, the spectrum of the cortical receptive field, and the receptive field. The fourth column is equal to the product of the first three columns, and the last column is the inverse Fourier transform of the fourth column. Rows from top to bottom show levels from 0 to 3. There is no pooling kernel at level 0. Parameters are $r = 1$, $q = 6$, $s = 0.5$. Dimensions of each image are 64λ.

Hyperchexagons. The process of generating larger and larger cells must stop somewhere. The number of levels corresponds to what have elsewhere been called channels, which have been estimated psychophysically to number between three and eight (Wilson & Bergen, 1979; Watson, 1982). At the top of the pyramid, the receptive fields will have a particular size. It is useful to be able to talk about all the receptive fields in the area occupied by this largest receptive field, so I will call them collectively a *hyperchexagon*. Each hyperchexagon is itself a pyramid which analyzes a sub-region of the visual field.

Efficiency. Although we do not demonstrate it here, it is worth noting that the simple chexagon pyramid provides a complete representation of the image pro-

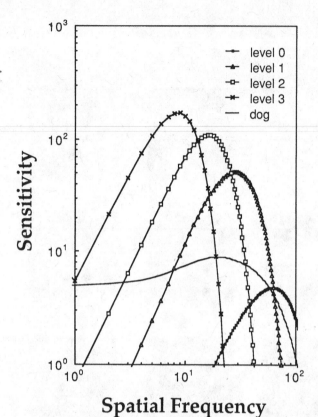

Fig. 35.7. 1D frequency spectra for four levels of the simple chexagon receptive field. The spectrum of the retinal input DOG is also shown. Sensitivity is expressed in signal/noise terms. Parameters are $\varkappa = 10$, $r = 1$, $q = 6$, $s = 0.5$. Frequency is in units of $1/(256\lambda)$.

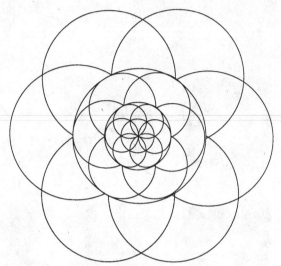

Fig. 35.8. Three levels of the simple chexagon pyramid. The smallest circles represent receptive field centers of retinal ganglion cells. The larger circles represent pooling units. Only one chexagon is shown at each level.

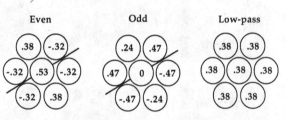

Fig. 35.9. Orthogonal chexagon kernels. The oblique lines indicate one axis of symmetry for the high-pass kernels.

vided by the input ganglion cells. In fact, as might be suspected from the multiplication by four of the total number of cells, the representation is redundant. Elsewhere we have noted that the cortex as a whole greatly expands the number of cells, relative to the retinal input. This over-representation may in part serve to immunize the system against noise and loss of cells, and so we should not necessarily expect a cortical representation that is highly efficient. Nevertheless, it is worth considering the form such an efficient code might take, if only to understand the redundancy imposed by less efficient codes. This leads us to the second form of chexagon pyramid.

Orthogonal chexagons
Kernels. In this case we have sought a set of kernels that are band-pass and oriented as above, but that are also orthogonal, and that form odd–even (quadrature) pairs. One consequence of orthogonality is that the number of cells constructed is equal to the number of input cells, hence the code is maximally efficient in this sense. The orthogonal code is complete, and thus permits exact reconstruction of the input samples. In addition, reconstruction of the image employs the same kernels used in coding. The derivation of the kernels is described elsewhere (Watson & Ahumada, 1987). The resulting kernel values are shown in Fig. 35.9.

There are seven kernels, of which only three are shown in Fig. 35.9. They are even, odd, and low-pass. The four not shown are produced by rotations of even and odd kernels by angles of 60° and 120°. The receptive fields are shown in Fig. 35.10.

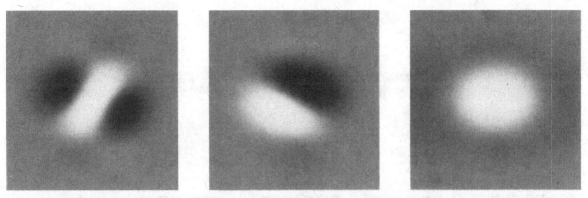

Fig. 35.10. Receptive fields generated by orthogonal chexagon kernels. From left to right they are: even, odd, and low-pass. Dimensions of each image are 8λ.

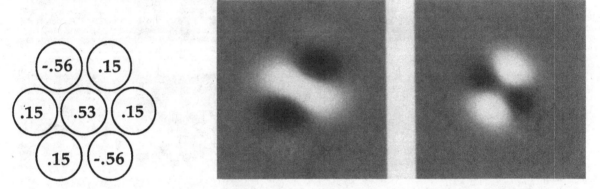

Fig. 35.11. Alternate form for the even kernel, with corresponding receptive field and frequency transform.

Alternate even kernel. We define the *orientation* of a receptive field as the orientation of the peak of the frequency spectrum, that is, the orientation of a sinusoidal input at which the kernel gives the largest response. An interesting feature of the resulting kernels is that while the axis of symmetry was fixed at 30°, the orientation of the even kernel is actually orthogonal to this axis at 120°. This places its orientation axis on the hexagonal lattice. The constraints under which the kernels were derived (essentially orthonormality, completeness, and quadrature pairs) generate another alternate solution for the even kernel (Fig. 35.11).

Calling the first solution type 0 and the second type 1, the latter has an orientation of 30°, equal to that of the odd receptive field. Thus if it is desired to have quadrature pairs with equal orientation, the type 1 even kernel must be used. But as can be seen in Fig. 35.11, the type 1 kernel suffers relative to the type 0 in having substantially greater sensitivity at the non-preferred orientation.

Pooling. In this scheme, the pooling is done by the low-pass kernel. The next level of the pyramid is constructed from these pooling units. Because the low-pass kernel is orthogonal to all six high-pass kernels, the high-pass kernels at level 1 will be orthogonal to the high-pass kernels at level 0 (since they are linear combinations of the low-pass kernel). By extension of this argument, it is clear that all kernels in the pyramid are orthogonal.

Receptive fields and spectra. The kernels at each level are self-similar. The receptive field will be only approximately self-similar, because while the kernels scale in size at each level, the retinal DOG function with which they are convolved remains fixed in size. Figure 35.12 illustrates an even receptive field and its spectrum at four scales. The spectra are approximately band-pass in frequency and orientation, with bandwidths similar to those encountered physiologically. For this even filter, there is substantial sensitivity at 90° to the preferred orientation. Such secondary peaks in

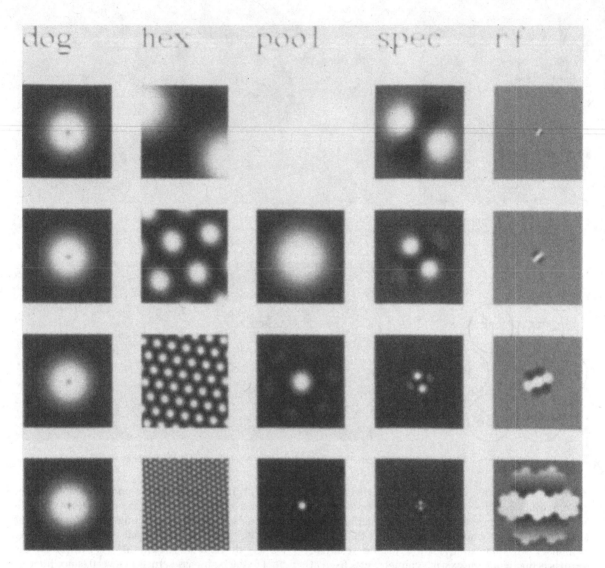

Fig. 35.12. Receptive fields and frequency transforms for four levels of the orthogonal chexagon pyramid. Only the even type 0 receptive field at one orientation is shown. From left to right, the columns show the spectrum of the retinal inputs (DOG), the spectrum of the kernel of weights, the spectrum of the pooling kernel, the spectrum of the cortical receptive field, and the receptive field. The fourth column is equal to the product of the first three columns, and the last column is the inverse Fourier transform of the fourth column. Rows from top to bottom show levels from 0 to 3. There is no pooling kernel at level 0. Parameters are $r = 1$, $q = 6$, $s = 0.5$. Dimensions of each image are 64λ.

orientation tuning are quite often found in cortical cells, but may not be a general feature (De Valois, Yund & Hepler, 1982). A closer look at a one-dimensional cross-section through each filter at the optimal orientation (Fig. 35.13) shows considerable ringing in the higher order filters.

Since the filters are orthogonal, this creates no problems for coding or reconstruction, but does

render this exact form of the filters less like cortical cells. However, only the ringing in the highest level cell would be detectable in physiological measurements, due to their limited precision. This ringing can be reduced to some extent through judicious choice of filter parameters, but is an inherent property of these filters attributable to the small area and abrupt borders of the pooling region. It is not evident in the previous

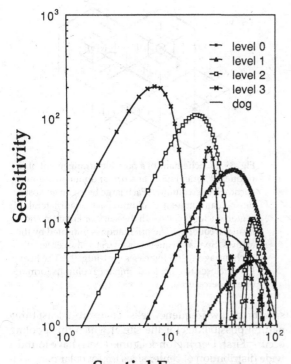

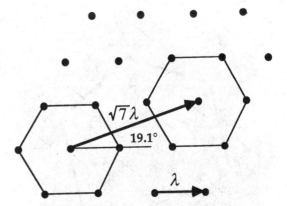

Fig. 35.14. Construction of receptive fields at level 0. Each point is the center of a retinal ganglion cell receptive field. Each hexagon shows a set of inputs that are combined to form the level 0 receptive fields.

Spatial Frequency

Fig. 35.13. 1D frequency spectra for four levels of the orthogonal chexagon receptive field. The spectrum of the retinal input DOG is also shown. Sensitivity is expressed in signal/noise terms. Parameters are $x = 10$, $r = 1$, $q = 6$, $s = 0.5$. Frequency is in units of $1/(256\lambda)$.

scheme (Fig. 35.5) because there pooling employs a Gaussian extending over a larger area.

Subsampling. Since the information in each hexagonal neighborhood of seven retinal inputs is completely captured in the seven cortical receptive fields constructed therefrom, there is no need for overlap of adjacent kernels. We therefore tesselate the retinal input lattice with hexagonal kernels, as illustrated in Fig. 35.14. Because each kernel consumes exactly seven inputs, the number (or density) of receptive fields of a given type (e.g. odd at 60°) will be one seventh the number (or density) of retinal inputs. The kernel centers form a new hexagonal lattice with a sample distance of $\sqrt{7}\,\lambda$. The lattice is rotated by an angle of $\tan^{-1}(\sqrt{3/5}) \approx 19.1°$ relative to the retinal sample lattice. The kernels of level 1 are constructed from this new lattice, using the low-pass cells of level 0. Likewise at each successive level new kernels are constructed from the low-pass units at the previous

stage, on a hexagonal lattice whose sample distance increases by $\sqrt{7}$ at each level, and which rotates by $\pm 19.1°$ at each level. After n levels, there are n sizes (spatial frequencies) of receptive field, and the total number of receptive fields is equal to the number of retinal inputs. The complete pyramid is illustrated in Fig. 35.15.

Discussion

In this section I will make some observations that apply to all of the schemes described above.

Hypercolumns. In the first scheme, the radius of the kernel increases by a factor of two at each level, so that at level n it is $\lambda 2^n$. This defines the size of the hyperchexagon. For example, if $n=4$, (5 levels), and $\lambda = 0.01°$ (Hirsch & Miller, 1987), then a single hyperchexagon has a radius of about 16 receptors or 0.16°. Foveal cortical magnification has been estimated in macaque at between 5 and 13 mm/°, so that a single hypercolumn of radius 1 mm corresponds to about 0.11°. While the numbers used in this calculation are not known with precision, and are further confused by the change in scale with eccentricity, they nevertheless suggest an identity between the hyperchexagon and the hypercolumn. This in turn suggests a speculation concerning the topography of cells within a hypercolumn.

Hypercolumn Architecture. In the pyramid schemes the number of cells per level is in proportion to the pass-band of that level, many for high-frequency levels, few for low-frequency levels. Adding to this the observation that the cortex is relatively homogeneous

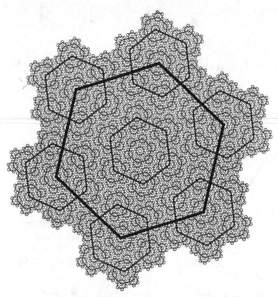

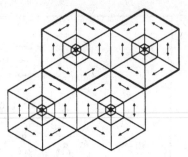

Fig. 35.16. Schematic of a possible arrangement of frequency, orientation, and ocular dominance among cortical hypercolumns. Each large hexagon encloses one ocular dominance column. Each quadrilateral region encloses cells with the same orientation and spatial frequency. The orientation is indicated by the arrows. Spatial frequency is lowest at the center of each hexagon, and increases centrifugally. The heavy line encloses two ocular dominance columns forming one hypercolumn.

Fig. 35.15. Orthogonal chexagon pyramid. The level 0 kernels are represented by the smallest hexagons. The vertices of these smallest hexagons correspond to centers of the retinal ganglion cell receptive fields (and hence to receptors). Kernels at successive levels correspond to larger and larger hexagons. The vertices of each hexagon at each level coincide with the centers of the hexagons at the previous level. At each level, the kernels are applied to the low-pass responses from the previous level. This hexagonal fractal was constructed by first creating the largest hexagon, then placing at each of its vertices a hexagon rotated by $\tan^{-1}(\sqrt{3/5}) \approx 19.1°$ and scaled by $1/\sqrt{7}$. The same procedure is then applied to each of the smaller hexagons, down to a terminating level of 5. The sample lattice (defined by the vertices and centers of the smallest hexagons) is then a finite-extent periodic sequence on a hexagonal sample lattice. The sample lattice has 7^6 points, the same as a rectangular lattice of 343^2. The perimeter is a 'Koch curve' with a fractal dimension of $\log 3/\log \sqrt{7} \approx 1.19$ (Mandelbrot, 1983, p. 46). The program used to create this image is given in Watson & Ahumada (1987).

in cell density, we confront the problem of how to arrange the cells within each hypercolumn. A simple solution is to arrange them as a replica of the spectrum itself, as shown in Fig. 35.16. This would lead naturally to the orientation columns found anatomically, as well as to the progressive changes in orientation found along certain tangential electrode tracks. This is speculative, of course, but amenable to test.

Pooling units. The pooling process described in the above schemes is essential to generate narrowband

spectra for low-frequency cells. There are at least three natural possibilities for the site at which this pooling occurs. First, Derrington & Lennie (1984) have found a wide distribution of center sizes for foveolar parvocellular geniculate cells. While they suggest this may be due to measurement errors, it may reflect a pooling operation within the geniculate. A second and perhaps more likely possibility is that the pooling units may be the various non-oriented cortical cells such as those found in the cytochrome oxidase blobs at the center of each hypercolumn in layers 2 and 3 (Livingstone & Hubel, 1984), or the non-oriented cells found in layers $4c\beta$ (Hawken & Parker, 1984). A third possibility is that the pooling may be at the level of the oriented cell itself, although, for a low-frequency cell, this calls for the convergence of very large numbers of geniculate cells upon a single cortical cell.

Multiplexing of luminance and color information.   To this point I have spoken of retinal and geniculate inputs as being of two types: on- and off-center. But Derrington & Lennie have shown that the parvocellular geniculate cells are chromatically, as well as spatially opponent. They are of two types. By far the more numerous are R–G cells, in which center and surround receive opposed contributions from R and G cones (red on-center, red off-center, green on-center, green off-center). Much rarer are B–(R&G), in which B cones, in either center or surround, are opposed by some combination of R and G cones in the other spatial region. Furthermore, from the ratio of receptors to ganglion cells it appears that foveal retinal ganglion cell centers are driven by a single cone. Thus the lattice of inputs, at least in the fovea, is presumably color opponent. Since oriented cortical cells are generally found to have negligible color opponency, we may ask how they are constructed from these color opponent inputs.

The simplest answer is to combine spatially coincident inputs of opposite center color before forming the kernel. For example, if a retinal input in a previous scheme was assigned a weight of 1, we now assign weights of 1 to both a red on-center cell and a coextensive green on-center cell. The resulting cortical receptive field will have no color opponency. It has been argued that retinal and geniculate cells multiplex both luminance and color information (Ingling & Martinez, 1983; Derrington, Krauskopf & Lennie, 1984). By combining chromatically opponent cells we 'de-multiplex' the luminance information.

At level 0 of the pyramid, this scheme is problematic, since it requires both R and G centers at each point in the initial hexagonal sample lattice. But as noted above, for foveal ganglion cells there is evidently *only* an R *or* a G center at each point, but not both. This is only a problem for the highest-frequency cells (level 0), and it may be that without the demultiplexing operation, chromatic abberation and the quasi-random assignment of cone types to input nodes renders these highest-frequency cells effectively achromatic.

Push–pull inputs. Assigning a positive weight to an input may mean any of three things: excitatory input from an on-center cell, inhibitory input from an off-center cell, or both. The last scheme has the advantage of rejecting certain nonlinearities common to both on- and off-center cells (Derrington, this volume). It also has the advantage of rejecting noise common to both cells that arises distal to the image. In the present case, use of push–pull inputs would mean that each of the seven nodes in the hexagon of inputs would receive four spatially coextensive inputs: on- and off-centers of both R and G types. Whether push–pull inputs are used in the construction of cortical cells is not yet known, though they appear to be used in the retina (Sterling, 1983).

Spatial inhomogeneity and disorder. The constructions above are based on a hexagonal lattice with spacing λ, identified with the cone spacing. As noted above, in the primate retina this spacing increases with distance from the fovea (Hirsch & Miller, 1987; Perry & Cowey, 1985). There is also a general increase in the disorder of the cone lattice, proceeding from foveal sections of nearly perfect hexagonal packing to peripheral sec-

tions with high disorder. There are several ways to generalize the chexagon models to the case of an inhomogeneous, disordered retina. One is to establish cortical connections with an ordered, homogeneous retina, and to preserve these connections during a process of retinal warping and perturbation. A second is to apply the chexagon construction to the six nearest neighbors, regardless of their precise locations. These speculations are perhaps better deferred until a clearer picture of retinal and cortical development is available.

The chexagon constructions described above specify a fixed convergence from receptors to ganglion cells, to geniculate, and to cortex. But it is known that the ratio of numbers of these four cell types devoted to a given retinal area vary considerably with eccentricity. Specifically, the ratio of cones to ganglion cells is about 1 within 5 mm (about 20°) of the fovea, increasing to 2 or 3 in the far periphery (Perry & Cowey, 1985). In contrast, the ratio of parvocellular geniculate cells to the P_β ganglion cells (anatomically distinct cells believed to be the inputs to the parvocellular pathway in the geniculate) is approximately 1 throughout the visual field (Perry & Cowey, 1985). Finally, the ratio of cortical cells to retinal cells is much higher in the fovea than in the periphery. The cortex devotes about 35% of its cells to the central 10 degrees, while the retina devotes only about 7%. These spatial variations in the pattern of convergence are a challenge for future models.

Conclusions

I have reviewed a number of the facts and principles that must be observed by a theory of operation of striate visual cortex. This list has necessarily been fragmentary. I have presented a general scheme in which oriented, band-pass cortical receptive fields are constructed from hexagonal kernels of weights applied to retinal or geniculate inputs. Two specific schemes were considered: one with greater physiological plausibility, the other with greater mathematical elegance. We may hope that a future scheme will combine both virtues. Both schemes are successful, however, in producing the general features of cortical processing, in particular band-pass receptive fields with moderate bandwidths in frequency and orientation. In the case of the orthogonal filters, quadrature pairs are also produced. Both schemes are exciting in that they suggest a wealth of questions and experiments, as well as refinements of the theory. A natural direction for future development is to consider kernels of more than seven inputs. This would allow greater degrees of freedom in design of the receptive field, and hence a better match to physiological data. Another research direction is to consider how the construction of chexagon receptive fields might be manifest in the microcircuitry of the cortex (Gilbert, 1983).

In exploring this domain we frequently experience a tension between mathematical simplicity and biological complexity. We are reminded of Niels Bohr's dictum that 'truth' is the variable complementary to 'clarity'. It may help to consider two possible states of nature. In one, the visual brain obeys some simple architectural principle, and the variability and imperfection we observe are merely developmental perturbations. In this case, there is good reason to search for the guiding principle. In the second case, cortical 'structure' is a byproduct of some mindless evolutionary and developmental process. But while

such a process may result in a less orderly structure, it is not random and can also be probed for its 'principle'. Thus in both cases it is worth searching for a canonical algotecture.

The cortical code poses an exciting and fundamental challenge for neuroscience, for cognitive science, and for vision science. It is a game that must be played by the rules, from experimental data to abstract principles of visual coding. A solution to the puzzle must work on all levels, physiological, anatomical, mathematical, perceptual and functional. The scheme I have proposed, while it does not fit every aspect of the data, at least provides an example of an hypothesis that works at every level, and that may encourage newer and better proposals. We will not solve the puzzle until we start to put the pieces together.

References

Ahumada, A. J., Jr. & Poirson, A. (1987) Cone sampling array model. *J. Opt. Soc. Am. A*, **4**, 1493–502.

Barlow, H. B. (1983) Understanding natural vision. In *Physical and Biological Processing of Images*, ed. O. J. Braddick & A. C. Sleigh, pp. 2–14. New York: Springer-Verlag.

Blakemore, C. B. & Vital-Durand, F. (1981) Distribution of X- and Y-cells in the monkey's lateral geniculate nucleus. *J. Physiol. (Lond.)*, **320**, 17–18P.

Blasdel, G. G. & Lund, J. S. (1983) Terminations of afferent axons in macaque striate cortex. *J. Neurosci.*, **3**, 1389–413.

Boycott, B. B. & Dowling, J. E. (1969) Organization of primate retina. *Phil. Trans. Roy. Soc.*, B255, 109–84.

Buchsbaum, G. (1987) Image coding in the visual system. *Optic News*, **13**, 16–19.

Burt, P. J. & Adelson, E. H. (1983) The laplacian pyramid as a compact image code. *IEEE Transactions on Communications*, COM-31, 532–40.

Chellappa, R. & Sawchuck, A. (ed.) (1985) *Digital Image Processing and Analysis Volume 1: Digital Image Processing.* Silver Spring, MD: IEEE Computer Society Press.

Crick, F. H. C., Marr, D. C. & Poggio, T. (1981) An information processing approach to understanding the visual cortex. In *The Organization of the Cerebral Cortex*, ed. F. O. Schmitt, F. G. Worden, G. Adelman & S. G. Dennis. Cambridge, Mass.: MIT Press.

Daniel, P. M. & Whitteridge, D. (1961) The representation of the visual field on the cerebral cortex in monkeys. *J. Physiol. (Lond.)*, **159**, 203–21.

Daugman, J. G. (1985) Uncertainty relation for resolution in space, spatial frequency and orientation optimized by two-dimensional visual cortex filters. *J. Opt. Soc. Am. A*, **2**, 1160–9.

De Monasterio, F. M. (1978) Properties of concentrically organized X and Y ganglion cells of macaque retina. *J. Neurophysiol.*, **41**, 1394–417.

Derrington, A. M. & Lennie, P. (1984) Spatial and temporal contrast sensitivities of neurones in lateral geniculate nucleus of macaque. *J. Physiol. (Lond.)*, **357**, 219–40.

Derrington, A. M., Krauskopf, J. & Lennie, P. (1984) Chromatic mechanisms in lateral geniculate nucleus of macaque. *J. Physiol. (Lond.)*, **357**, 241–65.

De Valois, R. L., Albrecht, D. G. & Thorell, L. G. (1982) Spatial Frequency Selectivity of Cells in Macaque Visual Cortex. *Vision Res.*, **22**, 545–59.

De Valois, R. L., Yund, E. W. & Hepler, H. (1982) The orientation and direction selectivity of cells in macaque visual cortex. *Vision Res.*, **22**, 531–44.

Dudgeon, D. A. & Mersereau, R. M. (1984) *Multidimensional Digital Signal Processing.* Englewood Cliffs, NJ: Prentice-Hall.

Enroth-Cugell, C., Robson, J. G., Schweitzer-Tong, D. & Watson, A. B. (1983) Spatio-temporal interactions in cat retinal ganglion cells showing linear spatial summation. *J. Physiol. (Lond.)*, **341**, 279–307.

Field, D. J. (1987) Relations between the statistics of natural images and the response properties of cortical cells. *J. Opt. Soc. Am. A*, **4**(12), 2379–94.

Field, D. J. & Tolhurst, D. J. (1986) The structure and symmetry of simple-cell receptive-field profiles in the cat's visual cortex. *Proc. Roy. Soc. Lond.*, **228**, 379–400.

Foster, K. H., Gaska, J. P., Nagler, M. & Pollen, D. A. (1985) Spatial and temporal frequency selectivity of neurones in visual cortical areas V1 and V2 of the macaque monkey. *J. Physiol. (Lond.)*, **365**, 331–63.

Geisler, W. S. & Hamilton, D. B. (1986) Sampling-theory analysis of spatial vision. *J. Opt. Soc. Am. A*, **3**, 62–70.

Gilbert, C. D. (1983) Microcircuitry of the visual cortex. *Ann. Rev. Neurosci.*, **6**, 217–47.

Green, D. M. & Swets, J. A. (1966) *Signal Detection Theory and Psychophysics.* New York: Wiley.

Hawken, M. J. & Parker, A. J. (1984) Contrast Sensitivity and orientation selectivity in lamina IV of the striate cortex of old world monkeys. *Exp. Brain Res.*, **54**, 367–72.

Hawken, M. J. & Parker, A. J. (1987) Spatial properties of neurons in the monkey striate cortex. *Proc. Roy. Soc. Lond.*, B**231**, 251–88.

Hendrickson, A. E., Wilson, J. R. & Ogren, M. P. (1978) The neuroanatomical organization of pathways between the dorsal lateral geniculate nucleus and visual cortex in old and new world primates. *J. Comp. Neurol.*, **182**, 123–36.

Hirsch, J. & Miller, W. H. (1987) Does cone positional disorder limit resolution? *J. Opt. Soc. Am. A*, **4**, 1481–92.

Hubel, D. H. & Wiesel, T. N. (1968) Receptive fields and functional architecture of monkey striate cortex. *J. Physiol. (Lond.)*, **195**, 215–43.

Hubel, D. H. & Wiesel, T. N. (1972) Laminar and columnar distribution of geniculo-cortical fibres in macaque monkey. *J. Comp. Neurol.*, **146**, 421–50.

Hubel, D. H. & Wiesel, T. N. (1977) Functional architecture of the macaque monkey visual cortex. Ferrier Lecture. *Proc. Roy. Soc. Lond. (Biology)*, **198**, 1–59.

Hughes, A. (1981) Cat retina and the sampling theorem; the relation of transient and sustained brisk-unit cut-off frequency to a- and b-mode cell density. *Exp. Brain Res.*, **42**, 196–202.

Ingling, C. R. & Martinez, E. (1983) The spatiochromatic signal of the r–g channel. In *Colour Vision*, ed. J. D. Mollon & L. T. Sharpe, pp. 433–44. London: Academic Press.

Jerri, A. J. (1977) The Shannon sampling theorem – its various extensions and applications: a tutorial review. *Proceedings of the IEEE*, **65**, 1565–96.

Kaplan, E. & Shapley, R. M. (1982) X- and Y-cells in the lateral geniculate nucleus of macaque monkeys. *J. Physiol. (Lond.)*, **330**, 125–43.

Kaplan, E. & Shapley, R. M. (1986) The primate retina contains two types of ganglion cells, with high and low contrast sensitivity. *Proc. Natl. Acad. Sci. USA*, **83**, 2755–7.

Koenderink, J. J. & van Doorn, A. J. (1987) Representation of local geometry in the visual system. *Biol. Cybern.*, **55**, 367–75.

Kulikowski, J. J., Marcelja, S. & Bishop, P. O. (1982) Theory of spatial position and spatial frequency relations in the receptive fields of simple cells in the visual cortex. *Biol. Cybern.*, **43**, 187–98.

Lennie, P. (1980) Parallel visual pathways: a review. *Vision Res.*, **20**, 561–94.

Livingstone, M. S. & Hubel, D. H. (1984) Anatomy and physiology of a color system in the primate visual cortex. *J. Neurosci.*, **4**, 309–56.

Maloney, L. T. & Wandell, B. A. (1986) Color constancy: a method for recovering surface spectral reflectance. *J. Opt. Soc. Am. A*, **3**, 29–33.

Mandelbrot, B. B. (1983) *The Fractal Geometry of Nature*. New York: Freeman.

Marcelja, S. (1980) Mathematical description of the responses of simple cortical cells. *J. Opt. Soc. Am.*, **70**, 1297–300.

Marr, D. & Hildreth, E. (1980) Theory of edge detection. *Proc. Roy. Soc. Lond.*, B**207**, 187–217.

Movshon, J. A., Thompson, I. D. & Tolhurst, D. J. (1978a) Spatial summation in the receptive fields of simple cells in the cat's striate cortex. *J. Physiol. (Lond.)*, **283**, 53–77.

Movshon, J. A., Thompson, I. D. & Tolhurst, D. J. (1978b) Spatial and temporal contrast sensitivity of neurones in areas 17 and 18 of the cat's visual cortex. *J. Physiol. (Lond.)*, **283**, 101–20.

Perry, V. H. & Cowey, A. (1981) The morphological correlates of X- and Y-like retinal ganglion cells in the retina of monkeys. *Exp. Brain Res.*, **43**, 226–8.

Perry, V. H. & Cowey, A. (1985) The ganglion cell and cone distributions in the monkey's retina: implications for central magnification factors. *Vision Res.*, **25**, 1795–810.

Perry, V. H., Oehler, R. & Cowey, A. (1984) Retinal ganglion cells that project to the dorsal lateral geniculate nucleus in the macaque monkey. *Neurosci.*, **12**, 1101–23.

Pollen, D. A. & Ronner, S. F. (1981) Phase relationship between adjacent simple cells in the visual cortex. *Science*, **212**, 1409–11.

Robson, J. G. (1983) Frequency domain visual processing. In *Physical and Biological Processing of Images*, ed. O. J. Braddick & A. C. Sleigh, pp. 73–87. Berlin: Springer-Verlag.

Sakitt, B. & Barlow, H. B. (1982) A model for the economical encoding of the visual image in cerebral cortex. *Biol. Cybern.*, **43**, 97–108.

Schiller, P. H., Finlay, B. L. & Volman, S. F. (1976) Quantitative studies of single cell properties in monkey striate cortex. III. Spatial frequency. *J. Neurophysiol.*, **39**, 1334–51.

Shannon, C. E. (1949) Communication in the presence of noise. *Proceedings IRE*, **37**, 10–21.

Shapley, R. M. & Lennie, P. (1985) Spatial frequency analysis in the visual system. In *Annual Review of Neuroscience*, Vol. 8, ed. W. M. Cowan, pp. 547–83. Palo Alto, CA: Annual Reviews, Inc.

So, Y. T. & Shapley, R. (1981) Spatial tuning of cells in and around lateral geniculate nucleus of the cat: X and Y relay cells and perigeniculate interneurons. *J. Neurophysiol.*, **45**, 107–20.

Sterling, P. (1983) Microcircuitry of the cat retina. *Ann. Rev. Neurosci.*, **6**, 149–85.

Tanimoto, S. & Pavlidis, T. (1975) A Hierarchical data structure for picture processing. *Computer Graphics and Image Processing*, **4**, 104–19.

Van Essen, D. C., Newsome, W. T. & Maunsell, J. H. R. (1984) The visual field representation in striate cortex of the macaque monkey: asymmetries, anisotropies, and individual variability. *Vision Res.*, **24**, 429–48.

Watson, A. B. (1982) Summation of grating patches indicates many types of detector at one retinal location. *Vision Res.*, **22**, 17–25.

Watson, A. B. (1983) Detection and identification of simple spatial forms. In *Physical and Biological Processing of Images*, ed. O. J. Braddick & A. C. Sleigh, pp. 100–14. Berlin: Springer-Verlag.

Watson, A. B. (1986) *Ideal Shrinking and Expansion of Discrete*

Sequences. NASA Technical Memorandum 88202. Washington DC: NASA.

Watson, A. B. (1987a) The cortex transform: rapid computation of simulated neural images. *Computer Vision, Graphics, and Image Processing,* **39**, 311–27.

Watson, A. B. (1987b) Efficiency of an image code based on human vision. *J. Opt. Soc. Am. A,* **4**, 2401–17.

Watson, A. B. & Ahumada, A. J., Jr. (1987) *An Orthogonal Oriented Quadrature Hexagonal Image Pyramid.* NASA Technical Memorandum 100054. Washington DC: NASA.

Watson, A. B., Ahumada, A. J. Jr. & Farrell, J. (1986) Window of visibility: psychophysical theory of fidelity in time-sampled visual motion displays. *J. Opt. Soc. Am. A,* **3**, 300–7.

Webster, M. A. & De Valois, R. L. (1985) Relationship between spatial-frequency and orientation of striate-cortex cells. *J. Opt. Soc. Am. A,* **2**, 1124–32.

Williams, D. R. (1985) Aliasing in human foveal vision. *Vision Res.,* **25**, 195–205.

Wilson, H. R. & Bergen, J. R. (1979) A four mechanisms model for threshold spatial vision. *Vision Res.,* **19**, 19–33.

Woods, J. W. & O'Neil, S. D. (1986) Subband coding of images. *IEEE Transactions on Acoustics, Speech, and Signal Processing ASSP-34,* 1278–88.

Yellott, J. I. (1982) Spectral analysis of spatial sampling by photoreceptors: typological disorder prevents aliasing. *Vision Res.,* **22**, 1205–10.

Yellott, J. I. (1983) Spectral consequences of photoreceptor sampling in the Rhesus retina. *Science,* **221**, 382–5.

Young, R. A. (1985) *The Gaussian Derivative Theory of Spatial Vision: Analysis of Cortical Cell Receptive Field Line-Weighting Profiles.* General Motors Research Report GMR-4920. Warren MI: General Motors.

36
The iconic bottleneck and the tenuous link between early visual processing and perception

K. Nakayama

Introduction

Late 19th century studies of the brain provided evidence that part of the cerebral cortex was made up of primary sensory receiving areas and primary motor areas. These comprised a relatively small portion of the total surface area of the cortex and with the exception of some specialized regions (such as Broca's area), the functional relevance of the other parts of the cortex remained a mystery. Vision was relegated to a small portion of the human cortex, occupying about 15 per cent of the total surface. Surrounding this primary area were secondary and tertiary zones, often referred to as 'association cortex'.

Very recent advances in neuroanatomy and neurophysiology, however, have changed this picture dramatically. Thanks to the pioneering work of Allman & Kaas (1974), Zeki (1978), and Van Essen (1985), we now know that monkey visual cortex contains at least 19 separate maps of the visual field and according to a recent review by Maunsell & Newsome (1987) visual processing occupies about 60 per cent of the cortical surface!

This overwhelming dominance of vision in relation to other functions should serve as a reminder that, as generally practiced, the current subdisciplines of visual perception and psychophysics may be too narrow to capture the wealth of processing involved. Threshold psychophysics, especially, has been preoccupied with just the earliest aspects of vision. It has neglected the seemingly intractable questions such as the nature of visual experience, pattern recognition, visual memory, attention, etc.

Meanwhile the neurophysiologists have been making recordings from diverse regions of the visual cortex which could be closely related to these higher functions. For example, in V2, just one synapse beyond the primary receiving area, it appears that the firing of some neurons is related to the formation of 'illusory' contours (von der Heydt et al., 1984). In area V4 the receptive field organization of cells is very specifically and profoundly altered by the attentional state of the monkey (Moran & Desimone, 1985). Finally, in infero-temporal cortex, many laboratories find that some cells only fire when the complex image of a face appears in the visual field (Gross, 1973; Perrett et al., 1982, 1987). So now it is the physiologists who seem to be leading the way, at least as far as higher visual functions are concerned; their observations show that many complex functions are being performed in these newly identified regions of visual cortex.

To begin to redress this imbalance between psychology and neurophysiology we offer a frankly speculative theory as to the overall functional organization of the visual system. It postulates an associate memory for image fragments (icons) adapted from cognitive psychology (Lindsay & Norman, 1977; Rumelhart & McClelland, 1986) and couples this with the emerging notion of a multi-resolution pyramid representation for early vision as suggested by workers in psychophysics, physiology and artificial intelligence. Because it is so very general and covers such a large range of phenomenon and possible mechanisms, the theory will probably resist verification or falsification. We present it nonetheless, mainly because of the paucity of plausible ideas in this area. Hopefully such a skeletal framework will open the door for more precisely formulated ideas, and ones that can be more easily tested.

In essence, our theory divides the visual system in two: early vision consisting of a feature pyramid followed by visual memory. We describe each in turn.

The feature pyramid – an overview

Closest to the input is a massively parallel feature pyramid which comprises striate cortex and those portions of extrastriate cortex which are organized more or less retinotopically. This system is organized as a multi-resolution multi-feature pyramid. For example, such a system contains neurons sensitive to a variety of features, including disparity, motion, color, line orientation, line termination etc., each of which can be represented at a variety of scales.

The usefulness of a generic and multi-purpose pyramid has been suggested by Rosenfeld (this volume) and the specific notion of a multi-resolution pyramid for early cortical representation has been proposed on empirical and theoretical grounds (Burt & Adelson, 1983; Sakitt & Barlow, 1982). Moreover, the general idea is consistent with the physiological findings (DeValois *et al.*, 1982). The essence of the idea is a retinotopic representation of the image at varying degrees of scale or coarseness. So with each ascending level of the pyramid (as shown in Fig. 36.1), the image is represented with less and less spatial precision and resolution. It should be obvious that the different levels differ in information content with the coarsest representation of the image requiring fewer bits of information than the finest level.

For illustrative purposes we will make this more concrete by estimating the relative information content at the various levels, recognizing that such numerical estimates are subject to error and acknowledging that they gloss over the actual details of the encoding process. The empirical basis of such estimates does not match the specificity suggested by the numbers themselves, and we do not mean to imply by assigning numbers that the entities denoted are physically discrete or quantized. Yet despite these limitations, it is possible that the use of such estimates can help us focus on otherwise difficult issues. For purposes of illustration we adopt the fiction that the system encodes the image in terms of pixels of varying size with a roughly constant number of bits per pixel. So the number of pixels becomes an intuitively reasonable index of information content. Again, we are aware that a very different type of coding than single pixel representation occurs. Thus in terms of contrast, it is likely that the system encodes the image in terms of oriented receptive fields of various sizes (DeValois *et al.*, 1982; Wilson & Bergen, 1979; Watson, this volume).

As an example, we provide an estimate as to the number of pixels required for the coding of contrast. First we need to remove the complication introduced by the cortical magnification factor. We take a functional approach by noting how ordinary visual acuity varies with retinal eccentricity. Consistent with the complex logarithm description of the retino-cortical projection (Schwartz, 1977), the typical function relating letter acuity to eccentricity increases linearly with eccentricity (Weymouth, 1958). Using this data to calculate (by numerical integration) the number of such recognizable letters that could be squeezed into the visual field, we come up with a figure of about 1000. Assuming that each letter comprises a 5×5 pixel array, roughly consistent with data indicating that 2 sinusoidal cycles/letter is adequate for letter recognition (Ginsburg, 1981), we arrive at a total of about 25 000 pixels in the whole visual field. This is roughly the equivalent of a 160×160 pixel grid.

This describes the image as it is represented at the highest level of detail that can be encoded. But because it is a pyramid, the image is also represented at progressively coarser degrees of visual resolution. Thus, if at each level, we get coarser by a scale factor of two, we can see that a system of just five levels will have at its most coarse representation, a pixel grid of about 10×10 pixels. To get a pictorial understanding of the hypothesized number of pixels, at least for the coding of achromatic contrast, five such representations are schematized in Fig. 36.1 where each definable square represents 100 pixels (a 10×10 pixel grid).

So far, we have depicted the pyramid as if it operated at different scales analogous to banks of spatial frequency filters (Burt & Adelson, 1983; Sakitt & Barlow, 1982). This is misleading, however, since we would not want to exclude dots, edges and lines which only contain high spatial frequency information from being represented at the coarsest level of representation. Thus Craik–Cornsweet edges and difference of Gaussian dots (Carlson *et al.*, 1984) are represented similarly as ordinary edges and dots. So the early vision pyramid is far more abstract than simple spatial frequency scaling insofar as it represents edges, lines, etc. at different scales. Thus some form of appropriate communication between high spatial frequency mechanisms and the coarse level of representation in the pyramid is required. Interactions of this sort have been suggested by Rosenfeld (this volume) and Grossberg & Mingolla (1985) among others.

Visual memory – an overview

At the other extreme, farthest removed from the eye, is visual memory. Such a system contains tiny pattern

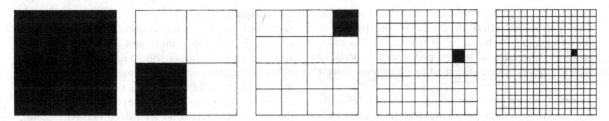

Fig. 36.1. Schematic representation of the multi-level pyramid. Coarsest representational level is shown at left. Finest representation shown on extreme right. Three intermediate representations are also shown. Note the existence of one shaded square at each level of the pyramid. This represents the size of the visual field that can be utilized for a hypothetical elementary pattern recognition operation at that level of representation in the pyramid.

recognition templates or icons[1] which are associatively linked. Thus they can be activated or potentiated by two different routes. First, by the process of pattern matching with incoming visual signals from the feature pyramid. Second, by the activation of other icons through associative learning. This memory system is situated in regions of visual cortex which shows the least evidence of retinotopic order and is most likely to be localized in the temporal lobes (Mishkin & Appenzeller, 1987). A small schematized subsection of this memory is shown in Fig. 36.2, illustrating at least two types of connections to these icons: afferent (from the pyramid) and associative (from within the memory itself).

The experience of seeing is dependent on the activation of these nodes or icons in visual memory. *Without such activation, visual perception cannot exist.* Essential to the theory as it is proposed is the assertion that these icons or templates contain surprisingly small amounts of information and that they capture the essential properties of an image fragment with very few bits. To keep our argument as numerically concrete as possible and to emphasize their small size, we assert that such icons contain only 100 pixels. Thus if such a template were to be roughly square it would comprise about 10×10 pixels.

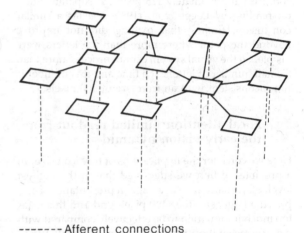

------- Afferent connections

——— Associative connections

Fig. 36.2. Schematic description of a very small subsection of visual memory. Each icon or node has two types of possible connections, one set from within visual memory itself (solid lines) and one set to the output of the early vision pyramid (dashed lines).

Evidence that icons are low resolution

Perhaps the most seemingly arbitrary single aspect of the theory is this assertion that the templates or icons have very low information content. Less controversial is the assertion that visual memory is made up of an associative network of such elements. To provide some plausibility to this idea of the very small icon size, we note data obtained from reading performance. If the visual system could pattern process only a small amount of pixels per unit time, then one should be able to drastically reduce the effective information available in certain visual tasks, and one should see no decrement in performance. This is a difficult experi-

---

[1] Note that our use of the term 'icon' is very different from that used in the past in cognitive psychology. Neisser (1967) coined the term to refer to short term visual storage (as originally described by Sperling, 1960) and it is synonymous with what could be called early cortical after discharge, specifically residual activation in the early vision pyramid after a brief flash. Our use of the term establishes the icon as a very small learned visual template, a constituent of visual memory.

ment to design in most free viewing tasks because one does not know where in the array the person is attending nor at what level of resolution. Reading, however, provides a stereotyped visual procedure which requires systematic attentional fixations along a line of print. Rayner (1978) has developed a computerized technique to limit the amount of intelligible text that is on a page by monitoring eye movements and replacing all but a small number of letters around the fixation point with meaningless symbols. They find that if one makes more than about 5 letters visible, then reading is not substantially improved. This tallies reasonably well with our 100 pixel limit since 5 letters comprise approximately 125 pixels. A separate study on reading by Legge *et al.* (1985) reaches a similar conclusion, finding that reading did not improve beyond the point where more than 3.5 letters were visible. So the visual system cannot process more than a small number of letters at a time and this number is not inconsistent with an icon size of 100 pixels.

Focal attention: limited readout from the early vision pyramid

Here we consider the implications of tiny icon size. In a previous section we suggested that at the highest level of resolution, the image representation comprised a large, say 160×160 pixel, grid and this is far too much information to be effectively compared with pattern recognition templates having a small 10×10 pixel extent. The amount of information that can be sampled from the pyramid in the process of pattern recognition cannot exceed the size of the templates or icons themselves.

From this it follows that pattern recognition from the whole pyramid is not feasible in one single step. Many such steps which we call attentional fixations or elemental pattern matching operations will be required. In quantitative terms and if our estimates and ideas are reasonable, the sampling of the whole field will require about 250 of these elemental pattern matching operations because the 10×10 pixel arrangement can only cover 1/256th of the high-resolution map (see Fig. 36.1). If one were to sample the representation of the visual field at the coarsest 10×10 level of resolution, however, only a single elemental pattern matching operation will be required.

Because of these quantitative considerations, it would seem that for the purposes of elementary pattern recognition, the visual system is faced with a trade-off. It can sample from the pyramid at lower levels of spatial resolution to obtain an overview of the visual scene whilst sacrificing detail. Alternatively, it can sample at a very high level of resolution to get detail but sacrificing the overview. The shading of squares in Fig. 36.1 illustrates the very different amounts of coverage of the visual field that can be obtained as one conducts an elemental pattern matching operation at different levels of the pyramid. The existence of selective attention to particular portions of the visual field has been well documented (Posner, 1980, 1987). See also Nakayama & Mackeben, 1989. Selective attention to one spatial scale vs. another is less well documented but preliminary evidence to support such mechanism has been obtained by Sperling & Melcher (1978).

Figure 36.3 schematizes the visual system as a whole. Closest to the input end is the massively parallel pyramid, comprising the machinery of early vision and receiving parallel input from the retina. Farthest from the input is visual memory, also a massively parallel system, associatively linked and composed of tiny icons having very low informational capacity. Although the connections and consequent quantity of information shared within each of these massively parallel systems is great, the connection *between* these systems is not. This link is extremely band-limited and constitutes a critical bottleneck in the visual system.

So how does vision occur in ordinary circumstances? We argue that for normal scenes, vision involves a serial sequencing of elementary pattern matches (attentional fixations) from different loci in the pyramid. The net result of such matches is residual activity in those icons which have been recently activated by feature pyramid output and also those which have been associatively linked or potentiated by such icons. Thus we argue that the conscious act of perception is directly related to aggregate activation of these icons in visual memory.

As an illustrative example, consider the visual system confronted with a mountain landscape scene which is very briefly presented in a tachistoscope but with sufficient time to allow for three attentional fixations. First the system does a pattern match to the whole scene at lowest resolution and gets a memory activation capturing the gross outline of the mountain. Then it makes a second more detailed attentional fixation at a lower level of the pyramid centered at the mountain peak. Finally, one other fixation is directed downward towards the house near the base. We argue, however, that other icons may also be partially activated, not through visual input but by associative linkage of those icons which have received visual input. So from the perspective of capturing specific input from the retina, only three very low resolution

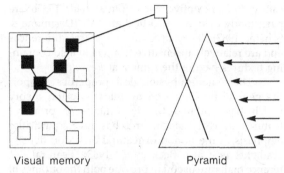

Visual memory   Pyramid

Fig. 36.3. Overview of the visual system. On the left is visual memory, containing tiny icons linked associatively. On the right is the multi-resolution pyramid which receives afferent visual input. The linkage between these two massively parallel systems is a narrow bandwidth channel having a capacity of the order of a single icon.

Shaded squares in visual memory provide a schematic representation of a number of icons which have residual activation from previous pattern matches from the early visual pyramid and which constitute the 'contents' of conscious visual experience.

'snapshots' at three different scales have been taken, yet it is sufficient for the observer to capture the essentials of the scene. The total set of activated icons is enough to convey the 'meaning' of the scene, and the observer is unaware of the essentially serial nature of the construction process nor of its tenuous relation to visual input. As far as the observer is concerned he was presented with a scene and he has grasped it all at once.

What we are saying is that our own introspective understanding of vision is somewhat of an illusion. We regard our visual world as 'just there', not as something which is only acquired after sequential sampling and reconstruction. It appears that vision occurs in parallel yet our actual contact with the world is essentially serial,[2] constructed by a sequence of low bandwidth pattern recognition matches. Thus the actual amount of visual information that is explicitly

---

[2] At the same time that we have the phenomenologically naive belief that visual perception is conducted in parallel, it can also be argued that the phenomenology associated with eye fixations supports something much closer to the present theory. As we make a set of eye fixations we know that very fine detail can only be made in central vision. Yet the scene remains remarkably 'seamless' and 'there'. Thus we are forced to conclude that the pick-up is serial yet something endures (the activation of visual memory), to preserve the scene.

used as part of the pattern recognition process is but a tiny fraction of the information available at any instant in the feature pyramid.

Need for a controller?

The most distinguishing feature of the theory is the notion of a limited attentional bandwidth (limited pattern recognition capacity) coupled with the complementary notion of a multi-scale pyramidal representation of early vision. The organization of the pyramid as a data structure is well suited for the tasks we suggest because it enables the system to scan the image for its essential properties in an efficient manner, appropriately switching levels of resolution to get both the overview and the necessary details.

As described, however, the process might seem to require an 'agent' or 'genie', to direct these attentional fixations so as to optimize the pickup of information. This is likely to be the case for a certain fraction of the time, but at others, the control of attention could be determined at a very low level. This has been suggested by Julesz (1984) who concluded that texton or feature gradients draw attention. Koch & Ullman (1985) say much the same in their description of the saliency map which directs the spotlight of attention. In particular, Koch & Ullman suggest a winner-take-all network based on some plausibly hypothetical properties of early feature maps which is adequate to direct some aspects of attention. Beyond this selection, Koch & Ullman suggest that the system may shift to the next most salient feature, based on its proximity or similarity to the previous feature.

Such low level schemes will not be sufficient for many aspects of attentional control and other mechanisms will be required. Again this may not require as much centralized control as one might think. It is conceivable that attentional fixation instructions could be distributed and linked to the visual memory itself. One possibility is to attach the fixational routines to particular icon sets in visual memory. A low resolution icon representing the gross features of an object might contain 'pointers' to other appropriate fixations. Thus the outline of a face might activate attentional 'fixations' at finer levels of detail to recognize eyes, nose and mouth, thus providing information to recognize a specific face (see Noton & Stark, 1971). Such an approach might be analogous to object oriented algorithms more familiar to specialists in computer science.

In addition to the controller function we speculate that there also needs to be an 'addresser'. Such a mechanism will register the address or locus of sampling from the pyramid and create a corresponding address and size for an activated icon in a more generalized body-centered coordinate system. Such organization is necessary to preserve the spatial relations of the sampled image fragments in the scene and also to provide a coordinate reference for motor behavior.

Finally a comment about neural implementation. The model as proposed implies that the connections between visual memory and the outputs from early vision are constantly changing. At one moment, visual memory is connected to, and thus samples from, say, the lowest level of the pyramid. Then later it may sample from a restricted region of the visual field from a high-resolution section. As yet there is no obvious circuitry to mediate these processes which would seem to require the formation of temporary yet orderly sets of connections. But it is perhaps interesting to note that the existence of temporary synapses has been proposed (Crick, 1984) and that more recently 'shifter-circuits' have been suggested (Anderson & Van Essen, 1987) which could temporally connect one two-dimensional representation to another, preserving local retinotopic order.

Extensive preprocessing in the pyramid

Our discussion so far has purposely oversimplified the nature of the multi-feature pyramid so as to stress the main features of the theory. Now, however, we must mention several properties of the pyramid which are of critical importance to guide the pattern recognition process. Thanks to the work of many, most notably Barlow (1960, 1961) and Marr (1982) it has become increasingly clear that the processing in early vision is highly sophisticated and captures visual information in a seemingly 'intelligent' manner without recourse to cognitive top-down processing. Two properties of the pyramid seem particularly important in this regard: feature differencing and feature grouping.

With respect to featural differencing, we envision that for each feature map, there exist inhibitory networks to enhance differences in that particular feature. Thus for the representation of motion, neural networks are organized so that velocity differences rather than absolute velocities are registered (Allman et al., 1985a; Frost & Nakayama, 1983). Likewise, orientation (Blakemore & Tobin, 1972; Nelson & Frost, 1978), as well as other features, is organized so that spatial differences in that feature are emphasized rather than the features themselves. These mechanisms, consisting of connections outside of the classi-

cally defined receptive fields (Allman et al., 1985b) are particularly evident in cortical area V4 (Desimone & Schein, 1987). They accentuate featural differences and are relatively insensitive to a whole field containing textures having the same features.

These neurophysiological properties support the general points raised by Julesz's texton theory which has outlined the importance of primitive features in early vision and has given particular emphasis to the notion of featural or texton density gradients (see also Beck et al., 1983). Featural difference maps are useful to provide both the outlines of a two-dimensional image to be compared with templates in visual memory (such outlines may be analogous to Marr's place tokens) as well as providing potential loci for the direction of visual attention (as suggested by Julesz, 1984).

In addition to feature differencing, the pyramid must also support grouping algorithms. These have at least two major functions: (1) to appropriately link and enhance different portions of the image for the purposes of pattern recognition; (2) to suppress all other parts of the image so that pattern matching is only applied to the appropriate portion of the image. Grouping is a process which pre-organizes information in the feature pyramid to make it amenable for pattern recognition. This is the familiar figure-ground process and one that is essential if pattern recognition is to occur.

Many grouping laws are well known as they are embodied in various Gestalt laws of perception. Furthermore, they have also received some attention in recent times. The work of Julesz, Grossberg and others, for example, are partially devoted to characterizing the cooperative and competitive networks underlying this grouping process. One of the most important process is similarity of grouping, i.e. those elements which have the same color, orientation, disparity, motion, etc. are linked (see Barlow, 1981). It is suggested that grouping requires an excitatory linkage between the representation of like features and inhibiting coupling between unlike features and that the network parameters of excitation and inhibition can increase or decrease as a function of experience (plasticity) or the demands of the moment (modulation).

The existence of feature differencing and similarity grouping is particularly helpful in interpreting the results of visual search experiments, where it is the task of the observer to identify a target from amongst a set of distractors. Treisman (1985) found that the search for a target differing by a single feature was easy and conducted in parallel (search time

A   B

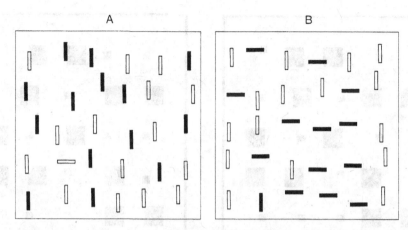

Fig. 36.4. Two types of visual search task. In (A) the observer has to find the target defined by a single feature difference, namely he needs to find the target having the horizontal orientation. We argue that feature differencing mechanisms (in the domain of orientation for this particular case) automatically mark the spot at which an elementary pattern matching operation will occur. Consequently, the search for such a single target will be rapid and will not be slowed by increasing the number of distractors (vertical bars). In (B) the observer must find the target defined by the conjunction of orientation and color. The observer must find either a white horizontal bar or a dark vertical bar amongst the distractors. We argue that, for this situation, feature differencing operations (either for color or orientation) will fail to select a unique site for pattern matching. As a consequence, pattern matching will be made at a number of wrong sites before the correct target is found. As such, search time will increase for greater number of distractors.

independent of number of distractors) whereas the search differing in a conjunction of two features was serial (search time increased for larger number of distractors). See Fig. 36.4 for an illustration of these two types of visual search displays.

We have confirmed this for a number of conjunctions (in particular, the conjunction of orientation and color), but for many other conjunctions including any dimension linked to disparity (Nakayama & Silverman, 1986a,b), the search can be conducted in parallel. Furthermore, with extended practice, it has been claimed that the conjunction of virtually any pair of dimensions can be made to occur in parallel (see Steinman, 1987; also Wolfe *et al.*, 1989 and personal communication).

The ideas proposed here provide an interpretative framework to understand these rather puzzling results. In such multi-element search arrays the system is faced with two problems. First is the capacity limitations of learned pattern recognition templates. We have postulated that such icons have only very limited information content. Thus it is not feasible to sample the whole target display with a single template match at the lowest level of resolution because the targets are too small and are thus indistinguishable at the lowest level of resolution. The pattern matching operation needs to be directed to a higher resolution level in the pyramid and to a particular locus. This

leads to the second problem. How is this site to be selected? In the case of a simple search for a single deviant feature, the problem is relatively easy. Feature differencing mechanisms can designate the single site for pattern recognition. For the case of feature conjunctions, however, the problem is more complex since feature differences on any given dimension are present in many sectors of the array and no single obvious site emerges for the more specialized pattern matching process. The system is forced to pattern match at a variety of wrong sites before finding the target. This could account for the increased search time for some conjunctions.

As mentioned earlier, however, the search for many feature conjunctions can be conducted in parallel (Nakayama & Silverman, 1986a,b). To explain this ease by which many conjunctions are searched, we invoke similarity grouping. This process takes like features, say those sharing a common disparity and links them, suppressing all others,[3] see Fig. 36.5. Then feature differencing operations on the remaining targets (those not suppressed) enable a single site to be marked for pattern recognition and the search task

[3] Although designed to solve the lower level problem of stereo-matching, the postulation of such a cooperative process has been suggested earlier (Nelson, 1975; Marr & Poggio, 1976).

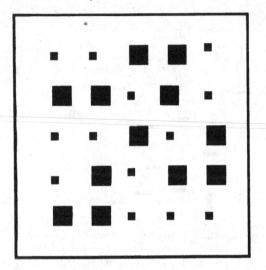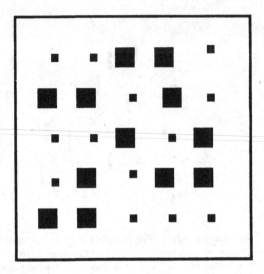

Fig. 36.5. Hypothetical feature grouping processes in the search for the conjunction of stereoscopic depth and size. If this pair of images are fused stereoscopically, all the distractors in one stereo-plane will be of one size and the distractors in the other plane will be of the other size. Task of the observer is to find the odd size in a given depth plane. For the usual case of crossing one's eyes (so that the right image is viewed by the left eye) the odd target is a large square in the front plane. We argue that feature grouping algorithms link targets of the same disparity and suppress targets of other disparities. Then feature differencing algorithms can pick out the odd size target from within a given stereoscopic plane. As such, search times are not influenced by the number of distracting targets (see text, also Nakayama & Silverman, 1986a).

appears as essentially effortless. To deal with the often marked improvement in performance with extended practice (Steinman, 1987), we suggest that the coupling parameters of the underlying neural networks can become modified to enhance grouping along particular feature dimensions.

Object representation

The theory concentrates on the pick-up of information from the pyramid, emphasizing the very small size of the visual icon and the consequent bottleneck in visual information transmission. Thus vision proceeds by a set of sequential pattern matches from different levels of the pyramid, grabbing information from the pyramid at varying scale and position and activating icons corresponding to various sizes and position in the visual field. In this section we suggest how this process of sampling from a multi-resolution pyramid could dictate the basis of object representation in visual memory.

Most important to consider is the very small amount of information contained in an icon in comparison to the detailed visual knowledge that we have of most real objects. Thus the icon itself cannot be the fundamental unit of object representation but is only a component. So we suggest that visual objects are assemblies of icons, associatively linked through visual experience. These correspond to the set of samplings or attentional fixations taken from the multi-level pyramid. For each object, therefore, there are various iconic shapshot representations taken at varying degrees of size (relative to the object). Thus, object representation consists of the aggregate of icons activated by a given object. For example the representation of an elephant might consist of some whole body icons showing typical side, rear, front and three-quarter views. Associatively linked to each of these views might be more detailed representation of head, trunk, tusks, mouth, eyes, feet, tail, etc. We suggest that these views at different scales (corresponding to attentional fixations) represent canonical representations of object parts and they are linked associatively. Hoffman & Richards (1985) suggest, for example, that distinct 'parts' of an object are almost invariably delineated by regions of negative intrinsic curvature in the object and are correlated with concavities in the image. It is possible that such 'parts' plus whole views of an object comprise the canonical views or canonical representations of an object. The plausibility of such canonical views and of their dominant role can be appreciated by introspection.

For example, it is far more difficult to visualize in one's imagination anything other than such canonical views. This point becomes more convincing as one tries to conjure up in one's imagery, sections of an object which are just partial views of several canonical icons. For example, imagine a whole frontal view of a very familiar friend, or just the face, each of which corresponds to a hypothetical canonical fixation or attentional snapshot. This is relatively easy in most cases. Compare this with the greater difficulty in imagining the combined partial samplings of two canonical views. For example, it is far more difficult to imagine an arbitrary 'section' of one's friend, and not coincident with such canonical views, say a view which extends from his nose to his waist.

So we suggest a rather frankly viewer-centered approach and stress that the representation of an object consists of an aggregate of canonical viewer-centered icons. As a consequence, the present theory is somewhat different from the notion of an object-centered coordinate representation as suggested by others (Marr & Nishihara, 1978; Biederman, 1985; Shephard, 1975). As such, the theory proposed shares some similarities with ideas proposed by Kosslyn (1980) who has argued that visual imagery is a computationally legitimate form of knowledge representation. The present theory differs, however, in its explicit representation of objects as associatively linked image fragments (or icons) of differing scales, corresponding to specific attentional fixations from the early vision pyramid.

Subjective experience

Here we make a number of interpretations of subjective experience in the context of the theory. First we divide visual experience for most normal observers into three categories: (1) dreams, hallucinations and hypnogogic imagery; (2) waking visualization and imagining; (3) ordinary seeing.

Dreams, hallucinations and hypnogogic imagery are very vivid and one is rather hard pressed to say that they are entirely different from ordinary vision in terms of their perceptual quality. Hallucinatory visions are also seen during long episodes of sensory deprivation (Bexton *et al.*, 1954), under drugs and in certain forms of psychoses. We argue that the similarity of these states and ordinary vision is not accidental (see also Neisser, 1967; Hebb, 1968). All are based on related states of activation in visual memory. With these endogenously generated perceptions, it is likely that the original excitation of the icons arises independent of the feature pyramid and must be a consequence of interconnections between the icons themselves or from other brain centers. Since we do not have such vivid non-visually driven impressions during our ordinary waking state it suggests that these associative connections within visual memory are probably facilitated when dreaming or hallucinating. Conversely, we speculate that these associative connections are relatively dampened in the ordinary waking state so as not to compete excessively with visual inputs.

The act of visualization or visual imagination is rather different. Here it is the experience of most observers[4] that one's powers of visualization are less acute in the ordinary waking state, certainly they pale in intensity and clarity when compared with visual perception or dreams. Suppose that only one icon is activated at a time during the course of 'imagining' and this one icon can represent only the simplest visual 'object' with any clarity. More complicated objects therefore must be represented as the activation of many such elementary icons. To provide some plausibility for this speculative assertion, close your eyes and imagine the capital letter E as it appears typographically, say as in a Snellen eye chart. For most observers, this process of imagination yields a rather clear image of the letter E with relatively sharp edges and some can even visualize the little serifs at the same time. On the other hand, now imagine a more complicated typographic image, say the word 'England'. Most people can image such a word as it appears on the printed page but cannot see both the whole word and the details of the individual letters at the same time.

A similar 'vision experiment' can be done with non-typographic images as well. Imagine an elephant seen from the side. If one imagines the whole elephant its hard to visualize the trunk with maximum clarity. To do this requires one to 'zoom up' and to visualize a much clearer image of the trunk, yet now one cannot image the whole elephant at the same time. This is rather different from ordinary visual perception where if we were viewing a real elephant, we would see his trunk sharply and also see the whole body as well – all with apparent simultaneity.

So ordinary vision has the appearance of being

---

[4] Although most people experience ordinary waking imagery with much less detail and vividness than ordinary perception, many exceptions have been reported. Some children have been reported to have much more vivid and detailed imagery (see Haber & Haber, 1964) and anecdotes and case histories indicate that in rare instances, adults can have astonishing powers of visual imagination (see Luria, 1968).

very rich and one thinks one is seeing both the 'forest and the trees' simultaneously. Waking visualization, on the other hand, is highly impoverished, providing only a vague impressionistic representation and one must alternate 'views' to see both the forest and the trees. Again, we explain this difference by speculating that for the case of ordinary seeing, many icons in visual memory can be simultaneously activated, but that only one or very few of such icons can be activated in the case of waking visualization.

Computational advantages

We argue that the proposed theoretical framework has at least two significant biological and computational advantages. First by restricting the scope of the elementary pattern recognition (template matching) to a very small portion of the early image representation, it removes much of the criticism that has generally been directed to pattern recognizers which are formally equivalent to perceptrons (Rosenblatt, 1962; Minsky & Papert, 1969). Perceptrons are units which had the ambitious job of detecting learned patterns anywhere in the visual field by using parallel processing. One major problem with such schemes was combinatoric, they required too many intermediate 'hidden units'. Thus recognition units or demons had to be replicated for many positions in the visual field. A second problem associated with such schemes is that once such a target was recognized, there was no way to determine its location. Since the present scheme abandons the possibility of complex pattern recognition occurring in parallel over the whole of the visual field, these combinatoric problems are eliminated.

A second advantage of the theory is that by suggesting scale invariant icons in visual memory linked through associative learning, the stored visual representation of objects is more compact and thus allows the needed opportunity for 'top-down' processing. It is well known that prior knowledge, context, and expectancy can assist in the pattern recognition process. Yet such a system of associations would be combinatorically implausible if such icons were replicated and distributed for each region in the visual field. By having them organized as scale invariant entities relatively independent of retinotopic order, however, previously activated icons can potentiate other icons through associative connections so that the 'correct' activation is assured, even in the face of incomplete input, distorted input or noise.

Concluding summary

A speculative theoretical framework regarding the overall organization of the visual system has been outlined, emphasizing the need to recognize a vast number of learned objects. It is assumed that the visual system can be subdivided into two major subsections: (1) early visual processing, (2) visual memory.

Early visual processing is organized as a multilevel multi-feature pyramid, analyzing the incoming image into feature representations of differing scales. It is a massively parallel, retinotopically organized system. Visual memory consists of a very large number of low-resolution scale-invariant pattern recognition icons (templates) organized as a massively parallel associatively linked system. It is assumed that for ordinary perception to occur, sets of icons in visual memory must be activated. Most critical is the very small size of these icons and the correspondingly limited transmission bandwidth between the features pyramid and individual icons in visual memory. The existence of this 'iconic bottleneck' means that the system can sample or perform an elementary pattern match from a large fraction of the whole visual field but at the cost of doing this at a lower resolution level of the pyramid. Alternatively, it can sample at high resolution but at the expense of doing this for only a small subsection of the visual field. So to capture information from ordinary visual scenes, the system needs to conduct a sequence of elementary pattern matching operations from a variety of levels and lateral positions in the early vision pyramid. Feature differencing and feature grouping algorithms in the pyramid are of major importance in guiding the sampling process.

Acknowledgements

We acknowledge support from grants 83-0320 from AFOSR. Thanks to Gerald Silverman for early discussions and to Shinsuke Shimojo for helpful comments on the manuscript.

References

Allman, J. & Kaas, J. (1974) The organization of the second visual area (V II) in the owl monkey: a second order transformation of the visual hemifield. *Brain Res.*, **76**, 247–65.

Allman, J., Miezin, J. & McGuiness, E. (1985a) Direction- and velocity specific responses from beyond the classical receptive field in the middle temporal visual area (MT). *Perception*, **14**, 105–26.

Allman, J., Miezin, J. & McGuiness, E. (1985b) Stimulus specific responses from beyond the classical receptive field: neurophysiological mechanisms for local–global comparisons in visual neurons. *Ann. Rev. Neurosci.*, **8**, 407–29.

Anderson, C. H. & Van Essen, D. C. (1987) Shifter circuits: a computational strategy for dynamic aspects of visual processing. *Proc. Natl. Acad. Sci. USA*, **84**, 6297–301.

Barlow, H. B. (1960) The coding of sensory messages. In *Current Problems in Animal Behaviour*, ed. W. H. Thorpe & O. L. Zangwill, pp. 331–60. Cambridge: Cambridge University Press.

Barlow, H. B. (1961) Possible principles underlying the transformation of sensory messages. In *Sensory Communication*, ed. W. A. Rosenblith, pp. 217–34. Cambridge, Mass: MIT Press.

Barlow, H. B. (1981) Critical limiting factors in the design of the eye and the visual cortex (The Ferrier Lecture, 1980). *Proc. Roy. Soc. Lond.*, **B212**, 1–34.

Beck, J., Prazdny, K. & Rosenfeld, A. (1983) A theory of textural segmentation. In *Human and Machine Vision*, ed. J. Beck, B. Hope & A. Rosenfeld. New York: Academic Press.

Bexton, W. H., Heron, W. & Scott, T. H. (1954) Effects of decreased variation in the sensory environment. *Canadian J. Psychol.*, **8**, 70–6.

Biederman, I. (1985) Human image understanding: recent research and a theory. *Computer Vision, Graphics, and Image Processing*, **32**, 29–73.

Blakemore, C. & Tobin, E. A. (1972) Lateral inhibition between orientation detectors in the cat's visual cortex. *Exp. Brain Res.*, **15**, 439–40.

Burt, P. & Adelson, E. (1983) The Laplacian Pyramid as a compact image code. *IEEE Transactions on Communication. COM–31*, pp. 532–40.

Carlson, C. R., Mueller, J. R. & Anderson, C. H. (1984) Visual illusions without low spatial frequencies. *Vision Res.*, **24**, 1407–13.

Crick, F. (1984) Function of the thalamic reticular complex: the searchlight hypothesis. *Proc. Natl. Acad. Sci. USA*, **81**, 4586–90.

Desimone, R. & Schein, S. J. (1987) Visual properties of neurons in area V4 of the macaque: sensitivity to stimulus form. *J. Neurophysiol.*, **57**, 835–68.

DeValois, R. L., Albrecht, D. G. & Thorell, L. (1982) Spatial frequency selectivity of cells in macaque visual cortex. *Vision Res.*, **22**, 545–59.

Frost, B. J. & Nakayama, K. (1983) Single visual neurons code opposing motion independent of direction. *Science*, **220**, 744–5.

Ginsburg, A. (1981) Spatial filtering and vision: implications for normal and abnormal vision. In *Clinical Applications of Visual Psychophysics*, ed. L. Proenza, J. E. Enoch and A. Jampolsky, pp. 70–106. Cambridge: Cambridge University Press.

Grossberg, S. & Mingolla, E. (1985) Neural dynamics of perceptual grouping: Textures, boundaries, and emergent segmentations. *Perception and Psychophysics*, **38**, 141–71.

Gross, C. G. (1973) Inferotemporal cortex and vision. *Prog. Physiol. Psychol.*, **5**, 77–115.

Haber, R. N. & Haber, R. B. (1964) Eidetic imagery. I. Frequency. *Pereceptual & Motor Skills*, **19**, 131–8.

Hebb, D. O. (1968) Concerning Imagery. *Psychological Review*, **75**, 466–77.

Hoffman, D. D. & Richards, W. (1985) Parts of recognition. *Cognition*, **18**, 65–96.

Julesz, B. (1984) Toward an axiomatic theory of preattentive vision. In *Dynamic Aspects of Neocortical Function*, ed. G. M. Edelman, W. E. Gall & W. Cowan. New York: Neurosciences Research Foundation.

Koch, C. & Ullman, S. (1985) Shifts in selective visual attention: towards the underlying neural circuitry. *Human Neurobiol.*, **4**, 219–27.

Kosslyn, S. M. (1980) *Image and Mind*, Cambridge, Mass: Harvard University Press.

Legge, G., Pelli, D., Rubin, G. S. & Schleske, M. M. (1985) Psychophysics of reading – I. Normal vision. *Vision Res.*, **25**, 239–52.

Lindsay, P. H. & Norman, D. A. (1977) *Human Information Processing: an Introduction to Psychology*. 2nd edn. New York: Academic Press.

Luria, A. R. (1968) *The Mind of a Mnemonist: a Little Book About a Vast Memory*. New York: Basic Books.

Marr, D. (1982) *Vision*. San Francisco: Freeman.

Marr, D. & Nishihara, H. K. (1978) Representation and recognition of three dimensional shapes. *Proc. Roy. Soc. Lond.*, **B200**, 269–94.

Marr, D. & Poggio, T. (1976) Cooperative computation of stereo disparity. *Science*, **194**, 283–7.

Maunsell, J. H. R. & Newsome, W. T. (1987) Visual processing in monkey extrastriate cortex. *Ann. Rev. Neurosci.*, **10**, 363–401.

Minsky, M. & Papert, S. (1969) *Perceptrons*. Cambridge, Mass: MIT Press.

Mishkin, M. & Appenzeller, T. (1987) The anatomy of memory. *Sci. Am.*, **256**, 80–9.

Moran, J. & Desimone, R. (1985) Selective attention gates visual processing in the extrastriate cortex. *Science*, **229**, 782–4.

Nakayama, K. & Mackeben, M. (1989) Sustained and transient aspects of focal visual attention. *Vision Res.*, **29**, 1631–47.

Nakayama, K. & Silverman, G. H. (1986a) Serial and parallel processing of visual feature conjunctions. *Nature*, **320**, 264–5.

Nakayama, K. & Silverman, G. H. (1986b) Serial and parallel encoding of visual feature conjunctions. *Invest. Ophthal. and Vis. Sci.*, **27**, 82.

Neisser, U. (1967) *Cognitive Psychology*. New York: Appleton Century Crofts.

Nelson, J. I. (1975) Globality and stereoscopic fusion in binocular vision. *J. Theor. Biol.*, **49**, 1–88.

Nelson, J. I. & Frost, B. J. (1978) Orientation selective inhibition from beyond the classical receptive field. *Brain Res.*, **139**, 359–65.

Noton, D. & Stark, L. (1971) Eye movements and visual perception. *Sci. Am.*, **224**(6), 34–43.

Perrett, D. I., Rolls, E. T. & Caan, W. (1982) Visual neurons responses to faces in the monkey temporal cortex. *Exp. Brain Res.*, **47**, 329–42.

Perrett, D. I., Mistin, A. J. & Chitty, A. J. (1987) Visual neurons responsive to faces. *Trends Neurosci.*, **10**, 358–64.

Posner, M. L. (1980) The orienting of attention. *Q. J. of Exp. Psychol.*, **32**, 3–25.

Posner, M. L. (1987) Selective attention and cognitive control. *Trends Neurosci.*, **10**, 13–17.

Rayner, K. (1978) Eye movements in reading and information processing. *Psychol. Bull.*, **85**(3), 618–60.

Rosenblatt, F. (1962) *Principles of Neurodynamics*. New York: Spartan Books.

Rumelhart, D. E. & McClelland, J. L. (1986) *Parallel Distributed Processing: Explanations in the Microstructure of Cognition.* Vol. 1. Cambridge, Mass: MIT Press.

Sakitt, B. & Barlow, H. B. (1982) A model for the economic encoding of visual image in cerebral cortex. *Biol. Cybern.*, **43**, 97–108.

Schwartz, E. L. (1977) Spatial mapping in the primate sensory projection: analytic structure and relevance to perception. *Biol. Cybern.*, **25**, 181–94.

Shepard, R. N. (1975) Form, formation and transportation of internal representations. In *Information Processing and Cognition, the Loyola Symposium*, ed. R. Solso, pp. 87–117. Hillsdale, NJ: Erlbaum.

Sperling, G. (1960) The information available in brief visual presentations. *Psychological Monographs*, 74 (11, Whole No. 498).

Sperling, G. & Melcher, M. J. (1978) The attention operating characteristic: examples from visual search. *Science*, **202**, 315–18.

Steinman, S. B. (1987) Serial and parallel search in pattern vision? *Perception*, **16**, 389–98.

Treisman, A. (1985) Preattentive processing in vision. *Computer Vision, Graphics and Image Processing*, **31**, 156–77.

Van Essen, D. C. (1985) Functional organization of primate visual cortex. In *Cerebral Cortex, Volume 3*, ed. A. Peters & E. G. Jones. New York: Plenum Publishing Corporation.

von der Heydt, R., Peterchase, E. & Baumgartner, G. (1984) Illusory contours and cortical neuron responses. *Science*, **224**, 1260–2.

Weymouth, F. W. (1958) Visual sensory units and the minimal angle of resolution. *Am. J. Ophthal.*, **46**, 102–13.

Wilson, H. R. & Bergen, J. R. (1979) A four mechanism model for spatial vision. *Vision Res.*, **19**, 19–32.

Wolfe, J. M., Cave, K. R. & Franzel, S. L. (1989) Guided search, an alternative to the feature integration theory for visual search. *J. Exp. Psychol.: Human Perception and Performance* (in press).

Zeki, S. (1978) Functional specialization in the visual cortex of the rhesus monkey. *Nature*, **274**, 423–8.

37
Pyramid algorithms for efficient vision

A. Rosenfeld

Introduction

This paper describes a class of computational techniques designed for the rapid detection and description of global features in a complex image – for example, detection of a long smooth curve on a background of shorter curves (Fig. 37.1).

Humans can perform such detection tasks in a fraction of a second; the curve 'pops out' of the display relatively immediately. In fact, the time required for a human to detect the curve is long enough for at most a few hundred neural firings – or, in computing terms, at most a few hundred 'cycles' of the neural 'hardware'. If we regard the visual system as performing computations on the retinal image(s), with (sets of) neuron firings playing the role of basic operations, then human global feature detection performance implies that there must exist computational methods of global feature detection that take only a few hundred cycles.

Conventional computational techniques of image analysis fall far short of this level of performance. Parallel processing provides a possible approach to speeding up the computation; but some computations are not easy to speed up. For example, suppose we input the image into a two-dimensional array of processors, one pixel per processor, where each processor is connected to its neighbors in the array; this is a very natural type of 'massive parallelism' to use in processing images. Unfortunately, if we try to use it for global feature detection, we find that (because of the time needed for communication across the array, from processor to processor) it requires a number of processing steps that grows linearly with the size of the feature, so that it takes hundreds of cycles to detect a curve that is hundreds of pixels long.

In this paper we describe a class of parallel processing techniques that can detect global features and measure their properties in a number of steps that does not grow linearly, but only logarithmically, with the feature size. The techniques are designed to be implemented on a 'pyramid' of processors – an exponentially tapering stack of processor arrays – with the image input to the base of the pyramid, one pixel per processor. The pyramid architecture allows us to employ 'divide and conquer' techniques to collect

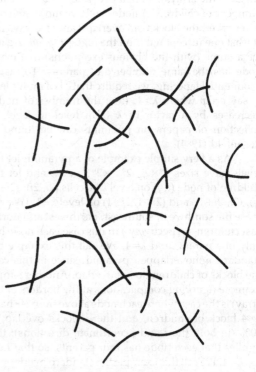

Fig. 37.1

global information about a feature in a logarithmic number of computational steps.

The next section of this paper describes the basic pyramid hardware architecture, as well as some alternative architectures that have the same capabilities. Later sections describe a collection of computational techniques that measure global properties of an image, or detect global features in an image, in numbers of steps proportional to the logarithm of the image or feature size, and also suggest how this approach might serve as a model for visual 'pop-out' phenomena.

The pyramid architecture

A pyramid is an exponentially tapering stack of square arrays of processors (which from now on we call 'nodes'). The arrays are called the *levels* of the pyramid; the largest array, level 0, is called the *base*. Each node is connected to its neighbors (e.g. north, south, east and west) on its own level (provided they exist). In addition, each node N above the base is connected to a block of nodes on the level below it; these nodes are called N's *children*, and N is called their *parent*. We assume, for simplicity, that the blocks all have the same size and shape (except possibly at the edges of the arrays), so that every node has the same number c of children. A node can have more than one parent (i.e., the blocks can overlap), and it always has at least one (except if it is on the highest level). Again, we assume (with the obvious exceptions) that every node has the same number p of parents. To insure exponential tapering, we require that c is a multiple of p, say $c = \lambda p$ where $\lambda > 1$; thus the number of nodes decreases by a factor of λ from level to level. A collection of papers on pyramids can be found in Rosenfeld (1984).

As a very simple example of a pyramid, let the levels have sizes $2^n \times 2^n$, $2^{n-1} \times 2^{n-1}$, . . ., and let the children of node (i, j) on level k be cells $(2i, 2j)$, $(2i+1, 2j)$, $(2i, 2j+1)$, and $(2i+1, 2j+1)$ on level $k-1$. (We call these the southwest, southeast, northwest and northeast children, respectively.) In this case each node has only one parent, and $\lambda = 4$. We call this example the standard nonoverlapped pyramid, since in this case the blocks of children do not overlap. Another simple example (ignoring complications at the borders of the array) is the case where each node above the base has a 4×4 block of children, and these blocks overlap by 50% (in both the i and j coordinate directions); this implies that each node has four parents, so that here too $\lambda = 4$. We call this example the standard overlapped

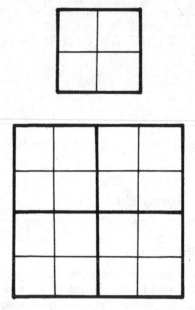

Fig. 37.2a.

pyramid. Small pieces of both of these examples are illustrated in Figs. 37.2a and 37.2b.

When we process an image using a pyramid, we input the image to the base of the pyramid, one pixel per node. (We can imagine that each node in the base incorporates a photosensor, and that the base lies in the image plane of a camera.) We shall think of the processing as consisting of a series of synchronized steps, where at each step every cell obtains information from its children, neighbors, and parents (a bounded amount of information from each) and performs some computation on this information. In most of the algorithms that we will describe, at a given step only the nodes on one level of the pyramid are actively computing; the others are inactive.

Our algorithms are designed to be implemented on a pyramid, but they can also be implemented on a number of other computational structures. One example is a *prism* (Rosenfeld, 1985), which is a stack of $n+1$ arrays all of the same size 2^n by 2^n. Here node (i, j) on level k is connected to its siblings and also to nodes (i, j), $(i+2^k, j)$, and $(i, j+2^k)$ on level $k+1$ (where the additions are modulo 2^n). Each computational step on a (standard nonoverlapped) pyramid can be simulated by a few steps of computation on a prism; see Rosenfeld (1985) for the details. Another important example is a *hypercube* having 2^n nodes. We assign to each node a distinct n-bit binary number, and connect each node N to the n nodes whose numbers differ from N's in

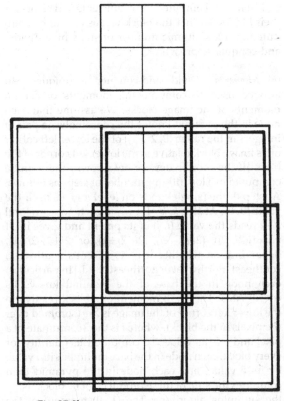

Fig. 37.2b.

exactly one binary place. It is not hard to see (Rosenfeld, 1985) that a hypercube can simulate a prism. Many pyramids and hypercubes have been designed or built; for examples see Hillis (1985) and Cantoni & Levialdi (1986).

The architectures considered in this paper are regularly structured; for example, in our pyramids, the blocks of children are all congruent (e.g. 2×2 or 4×4) and are regularly spaced (e.g., their centers are distance 2 apart horizontally and vertically). From a biological standpoint, such regularity would be very unrealistic. As it turns out, however, some of the basic pyramid operations can be carried out adequately using a 'noisy' pyramid in which the block sizes and spacing vary randomly (within limits) (Baugher *et al.*, 1986). It would be of interest to extend the algorithms described in this paper to such noisy pyramids.

Statistical computations

In this section we describe a set of algorithms for computing 'statistical' information about the input image, using the standard nonoverlapped pyramid. In

this pyramid each node N on level k has a block of 4 children on level $k-1$, a block of 16 grandchildren on level $k-2$, . . ., and a block of $2^k\times2^k$ descendants on level 0 (the base); we call this last block N's block of the image. To compute statistical information about the blocks of size $2^k\times2^k$, our algorithms perform k computational stages, each of which involves only a bounded amount of computation. In this sense, we can say that the total amount of computation is proportional to the logarithm of the block size.

Our algorithms can operate either on the original input image, or on images generated from the input image using local operations (in which the new value of a pixel depends only on the old values of that pixel and a set of its neighbors). Evidently any local operation can be performed on the input image, using the neighbor connections in the base of the pyramid, in a bounded number of steps. An important class of examples are those in which the local operations detect the presence of local features in the input image and measure properties of these features – for example, they detect the presence of short edge segments and measure their slopes. The result of such a process will be called a *feature map*, and will generally be sparse – i.e., features will be present only at some of the pixels.

Basic operations

(a) Summing.   In our first basic algorithm, each node simply computes the sum of the values in its block of the image. (When the image is a feature map, it is convenient to assign the value 0 to pixels at which no feature is present; thus when we apply the summing algorithm to a feature map, it adds the values of the properties of the features that are present in each image block.) Initially, the value of a node on level 0 is its input value or its feature property value (if any). At the first step of the algorithm, each node on level 1 adds the values of its four children; at the second step, each node on level 2 adds the values of its four children; and so on. Evidently, after k steps, the nodes on level k have computed the sums of the values in their $2^k\times2^k$ image blocks. This style of computation is called 'divide and conquer'; the task of adding 4^k numbers is recursively decomposed into k subtasks – i.e., a number of subtasks proportional to $\log(4^k)$ – each of which involves adding only four numbers (so that each subtask involves only a bounded amount of computation).

(b) Counting.   A simple variation on the summing algorithm allows each node to count the number of

occurrences of a specified value v in its image block. Here, at the initial step, each node in the base gives itself value 1 if its original value was v, and 0 otherwise. We then perform the summing algorithm on the resulting two-valued images. The same idea allows each node to count the number of features in its image block; we need only, in detecting the features, give all feature pixels value 1 and all nonfeature pixels value 0.

(c) The mean. Each node at level k can compute the average pixel value in its image block by adding the values, as in (a), and dividing the sum by 4^k. Note that the nodes at level k have thus computed a reduced-resolution version of the image; we will make extensive use of this when we consider 'coarse' feature detection. Similarly, each node can compute the average feature value in its block by adding the feature values as in (a), counting the features as in (b), and dividing the sum of values by the number of features.

(d) The variance. In order for each node to compute the variance of its pixel values, we proceed as follows: each node computes the average of the values in its block as in (c), and squares this average to obtain $(\bar{v})^2$. We also square the values (this is a single operation performed by each node in the base), and each node then computes the average $\overline{v^2}$ of the squared values in its block. The variance is then just $\overline{v^2} - (\bar{v})^2$. The variance of feature values can be computed similarly in terms of the values, the squared values, and the numbers of features.

Extensions

(a) Least squares polynomial fitting. The mean of a set of data is the constant value that best 'fits' the data in the least squares sense, and the variance of the set is the (average) squared error of the fit. We have just shown how the mean and variance can be computed for the set of values in each image block in a logarithmic number of steps. More generally (Burt, 1979), it can be shown that the bivariate polynomial of a given degree d that best fits the data in each image block can also be computed in a logarithmic number of steps. (Note that a constant is a polynomial of degree zero.) In fact, given the coefficients of the degree-d polynomials that best fit the four quadrants of a block, and the squared errors of the fits, in a bounded number of steps we can compute the coefficients and error for the entire block. Thus each node in a (standard nonoverlapped) pyramid can compute the coefficients and error for its image block in a bounded number of steps (though as d increases, the number of steps grows), once its

children have computed the coefficients and errors for their blocks, so that the block values can all be computed in a logarithmic number of steps by a divide-and-conquer approach.

(b) Moments. Divide-and-conquer techniques can also be used to compute the moments or central moments of the image blocks. We assume that each node in the pyramid knows the coordinates [a pair of integers in the range $(0, 2^n - 1)$] of the lower left corner of its image block relative to the lower left corner of the base. [If the coordinates are not known, they can be computed in a logarithmic number of steps as follows: At step 0, the (single) node on level n gives itself the value $(0, 0)$. At step k, $k = 1, \ldots, n$, each node on level $n - k$ reads the value (i, j) of its parent and gives itself value $(2i, 2j)$, $(2i+1, 2j)$, $(2i, 2j+1)$, or $(2i+1, 2j+1)$, depending on whether it is its parent's southwest, southeast, northwest or northeast child.] In particular, each node in the base of the pyramid knows its coordinates. The $(1, 0)$ moment of a block relative to the lower left corner of the image is Σiv (summed over the pixels in the block), where i is the i-coordinate of a pixel and v is its value. To compute this quantity for every block, each node in the base multiplies its i value by its v value, and each node in the pyramid then computes the sum of these products for its block using the summing algorithm. The $(1, 0)$ moment of the block relative to its own lower left corner is then given by $\Sigma(i - i_0)v$, where i_0 is the coordinate of the lower left corner; but this is just $\Sigma iv - i_0 \Sigma v$, and can be computed by a node as soon as it has computed Σiv and Σv. Computation of higher order moments, or of central moments, is similar; of course, it is more complicated, but it still requires only a bounded amount of computation (depending on the order of the moments) at each stage.

(c) Bimodality detection. If a set of data has a strongly bimodal distribution of values, it can be partitioned into two subsets each of which has a relatively low variance (compared to that of the entire set). The nodes in a pyramid can detect sufficiently strong bimodality of their image blocks in a logarithmic number of steps as follows: each node at level 1 finds the best partition of its block; this involves only a bounded amount of computation, since the blocks are small. Each node at level 2 examines its children's partitions and groups them into a 'best' partition for its block; and so on. (A node can compute the variance of a union of subsets in a bounded number of steps, given the sizes, means, and variances of the subsets.) Note that the partitions obtained at level k are not necess-

arily optimal (Dunn *et al.*, 1983); if a node's partition is bad, this limits the quality of the best partition obtainable by its parent. However, a node can still detect bimodality in its image block if it is sufficiently strong. Detection of bimodality may play a role in the perception of 'similarity grouping' in a feature map, where an image block contains (randomly placed) features having two strongly differing (ranges of) values.

(d) Anomaly detection. Similarly, a node can find a 'best' partition of the values in its image block into two subpopulations – a 'typical' population and 'outliers' – in a logarithmic number of steps by combining the partitions provided by its children. In particular, a node can determine the most 'anomalous' value(s) (i.e., the farthest outlier(s)) in its image block. The node can compute statistics of its 'typical' population, but for an 'anomaly' it can preserve more detailed information, including its value and position, as long as the number of anomalies allowed is limited. Note that an anomalously-valued feature in a feature map tends to 'pop out'; this suggests that it is possible to identify and locate it very rapidly. We suggest that a feature pops out if it remains anomalous up to the top level of the pyramid.

'Coarse' feature detection

As pointed out earlier (p. 426), when the pyramid nodes compute the means of their image blocks, we obtain a set of reduced-resolution versions of the input image; in fact, the values in the nodes at level k are averages of adjacent, nonoverlapping $2^k \times 2^k$ image blocks, so that level k contains a version of the image that has been averaged over a $2^k \times 2^k$ neighborhood of each pixel and then sampled at a spacing of 2^k horizontally and vertically.

More generally, each node can compute a *weighted* average of its children's values – i.e., it can multiply their values by a set of coefficients that sum to 1, and add the resulting products. When this is done successively at levels 1, 2, . . ., the nodes at each level have computed weighted averages of their image blocks. (This is true even if the children of different nodes can overlap.) If the weights are properly chosen (and the number of children per node is sufficiently large, e.g., each node has at least a 4×4 block of children), then (Burt, 1981) the weights in these weighted averages are good approximations to samples of a Gaussian weighting function. Thus the values at a given level constitute a version of the image that has been convolved with an approximately Gaussian kernel and then sampled. In other words, a pyramid can compute sampled large-kernel Gaussian convolutions of an image in a number of stages that grows only logarithmically with the kernel size.

If we perform local operations on reduced-resolution versions of an image (whether based on unweighted or weighted averaging), the result is the same as if we had performed 'coarse' operations on the original image in sampled positions. In this way we can compute sampled 'coarse' first or second differences in various orientations, which can be used to detect large-scale edges or bars in the image, or we can compute sampled difference-of-Gaussian convolutions (by subtracting the results of Gaussian convolutions at two different scales). Note that once the reduced-resolution images have been computed, this requires only a few additional computational steps.

'Coarse' convolutions (with Gaussians, differences of Gaussians, bar masks, etc.) are commonly used to process images and to model the processing that takes place in the early stages of biological visual systems. Pyramids can compute such convolutions efficiently in a logarithmic number of steps, each involving only small numbers of arithmetic operations. By applying nonlinear local operations to the reduced-resolution images, we can perform other types of 'coarse' operations, such as 'gated' convolutions, which can be used for more selective detection of large-scale image features such as bars, spots, etc. (Rosenfeld & Thurston, 1971). By using a (small-scale) feature map as input instead of the original image, we can detect large-scale features that differ texturally, rather than simply in average gray level, from their backgrounds. (Statistics of the (small-scale) feature values that define a large-scale feature can also be computed, if desired, using the methods described in the previous section.) A pyramid computes only sampled versions of these operations, but other architectures such as the prism can compute unsampled versions, if needed.

Edge and curve description

We have seen that the nodes in a pyramid can efficiently compute various types of statistical descriptions (weighted averages, moments, etc.) of the data in the image blocks, and can efficiently perform 'coarse' operations on an image by combining these descriptions. In this section we describe a more unconventional use of pyramids to compute geometrical descriptions of the edges or curves contained in image blocks, in numbers of stages that grow only logarithmically with the block size. For simplicity, we first assume that we are dealing with 'perfect' data, i.e., with high-contrast edges or one-pixel thick high-contrast curves. In the remainder of this section we will speak only about curves, but a similar discussion applies to edges.

At the first stage, each node on the first level of the pyramid examines its image block. The pixels in the block that lie on curves (away from junctions where curves cross or branch) are detected by suitable local operations, and connected components of these pixels are labeled; we call these components 'arcs'. Junctions are also detected by local operations, and pairs of arcs that have local good continuation at a junction are linked into a single arc. Pairs of arcs that have local good continuation across a small gap are also linked into a single arc. A set of properties is computed for each arc; these might include its length, its mean slope, its mean curvature, and the positions and slopes of its endpoints. (In the case of an edge, we also compute the mean gray level of the pixels adjacent to the edge on each side of it.) In addition, we least-squares fit a straight line segment to the arc (i.e., we compute its principal axis of inertia); if the error is high, we break the arc into a limited number of subarcs such that the least-squares fits to the subarcs are good, i.e., we fit a polygonal line to the arc. Note that since the image blocks of the first-level cells are of bounded size (e.g., 4×4), all of these operations require only a bounded (though large) amount of computation, and the number of arcs in a block is limited.

At the next stage, each node on the second pyramid level receives from its children the descriptions of the arcs (if any) in their image blocks. It combines arcs that continue one another (possibly across small gaps), and consolidates their property values – i.e., it adds their lengths; computes the weighted average of their means, slopes or curvatures, weighted by their lengths; and so on. It also combines their polygonal lines; if the combination has too many segments, it merges segments until the number is small enough, choosing segments to merge that add the least to the error when they are fit by a single segment. Since a node has only a limited number of children, this too requires only a bounded amount of computation. The result is a description of the arcs in the node's image block.

At subsequent stages, the nodes on successively higher levels of the pyramid combine the descriptions of the arcs in their children's image blocks. This can be done with a bounded amount of computation even when the blocks are very large, as long as the number of arcs in a block remains limited. If, for a given node, the number of arcs in its block exceeds the permissible limit, the node does not attempt to keep a description of every arc, but only a statistical description of the population of arcs – i.e., the number of arcs, the means of their property values, etc. If the population is strongly bimodal (e.g., some of the arcs are short and some are long, some are straight and some are curved, etc.), the node keeps statistical descriptions of both subpopulations. If a few of the arcs are outliers, the node keeps individual descriptions of those arcs, and a statistical description of the remaining arcs. Nodes at higher levels can then combine the statistical (and individual) descriptions provided by their children, as described earlier (pp. 426–7). Here again, the nodes at each level only need to perform a bounded amount of computation.

The procedure just outlined yields, for each node at level k of the pyramid, descriptions of the curves contained in its image block, or (if the number of curves exceeds some limit) a statistical description of the set of these curves. Note that if the input image contains only a few curves (and they do not double back on themselves too many times), descriptions of these curves are thus computed in a number of steps that does not grow with the lengths of the curves, but only with the logarithm of the image size. If the image contains an 'outlier' curve that differs greatly from all the other curves in the image, as in Fig. 37.1, then at the top level of the pyramid the individual description of that curve is preserved while the other curves are described only as a statistical ensemble; thus the outlier curve 'pops out'.

The discussion so far has assumed that the input curves are 'perfect' – high-contrast and thin. If their contrast is low and the image is noisy, we may only be able to detect them fragmentarily; but the techniques described in this section should be able to handle (small) gaps. To handle thickness variations, we use the pyramid techniques of the previous section to reduce the resolution of the image, and apply line detection operations to each level of that pyramid (which is equivalent to applying bar detection operations to the original image). This yields a set of fragmentary detections at various pyramid levels. We assume that the positions and slopes (and thicknesses) of these detections are all input to the base of another pyramid that computes curve descriptions using the techniques outlined in this section. Pyramid techniques for the detection of curves of varying thickness are described in Connelly & Rosenfeld (1987), and initial work on pyramid curve description can be found in Meer *et al.* (1986).

Blob and ribbon detection

Finally, we briefly sketch how pyramid computational techniques can be used to rapidly detect compact regions ('blobs') and elongated regions ('ribbons') in an image, in numbers of computational steps that grow only logarithmically with the region size.

A simple pyramid approach to blob detection is to regard a blob as a coarse feature. If the blob contrasts with its background, and we reduce the resolution of the image sufficiently (namely, by a factor about equal to the blob diameter), the blob becomes a bright or dark spot in the reduced image, and can be detected using a local spot detection operator. (Note that this method only detects the blob's presence; we know its position only approximately, and we know nothing about its shape beyond the fact that it is compact, i.e., non-elongated. Pyramid methods of precisely extracting a detected blob are described in Baugher & Rosenfeld (1986) and Gross & Rosenfeld (1986).)

An objection to this simple approach is that humans can detect a blob even when it does not contrast with its background, provided local contrast is present around its edge. The Craik–O'Brien–Cornsweet illusion (Cornsweet, 1970) demonstrates that a region surrounded by a locus of local contrast change looks like a uniformly dark region on a uniformly light background (or vice versa), even though the brightness of the region's interior is exactly the same as that of its surround. Evidently, the coarse feature detection approach will not detect such a blob.

An alternative pyramid-based approach to blob detection is to detect the edges of the blob (locally) on the input image; use the techniques of the previous section to construct successively coarser (polygonal) approximations to these edges; and at each stage, check for the presence of approximated edges that *locally* surround a point. This will happen at a pyramid level where the nodes are somewhat smaller than the blob diameter, so that the approximated blob edges will all be contained in a small (e.g., 3×3) block of nodes. As indicated in the previous section, our description of an approximated edge includes information about the mean gray levels adjacent to the edge (on both sides) in the original image; thus we can also check that the locally surrounding edges have the same mean gray levels on their interior and exterior sides, and we can associate these mean gray levels with the detected blob's interior and exterior. These levels will be the same whether the blob actually contrasts with its background or is merely surrounded by a locus of local contrast change; this might serve as a

basis for explaining the Craik–O'Brien–Cornsweet illusion. (Note that when we detect a blob in this way, we only have approximate information about its location and shape, based on the approximate descriptions of its edges. A pyramid method of precisely locating the edges of a detected blob, and 'coloring in' its interior with the associated gray level, is described in Hong *et al.* (1982).)

We can similarly define a pyramid approach to the detection and description of ribbons, based on approximations of their edges. At each stage of the edge approximation process, we check *locally* for antisymmetric pairs of edges. We will find such pairs at a pyramid level where the nodes are somewhat smaller than the ribbon width. ['Antisymmetric' means that the edge arcs are approximately mirror images of one another with respect to some axis, and that their contrasts have opposite sign (i.e., their sides that face one another are both dark or both light).] When we find them, we have detected pieces of ribbon having straight axes of approximate symmetry. To find an entire ribbon, we look for such pieces of symmetry axis that continue one another; in other words, we regard the pieces of axis (detected at various pyramid levels) as inputs to another pyramid which attempts to group them into curves, as in the previous section.

Concluding remarks

We have described a collection of pyramid-based algorithms that can detect and describe global image features such as blobs, curves, and ribbons. These algorithms involve numbers of computational stages which grow only logarithmically with the feature size, and where each stage involves only a bounded (though possibly large) amount of computation. It would be of interest to investigate whether computational processes of this type play a role in the rapid detection and description of global features by humans.

Global features constitute a rich set of primitives that can serve as clues to the presence of given types of objects in an image. The ability to detect them quickly thus provides a possible basis for rapid object recognition (Rosenfeld, 1987); but a discussion of this topic would be beyond the scope of this paper.

Acknowledgements

The support of the National Science Foundation under Grant DCR-86-03723 is gratefully acknowledged, as is the help of Barbara Bull in preparing this paper.

References

Baugher, S., Meer, P. & Rosenfeld, A. (1986) *Effects of Structural Noise on Image Pyramids*. TR 1703, Center for Automation Research. College Park: University of Maryland. (August)

Baugher, S. & Rosenfeld, A. (1986) Boundary localization in an image pyramid. *Pattern Recognition*, 19, 373–95.

Burt, P. (1979) *Hierarchically Derived Piecewise Polynomial Approximations to Waveforms and Images*. TR 838, Computer Vision Laboratory. College Park: University of Maryland. (November)

Burt, P. (1981) Fast filter transforms for image processing. *Computer Graphics Image Processing*, 16, 20–51.

Cantoni, V. & Levialdi, S. (eds.) (1986) *Pyramidal Systems for Computer Vision*. Berlin: Springer.

Connelly, S. & Rosenfeld, A. (1987) *A Pyramid Algorithm for Fast Curve Extraction*. TR 1790, Center for Automation Research. College Park: University of Maryland. (February)

Cornsweet, T. (1970) *Visual Perception*, pp. 270–5. New York: Academic Press.

Dunn, S., Janos, L. & Rosenfeld, A. (1983) Bimean clustering. *Pattern Recognition Letters*, 1, 169–73.

Gross, A. D. & Rosenfeld, A. (1986) Multiresolution object detection and delineation. *Computer Vision, Graphics, Image Processing*, 39, 102–15.

Hillis, W. D. (1985) *The Connection Machine*. Cambridge, MA: MIT Press.

Hong, T. H., Shneier, M. & Rosenfeld, A. (1982) Border extraction using linked edge pyramids. *IEEE Trans. Systems, Man, Cybernetics*, 12, 660–8.

Meer, P., Baugher, S. & Rosenfeld, A. (1986) *Hierarchical Processing of Multiscale Planar Curves*. TR 1748, Center for Automation Research. College Park: University of Maryland. (December)

Rosenfeld, A. (ed.) (1984) *Multiresolution Image Processing and Analysis*. Berlin: Springer.

Rosenfeld, A. (1985) The prism machine: an alternative to the pyramid. *J. Parallel Distributed Computing*, 2, 404–11.

Rosenfeld, A. (1987) Recognizing unexpected objects: a proposed approach. *Intl. J. Pattern Recognition Artificial Intelligence*, 1, 71–84.

Rosenfeld, A. & Thurston, M. (1971) Edge and curve detection for visual scene analysis. *IEEE Trans. Computers*, 20, 562–71.

38
High level visual decision efficiencies

A. E. Burgess

Introduction

It seems only fitting to begin this chapter with a quote from Horace Barlow (1980).

> Our perceptions of the world around us are stable and reliable. Is this because the mechanisms that yield them are crude and insensitive, and thus immune to false responses? Or is it because a statistical censor who blocks unreliable messages intervenes between the signals from our sense organs and our knowledge of them? This question can be answered by measuring the efficiency with which statistical information is utilized in perception.

In this chapter, I describe some experiments done in the spirit of Barlow's suggestion. The results agree with his findings (1978, 1980) of very high human efficiency and are consistent with the view that humans can take a Bayesian approach to perceptual decisions. In this approach one combines a priori information (expectations) about what might be in the image and where together with image data. One does a detailed comparison (cross-correlation) of expectations with the new data and makes decisions based on a posteriori statistical probabilities (or likelihoods). This model gives a rather good explanation of human performance provided that one includes a number of limitations of the visual system. The efficiency method also allows one to investigate those sources of human inefficiency.

The experimental tasks all deal with high contrast signals in visual noise. The observer's task is therefore one of deciding whether one sees a signal in easily visible noise. The noise limits signal detection performance in a well known way and one can determine the best possible decision performance for the task. The hypothetical device that operates at this best possible performance is referred to as the *ideal observer*. One measures human performance and compares it to the ideal observer to calculate human efficiency. This approach was suggested by Tanner & Birdsall in 1958 but was neglected until revived by Barlow in 1978. About the same time, Wagner (1978) introduced the concept of the ideal observer to the medical imaging field. A number of experimental results give efficiencies in the range between 10% and 80% depending on the particular visual task.

The ideal observer

The ideal observer performance depends on the signal and noise properties, the nature of the task and the amount of *a priori information* about signal parameters. The dependence on prior information should be carefully noted because it is neglected in many discussions about signal detection. This fact forces one to acknowledge that *signal-to-noise ratio (SNR) by itself* does not completely determine task performance accuracy. The ideal observer calculates the a posteriori conditional probabilities of all the alternative hypotheses, H_i, using Bayes theorem (Van Trees, 1971) given by

$$P(H_i \text{ given data}) = P(H_i)P(\text{data given } H_i)/P(\text{data})$$

The optimum decision method under uncertainty is to select the alternative decision that has the maximum a posteriori probability (MAP). In order to make the MAP decision the observer needs to combine the a priori probabilities, $P(H_i)$, of each alternative hypothesis with the conditional probability of the image data given that alternative. For simple tasks the conditional probability, $P(\text{data given } H_i)$, is obtained by cross-correlation. The signal detection SNR is simply the ensemble average of normalized cross-

432 A. E. Burgess

correlation values. The SNR implies one particular weighted integral over the noise power spectrum – namely the signal spectrum is used as a weighting function; which implies a strong weighting toward the low frequency end of the spectrum. Hanson (1983) showed that high frequency information content has increased importance for more complex tasks since the observer is really discriminating between different alternative amplitude profiles. Hanson showed that the integrands for higher order tasks are weighted by u^{2n}, where u is spatial frequency and the exponent, n, depends on the task. For simple detection n equals zero. Example tasks included signal width estimation and position estimation (u^2 dependence) and estimation of the separation of binary objects (u^4). Hanson also pointed out that similar high frequency emphasis occurs for 'simple' detection with variable or unknown backgrounds. Given these theoretical results, one concludes that one must be careful not to put excessive emphasis on observer results for simple tasks such as detection of completely specified signals in uniform backgrounds.

Signal detectability and SNR

This topic is covered in many texts (Van Trees, 1971) and will only be outlined. We wish to characterize two things. One is a measure of relative 'intensities' of the signal and noise and the other is a measure of detector performance (detectability index, d'). The first measure will be referred to as 'signal-to-noise ratio' (SNR). Unfortunately, this term is used with a wide variety of meanings. We use a special definition that is based on the ideal observer itself with the signal completely specified. With this definition one finds (for the special case of uncorrelated noise)

$$(\text{SNR})^2 = \frac{E}{N_0} = \frac{1}{N_0} \iint_{-\infty}^{\infty} S(u,v)S^*(u,v)\mathrm{d}u\mathrm{d}v$$

when $S^*(u,v)$ is the complex conjugate of the signal spectrum, E is the signal energy, and N_0 is the noise spectral density. If the task is simple detection, then $S(u,v)$ is the signal to be detected. If the task is discrimination between two signals s_1 and s_2 then $S(u,v)$ is the difference signal (s_1-s_2). There are two common measures of detector performance. One is the percentage of correct responses, P, which will be between $1/M$ and 1 for a multiple alternative forced choice (MAFC) task (M=number of alternatives). The other measure is signal detectability, d' which is determined from P by a calculation that depends on the detailed nature of the task (Elliot, 1964). The detectability index, d', is in

fact the SNR that an ideal detector would require to achieve the percentage correct score of the observer in the experiment.

Statistical efficiency

One compares the human detectability index, d'_H, for a task with that of the ideal observer, d'_I, and obtains a statistical efficiency $\eta = (d'_I/d'_H)^2$. You may find it easier to think about efficiency in SNR terms. The ideal observer's index, d'_I, is actually the physical SNR of the signal as defined above and the human observer's index, d'_H, is actually the SNR required by the ideal observer to achieve the same performance accuracy as the human. For example, assume the signal SNR is 3.0 in a 2AFC task and the human achieves 92% correct. The ideal observer would need SNR=2.0 for 92% correct so the statistical efficiency is $(2.0/3.0)^2=0.44$.

The power of the efficiency approach lies in the fact that one does not have to resort to model-building and curve-fitting to analyze results. Given the enormous complexity of vision, any model is probably wrong. Given the high efficiencies one finds under best conditions, the simplest experimental strategy is to identify and study sources of *inefficiency*.

Human strategy

My view is that the suprathreshold detection and decision tasks that the observers are asked to do are performed at a high (cognitive) level in the brain. I believe that the observers are attempting to use a maximum a posteriori decision strategy employing any a priori and image information that is available. This decision strategy is clearly adaptive in the sense that the observer has to adjust where he looks and what he looks for on the basis of information provided. When the observer is looking for two-cycle sine waves he sees chance correlations in the noise that look like two-cycle sine waves. If he is looking for disc signals (with either positive or negative contrast) he sees similar correlated regions in the noise. The a priori information about signal location and phase allow the observer to discount or ignore those chance correlations that are in the wrong place in the image or have the wrong phase. When signal location or phase information is incomplete or unavailable the observer has to consider all chance correlations that are consistent with the available signal information.

What might be the sources of reduced human performance? There are a large range of possibilities but they can, for convenience, be grouped into four categories – inefficient sampling or filtering, signal parameter uncertainty effects, non-linear or thresholding operations in the visual system, and internal noise.

Can humans do cross-correlation detection?

There is a long standing controversy in the psychophysics literature about whether humans can do cross-correlation detection. A number of experiments have demonstrated that detectability is directly related to SNR. This does *not* confirm cross-correlation because *suboptimal signal energy* detection strategies such as auto-correlation (Uttal, 1975) predict a similar relationship between d' and SNR. In fact the auto-correlation model gives a *better* fit to some d' versus SNR data if one ignores *absolute* normalization factors (as most authors do).

A number of experiments have been done that can be interpreted as supporting one view or the other. Unfortunately the interpretation has been invariably based on a *model* of how the visual system works. We did an experiment (Burgess & Ghandeharian, 1984a) designed as a model-free test of cross-correlation capability using a two-cycle sine-wave pattern because the detectability of such a pattern is particularly sensitive to the detection method used.

The experimental results are summarized in Fig. 38.1. The best possible cross-correlation and auto-correlation (i.e. energy) detector performances are shown. Humans did the task in two ways – in some trials they were given complete knowledge of signal phase while on other trials phase information was not given. There was a very significant difference in results for the two situations. More importantly the phase-known results were superior to the *very best* possible results for an observer that could not use phase information. We concluded that well trained humans can perform cross-correlation detection when sufficient a priori information is available.

Prior knowledge

Many theories (Uttal, 1975) of the human visual system do not include the ability to use prior information. Other researchers such as Gregory (1981a,b) have emphasized the rôle of prior knowledge in human vision. The ideal observer is able to effectively use all available prior knowledge about signal characteristics. Detection probability decreases, however, if any signal parameter information is not available. This is also true for human observers.

We also did experiments on the effect of signal location uncertainty (Burgess & Ghandeharian, 1984b)

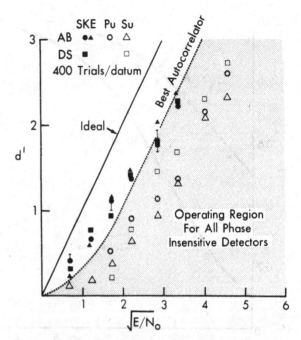

Fig. 38.1. Detectability (d') for two-cycle sine waves in visual noise. The ideal observer has d' equal to the signal-to-noise ratio ($\sqrt{E/N_0}$). The dotted line is the best possible performance for a phase-insensitive observer. The solid data points are for human observers who were provided with signal phase information on each trial (SKE). The open symbols are for humans with either sine-wave phase uncertainty (Pu) or starting position uncertainty (Su). The results demonstrate that humans must be able to do phase-sensitive detection when signal phase information is available (from Burgess and Ghandeharian, 1984a).

and on the identification of one of M orthogonal (Hadamard) signals (Burgess, 1985). We found efficiencies of 50% and 35% for the two situations. In both cases the human M-alternative performance could be predicted from 2-alternative detection performance. The identification results are shown in Fig. 38.2. Human efficiency did not change as the number of decision alternatives increased. This demonstrates that the additional uncertainty had exactly the same effect on humans as it did on the ideal observer and suggests that humans are able to use a Bayesian decision strategy.

Inefficient filter or sampling

The ideal observer is able to precisely use the signal as a template for cross-correlation. Any observer that

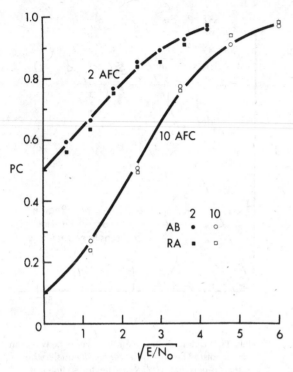

Fig. 38.2. Percentage of correct responses for 2AFC detection and 10AFC identification of Hadamard signals in noise as a function of signal-to-noise ratio ($\sqrt{E/N_0}$). The solid lines are for observers with efficiencies of 33% and 40% for 2AFC and 10AFC respectively. The difference in efficiencies is not statistically significant (from Burgess, 1985).

cycles and a marked drop at four cycles. Similar results have been reported by Watson, Barlow & Robson, (1983) for noiseless sine waves and by Kersten & Barlow (1984). These results can be interpreted in the spatial frequency domain as showing lower limits to visual system bandwidth with the bandwidth being a fixed proportion of centre frequency (constant Q filters) at higher spatial frequency.

How does one measure human filter or sampling efficiency? The first step is to eliminate parameter uncertainty effects. This can be done using a 2AFC amplitude discrimination task in which two signals are present and one has a higher amplitude, the lower amplitude signal (called the pedestal) should be moderately detectable (d' around 2 which gives a 90% pedestal detection probability). Discrimination performance can then be plotted for a number of image noise levels as shown in Fig. 38.3. Internal noise is estimated from the intercept on noise spectral density axis. The slope of the best fit line is used to estimate a lower limit sampling (or filter) efficiency. In this way, we found sampling efficiencies (Burgess et al., 1981) ranging from 0.5 for disc signals to as high as 0.8 for a 4.6 cycle per degree sine wave with a gaussian envelope. The highest sampling efficiencies were reported by Burgess & Barlow (1983) for random dot images. In that case, absolute efficiency went as high as 50% and all the inefficiency was accounted for by internal noise. Sampling efficiency was unity within experimental error.

Parameter uncertainty

It is well known that reduction in prior information about signal parameters reduces ideal observer decision performance. This occurs because the observer must consider a wider range of possible signals which in turn increases the probability that chance correlations in the noise will look like one of the possibilities. The theory of signal detectability (Van Trees, 1971) can be used to rigorously determine the effect of parameter uncertainty on the ideal observer. Observers require increased SNR to maintain a given decision accuracy. What happens if humans are given signal parameter information but are unable to use it effectively? In other words, the observer has intrinsic uncertainty. The experimentally observable result would usually be a reduced decision performance and in some cases a non-linear psychometric function (plot of d' versus SNR). Intrinsic uncertainty was suggested by Tanner in 1958 and was discussed recently in great detail by Pelli (1985).

What might humans be uncertain about? The

uses an inappropriate filter or sampling strategy will have reduced efficiency. Sampling errors can be of two kinds, random and systematic. Systematic errors will be considered first. Random sampling error effects will be considered in detail in a later section. For example, consider a disc signal. If the observer systematically cross-correlates with a larger disc then additional external noise will be introduced into the decision process and efficiency will go down. Alternatively, if the observer has a restricted integration area or sampling aperture diameter then he will not completely sample and sum the signal energy. The upper limits of human sampling apertures seem to be signal dependent. Disc signal detection efficiency drops off rapidly for diameters larger than about one degree of visual angle. The size limit for sine-wave detection seems to be determined by the number of cycles rather than absolute visual angle. In our preliminary work (Burgess et al., 1981) with static noise images, we found high efficiencies for one and two

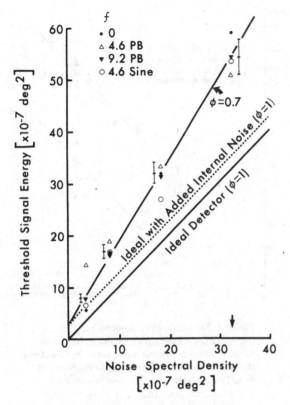

Fig. 38.3. Contrast energy threshold (at $d' = 1$) as a function of image noise spectral density. The task was 2AFC amplitude discrimination of disc ($f = 0$ in legend) and sinusoidal signals (PB = Gabor function, Sine wave is two cycles) at 4.6 and 9.2 cycles per degree. (Averages for two observers.) The solid line through the human observer data is for a model including both internal noise and sampling efficiency (70%). The highest noise level used (arrow) had a standard deviation per pixel of 0.13 of mean luminance (from Burgess et al. 1981).

possibilities include signal amplitude, shape, extent and location. More subtly, as suggested by Pelli, cells at a high level in the visual system may be uncertain about which spatial frequency or orientation channels to attend to. The problem can be stated in a general way by considering that visual input is represented by coefficients in a basis function set (n-dimensional feature space). Intrinsic uncertainty can then be modelled as a maximum likelihood decision device which is uncertain about how to assign weights to different basis functions or signal features.

What are the observable effects of intrinsic observer uncertainty? One example is the commonly found non-linear psychometric function (d' versus

SNR) which is present in any situation that produces a non-gaussian probability density function (PDF) for the decision variable. Any random variation in filter or template selection also acts as a source of 'induced' internal noise because the observer will not reach the same decision on repeated trials with the same input data. This will be discussed below.

What do human experimental results show? Detection experiments done with completely defined signal parameters should give linear psychometric functions. This is almost never the case with humans. Almost invariably one sees an accelerating non-linearity (Pelli, 1985). The closest approach to linearity is with aperiodic signals (discs, squares, rectangles) in static noise where the best fit line to the d' versus SNR data intercepts the horizontal axis at an SNR of about 0.4. For detection of sine waves in noise, the intercept increases with spatial frequency and also increases as the ratio of noise field area to signal area increases. The intercept also increases if the experimenter does not provide the observer with good cues as to the location of the specified signal position. Pelli (1985) has used fitted psychometric functions to signal known exactly (SKE) data and has interpreted results for pulsed, noiseless and sine waves to indicate an intrinsic uncertainty of 1000 orthogonal channels. I have used a Hadamard signal task (SKE and uncertain conditions) to argue (Burgess, 1985) that the upper limit of channel uncertainty is about 10.

Observer inconsistency

Human observers are inconsistent decision-makers. This inconsistency is usually interpreted by attributing internal noise to the observer.

We have found (Burgess, 1986; Burgess & Colborne, 1988) that internal noise has two components, one N_c, that is independent of external noise and one, N_i, that is 'induced' and is proportional to external noise. The independent component will be discussed first.

Constant internal noise component

One might naively expect that the detectability of noiseless visual signals would abruptly go from zero to 100% at some 'visibility threshold'. It has been known for over a century that the transition is not abrupt but in fact usually has a sigmoid shape. Jastrow suggested in 1888 that this effect was due to 'lapses of attention, slight fatigue and all the other numerous psychological fluctuations . . .'. Cattell (1893) suggested adding variations in the conductivity of neural pathways to the list. There have been suggestions of fluctuation

sources at various levels in the visual system beginning at the retina and ending at high levels. Internal
noise, as pointed out by Thurstone (1927), causes
fluctuations in the sensory effect of a fixed signal from
one judgement to the next. It is this fluctuation that
gives one a method of measuring internal noise.

Most estimates of internal noise (Nagaraja, 1964;
Pelli, 1981) have been based on the slope and intercept
method outlined in Fig. 38.3. Nagaraja (1964) used this
method to show that signal threshold energy
increased linearly with display noise spectral density
and that internal noise varied inversely with display
mean luminance. Unfortunately this analysis method
will not detect internal noise that is proportional to
external noise.

Induced internal noise

Consider an observer taken twice through a sequence
of noisy signal trials. An ideal observer will always
make the same decision given the same input data
(signal plus noise). Similarly, an observer with a systematic source of inefficiency (e.g. fixed inappropriate
filter, or maximum likelihood search over a region of
signal parameter space) will make the same decisions
on the two passes. Any non-systematic source of
inefficiency will reduce the probability of agreement
between the responses on the two sets of trials. The
reduced probability of agreement can be used together
with the probability of correct response to estimate the
ratio of standard deviations of internal noise to the
external noise *as measured through the filter used by the
observer*.

Human observer internal/external noise ratios
were estimated by the two-pass method for a number
of external noise amplitudes (Burgess, 1986; Burgess &
Colborne, 1988) and results are shown in Fig. 38.4. For
high noise levels, internal noise is directly proportional to external noise and the ratio is approximately
0.8. At low external noise levels it would appear that
internal noise *spectral* density is approaching a lower
limit. The transition appears to be near the point
where the external noise is just barely visible. We
suggested that this 'induced internal noise' could be
due to decision variable fluctuation. We showed that
this source of internal noise would have an effect
proportional to external noise if the standard deviation
of the decision variable fluctuations was proportional
to the signal-to-noise ratio. This is an intuitively
reasonable assumption and it represents a 'Weber's
law effect' limiting the precision with which an
observer could apply a decision criterion.

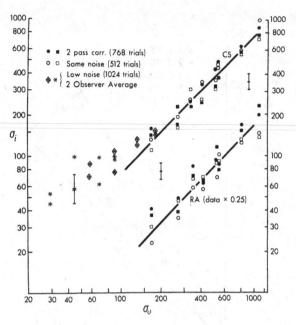

Fig. 38.4. human observer internal noise, σ_i,
dependence on external image noise, σ_0, in relative
units. If observer internal noise were constant then
the best fit line would be parallel to the horizontal
axis. There is a trend in this direction for barely
visible external noise ($\sigma_0 < 100$). However internal
noise is directly proportional to external noise when it
is easily visible. Two different measurement
techniques were used: comparison of responses for
two passes through stored image sets and 2AFC trials
with the same noise in both alternative fields. The
data for RA is displaced downward for clarity and
agrees with the data for CS (from Burgess, 1986).

Channels and codes

How do these high visual efficiencies relate to the
popular view that the visual system consists of a
number of independent transmission channels. This
issue can be best understood by considering the task
of detection of a small disc-like object, for example a
star. Since the object is small its two-dimensional
amplitude spectrum is very broad. Now consider a
visual spatial frequency channel which may be
represented by an elliptical region (1 octave by 30
degrees) in the 2-D frequency domain. It is usually
supposed that each point on the retina is served by a
large number of such channels covering the spatial
frequency domain (Sakitt & Barlow, 1982; Watson,
1983). It would be reasonable to assume that the
information about the star is therefore carried by some
50–100 separate channels. Now consider a typical

human observer model of the 1970s. It was assumed that the channels could be represented by an array of parallel spatial frequency filters followed by an 'exclusive OR' detection device. This detector would respond 'Yes' if the output of any one of the channels exceeded a pre-determined threshold. The models also had to deal with the possibility (as in the case of the star) that signal information was carried on more than one channel. It was commonly assumed that the output of the multiple channels was combined using the statistical procedure of probability summation. It should be immediately clear that this particular procedure would not be particularly efficient for detecting stars. I have done a Monte Carlo simulation of this model. The task was 2AFC detection of a signal in white noise. One alternative consisted of N independent samples with equal fractions of the signal added to noise samples from a gaussian distribution. The other alternative consisted of N noise samples. The observer selected the alternative that contained the *single* largest sample. The performance of this model was compared to the ideal observer which used a weighted sum of all samples in each alternative. The statistical efficiency of the N-channel, probability-summation model is approximately $1/\sqrt{N}$. So the maximum model efficiencies are about 15% and 10% for 50 and 100 channels respectively. This is well below the 50% efficiency found for detection of small disc signals in noise.

Now consider visual channels from the prospective of the 1980s. Suppose we regard the channels as a convenient method of preliminary coding of the visual information and subsequently a method of transmission to higher levels. The information about the star in this model is carried as coefficients of a basis-function set; Gabor functions or DOG functions for example. Since the retina samples the visual scene and transmits data to the visual cortex, it is mandatory that some basis function set be used as a communication device. There are a large number of possible basis function sets including the outputs of individual photoreceptors. It is assumed that the set (or sets) used by the visual system are chosen to optimize data representation in some way. The high efficiencies for signal detection and discrimination imply that this communication is very efficient. Our first experiments suggested that this sampling efficiency was in the range of 50 to 80% (see Fig. 38.3). However, the induced internal noise results show that we seriously underestimated sampling efficiency. Most of the increased slope in Fig. 38.3 can be attributed to induced internal noise, so it is possible that sampling efficiency is close to 100%. This implies that *all* the

basis-function coefficients required to represent a signal (such as a star) are suitably weighted and combined at some high level in the visual system. This should not be surprising. By analogy, one does not care how the telephone company encodes or transmits a conversation from London to San Francisco. The telephone company could select a basis-function set and transmit the coefficients separately over a large number of independent channels. As long as the coefficients get associated correctly at the receiving end no information is lost.

Simple sub-optimal observer model

Several years ago we proposed a simple model (Burgess *et al.*, 1981) for an observer that did sub-optimal cross-correlation detection and had internal noise. The model is outlined as follows. The signal to be detected is $s(x,y)$ and has a Fourier transform $S(u,v)$. The observer is assumed to have a fixed pre-detection filter with frequency response $F(u,v)$. This pre-detection filter corresponds to spatial filtering operations in early stages of the visual system (lens, retina, etc.). The observer was also assumed to be able to attempt adaptive matched filtering using an adjustable filter with frequency response $M(u,v)$. The model observer also added intrinsic noise with spectral density $N_1 G^2(u,v)$. The detectability index for this observer is

$$(d')^2 = I^2_2/(I_3 N_0 + I_4 N_1)$$

with
$$I_2 = \iint S(u,v)F(u,v)M(u,v)\,du\,dv$$
$$I_3 = \iint F^2(u,v)\ M^2(u,v)\,du\,dv$$
$$I_4 = \iint G^2(u,v)\,du\,dv$$

We defined sampling efficiency as the ratio $f = I^2_2/EI_3$ where E is the signal energy $E = \iint S^2(u,v)\,du\,dv$ and we also defined the observer's effective 'constant' noise spectral density as $N_c = N_1 I_4/I_3$. Experimental results to date suggest that external noise and internal noise are 'seen' through the same filter so $I_3 = I_4$. So our initial model reduces to $(d')^2 = fE/(N_0 + N_1)$. This equation can be rephrased in terms of a 'threshold' as follows. Let us define a threshold using the signal energy, E_T, required to give a selected value of d' (usually 1 or 2). Then $E_T = (d')^2(N_0 + N_1)/f$. This first model did not include the induced noise effect. Induced noise can be included by noting that the observer performs as if the total noise spectral density is $(1+b)N_0 + N_c$ where b is the ratio of the induced internal to external noise densities and N_c is the 'constant' component of internal noise. Note that the induced internal noise is 'seen' through the same filter as the external noise so the noise density ratio equals the

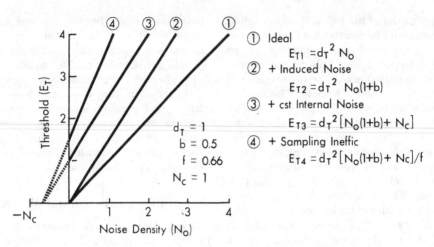

Fig. 38.5. Predicted energy thresholds (at $d' = 1$) for four model observers to illustrate the cumulative effect of three sources of inefficiency (induced internal noise, constant internal noise, and sampling inefficiency). Note that the extrapolation method underestimates the constant component of internal noise (N_c) (from Burgess, 1986).

noise variance ratio (b is approximately 0.6). This approach can be used to predict the relationship between threshold energy and external noise spectral density for a variety of conditions as shown in Fig. 38.5. Four examples are illustrated with the simplified equations together with a plot ($d'_T=1$, $b=0.5$, $f=0.66$ and $N_c=1$). It should be noted that the extrapolated lines do not pass through $-N_c$ but rather at $-N_c/(1+b)$.

Conclusions

A review of the literature indicates that one could have predicted high efficiencies 30 years ago when the concept of observer efficiency was first suggested by Tanner & Birdsall. The clue to the high efficiency lies in early results on detection of discs in photon noise limited images by de Vries in 1943 and Rose in 1948. Rose analyzed the experimental results using a fluctuations theory approach that is described in his recent book (1973). In his theory, the observer is assumed to integrate over the complete area of disc-shaped signal and decide that a signal is present if the signal-to-noise ratio is above some threshold value 'k'. Note that since the signals were flat-top discs, integration is equivalent to cross-correlation. Rose considered the possibility of false positive responses and concluded that observers would use a value of k in the range from 3 to 5. There was a 20 year discussion about the appropriate value of k with suggestions ranging from 2.5 to 5. Considering these results in retrospect, one immediately notices that the decision part of the Rose theory was based in fact on an ideal observer. If human performance were not very good, the

estimates of k in the range from 2.5 to 5 would have been immediately regarded as absurd. Human efficiency of 1% would have led to suggestions of 'k' in the range from 25 to 50 for humans. This did not happen, so one should have been led to suspect that human decision efficiency is very high.

Experimental results to date allow one to make a number of substantial statements about human observer performance. This is of practical importance for medical images which are invariably noise limited. If observers are given complete freedom to control display conditions, they definitely rank images in order of increasing SNR and measured human performance for detection and discrimination tasks seems to be rather close to the fundamental limits determined by statistical decision theory. Humans do have fundamental contrast sensitivity limits which can be represented theoretically as a source of constant observer internal noise. This inherent contrast sensitivity causes problems for images displayed with low contrast gain. However, as the display gain is increased the observer contrast sensitivity limit becomes less and less important and observer performance approaches a limit that requires an SNR $\sqrt{2}$ higher than that of the ideal detector. It appears that for relatively small signal areas humans can do maximum likelihood signal detection. However, there is an upper limit to signal size for this sort of processing. However, this is usually not a problem because observers automatically adjust their viewing distance to compensate. Another human limitation seems to be the inability to compensate for inherent correlations in image noise (Myers et al., 1985). This inability causes a significant decrement in performance for images that are produced by reconstruction from projections as is done in computer tomography and in some modes of magnetic resonance imaging.

A number of experiments give human visual efficiencies of about 50%. One naturally asks why this might be so. Why is it 50% rather than some other number, 90% or 15%, for example. There are several possible answers to this question. One possibility is that humans do not make *absolute* judgements based solely on image information within the signal boundary. The ideal observer knows exactly where to look and ignores all image data outside the signal boundary by setting the cross-correlation weighting function to zero. By contrast, humans may have to compare the signal region with nearby regions in order to reach a decision. Such a comparison would 'mix' more image noise into the decision. This comparative process would appear in the experimental results as an apparent 'differentiation' process. The induced internal noise results suggest another alternative. The

induced observer variance is about 64% of the external noise variance. This gives an upper performance limit of about 60% efficiency.

All results to date suggest that humans can be modeled as a sub-optimal Bayesian decision maker. The list of human limitations includes the following – internal noise that is dependent on image noise, inability to precisely use location information, reduced (cross-correlation) sampling efficiency because of spatially and temporally local comparisons (quasi-differentiation) of image amplitudes, limited range of integration in space and time, probably the inability to compensate for correlations in image noise (i.e. cannot 'rewhiten' coloured noise), and losses due to masking by deterministic structure. These limitations have surprisingly small effects on task performance and sophisticated image users are able to adopt a variety of strategies for minimizing their effects. Given complete control of display conditions, humans are able to get within factors of 2 to 4 of ideal performance.

References

Barlow, H. B. (1978) The efficiency of detecting changes in density in random dot patterns. *Vision Res.*, **18**, 637–50.

Barlow, H. B. (1980) The efficiency of perceptual decisions. *Phil. Trans. Roy. Soc. (Lond.)*, B**290**, 71–82.

Burgess, A. E. (1986) On observer internal noise. *S.P.I.E. Proc.*, **626**, 208–13.

Burgess, A. E. (1985) Visual signal detection III, on Bayesian use of prior knowledge and cross-correlation. *J. Opt. Soc. Am.*, **A2**, 1498–507.

Burgess, A. E. & Barlow, H. B. (1983) The efficiency of numerosity discrimination in random dot images. *Vision Res.*, **23**, 811–29.

Burgess, A. E. & Colborne, B. (1988) Visual signal detection IV – observer inconsistency. *J. Opt. Soc. Am.*, **A5**, 617–27.

Burgess, A. E. & Ghandeharian, H. (1984a) Visual signal detection I: phase sensitive detection. *J. Opt. Soc. Am.*, **A1**, 900–5.

Burgess, A. E. & Ghandeharian, H. (1984b) Visual signal detection II: effect of signal-location uncertainty. *J. Opt. Soc. Am.*, **A1**, 906–10.

Burgess, A. E., Wagner, R. F., Jennings, R. J. & Barlow, H. B. (1981) Efficiency of human visual discrimination. *Science*, **214**, 93–4.

Cattell, J. M. (1893) On errors of observation. *Am. J. Psychol.*, **5**, 285–93.

deVries, H. (1943) *Physica*, **10**, 553–64.

Elliot, P. (1964) Forced choice tables (Appendix 1). In *Signal Detection and Recognition by Human Observers*, ed. J. A. Swets, pp. 679–84. New York: Wiley.

Gregory, R. L. (1981a) *The Intelligent Eye*. London: Weidenfeld and Nicolson.

Gregory, R. L. (1981b) *Mind in Science*, pp. 383–415. London: Weidenfeld and Nicolson.

Hanson, K. M. (1983) Variations in task and the ideal observer. *S.P.I.E. Proc.*, **419**, 60–7.

Jastrow, J. (1888) A critique of psycho-physic methods. *Am. J. Psychol.*, **1**, 271–309.

Kersten, D. & Barlow, H. B. (1984) Searching for the high-contrast patterns we see best. *Suppl. Invest. Ophthal. and Vis. Sci.*, **25**, 313.

Myers, K. J., Barrett, H. H., Borgstrom, N. C., Patton, D. D. & Seeley, G. W. (1985) Effect of noise correlation on detectability of disc signals in medical imaging. *J. Opt. Soc. Am.*, **A2**, 1752–9.

Nagaraja, N. S. (1964) Effect of luminance noise on contrast thresholds. *J. Opt. Soc. Am.*, **54**, 950–5.

Pelli, D. G. (1981) Effects of visual noise, Ph.D. Thesis, Cambridge University (unpublished).

Pelli, D. G. (1985) Uncertainty explains many aspects of visual contrast detection and discrimination. *J. Opt. Soc. Am.*, **A2**, 1058–532.

Rose, A. (1948) The sensitivity performance of the human eye on an absolute scale. *J. Opt. Soc. Am.*, **38**, 196–208.

Rose, A. (1973) *Vision – Human and Electronic*. New York: Plenum Press.

Sakitt, B. & Barlow, H. B. (1982) A model for the economical encoding of the visual image in cerebral cortex. *Biol. Cybern.*, **43**, 97–108.

Tanner, W. P. & Birdsall, T. G. (1958) Definitions of d' and η as psychophysical measures. *J. Acoust. Soc. Am.*, **30**, 922–8.

Thurstone, L. L. (1927) Psychophysical analysis. *Am. J. Psychol.*, **38**, 368–89.

Uttal, W. R. (1975) *An Autocorrelation Theory of Form Detection*. Hillside, NJ: Erlbaum.

Van Trees, H. L. (1971) *Detection, Estimation, and Modulation Theory*, Part III, pp. 8–55. New York: Wiley and Sons.

Wagner, R. F. (1978) Decision theory and the detail signal to noise ratio of Otto Schade. *Photog. Sc. Engr.*, **22**, 41–6.

Watson, A. B. (1983) Detection and recognition of simple spatial forms. In *Physical and Biological Processing of Images*, ed. O. J. Braddick & A. C. Sleigh. Berlin: Springer-Verlag.

Watson, A. B., Barlow, H. B. & Robson, J. G. (1983) What does the eye see best? *Nature*, **302**, 419–22.

Index

Printed in the United States
By Bookmasters